Handbook of Experimental Pharmacology

Continuation of Handbuch der experimentellen Pharmakologie

Vol. 77

Chemotherapy of Gastrointestinal Helminths

Contributors

J. H. Arundel · J. H. Boersema · C. F. A. Bruyning · J. H. Cross
A. Davis · A. De Muynck · P. G. Janssens · W. S. Kammerer
J. F. Michel · M. H. Mirck · M. D. Rickard · F. Rochette
M. M. H. Sewell · H. Vanden Bossche

Editors

H. Vanden Bossche · D. Thienpont · P. G. Janssens

Springer-Verlag Berlin Heidelberg New York Tokyo

HUGO VANDEN BOSSCHE
Department of Comparative Biochemistry
Janssen Pharmaceutica, Research Laboratories
Turnhoutseweg 30, 2340 Beerse, Belgium

DENIS THIENPONT
Department of Chemotherapy
Janssen Pharmaceutica, Research Laboratories
Turnhoutseweg 30, 2340 Beerse, Belgium

PIETER G. JANSSENS
Vogelsanck 12, 2232 Gravenwezel, Belgium

With 62 Figures

ISBN-13:978-3-642-69529-2 e-ISBN-13:978-3-642-69527-8
DOI: 10.1007/978-3-642-69527-8

Library of Congress Cataloging in Publication Data. Main entry under title: Chemotherapy of gastrointestinal helminths. (Handbook of experimental pharmacology; vol. 77) Includes bibliographies and index. 1. Anthelmintics. 2. Helminthiasis – Chemotherapy. I. Arundel, J. H. II. Bossche, H. Vanden. III. Thienpont, D. IV. Janssens, P. G. V. Series: Handbook of experimental pharmacology; v. 77. [DNLM: 1. Anthelmintics – therapeutic use. 2. Helminthiasis – drug therapy. W1 HA51L v. 77 / WC 800 C517] QP905.H3 vol. 77 [RM356] 615.1 s [616.9'62061] 84-26781
ISBN-13:978-3-642-69529-2 (U.S.)

2122/3130-543210

List of Contributors

J. H. Arundel, School of Veterinary Science, Veterinary Clinical Centre, University of Melbourne, Princes Highway, Werribee, Victoria 3030, Australia

J. H. Boersema, Department of Veterinary Helminthology and Entomology, State University Utrecht, Yalelaan 1, 3584 CL Utrecht, The Netherlands

C. F. A. Bruyning, Laboratorium voor Parasitologie, Rijksuniversiteit Leiden, Wassenaarseweg 62, 2333 AL Leiden, The Netherlands

J. H. Cross, Tropical Public Health, Department of Preventive Medicine/Biometrics, Uniformed Services University of the Health Sciences, School of Medicine, 4301 Jones Bridge Road, Bethesda, MD 20814, USA

A. Davis, Director, Parasitic Disease Programme, World Health Organization, 1211 Geneva 27, Switzerland

A. De Muynck, Instituut voor Tropische Geneeskunde, Nationalestraat, 155, 2000 Antwerpen, Belgium

P. G. Janssens, Vogelsanck 12, 2232 Gravenwezel, Belgium

W. S. Kammerer, Division of Internal Medicine, The Milton S. Hershey Medical Center, The Pennsylvania State University, Hershey, PA 17033, USA

J. F. Michel, King John House, Gomshall, Guildford, Surrey GU5 9LG, Great Britain

M. H. Mirck, Department of Veterinary Pathology, State University Utrecht, Yaleaan 1, 3584 CL Utrecht, The Netherlands

M. D. Rickard, School of Veterinary Science, Veterinary Clinical Centre, University of Melbourne, Prince Highway, Werribee, Victoria 3030, Australia

F. Rochette, Janssen Pharmaceutica, Turnhoutseweg 30, 2340 Beerse, Belgium

M. M. H. Sewell, Department of Tropical Animal Health, University of Edinburgh, Easter Bush, Roslin, Midlothian EH25 9RG, Great Britain

H. Vanden Bossche, Laboratory of Comparative Biochemistry, Research Laboratories, Janssen Pharmaceutica, Turnhoutseweg 30, 2340 Beerse, Belgium

Preface

Parasitic diseases are the most widespread of all the major diseases, currently affecting about 3×10^9 people and innumerable domestic animals. There is no doubt that among these parasitic diseases, the helminthic infections of the gastrointestinal tract are about the most important because of their global distribution, their high prevalence, their effects on the nutritional status of men and animals, their effects on the physical and mental development of children, and their economic effects on the production of animals.

Anthelmintics are important elements in the control of these gastrointestinal helminthic infections. In this volume the editors and authors have tried to find a way through the immense amount of information on anthelmintic drugs that is scattered throughout the literature. Different authors have critically examined this information from different angles. However, the aim of all has been to provide the information needed by veterinarians, physicians, and public health workers to select the most suitable drug for a given situation.

This review is not limited to an evaluation of the therapeutic efficacy of the more important anthelmintics, but also includes information on their pharmacology, pharmacokinetics, toxicity, and mode of action. Control strategies using mass chemotherapy or selective population chemotherapy are also covered. Since a rational basis for the use of anthelmintics is provided by a study of the epidemiology of intestinal helminths, introductory chapters on their epidemiology in human populations and in domestic animals have also been included. In the latter chapter attention is focused on the gastrointestinal nematodes of sheep and cattle.

The editors express the wish that this book might contribute to a rational use of anthelmintic drugs in order to improve human health and to reduce the wastage of livestock products.

We take this opportunity to thank A. Nuyts and her staff for all the secretarial work and typing during the past years.

Hugo Vanden Bossche
Pieter G. Janssens
Denis Thienpont

Contents

CHAPTER 4

Pharmacology of Anthelmintics. H. VANDEN BOSSCHE. With 37 Figures

CHAPTER 10

Chemotherapy of Gastrointestinal Nematodiasis in Birds. J. H. BOERSEMA

CHAPTER 11

Chemotherapy of Intestinal Trematodiasis in Mammals and Birds
M. M. H. SEWELL

CHAPTER 12

Chemotherapy of Intestinal Trematodiasis in Man. J. H. CROSS

CHAPTER 13

Chemotherapy of Tapeworm Infections in Animals
M. D. RICKARD and J. H. ARUNDEL. With 5 Figures

CHAPTER 14

Chemotherapy of Tapeworm Infections in Man. W. S. KAMMERER

CHAPTER 15

Mass Treatment. P. G. JANSSENS and A. DE MUYNCK

There is no such thing as applied science. There is only science and its applications, standing in relation to each other as is the fruit of the tree that bore it.

LOUIS PASTEUR

Feedback from the applications to the science often supplies key insights and tools so that science is nourished by its applications.

G. H. HITCHINGS

CHAPTER 1

Introduction

A. Davis

The subject of gastrointestinal helminthic infections constitutes an excellent example of the interlacing links and relationships existing within the more general fields of parasitology and medicine. Gastrointestinal helminthiases are of absorbing interest to practitioners of many disciplines and provide a common bridge between human and veterinary medicine since principle and practice applicable to organisms in one area can be adapted usefully to organisms in the other area.

A. Pathogenic Mechanisms in Man

The helminthic infections of the human gastrointestinal tract are, in most areas of the world, a mirror of socioeconomic conditions. In medical practice, their public health importance is obvious because of their high prevalences, their virtually global distributions, and their effects on both the nutritional and the immune status of populations, particularly those living in the tropics and subtropics. Where food is in short supply, where crop failures occur, or where intake of proteins, calories, vitamins, and trace elements is at best only marginal, then the presence of these infections may be the critical variable which transfers a population from a barely satisfactory nutritional state to an undernourished state.

Immunosuppression may lower resistance to other infections and render active immunization procedures less effective than in those in a nonparasitized state. Yet the phenomenon of immunosuppression is not confined to endemic areas in relation to gastrointestinal helminthiasis. Secondary immune deficiency resulting from drug therapy, X-irradiation, and during transplant surgery is well documented and the subsequent effects on the pathogenicity of *Strongyloides stercoralis* pose problems in clinical management. Indeed, ideally, all such candidate patients should be screened for strongyloidiasis before commencing therapy for the original condition.

While intestinal parasitic infections are maximally prevalent in children, that most vulnerable section of the population, they are also common in that most disadvantaged sector, the rural poor of the tropics, where polyparasitism is the rule, rather than the exception. By the production of adverse effects on physical and mental development they act as one of the major retarding influences in the progress of countries of the developing world.

B. Modes of Transmission

To the epidemiologist, the helminthic infections of the gut present numerous problems in their transmission cycles and, hence, in their control. Some can even be transmitted through polluted air as in enterobiasis, although in this case fecal-oral contamination via unclean hands is the usual route; some infections are acquired indirectly through ingestion of passive stages such as eggs of *Ascaris* or *Trichuris* which have matured outside the host; other infections result from the penetration of the skin by infective larval stages produced in the soil as in the strongyloid and hookworm infections. Yet others have larval stages in an intermediate host which are ingested by man, the definitive host, and can thus be classed as food-borne infections. Into this category fall *Taenia solium,* the pork tapeworm, which may produce the potentially serious human illness cysticercosis; *T. saginata,* the beef tapeworm; and *Diphyllobothrium latum,* due to consumption of insufficiently prepared fish, meat, liver, or hard roe, which rarely can result in that medical curiosity, tapeworm pernicious anemia, from vitamin B_{12} deficiency. In this transmission group are several nematodes with limited regional distributions; *Anisakis* and *Phocanema* spp., resulting from the consumption of raw or undercooked fish or shellfish; *Capillaria philippinensis,* an occupational infection in those areas where Philippine or Thai fishermen pursue their age-old eating habits; and the recently described *Angiostrongylus costaricensis,* where infection usually results from ingestion of food or water containing larvae eliminated with the mucosal secretions of slugs, which in turn have become infected by browsing on feces containing larvae expelled from the natural definitive rodent hosts.

The close relationships between zoonotic helminthic infections of man and animals is illustrated by the examples of those tissue parasites for which the gut is the portal for entry to the human organism, e.g., *Toxocara* spp., *Toxascaris leonina, Echinococcus* spp., *Angiostrongylus cantonensis,* and the special case of *Trichinella spiralis,* in which, although the adult reproductive stages live in the human gut, the pathological sequelae are produced in muscle by the larval stages.

To the mathematically-minded, the gastrointestinal helminths offer a fertile field for theory. All free-living organisms require space for living but little is known either of the size of a helminthic population in the gut that will invariably produce significant pathological change in a given host, or of the effects of crowding on the parasites themselves. In tapeworm infections, a crowding phenomenon has been described and in severe multiple infections individual worms are often stunted. As a general principle, worms in small numbers are relatively well tolerated, but "heavy" infections cause symptoms and signs characteristic of each particular parasite. The threshold population size determining these two outcomes has been determined only roughly for a few parasites in both veterinary and medical fields, but is seems important to attempt further studies. On the one hand, it is easy to visualize the physiological effects of a high population density in producing changes in normal feeding, mating, and other activities of worms while on the other hand further quantitation of worm burdens is essential in planning strategies for control. Regular anthelminthic use is practiced and is effective in the economic production of livestock. It has been shown, both in the veterinary field and from the experiences learned from the numerous hookworm control campaigns in man, that elimination of all worms from a definitive host by chemotherapy on a large scale is rarely achieved and in fact is not a reasonable goal. What is desired and what is probably attainable is the maintenance of worm burdens to levels below a threshold where the probability of causing pathology is high. However, this epidemiological type of thinking will not blind the more clinically attuned to the fact that, in man at least, there are no intestinal helminths which can be regarded as invariably harmless.

C. Clinical Sequelae of Infection

Even the common *Ascaris lumbricoides,* arguably the most prevalent parasite in the world, is responsible, through its enormous reproductive potential of some 240,000 eggs/day per female worm and a global daily contamination factor of 10^{14} eggs, for a not inconsiderable morbidity. Complications of ascariasis, due to migration of the adult worms or intestinal obstruction by a bolus of adults, are varied and have been well described in the medical literature. In the southeastern United States the approximate rate of intestinal obstruction per year is 2/1,000 in infected children aged 1–5 years (BLUMENTHAL and SCHULTZ 1975). In Capetown, South Africa, ascaris-associated complications constituted 10%–15% of all acute abdominal emergencies, were second in frequency only to acute appendicitis, and reached their highest incidence in children between 4 and 8 years of age (LOUW 1974). Hence even low case-fatality rates may mean thousands of deaths when considered against the hundreds of millions of infected people.

Clinical complications of heavy hookworm infections are well known to tropical physicians, and individual patients manifest the physical signs of a severe anemia which is hypochromic and microcytic through varying combinations of low iron intake and chronic blood loss. In some parts of the tropics a superadded folic-acid deficiency megaloblastic anemia is an accompaniment, while some degree of hypoalbuminemia is frequent. The observation that *Ancylostoma duodenale* larvae may become dormant in man (SCHAD et al. 1973; NAWALINSKI and SCHAD 1974) has important implications in the epidemiology, control, and treatment of human hookworm. Since dormant nematode larvae fail to respond to many anthelminthics, treatment may be complicated and the phenomenon also blurs the estimation of the life span of adult worms.

D. Epidemiological Considerations

In turn the public health official is aware of course that there are considerable variations in both the distributions and the seasonal occurrence of the gastrointestinal helminthiases due to the interplay of geographical and climatic factors and human behavioral practices. Yet there are still many questions to be answered on these variations in regional prevalences. Usually the pathology induced in the host is a function of the density of infection. Yet we are rarely clear why only some human hosts exhibit high worms loads. Biological life cycles in which there is no direct multiplication within the human host are characterized, in epidemiological terms, by greatly overdispersed parasite populations customarily described by a truncated form of the negative binomial distribution (Crofton 1971) in which a lethal effect is a function of the number of parasites in an individual host. In most gastrointestinal helminth infections, the majority of individuals harbour few parasites and only a small proportion of infected persons have high-intensity infections. This is of great practical importance in the theory and practice of control of these infections. In the human situation, what is required is the development of control strategies using population-based chemotherapy which will reduce worm burdens to generally low levels of minimal public health importance and maintain them there. This is a difficult task since the tactical variants may be based on periodic mass treatments, treatment of selected target population samples by age, sex, occupational group, etc., or simply selective population chemotherapy to high-density infections in attempts at disease control.

Whichever is selected for different epidemiological situations and areas, the prime need in practice is for cheap and easily applicable techniques of diagnosis which can be used by paramedical personnel in the peripheral areas of the health services in the tropics and subtropics. Fortunately such techniques are becoming more generally used in the form of various modifications of the thick fecal smear introduced by Kato and Miura (1954), and neither sensitivity nor specificity present any problems in an epidemiological sense. Yet there remains a necessity for easy identification of larval nematodes since many laboratories do not practice coproculture techniques. In particular the identification of the larvae of *Strongyloides stercoralis* and the various hookworms is at times essential for rational therapy.

E. Chemotherapy

Research on specific drug treatment for the many gastrointestinal helminthic infections is one of the success stories of modern chemotherapy and examples are numerous. Mebendazole is effective in the individual treatment of ascariasis, enterobiasis, trichuriasis and the hookworm infections. It is the drug of current choise for *Capillaria philippinensis* infections and has been used against both *Taenia solium* and *T. saginata* with, however, rather variable results. Flubendazole, a parafluor analogue of mebendazole, gives similar, but not superior, therapeutic results. Tetramisole and levamisole are in constant use for a broad range of nematode infections in animals, and levamisole is well known for its mass use in ascariasis. Presently it is under intensive clinical investigation for the treatment of immunodeficiency diseases and certain malignant conditions. Tiabendazole, one of the oldest benzimidazoles, remains in clinical usage and has not yet been displaced for strongyloidiasis and cutaneous larva migrans. Its more general utility is limited by the production of side effects in up to 50% of treated patients. The latest benzimidazole, albendazole, has a broad spectrum of activity and is effective in a single oral dose. It appears very promising for use at Primary Health Care level.

The tetrahydropyrimidine, pyrantel pamoate, is widely and successfully used as a single oral dose in the treatment of ascariasis and enterobiasis, but hookworm infections require a 3-day schedule.

Oxantel pamoate is used for *Trichuris trichiura* but, unlike its analogue pyrantel, is ineffective in ascariasis. The combination of oxantel and pyrantel shows promise as a wide spectrum anthelmintic, being effective against *Ascaris lumbricoides, Enterobius vermicularis, T. trichiura,* and the hookworms.

The advent of praziquantel, an effective antischistosomal agent, also markedly changed the therapeutic scene in cestodiasis for it is highly active against *Taenia solium, T. saginata, Hymenolepis nana,* and *Diphyllobothrium latum.* Cure rates after a single oral dose are very high and patient tolerance excellent. Furthermore, the drug is effective experimentally against cestode larval forms in the animal model, and initial trials in cerebral cysticercosis have given promising results. Praziquantel has been widely used in the therapy of animal cestode infections and seems effective in human trematodiasis; it is, indeed, a broad spectrum compound.

Praziquantel may well tend to eclipse niclosamide in the treatment of cestodiasis in man although the latter compound has a long history of successful use.

It can thus be appreciated that there are now many efficient, acceptable, well-tolerated compounds available for the treatment of the many gastrointestinal helminth infections of man and animals. Unfortunately, their regular use in developing countries is minimal and a major cause may be shortage of foreign exchange for their purchase. Among the tasks facing both international and national agencies and those interested and concerned sectors of the pharmaceutical industry is the provision of drugs which can be used in countrywide control programs at an affordable price. This may demand innovative solutions in the areas of drug pricing and drug purchase and the maintenance of the strictest standards of quality control.

F. Conclusion

Since there is now a real possibility that progress will be made rapidly in the adoption of programs of gastrointestinal helminth diagnosis and control, the advent of the present volume is particularly appropriate at this time, for the reviews of the recent advances in this broad field will undoubtedly aid, stimulate, and refresh the involved health and veterinary practitioners in many countries of the world.

References

Blumenthal DS, Schultz MG (1975) Incidence of intestinal obstruction in children infected with *Ascaris lumbricoides.* Am J Trop Med Hyg 24:801-805
Crofton HD (1971) A quantitative approach to parasitism. Parasitology 62:179–193
Kato K, Miura M (1954) Comparative examinations (in Japanese). Jpn J Parasitol 3:35
Louw JH (1974) Biliary ascariasis in childhood. S Afr J Surg 12:219–225
Nawalinski TA, Schad GA (1974) Arrested development in *Ancylostoma duodenale;* a course of self-induced infection in man. Am J Trop Med Hyg 23:895–898
Schad GA, Chowdhury AB, Dean CG, Kochar VK, Nawalinski TA, Thomas J, Tonascia JA (1973) Arrested development in human hookworm infection; an adaptation to a seasonally unfavourable external environment. Science 180:502–504

CHAPTER 2

Epidemiology of Gastrointestinal Helminths in Human Populations

C. F. A. BRUYNING

A. Introduction

Epidemiology is the study of the factors determining the distribution, frequency, and severity of disease in human populations. The epidemiologist measures the prevalences, intensities, distribution, and progression of disease in a specified human population. A study and assessment is made of the factors which affect the transmission and severity of disease, such as the environmental factors; the biology, ecology, distribution, and population dynamics of both the pathogenic agents and their vectors or intermediate hosts; the socioeconomic conditions of the human population; and the role of human behavior in the transmission and maintenance of disease. In cooperation with other disciplines, the epidemiologist studies the etiological factors in the pathology of disease. Epidemiological studies provide quantitative data on the present health status of the population and prognoses on the expected changes in distribution, prevalences, and severity of disease in a specified human population. The control of disease depends largely on a deep understanding of its epidemiology. Therefore, control and preventive measures must be based on data provided by epidemiological studies, which are essential to the planning and implementation of feasible programs. Moreover, the effects of control measures are evaluated mainly by epidemiological studies and, finally, the determination of health priorities must be based on the results of epidemiological surveys.

Some epidemiological data are available in routine health statistics, such as data on causes of death, occurrence of notifiable diseases, data from hospitals on morbidity and mortality, including records of outpatient clinics and data on absenteeism due to disease. However, these data are often unreliable, incomplete, and of limited value. More adequate information is required from well-defined epidemiological surveys, carried out by means of standardized methods and techniques.

The resources of the developing countries for health programs are limited and are not more than a fraction of what is needed. Often, not more than a few dollars per capita annually are available. Therefore, health programs require careful planning. Health authorities should utilize – where feasible – the techniques of cost-effectiveness and operational research as guides to the selection of health programs.

Several helminthic diseases are chronic, insidious diseases with a broad range of clinical symptoms and it is difficult to assess their impact on both the health and the economy of exposed human communities. Epidemiological studies, such as quantitative studies of the distribution of infections, their clinicopathological consequences, and the dynamics of transmission in whole human populations are a prerequisite for a better understanding of the importance to health and economic impact of helminthic diseases. The control of these diseases must be based on a comprehensive understanding of the epidemiology of their disease complex. The main aims of epidemiological studies are:

1. To enable the health authorities to define the groups in the human population which are at high risk
2. To provide information on the distribution and size of the disease problems, on alterations in transmission dynamics, and on potential epidemics
3. To provide data essential for planning and application of control measures in order to achieve effective control with respect to the local conditions
4. To evaluate the effectiveness of control measures

The use of chemotherapy in the control of helminthic diseases has become more important with the development of new, more effective drugs during the past decades.

In order to assess the ultimate results of control by chemotherapy in research-oriented pilot projects, extensive epidemiological studies should be employed.

The importance to human health of most intestinal helminthiases depends on: (a) the pathogenic activities of the parasite, (b) the intensity of the infection (worm load), (c) the prevalence in the human population, and (d) the immunological status of the patient.

Most prevalences of intestinal helminths reported in the literature are based on assessments of relatively small groups and are not representative of the whole population. Various techniques have been used and consequently the resulting data are often not comparable. Moreover, the prevalences of helminthic diseases may diverge strongly in different regions of a country, and without data on the worm loads they give limited information on the importance of the diseases as a public health problem. Therefore the prevalences which have been reported in the literature and the estimated number of global infections are of limited significance. Nevertheless, prevalences and estimates of the number of infected people will be mentioned in this chapter in order to give an impression of the problem.

B. Epidemiological or "Mathematical" Models and Control

The epidemiology of many helminthic diseases is very complex and depends on a large number of biological and environmental factors. Various authors have devised epidemiological or "mathematical" models in order to assess the effects of biological and environmental factors on prevalences, incidences, intensities of infections, and transmission of schistosomiasis. These models have been used to analyze regulation systems of the parasite population and to demonstrate the interplay of the variables and the responses of these systems to modifications of the inputs. All models have deficiencies because several factors have been omitted or simplified in order to make the models manageable. Thus, reliable, predictive models have not yet been formulated. In spite of their deficiencies, an attempt has been made to adjust the models to real situations in order to predict the outcome of the modifications of the inputs. Simplified "mathematical" models have been useful in clarifying the qualitative aspects of transmission dynamics and aid an objective evaluation of alternative control measures. Models have also been used to design control programs.

HAIRSTON (1965) and MACDONALD (1965) introduced mathematical models into the epidemiological studies of schistosomiasis. HAIRSTON constructed predictive models on the population regulation of *Schistosoma japonicum*. The models rely mainly on simple probability functions such as the probability of the hatching of an egg, of a miracidium being able to encounter and penetrate a snail, and of sporocysts being able to develop in a snail and produce cercariae. In the first model the rate of snail infection is predicted in a situation where the rate of egg production is known. The second model predicts the rate of mammalian infection. HAIRSTON analyzed the dynamics of the suprapopulation[1] of *S. japonicum* in the Philippines, where four species of mammals are epidemiologically important definitive hosts. His studies showed that the suprapopulation of *S. japonicum* could be maintained by infections in field rats. In this host, the turnover of the parasite is much higher than in man, due to the large host population and the very intensive rat-snail contact. If the human population in the area were replaced by an uninfected population, the infrapopulation of the parasite in the human population would reach the same level as a few years previously. However, HAIRSTON'S models were too simple and failed to fit the biological data accurately. MACDONALD constructed a mathematical model for schistosomiasis and studied the theoretical results of modifications of inputs to his model by computer simulation. His model also relies on probability functions.

The main features of MACDONALD'S model are:

1. Schistosomes are bisexual and the probability of the sexes meeting in the definitive host depends on the number of parasites infecting a host. MACDONALD considered the probability of the parasite mating within the vertebrate host as an important regulating factor. He concluded that in every environment there exists a critical number of worms to ensure survival in a human population. The presence of less worms leads to a progressive diminution of the infection. The mean load below which infection is unable to maintain itself is called the "breakpoint." The breakpoint theory had important consequences for the planning of control programs, since it was thought that by reducing the worm load in man beyond the breakpoint, the remaining worm population would die out naturally.
2. Superinfections of the snail intermediate host are possible but limited, due to the limited capacity of the snails. Considerable increases of miracidia beyond the saturation level of the snails do not increase the ultimate number of cercariae. Consequently, the parasite population can be regulated by infection saturation of the intermediate host.

The main predictions from MACDONALD'S model were that sanitation is an ineffective control method, but that reduction of contact with contaminated wa-

1 The suprapopulation includes all individuals of all stages of the parasite in its ecosystem, whether the free-living stages or the stages living in the definitive and intermediate hosts

ter, snail control, and effective case-finding and treatment are more effective means of control. A combination of these control methods is the best approach.

Several assumptions on which MACDONALD's model is based are not realistic. Therefore, the model has only a limited validity. BRADLEY and MAY (1978) have shown that the distribution of schistosome worms in man is not random (it deviates from the Poisson distribution), but that the worms aggregate together. Consequently, neither MACDONALD's breakpoint concept nor his epidemiological conclusions are valid. The expectation that a reduction of schistosome densities in man below a "breakpoint" level will spontaneously be followed by extinction is highly unlikely.

BRADLEY (1972, 1974) pointed out that endemic parasitic infections tend to combine an efficient transmission mechanism with a rather stable parasite population. This means that in these endemic situations the parasite has: (a) a reproduction potential which tends to increase its population and (b) a negative feedback which is adequate to prevent the increase of the parasite population.

BRADLEY (1972) divided the regulatory mechanisms of parasite populations into three types: regulation by the transmission process (type I); regulation by the host population by such means as host mortality or sterile immunity (type II); and regulation by the host individuals, often by premunition and similar forms of incomplete acquired resistance (type III). The last two types are density-dependent feedback processes. The three types are not exclusive and all three may be operating to regulate one parasite at one place and one time.

In experimental *S. mansoni* infections in some primates and mice, the parasite population can be regulated by the mechanism of concomitant immunity. The adult *S. mansoni* organisms of the established infection are antigenically disguised by incorporating host antigens in their tegument (CAPRON et al. 1980). In this way they manage to escape largely the immune responses of the host, whereas the schistosomula of superinfections are readily killed after penetrating into the host. This mechanism is capable of regulating large increases and falls in transmission of the parasite. In the parasitic infections, where the parasite population is regulated by density-dependent immune mechanisms, it is much more difficult to interfere with the transmission cycle by direct attacks on the vector or intermediate hosts. In type III, where the regulation depends on the partial immunity of the final host, control by immunizing the final host is more promising.

In most human intestinal roundworm infections the parasite populations are regulated mainly by mechanisms which are related to the transmission of the parasite from one host to another (first category of regulatory mechanisms of BRADLEY). At the host level partial immune processes may have a minor regulatory influence.

BRISCOE (1976) designed a "mathematical" model for hookworm transmission in a community in West Bengal, including behavioral as well as immunological factors. Through this model BRISCOE was able to correlate improvements in sanitation with changes in prevalences and intensities of infection in the community. The practical use of his model is limited since it does not enable any predictions on the effects of biological and environmental factors on prevalences and intensities of infections in other communities to be made. No mathematical models have been designed for other intestinal worm infections in man.

C. Nematodes

I. *Angiostrongylus costaricensis*

Clinical intestinal angiostrongyliasis was first described from Costa Rica in 1967 by MORERA and CÉSPEDES. In man the nematode *Angiostrongylus costaricensis* matures in the mesenteric arteries. The eggs cause eosinophilic granulomata in the lymphatic vessels of the intestinal wall. Intestinal angiostrongylosis is mainly a children's disease.

CHABAUD (1972) reclassified the Angiostrongylinae and placed *Angiostrongylus costaricensis* in a new genus *Morerastrongylus*, which includes two species: *M. costaricensis* and *M. andersoni.*

1. Geographical Distribution

Most cases of human abdominal angiostrongylosis have been reported from Costa Rica, but the disease has also been identified in other Central American countries, Venezuela, and the southern part of Mexico.

2. Life Cycle and Morphology

The natural definitive hosts of *A. costaricensis* are rodents (*Rattus rattus* or *Sigmodon hispidus*), and the natural intermediate host is a mollusk, *Vaginulus plebeius* (MORERA 1973). The adult parasite is found in the mesenteric arteries of its rodent definitive host, mainly in the cecum. The male worms are about 20 mm long with a maximum width of about 0.29 mm. The female worms have a body length of about 33 mm and a maximum width of 0.34 mm. The ova are oviposited in the intestinal wall. In man the unembryonated eggs degenerate inside the intestinal wall, inducing granulomatous reactions in the surrounding tissue. In the natural definitive hosts the eggs embryonate in the intestinal wall and the first-stage larvae (0.27 mm) migrate to the lumen and are then excreted in the feces. The mollusk intermediate hosts become infected by ingesting the first-stage larvae. The second and third-stage L3 larvae develop inside the mollusk and the L3 larvae reach complete maturity between 16 and 19 days. The final host becomes infected by eating the infected mollusk. Man may be infected also by larvae which have been excreted by the mollusk in mucous material.

After infection the nonmobile larvae are liberated in the stomach of the host from the two sheaths of the former larval stages and then become very active. Their length is 0.47 mm. They penetrate into the intestinal wall, mainly in the ileocecal region, and after two molts in the lymphatic nodes and vessels the young adult worms migrate to the mesenteric arteries of the ileocecal region. On the 10th day after infection, all the parasites are in the definitive habitat. In both the mesentery and the intestinal serosa multiple small hemorrhages develop around the arterioles. Yellowish-brown pigment indicates that the worms have ingested blood. Oviposition starts by the 18th day after infection.

The first clinical symptoms begin about 24 days after infection.

3. Epidemiology

LORÍA-CORTÉS and LOBO-SANAHUJA (1980) studied a group of 116 children with clinical angiostrongylosis. They observed that in Costa Rica the prevalences increased during the rainy season (September–November). In this period, the number of intermediate mollusk hosts, as well as their activities, increase strongly. The highest prevalences were observed in school children 6–13 years of age (53%). The second highest prevalence was found in the pre-school age group aged 2–6 years (37%). The infection rate was much higher in boys than in girls. Probably the boys have more outdoors activities with increased risk of contact with infected mollusk intermediate hosts or the mucous material excreted by them. The authors observed that a significant number of the children have a good socioeconomic background. Clinical angiostrongylosis has seldom been reported from adults.

4. Clinical Manifestations

The most evident symptom in patients is abdominal pain, which is usually localized in the right iliac fossa and the right flank. This symptom was observed in 85% of 116 children with abdominal angiostrongylosis by LORÍA-CORTÉS and LOBO-SANAKUJA (1980). Fever occurred in 80% of the children and lasted 2–4 weeks. Abdominal tenderness and anorexia were observed in 60%–65%, vomiting in 45%, and diarrhea in 35% of the children. In 50% of the cases an intra-abdominal mass was felt which may be confused with a malignant abdominal tumor.

The clinical picture is very similar to appendicitis and differential diagnosis may be difficult. In 75% of cases leukocytosis of 10,000–50,000 leukocytes/mm^3 and eosinophilia ranging from 11% to 82% was seen. Radiologic findings showed alteration of the intestinal wall, spasticity, filling defects, and irritability of the cecum and ascending colon.

II. *Anisakis marina*

Anisakiasis or herring worm disease was first described by VAN THIEL et al. (1960). The worm was discovered in an eosinophilic phlegmon of the intestinal wall of a patient in Rotterdam. In the Netherlands worms causing human infections appear to be the third-stage larvae of *Anisakis marina*.

1. Geographical Distribution

Cases of human anisakiasis have been reported mainly from the Netherlands and Japan and from among Alaskan Eskimos. VAN THIEL (1976) concluded that only one species of *Anisakis* has been found in the North Sea, viz., *A. marina*. Probably all cases of human anisakiasis which have occurred in Western Europe have been caused by *A. marina*. Larvae of the same species have been surgically removed from patients with clinical anisakiasis in Japan. *Anisakis marina* is the commonest species in cetaceans of the Japanese coastal waters, but *A. physeteris* also occurs there. Cases of clinical human anisakiasis caused by *Teranova decipiens* (*Phocanema decipiens*) have been reported by Japanese authors from Northern Japan. However, the larvae of this species have always been recovered from the stomach of patients by fibergastroscopic biopsies and have not been found in the human intestine.

2. Life, Cycle, and Morphology

Adult *Anisakis* and *Teranova* worms occur in the stomach of marine mammals, viz., whales (mainly toothed wales), dolphins, and occasionally seals. The eggs are excreted with the feces and sink to the seafloor. The second-stage larva hatches in 20–27 days at a water temperature of 5–7 °C. Planktonic crustacea, especially euphausids, are the first intermediate hosts. They become infected by ingesting the second-stage larvae. The planktonic crustacea remain near the seafloor during the day, but during the night they migrate toward the surface, where they may infect herring, which are pelagic feeders.

According to VAN THIEL (1976), the euphausids *Meganyctiphanes norvegica, Thysanoëssa inermis,* and *T. raschii* can be considered to be first intermediate hosts of *Anisakis* in the North Sea.

The second intermediate hosts are the fish and squids which feed on plankton. After the infected euphausids have been ingested, the *Anisakis* larvae pass through the stomach or intestinal wall into the body cavity and encyst.

The larvae invade the muscles after the death of the fish intermediate host. Removal of the entrails immediately after the fish have been caught may prevent invasion into the muscles. However, there is evidence that the larvae may penetrate into the tissues before the death of the fish host. It has been demonstrated that the percentage of larvae which have invaded the muscles increases considerably during the first days after catching.

Numerous fish species have been found infected by *Anisakis* larvae. OSHIMA (1972) found *Anisakis* larvae in 122 fish species from Japanese waters. BERLAND (1961) from Norway and KOBAYASHI et al. (1966) from Japan reported that squids may be infected and that high prevalences of infection have been observed, particularly in their main growing areas in the Japanese waters.

The larvae recovered from man measure 15–26 by 1 mm.

3. Epidemiology

The infection occurs by eating raw, slightly salted, or marinated fish. Since the distribution of the adult *Anisakis* worms and the infective larvae is cosmopolitan, infections may be expected in all areas where there is the habit of eating raw fish or squid.

In the Netherlands, infections used to result from eating slightly salted raw herrings (so-called green herrings), but infections were prevented after the Government issued regulations in 1968 which required the herrings to be frozen at −20 °C for at least 24 h. The last cases were reported in 1970.

In Japan anisakiasis is still a health problem. Many fishspecies are eaten raw in Japan and it has been proven that at least 12 species have caused anisakiasis infections.

VAN THIEL (1976) reviewed the global distribution of anisakiasis. Single cases have been demonstrated in Denmark, the Federal Republic of Germany, Belgium, and Chile; a few cases have probably also occurred in Britain and Norway.

All the cases of anisakiasis caused by *Teranova* have occurred in Northern Japan, where more raw cod is eaten by the inhabitants than elsewhere in Japan.

OSHIMA (1972) reported that in Japan the highest prevalences have been observed in adult males, probably because this group consumes more raw fish – in combination with alcoholic drinks – than adult females and children. Compared with the large numbers of anisakiasis larvae which must have been ingested by man, clinical anisakiasis is rather rare.

A Dutch research group has suggested (POLAK 1965) that the gastrointestinal lesions are due to a hypersensitivity reaction to a second infection near to the site where the first larvae penetrated into the intestinal wall. However, RUITENBERG (1970) demonstrated that in experimental infections severe lesions could be caused by a primary infection of a single *Anisakis* larva and no local hypersensitivity could be demonstrated around the site of penetration. The severe form of anisakiasis is supposed to be an allergic reaction following a secondary invasion, whereas mild anisakiasis would result from a primary infection.

OSHIMA (1972) explains the relatively low prevalence of clinical anisakiasis in Japan by the high resistance of the healthy gastrointestinal wall to invasions by the larvae.

Clinical manifestations and diagnosis are described in Chap. 5.

4. Prevention and Control

The second-stage *Anisakis* larvae are killed most effectively by keeping the infected fish at a temperature of −20 °C for 24 h or longer. The larvae are not killed by smoking the fish as long as the temperature does not exceed 50 °C. Marinating is only effective if the process lasts for some time (30 days) and with fairly high concentrations of acetic acid (7%) and sodium chloride (15%). In the Netherlands, control by freezing the herrings at −20 °C has been very successful. In Japan, control is more difficult, since many species of fish are eaten raw and more people have the habit of eating raw fish.

III. *Ascaris lumbricoides*

Ascaris or roundworm infection is one of the most common and most widespread helminthic infections in man.

1. Geographical Distribution and Prevalence

A. lumbricoides is cosmopolitan in its distribution. Both in the tropics and in temperate regions where ecological factors are favorable for the parasite and where standards of sanitation and hygiene are low, *A. lumbricoides* flourishes. Ascariasis is believed to occur in 25%–30% of the world's population. In countries with a low national prevalence of ascariasis, hyperendemic areas may occur with very high prevalences. Until after World War II, areas with very high prevalences were found in western Europe. According to the WORLD HEALTH ORGANIZATION (1967), in Italy 75% of children in the village of Rofrano and 40% of toddlers in Naples were found to be infected. In Portugal rates of 40%–80% were reported. In the period following World War II, high prevalences were reported among children in some rural communities in the Netherlands (up to 45%), Germany (52%), and France (46%).

In the developing countries, prevalences are higher. MÜLLER (1975) reported estimates of 83%–94% in Leyte (Philippines), 98% in children in central Iran, 75% in Java, 90% in Malaysia, 58% in Ethiopia, and 98% in children in southern Taiwan. Based on the epidemiological survey of 1965–1968 by the Ministry of Health (CHAIA 1980), it was estimated that 46 million people (68%) were infected by *A. lumbricoides* in Brazil. In these areas the standard of living and sanitary situation were very poor ("developing areas").

It may be concluded that in 1980 the number of people with *A. lumbricoides* infections amounted to at least 100 million in Africa; 90 million in Latin America; 640 million in Asia, out of which 335 million were in China; 6 million in Australia-Oceania; 32 million in Europe; and 20 million in the USSR, of which 13 million were in European and 7 million were in Asian republics. The grand total of the infected persons probably exceeded 980 million.

Assuming a mean worm load of six per infected person and an average weight of 6.75 g (4.5–9 g) per worm, the quantities and masses of *A. lumbricoides* in humans reach astonishing figures: 5,340 million *Ascaris* worms, with a weight of 36,075 tonnes, corresponding to 600,000 adults. Extending this parasitological arithmetic to the high egg production the figures are no less impressive: each female *Ascaris* worm produces 5 g eggs annually, which gives, for an initial sex ratio of nearly 1:1, a total egg mass of 13,350 kg (2,670 million female worms).

2. Life Cycle and Morphology

The adult worms normally lie free in the lumen of the small intestine. They are large nematodes and the body tapers at both ends. The length of the females ranges from 20 to 40 cm with a diameter of 3–6 mm, and the slightly smaller males measure from 15 to 30 cm with a diameter of 2–4 mm. The color is whitish or pale pink to pale yellow. The terminal mouth is surrounded by three lips, each bearing a pair of sensory papillae on the outer margins. The daily output of eggs in about 200,000–240,000. Repeated copulation is necessary to produce continuously fertilized eggs.

The duration of the maturation process of the fertilized eggs into the infective second-stage larvae depends on environmental factors like the temperature, moisture, protection against UV light, and other environmental factors. Under appropriate conditions the development into the infective stage is completed in about 4 weeks at 20 °C and 2 weeks at 30 °C (WORLD HEALTH ORGANIZATION 1967). The lowest temperature for embryonation is 18 °C, but the eggs remain viable when exposed to sub-freezing temperatures. Eggs exposed at −23 °C during a period of 40 days subsequently embryonated normally when the temperature was raised appropriately. Only eggs at the single blastomere stage continued development after an exposure of 90 days to temperatures of −12 °C to −15 °C. Eggs of this stage can survive the winter and may become infective during the next spring. In favorable conditions in temperate climates, the eggs may survive up to 7 years in the soil. The development and survival of the eggs in the soil are strongly affected by its structure and humidity. Sandy soils tend to be dry, but are well aerated. Clay soils retain more water, but are badly aerated, whereas silty soils are intermediate between clay and sandy soils in both respects. The size of the particles of the soil determines how deep the eggs penetrate. The eggs tend to settle on layers of particles in the soil that have a larger size than the eggs. Near the surface the eggs are not well protected against UV light and desiccation. Protection against these factors increases with the depths of the eggs. On the surface the surviving time is between 3 weeks and a month, whereas eggs at depths between 10 and 50 cm may survive for years.

The adults live from 9 months to a maximum of 2 years. The fertilized eggs are ovoid and have a thick, transparent eggshell, which is usually surrounded by an irregularly mammillated albuminous coat which is stained yellowish brown by bile pigments. The fertilized eggs measure 45–75 by 35–50 μm. Beside the fertilized eggs, smaller numbers of unfertilized eggs may be found in the feces. These are irregularly shaped, particularly their outer coating, and are longer and narrower with a thin shell. They measure about 90 × 40 μm. The fertile eggs are still in the blastomere when they are passed in the stool. Under favorable environmental conditions they develop inside the egg into the infective stage within 2–3 weeks. First a noninfective rhabditiform larva develops, which after molting is transferred into the second-stage infective rhabditiform larva. The eggs are now infective. After ingestion, the infective eggs hatch in the duodenum. The eggshell is dissolved under the conditions in the duodenum, viz., high CO_2 concentration, a pH around 7.0, a low oxidation-reduction potential, and a temperature of 37 °C. The larvae penetrate into the mucosa and are carried through the liver and heart into the lungs in 3 days. Here they molt twice and penetrate the alveolae, ascend the bronchotracheal tree, and pass through the esophagus to the ileum. Here they molt for the fourth time and develop into adult worms in 3 weeks. Usually eggs appear in the feces some 60–75 days after infection.

Immunological processes participate in the regulation of the parasite population at the individual host level (i.e., type III of Bradley's regulating mechanisms). However, the regulating mechanisms of the *Ascaris* population which are related to the transmission of the parasite (Bradley's type I) are more important than the immunological processes. The factors which influence transmission are mainly environmental and human behavioral factors. The percentage of the eggs which develop into the infective stage, as well as the duration of the development into infective eggs, is determined by environmental factors. Human behavioral factors determine the proportion of the infective eggs which are ingested by the population and the number of noninfective eggs which are deposited in the environment.

3. Epidemiology

Prevalences of ascariasis are high in most tropical countries, particularly in children of the dirt-eating age. The most frequent methods of infection are by ingesting polluted soil, ingesting unwashed polluted vegetables and fruit, and via fingers which are polluted by soil. Indiscriminate defecation is the main factor for intensive transmission. Most of the polluted soil, vegetables, and fruit are found around the house and in its yard, and therefore ascariasis is essentially a peridomiciliary infection. Young children become infected by crawling around the house and ingesting soil. They are also the main source of pollution by *Ascaris* eggs since they tend to have high worm loads and defecate indiscriminately. In some areas, infection rates of nearly 100% are found in children. In arid regions prevalences are generally lower. The high prevalences in children are probably due to differences in behavior between children and adults. Children tend to have more oral-fecal contact. Another factor may be the lack of immunological resistance against the parasite in uninfected persons. CHEN (1971) demonstrated that over a period of 2 years only 10% of infected children had an increase in their worm load. This may indicate that in infected children some resistance against reinfections gradually develops. The differences in prevalences between adults and children are less pronounced in populations with high infection rates.

Prevalences are high in all areas where night soil is used as an important organic fertilizer, without killing the eggs by special treatment. ANUAR and RAMACHANDRAN (1977) demonstrated that all samples of lettuces from 12 markets in Penang, Malaysia, were heavily contaminated with *Ascaris* eggs. SOH (1973) examined vegetables at a market in Korea and found *A. lumbricoides* eggs on 49% of the lettuce, 23.2% of the radish, and 91.9% of the cabbage. The farmers spray night soil mixed with water for manuring the vegetables. These may become polluted when the night soil is sprinkled on top of them, but pollution may also result from splashing up of eggs from the soil during heavy rains.

Experimentally it has been demonstrated that thorough washing removed only 40% of the eggs, whereas most of the eggs stick to the surface of the vegetables by means of the adhesive eggshells. Eggs could be removed by applying detergents or by soaking the vegetables for 10 min in 55°-60 °C hot water. In families with low standards of hygiene, transmission within the houses and peridomicilliary infections are common. Poor sanitary facilities, indiscriminate defecation, the use of night soil around the house, and intensive finger-soil contact lead to high prevalences within the family.

Dry seasons are generally unfavorable for the survival of *A. lumbricoides* eggs in the soil. Therefore, both the number of new infections and the worm loads diminish during the dry season. Since most of the adult worms in the human population have a life span of 9 months or more, they survive the dry season and consequently the prevalences of ascariasis in the human population remain at nearly the same level. After the rainy season sets in, the conditions for transmission of *A. lumbricoides* become more favorable, which results in more infections and increasing worm loads. About 2 months after the onset of the rainy season, the egg counts in the stools of the population begin to increase. The prevalences, however, show no or only minor seasonal fluctuations. GELPI and MUSTAFA (1967) observed a marked seasonal increase in the eosinophilia and in the number of cases of ascaris pneumonitis during the rainy season in Saudi Arabia.

Other environmental factors which exert an influence on the transmission of *A. lumbricoides* are: the wind, which increases the desiccation of the eggs; UV light, which kills the exposed eggs within a few hours; oxygen, which is necessary for the maturation of the eggs into the infective stage; and animals, which can disseminate the eggs over a wider area. *Ascaris* eggs are resistant against toxic agents such as formalin, acids, and alkaline solutions, but are sensitive to ethylalcohol, chloroform, methylbromide, and ammonia. In situations where polluted vegetables and fruits are mainly responsible for the transmission of ascariasis, the human population is evenly exposed and there are no great differences between the prevalences in adults and children. In situations with very poor sanitary conditions in and around houses, higher prevalences and worm loads are observed in children, particularly in the age group of between 5 and 10 years. These children have more contact with the heavily polluted soil in the yard and they also ingest more egg-infested soil than adults. Adult women who have more contact with polluted vegetables normally have higher prevalences and higher worm loads than adult males.

There is a great variation in the daily egg-output of *Ascaris* worms in the stool of the human host. Consequently, a single egg-count is a poor measure of the worm burden. Average egg counts on at least three consecutive days give much more reliable information on the worm burdens.

GHADIRIAN (1972–1973) observed that *Ascaris* prevalences in a group of Iranean nomads were extremely low. The parasite was nearly absent because they defecate in scattered sites and do not grow crops.

It is generally accepted that in human infections by *A. suum* the parasite does not complete its cycle in the host. The larvae may cause pulmonary symptoms but they do not develop into adult worms. TAKATA (1951), however, reported that in 7 out of 19 volunteers adult *A. suum* worms were observed after infections with infective eggs.

4. Clinical Manifestations and Intensity of Infections

The great majority of *Ascaris* infections are asymptomatic or the symptoms may be so slight that they are ignored by both the patients and the doctors. However, the presence of a few or even one worm may cause severe morbidity. Even very light infections are potentially dangerous. Next to direct pathological processes in the host, *Ascaris* infections also affect the nutritional status, particularly in children.

The morbidity caused by the impairement of nutrition may be of greater importance for the population than the direct effects caused by the worms. VENKATACHALAM and PATWARDMAN (1953) demonstrated that children harboring an average of 26 worms, and with a diet containing 35–50 g of protein daily, lose 4 g of protein due to the interference of the worms.

CHOWDURY (1980) observed that following fasting and a protein test meal, the average level of blood aminoacid nitrogen and the percentage of increase was significantly higher in a control group than in a group harboring *A. lumbricoides*.

The depressed aminoacid absorption in the infected group was corrected following deworming by chemotherapy. In other experiments it was demonstrated that the fecal and urinary nitrogen excretions in patients were significantly reduced after removal of the worms by chemotherapy. The absorption of fat and to a lesser extent also of carbohydrates are also impaired by *Ascaris* worms. Disturbance of vitamin A level, lowered retinol levels in infected children, and an association between ascariasis and xerophthalmia have been observed.

STEPHENSON (1980) concluded that in certain communities there is a relationship between childhood malnutrition and *Ascaris* infections. Deworming improved the growth of the infected children. She recommends periodic deworming by mass treatment in areas where ascariasis and protein malnutrition are highly prevalent.

LATHAM, LATHAM and BASTA (1977) studied the nutritional and economic implications of *Ascaris* infection in the Machakos District in Kenya. Groups of children were studied over a period of 10 months. The infected children as well as the uninfected control group received the same anthelmintic treatment twice at intervals of about 3 months. Skinfold thickness significantly increased in the infected group after treatment. Weight gain was significantly greater in the infected group after deworming when compared with the controls. Clinical signs of protein caloric malnutrition were significantly increased in children with *Ascaris* infections and decreased significantly after deworming. They concluded that ascariasis is an important health problem in Kenya. It retards the growth of children and is an important cause of morbidity.

Experiments carried out in Zaire demonstrated that the weight gain in a group of treated children (single dose of levamisole, 2.5 mg/kg, at 3-month intervals for 1 year) was 21% greater than in children receiving a placebo. Large number of worms increase the possibility of severe morbidity. Moreover, persons with large worm loads are more dangerous as a source of infection in the community. For these reasons it is important to estimate the worm load. The intensity of infection can be determined at autopsy by counting the worms. Following chemotherapy, the worm load can be estimated by counting the expelled worms. However, it is not sure that all worms have been evacuated and it is difficult to collect all the feces with voided worms. The most used method to estimate the worm load in epidemiological studies is an indirect one and is based on the number of eggs passed in the feces.

The direct smear is simple and rapid and can be used for egg counts since the egg output per female worm is high (about 240,000 eggs/day). The cellophane thick smear using stool samples of 50 mg can be used for estimations of the density of *Ascaris* eggs, but in heavy infections the egg output per worm is difficult to estimate because of the enormous numbers of eggs (often more than 100/mg feces). Another problem is that the egg output per worm varies with the age and size of the worm and that there are large daily differences. The mean output of eggs per gram formed stool per female worm has been estimated by several authors. The numbers reported vary from 1,500 to 3,645. The most reliable estimate (2,925) was made by MELLO (1974), who carefully studied 19 children. Nevertheless, there is a great variance in egg counts. For this reason it is recommended that the data on egg numbers is grouped into categories corresponding to light, moderate, and heavy infections, rather than making exact egg counts. Another method is the formalin-ether sedimentation method.

5. Control and Prevention

As in other intestinal roundworm infections, there are three main approaches of prevention and control:

a) Environmental Sanitation

The basic environmental control measures are: (a) safe disposal of human feces including night soil, (b) provision of safe household water in adequate quantities, and (c) prevention of contamination of food by fecal material.

Environmental sanitation will not be effective as long as the population concerned does not understand the meaning of the measures and does not, therefore, participate actively. In all areas with a marked improvement in the socioeconomic situation, the standards of sanitation rise and prevalences of *Ascaris* diminish quickly. In a population living under very poor socioeconomic conditions, control by environmental sanitation and health education will not be very successful.

Large-scale latrine construction may be efficient as a long-term control measure of *Ascaris*. However, in the short term it may not be expected to reduce the prevalences of ascariasis drastically. Young children, particularly pre-school age children, belong to the most heavily infected age groups and are too small and young to use pit latrines properly. They will continue to contaminate the soil with large amounts of eggs, since the daily egg-output per adult female *Ascaris* is enormous (about 240,000). Even a child with a relatively light infection can deposit millions of *Ascaris* ova peridomiciliary and keep transmission going on.

There are several reports (Arfaa et al. 1977; Chandler 1954; Eyles et al. 1953; Khalil 1926; Moore et al. 1965) on the influence of hygienic standards and sanitary facilities on the prevalences of ascariasis. In most cases it appeared that in families with higher hygienic standards and in villages with good sanitation the prevalence is significantly lower than in people living under poor hygienic conditions and poor sanitary facilities. Schliesmann et al. (1958) studied families with high, medium, and low hygienic standards and found significant differences in the prevalence of ascariasis between the three groups. Chandler (1954) found significantly lower infection rates in an Egyptian village with good sanitation than in a village with poor sanitation. In a community it appeared that the prevalence was lower in families with flush toilet facilities than in families with pit latrines. The hygienic and sanitary conditions, however, often reflect the socioeconomic situation of the population and it is difficult to assess each factor separately. The availability of sanitary facilities by themselves do not guarantee lower *Ascaris* prevalences. An unsanitary privy may be worse than no facilities at all. Sanitary facilities which remain unused are ineffective. It is therefore of great importance that the sanitary facilities are acceptable to the community. Flush toilets may become choked because the people cannot afford toilet paper. In some cases, sanitation has been successful, as on Réunion Island, where the prevalence of *Ascaris* infection diminished considerably in zones where facilities for sanitary disposal and potable water supplies had been provided a decade previously (Bonnefoy and Isautier 1978). However, the prevalence of *Trichuris trichiura* had changed but little. In Singapore squatter families became homeless after a severe fire and were transferred to modern flats with adequate sanitary facilities. Kleevens (1966) observed that after some time there was a much higher prevalence for ascariasis in the children in the squatter area than in the children from families which had been transferred to the flats. In the age group of 10–12 years 74.3% of the children in the squatter area and only 8.7% of the children in the flats were positive for ascariasis.

The differences between people with and people without good sanitary facilities are even more obvious when the mean worm loads and egg outputs are compared. Soh (1973) compared a group with bad sanitary facilities with a group with fairly good facilities and found 48.4% and 27.6% infected, respectively. The mean numbers of eggs in the two groups were 24,795 and 4,453.

b) Mass Chemotherapy

The primary objective of mass chemotherapy is the reduction of the community worm load below the level of clinical significance. It also reduces the environmental contamination with *Ascaris* eggs considerably. Deworming improves the growth of children and in areas with malnutrition and high prevalences of ascariasis, periodic deworming is a cost-effective control method. Latham, Latham, and Basta (1977) estimated that the total economic cost of ascariasis in Kenya in 1976 was over $5 million in a single year. The estimate includes the following costs: health care, $180,000; anthelmintic drugs purchased by the Government, $160,000; anthelmintic drugs purchased by the general public $199,000; and the value of food lost due to *Ascaris* infections $4,400,000. According to these authors, control by mass treatment is "the only way in which *Ascaris* and related helminthic infections can economically and significantly be reduced in Kenya in this decade." The cost of an effective dose schedule, based on wide spectrum anthelmintic treatment of every inhabitant, is estimated to be $800,000 annually in Kenya. A deworming program, based on an average of twice a year, is expected to result in a cost benefit ratio of 1 : 10.

In areas with high *Ascaris* prevalences, mass treatment may periodically be given to all persons in the vulnerable ago groups (target groups). In other areas, selective treatment of persons with positive stools may be preferred. In several experiments it has been demonstrated that, soon after treatment, the prevalence starts to rise again and that 12 months after a single treatment the prevalence returns to its original level. Therefore, the treatments should be repeated at 3-month intervals.

c) Health Education and Improvement of the Hygienic Standards of the Population

Health education should aim at motivating the population to participate in prevention and control measures by using the facilities offered by environmental measures, washing fruit, and cooking vegetables; to prevent promiscuous defecating, particularly in children's play areas; and to improve househould and personal hygiene.

IV. *Capillaria philippinensis*

Human intestinal capillariasis was first seen in a patient from Northern Luzon (Philippines) in 1962. No other definitive hosts than man have yet been discovered, but attempts are being made to find naturally infected mammals and birds (Cross et al. 1978, 1980).

1. Geographical Distribution

Human intestinal capillariasis has been reported from some coastal areas of the Philippines and several areas in Thailand. After the first report from Burguey in Northern Luzon, a severe epidemic of gastroenteritis in Tagudin was found to be caused by *C. philippinensis*. Other endemic foci have been reported from Luzon and northeastern Mindanao (Santiago). The first case in Thailand was reported in 1973 and new cases were observed in scattered areas throughout the country.

2. Life Cycle and Morphology

The life cycle has been established in experimentally infected laboratory animals and it is believed that in man the same cycle occurs. *C. philippinensis* is a very small intestinal nematode; the females are 2.3–5.3 mm in length and 29–47 μm wide at the widest part of the body. The males are smaller and measure 1.5–3.9 mm in length and 23–38 μm in diameter. The spicule is 230–300 μm long.

The parasites live in the lumen of the jejunum and throughout the jejunal tissue. In the uterus of the female worm, thick-shelled eggs, thin-shelled embryonated eggs, and first-stage larvae may be found. The characteristic lemon-shaped eggs measure 42 × 20 μm.

Eggs are excreted in human stools, and depending on the temperature they embryonate in water in 5–10 days. When the embryonated eggs are ingested by freshwater fish, the larvae hatch in the fish intestine. The newly emerged larvae measure 130–150 μm and in 2–3 weeks increase to 250–300 μm and become infectious. Several species of freshwater fish have been found to be suitable intermediate hosts. *Hypselotus bipartita* has been found naturally infected (CROSS et al. 1980). Infective larvae removed from the intestine of the fish intermediate host and fed by stomach tube to Mongolian gerbils developed into adult worms within 10–11 days. Within 13–14 days females produced larvae which developed into second-generation adults. The second-generation females produced eggs which were passed in the feces of the gerbil as early as 25 days after infection.

From gerbils which were fed with only two or three larvae, thousands of worms (as many as 7,000) were recovered at necropsy. Internal autoinfection is an integral part of the life cycle. As long as the infection persists, there are larviparous females present. By autoinfections the parasite is able to build up and maintain a large population in the final host, even when the initial infection was light.

3. Epidemiology

Gerbils, monkeys, and wild rats have been infected experimentally by feeding them infective larvae from fish (CROSS et al. 1980). Rats have a natural resistance and the infections were transient. Monkeys retained the infections for months and did not show severe symptoms, whereas the gerbils fell ill and died. Several fish-eating birds have also been found susceptible to infections with *C. philippinensis* and they may be reservoir hosts.

Since several species of freshwater fish are suitable intermediate hosts and many fish-eating birds could be infected, it may be expected that *C. philippinensis* has a wider geographical distribution than is known at present. Human infection depends on eating raw or undercooked fish.

During the epidemic which occurred in Tagudin, Philippines, in 1967–1968 over 1,300 people became infected, and 90 persons with parasitologically confirmed infections died.

Since 1968 a few hundred cases and 16 deaths have been reported. Several cases have been reported from scattered areas in Thailand, but so far only on fatal case is known from this country (CROSS et al. 1980). During the epidemic in Tagudin (1967–1968) most untreated patients with capillariasis died. Now mortality is very low provided that an early diagnosis is made and effective treatment is given. Capillariasis is characterized by diarrhea, abdominal pain, and borborygmi. If no treatment is given and the illness progresses, the symptoms become more severe and the patients experience weight loss, dehydration, muscle wasting, malabsorption, and cachexia. In the past, before the etiology of capillariasis was known, many cases of this disease probably occurred.

4. Control

Health education should be directed against the eating of raw or undercooked fish. Sanitary disposal of feces to prevent the infection of the fish intermediate host should also be included in the preventive control measures. At present treatment of capillariasis with mebendazole is the most effective method of control. In severe cases with malabsorption, protein-losing enteropathy, and electrolyte depletion, the treatment consists of antidiarrheal drugs, mebendazole, and electrolyte and protein replacement.

V. *Enterobius vermicularis*

Enterobius vermicularis (*Oxyuris vermicularis*) causes enterobiasis or oxyuriasis. Popular names for the infection are pinworm or threadworm infection (MAYERS and PURVIS 1970, MCDONALD and HOURIHANE 1972).

1. Geographical Distribution

Enterobius vermicularis is a cosmopolitan parasite of man and probably the commonest human helmintic infection. It is commoner in temperately countries than in the tropics.

2. Life Cycle and Morphology

The adult worms are small cylindrical nematodes which are pointed at both ends. They are whitish and have a smooth cuticle. The females measure 8–13 mm in length and 0.3–0.5 mm in diameter. The male worm measures only 2–5 mm in length and 0.1–0.2 mm in diameter. Three lips surround the mouth. The muscular esophagus has the characteristic posterior bulb. A pair of cervical alae on the cuticle arise just behind the nerve ring and continue as lateral projections almost to the anus in the female worm. Because of the lateral alae, *E. vermicularis* is easily recognizable in tissue sections in ectopic localizations. The female worms have a long, pointed tail. In the gravid females, the paired uterus is packed with eggs and nearly fills the whole body. The vulva is situated at one-third of the length of the body.

The posterior end of the male worm is curved ventrally. The males have a single, relatively long spicule.

Adults are found predominantly in the lumen of the cecum and appendix, but in heavy infections they may be present in the adjacent parts of the colon (ascending colon) and ileum. They lie free in the lumen or are attached with their head to the mucosa. They feed on the intestinal contents. The worms copulate in the cecum and the males die after copulation. The gravid females migrate through the colon and rectum, especially during the evening and the night and emerge via the anus to lay a large number of sticky eggs on the perianal and perineal skin. After oviposition the female worms die.

The ovoid eggs, which are flattened on one side, measure 50–60 by 20–32 μm and have a semitransparent shell. The outer albuminous layer of the egg is sticky and keeps most of the eggs attached to the skin. They are already partially embryonated and mature in about 6 h at body temperature in the presence of oxygen. At lower temperatures the embryonation requires more time. The total number of eggs per female is estimated to be 10,000. After the eggs have been swallowed by the host, the infective rhabditiform larvae hatch in the duodenum. The young juveniles molt two or three times and migrate slowly through the small intestine to the cecum, where they soon become sexually mature. The life span of the worms ranges from 35 to 53 days.

3. Epidemiology

Infection rates may be very high (up to 100%), particularly in children living in orphanages and boarding schools or attending kindergartens and crowded schools. High prevalences are also found in hospitals and in large families.

CHOBANOV and SALEKHOV (1979) compared the prevalences among urban and rural populations in Azerbaijan, USSR. Prevalences in the town and in the villages were similar, viz., 39.2% and 38.2%, respectively. Differences in prevalence could not be attributed to the level of personal hygiene or the local sanitary conditions. Children of the pre-school age who were brought up at home had low infection rates (9.4%–9.8%), but children of the age group of 4–7 years attending kindergartens had the highest prevalence rates (57.2%–60.9%).

The high prevalences in schoolchildren were mainly due to the introduction of the parasites by children who had previously attended kindergartens. Infection rates in adults were between 6.3% and 11.4%.

Childless families had low infection rates (4.2%), but infection rates increased in proportion to the number of children, reaching 70% in families with six children. Crowded and small spaces for the children's free activity increased transmission and infection rates. All these facts indicate that *Enterobius* is a group infection. In tropical countries the prevalences are generally lower, probably because clothes and bedclothes are important factors in the transmission of enterobiasis. Most new infections are brought by about dust infection, i.e., inhalation or ingestion of eggs in dust. Soiled bedclothes, nightwear, underwear, dust in bedrooms, lavatories, bedclothes, and bedpans are important sources of dust infections. The eggs become dislodged from the bedclothes, nightwear, etc. and large numbers of ova have been found in classroom dust and in lavatories (up to 465/m^2).

In an orphanage in Taiwan, ova were found on 85.7% of the bedpans, on 83.7% of the linen, on 78.5% of the toilets, and in 77.4% of the dust specimens but, on only 3.6% of the toys and 4.2% of the desks.

Below 23 °C, the eggs are unable to develop to the infective stage. In a moist environment the embryonated eggs may survive for 2 months. In dry conditions, the eggs are killed within a few days.

Most dust-borne infections are light. The heavier infections arise from direct or indirect anus to mouth transmission by finger contamination. Females and eggs in the perianal region can cause anal irritation and intense itching which lead to scratching and lodging of large numbers of eggs under the fingernails. The eggs are dislodged when the fingers are put in the mouth. Especially in small children this is the principal method of infection, leading to heavy infections. Indirect anal-oral infections result from food, cigarettes, and eating utensils which have been contaminated by fingers.

If the eggs hatch on the perianal skin, the infective larvae may migrate through the anus into the bowel and establish new infections. This method of infection is called retroinfection or retrofection. It is more common in adults than in children. Chronic infections in adults are mainly maintained by retroinfections, which are characterized by recurrent, short, mild infections at intervals of 40–50 days.

Clinical manifestations and diagnosis are described in Chap. 5.

4. Prevention and Control

Hygienic methods plus mass treatment of all infected persons is the best method of control. All members of a family group, orphanage, or school should be treated in order to prevent reinfections.

VI. *Gnathostoma spinigerum*

This enteric nematode is normally a parasite of cats and dogs, but has a very wide range of other fish-eating animals as final hosts. Human infections are normally contracted by eating raw, marinated, or poorly cooked freshwater fish.

In the human host the parasite does not develop into the adult stage, but migrates through the body, causing a visceral larva migrans syndrome. In normal hosts such as cats, dogs, and other felines, the adult parasites are located in the stomach. Other species belonging to the genus *Gnathostoma* have been reported as parasites in human beings, but it is believed that most of these specimens were *G. spinigerum*.

1. Geographical Distribution

The most important endemic areas of human gnathostomiasis are found in Thailand and Japan, but the disease has been observed throughout Southeast Asia up to Australia, including China, the Philippines, Malaysia, Indonesia, Bangladesh,

India, and Sri Lanka. Cases have also been reported from the Sudan and Israel (DAENGSVANG 1980).

2. Life Cycle and Morphology

The adult worms measure 20–30 mm in length. The anterior part of the worm is deeply embedded in the host's gastric wall, which forms a typical concave swelling consisting of hypertrophic mucosal tissue around the penetrated worm(s).

The eggs, which measure about 70 × 38.5 μm, are passed in the feces and hatch after 1 week in fresh water at an appropriate temperature. If the first-stage larvae are ingested by a compatible copepod (*Cyclops* spp.), they develop within 1–2 weeks into second-stage larvae. The second intermediate hosts are mainly freshwater fish which feed on copepods. The larvae penetrate into the gastric wall, migrate, grow, and finally encyst in skeletal muscles. This process requires at least 1 month. Inside the pale, yellow cysts, which have a diameter of 1 mm, lies the coiled larva which is 4 mm long. After the infected muscle is ingested by an appropriate final host, the third-stage larvae are set free by the gastric digestion of the cyst wall and then penetrate through the stomach wall into the abdominal cavity. During migration through several tissues the larvae reenter the stomach after 3½ months. Here they penetrate the gastric mucosa with their anterior part and develop into adult worms in about 6 months.

3. Epidemiology

The secondary infection of the second intermediate host seems to be more prevalent under natural conditions than the primary infection. MIYAZAKI (1960) reported that in Japan 32 species of animals, including fish, amphibians, reptiles, birds, and one mammal were found to be infected under natural conditions. Of the naturally infected animals, four species of fish and the domestic chicken are the main sources of human infections in Japan since they are frequently eaten raw by the Japanese people.

DAENGSVANG (1980) reported that in Thailand infective larvae occur in fermented food which is made of raw freshwater fish (*somfak*). This food is more often eaten by women than by men; therefore gnathostomiasis is more prevalent among women in Thailand. In Japan the main source of infection is raw, sliced meat of fish (*sashime*), particularly of *Ophicephalus* spp., but other fish as well as raw chicken may also cause infections.

For a description of the clinical manifestations, diagnosis, and treatment, see Chap. 5.

VII. Hookworms: *Ancylostoma duodenale* and *Necator americanus*

The two species of hookworms that affect man are *Ancylostoma duodenale* and *Necator americanus*. The disease caused by hookworms is called ancylostomiasis or uncinariasis. *N. americanus* infections are popularly called New World hookworm infection and *A. duodenale* infections Old World hookworm infections.

1. Geographical Distribution and Prevalence

The two main species of human hookworms have overlapping distributions. Both species have been spread widely by population movements. *N. americanus* is endemic in central Africa and Madagascar, and the tropical areas of the western hemisphere where it was introduced by the slave trade, including the West Indies and the southern United States, southern and eastern India, Indochina, Queensland, and the South Pacific Islands. This species has also been introduced into Turkey, Iran, and Portugal.

Ancylostoma duodenale is the dominant species in the more temperate areas. It is present in the Mediterranean area, north Africa, India, Burma, Indochina, Malaysia, Indonesia, China, Japan, the South Pacific Islands, Australia, and the Americas. However, *N. americanus* is more dominant in the western hemisphere.

In 1947 STOLL estimated the total number of people infected by hookworm at more than 450 million (STOLL 1947). Since then little if any improvement has been achieved in the control of hookworm, and consequently the number of infected people at present must be about 1.5 billion. Hookworm infection is mainly a rural problem. Many published surveys have been made in urban areas; most figures are therefore too low and not representative of the national prevalence. Reports have been made of prevalences of 89% in Ethiopian children and 27% –83% in adults; 50% in Egypt; 16%–85% in the Lake Victoria area in Uganda; 44% in Zambia; 30% in China; 86% in Delhi; 50%–70% in Bengal; 84% in the rural areas of Iran, but only 6% in the Nomads; 30% in Brazil; and 20% in Puerto Rico.

2. Life Cycle and Morphology

In both species the adult worms are located in the jejunum. *N. americanus* is found mainly in the second and third part of the jejunum and seldom in the duodenum. *A. duodenale* is found in the jejunum and not normally in the duodenum. Both species may be present as far back as the cecum in very heavy infections.

The adult worms are cylindrical with a smooth cuticle. In *N. americanus* the head is sharply curved dorsally. The large, spherical buccal capsule has a pair or semilunar cutting plates ventrally, two very small plates dorsally, and a tooth and short lancets at the bottom of the capsule. In *A. duodenale* the head is slightly curved dorsally. The large, elongated buccal capsule has two pairs of large curved teeth ventrally and a pair of smaller teeth at its bottom. Both species have a pair of glands which secrete anticoagulants into the buccal capsule.

The male worms measure 7–9 × 0.3 mm in *N. americanus* and 8–11 × 0.4–0.5 mm in *A. duodenale*.

The female measures 9–11 × 0.4 mm in *N. americanus* and 10–13 × 0.6 mm in *A. duodenale*.

The caudal bursa of the male in *N. americanus* is narrower than that of *A. duodenale* its dorsal ray is much more deeply cleft than that of *A. duodenale*.

The fertilized eggs of the hookworms are discharged with the feces. The daily egg output per *N. americanus* female has been calculated by BEAVER (1955) to be between 20,000 and 50,000, but the latter figure is probably too high. Other estimates for *N. americanus* egg output are between 15,000 and 32,000 eggs per day per female (NAWALINSKY et al. 1978 a, b). Egg production by *A. duodenale* is thought to be 2.5 times that of *N. americanus*. Estimates of the egg output by *A. duodenale* are between 30,000 (NAWALINSKY et al. 1978 a, b) and 100,000 eggs per day per female. In human hookworm infections the egg output is density dependent and egg production is lowered in medium and heavy infections. Only in the lightest infections is the egg output optimal. The eggs of *N. americanus* and *A. duodenale* are indistinguishable. They measure 60 × 40 µm. The eggs are unsegmented at laying and usually have reached a four- or eight-celled stage when they are discharged with the stools. When the eggs reach a soil with good ecological conditions, they hatch in 24–48 h and develop into the rhabditiform larvae. Favorable environmental conditions for rapid development are warmth (≧25 °C), shade (no UV light), moisture, and well-aerated soils.

The eggs and juveniles of hookworms do not develop under water. In apparently dry soils the larvae can survive and develop in capillary films of water. Oxygen is necessary for the hatching of the eggs as well as for the development of the larvae.

Clay soils are not well aerated, and consequently during the rainy season the survival rate of hookworm eggs and larvae is low in these soils. The rhabditiform larvae, which measure 280–300 × 17 µm, feed on fecal debris and other organic material in the earth and molt twice.

After the second molt, they are transformed into the infective-filariform larvae. Since the third-stage larva is ensheathed in the sheath of the previous second-stage larva, they are unable to take up food. In this stage the larvae of *N. americanus* and *A. duodenale* can be differentiated by several morphological characters, such as size, form of the esophagus, tail, and space between esophagus and intestine. The overall length is 660–720 µm, *A. duodenale* being somewhat longer than *N. americanus*.

3. Epidemiology

In favorable conditions the filariform larvae remain viable for several weeks. The optimal temperature range is 25°–30 °C. Most of the larvae live in the top soil providing moisture and oxygen are sufficient.

Optimal habitats are, shady, aerated soils covered by vegetation. In this type of soil, the filariform larvae can migrate horizontally over a distance of 60–90 cm. When the filariform larvae come into contact with the human skin, they become activated, penetrate the skin, enter the venules, and are carried by the circulation to the right heart and the lungs. Here they grow, penetrate through the wall of the alveoli, and ascend the bronchioli, bronchi, and trachea. Most of the larvae reach the jejunum. After molting twice, they become sexually mature. The fertilized females begin to oviposit 4–7 weeks after infection. Some authors (AKETAGAWA 1930; FÜLLEBORN 1926; KOIKE 1960; SAKURAI 1960; SHIRAI 1926; YOKOGAWA 1926) have claimed that oral infections with *A. duodenale* are more common than percutaneous infections. In human volunteers YANAGISAWA and MIZUNO (1963) demonstrated that in *N. americanus* the percutaneous "developing rates" are 10.3% and the oral infection rates only 0.09%, whereas in *A. duodenale* the percutaneous and the oral infection rates were 3% und 54.9% respectively. NAWALINSKY et al. (1978 a) compared the proportions of *A. duodenale* in groups of children with high and low prevalences of orally infecting helminths (*A. lumbricoides* and *Trichuris trichiura*). No correlation was found, however, which could support the hypothesis of the oral infection route of *A. duodenale*. The same authors (1978 b) calculated the percutaneous efficiency of *N. americanus* to be 17.5% and of *A. duodenale* to be 5.3% in West Bengal.

The hookworm infections are mainly confined to the humid tropical regions, but the geographical distribution of *A. duodenale* is larger than that of *N. americanus*, since the free-living stages can develop into the filariform larvae at lower temperatures. During the construction of the St. Gotthard tunnel (1877–1881) severe epidemics with many fatal cases of "tunnel anemia" broke out among the workers. Later these workers introduced ancylostomiasis into the coal mines. There it became an important health problem and many miners died of "cachexia montana".

Opinions on the life spans of adult *N. americanus* and *A. duodenale* are conflicting. Estimates of from a few months up to 20 years have been made. In a light *N. americanus* infection (25 *N. americanus* females), the egg production persisted for 15 years in a patient who was not exposed to reinfection. However, after the first 5 years the egg output diminished and the worms probably began to die at that time (PALMER 1955). Other observations confirm that the reduction of the egg output in patients with *N. americanus* infection occurs over a long period and that there are no seasonal fluctuations. NAWALINSKY et al. (1978 b) estimated a mean life span of 3–4 years for *N. americanus* in a group of children studied in West Bengal who were continuously exposed to reinfections. This may suggest that the potential life span of the adult hookworms in hosts which are not exposed to reinfections is much greater than the actual life span of worms in endemic areas under conditions of frequent reinfections. The mean life span of *A. duodenale* is much shorter than that of *N. americanus* and seasonal reductions in egg output are observed in patients with *A. duodenale* infection. In a group which was protected against reinfections a rapid decrease in the number of *A. duodenale* eggs was observed 15 months after the infection. According to NAWALINSKY et al. (1978 b) the adult *A. duodenale* in West Bengal lives for about 1 year under the prevailing conditions in this area.

Seasonal fluctuations have been reported from several endemic areas. NAWALINSKY et al. (1978 b) observed an increase of the intensity of hookworm infections during the premonsoon period and a decrease during the late monsoon period in West Bengal. They suggest that this seasonal increase is mainly the result of the maturation of latent *A. duodenale* larvae which were acquired 8–10 months previously during the previous wet season. Experimental infections with the same *A. duodenale* strain confirmed the long prepatent period (40 weeks) and an arrested development of the worms. The prepatent period in this strain is probably dependent on the reaction of the larvae to environmental conditions. Latent development of the worms in the definitive host does not occur in *N. americanus*.

Congenital human hookworm infections are suggested by observations of hookworm eggs in the feces of 6- and 7-day-old infants. Experimental congenital infections of dogs with *A. caninum* have been demonstrated.

By repeated infections with small doses of normal larvae or with large doses of irradiated larvae, dogs could be immunized against *A. caninum* infections. The immunization resulted in a high degree of resistance to the establishment of worms in challenge infections and an expulsion of adult worms. In man the infection intensities of *A. duodenale* are probably also affected by acquired resistance. In an experimentally infected volunteer who was immunized by infections with a total of 5,000 larvae of *A. duodenale* in gradually increasing doses, resistance was demonstrated against a large challenge dose of 5,000 filariform larvae. Immunity is also suggested by the fact that generally infections are relatively mild in the endemic areas.

The intensity of soil contamination with hookworm eggs is an important factor in the population dynamics of the parasite. A low socioeconomic level of the population, which is generally associated with poor sanitary facilities and ignorance, leads to promiscuous defecation and a high degree of contamination of the soil. Defecation often takes place in a limited number of sheltered sites which are used by families or groups of families. These sites become foci of intensive transmission, resulting in high prevalences and intensities of hookworm infection. In dry areas the preferred sites of defecation are often sheltered, shaded, and with a humid aerated soil, which provides appropriate ecological conditions for the development of the larvae and egg survival. In large areas night soil is used as an organic fertilizer. This practice promotes hookworm transmission unless the eggs are killed by proper treatment of the night soil.

A low prevalence of hookworm (6.1%) and other soil-transmitted helminths was observed in primitive nomadic shepherds in Iran (MOTABAR and MONTAZEMI 1978). This was attributed to poor climatic conditions, such as sub-zero temperatures during the winter and extremely hot and dry summers, as well as to the short time which the tribe spent at every camping site.

4. Intensity of Infections and Clinical Manifestations

The clinical manifestations during the stage of infection are absent or mild, viz., itching and burning at the site of penetration followed by vesicular eruptions ("ground itch"). During the migration through the lungs the larvae may cause coughing and eosinophilia. Bronchitis and pulmonary manifestations are infrequent and generally limited to heavy infections. The symptoms due to the adult worms depend mainly on the intensity of the infection. In mild hookworm infections there may be no clinical manifestations at all. In moderate infections the patient may suffer from abdominal discomfort, dyspepsia, pain, nausea, anorexia, and intermittent diarrhea or constipation. In moderate and heavy infections in which the blood loss is not compensated, a hypochromic microcytic anemia is the cardinal manifestation. In patients with light or moderate infections, anemia is the result of an insufficient iron uptake, due to a poor diet. In patients with heavy infections and significant losses of blood, even an adequate diet cannot compensate the loss of iron. A constant drain of the iron stores finally results in a hypochromic microcytic anemia. The anemia responds favorably to iron or liver therapy.

The amount of blood lost by a patient suffering from a hookworm infection is correlated with (a) the species of hookworm involved in the infection and (b) the number of worms (worm load). Therefore, there exists a correlation between the intensities of the infections and the severity of the anemia. The amount of blood lost by a hookworm-infected patient is estimated to be 0.03 ml per worm per day for *N. americanus* and 0.15 ml per worm per day for *A. duodenale*. Consequently, an infection with *A. duodenale* worms causes a blood loss which is five times larger than an infection with the same amount of *N. americanus* worms.

An infection with 100 adult *A. duodenale* worms causes a loss of 15 ml blood/day, which corresponds to about 7.5 mg iron in a patient with a normal hemoglobin level. A small amount of the hemoglobulin (about 12%) is reabsorbed from the intestine. In man an adult male absorbs about 0.6 mg iron from an adequate diet. In patients with a negative iron balance, the quantities of absorbed iron may increase. However, the quantity of lost iron exceeds the total amount of absorbed and reabsorbed iron in a heavy hookworm infection. Gradually the iron store in the body of the patient declines and if the deficit is only a few milligrams per day, it may take years before the anemia becomes overt. Poor diets with inadequate amounts of dietary iron accelerate the hookworm anemia.

In very heavy infections, acute symptoms may set in immediately after infection. Koshy et al. (1978) reported the clinical features in an unusually heavy infection of *A. duodenale* in a group of young males who had intensive body contact with the infected ground. Immediately after exposure to the soil a severe dermatitis with general urticaria set in. In *A. duodenale* infections dermatitis is less frequent than in *N. americanus* infections, and generally ground itch develops in less than 6% of the infected persons. After a period of 1 week the dermatitis subsided and a few days later nearly all the infected persons developed severe pulmonary symptoms which continued for months (average 3 months). Abdominal symptoms started 3–10 months (average 6.3) after exposure. Generally abdominal symptoms set in 6–7 weeks postinfection. Probably in this case the development of the larvae was arrested in the intestine (see Sect. C.VII.3).

The diagnosis of hookworm infection is discussed in Chap. 5.

5. Control

After the severe outbreaks of "tunnel anemia" during the construction of the St. Gotthard tunnel and the spread of hookworm by infected workmen into the countries of continental Europe, the medical authorities became aware of the hookworm problem. Studies demonstrated that hookworm disease had become a serious health problem, particularly among miners ("cachexia montana"). Before World War I (1903–1914) a well-organized control program was conducted in Germany. The main features of the program were: large-scale treatment of infected miners, prohibition of work underground for new employers with hookworm infection, installation of sanitary facilities in the mines, and health education of the miners. The control program was successful and was adopted by other European countries. In the western hemisphere, the Rockefeller Foundation and the International Health Board initiated hookworm control, first in Puerto Rico (1904) and the southern United States (1909) and later from 1913 onward in other parts of the world, mainly in the West Indies and Latin America and also in several Asian countries, New Guinea, and Australia. Basically, the concept of the control program was the same as that of the German control program:

1. Control by mass treatment
2. Control by the construction of sanitary facilities for safe disposal of human feces
3. Health education

Control by means of mass chemotherapy does not interfere strongly with transmission. As early as 1922 the Rockefeller Foundation made it clear that the objective of mass chemotherapy was not the elimination of all the hookworms in infected people (eradication), but considerable reduction of the worm loads and thereby a strong reduction of the severity of the clinical symptoms. Hookworms have a large output of eggs; frequent treatment is therefore a prerequisite for a reduction of transmission. Other negative factors of mass treatment are the inadequate coverage of the population and the lack of motivation of the people to follow the dosage scheme or to submit to chemotherapy repeatedly. Therefore, mass treatment should be combined with other control measures.

The excretal pollution of the soil is a crucial factor in the transmission cycle of all nematode infections which are transmitted by cutaneous larval penetration. Promiscuous defecation and the use of untreated nightsoil are the most important human factors in the transmission of hookworm. The sanitary disposal of the feces of the whole human community would break the transmission cycle. However, safe excretal disposal is not a simple problem. The introduction of environmental sanitation is not automatically followed by a decline in hookworm infections.

When environmental sanitation measures have been introduced in the community, the people continue to defecate in agricultural sites and maintain transmission of hookworm infection in these sites.

As long as the people are reluctant to use the sanitary facilities properly, control by environmental sanitation will fail. The community must be acquainted with the life cycle of the parasite, the dangers of hookworm infections, and the methods of preventing the infections. They must be motivated to participate and use the sanitary facilities provided. Health education should be simple and understandable for the community. It should explain and demonstrate individual prophylaxis, such as wearing shoes, avoiding contact with the soil, and washing the hands. An adequate diet should be propagated.

When mass chemotherapy, environmental sanitation, and health education are combined and integrated, the control program will be more successful. The results of the control measures must be evaluated by repeated quantitative measurements of the reduction of worm load as well as the anemia in the community.

VIII. *Oesophagostoma* spp.

Oesophagostomiasis in man is caused by strongylid nematodes, which are normally parasites of monkeys and apes. In many cases it has not been possible to determine the species involved in human infections. The most common species found in man is *Oesophagostomum apiostomum. O. stephanostomum,* which is normally found in gorillas in Africa, has been reported from human infections in Brazil and Uganda. It is a rare infection in man (HAAF and VAN SOEST 1964; KAMINSKY and NDINYA-ACHOLA 1977).

1. Geographical Distribution

Most cases of human oesophagostomiasis have been reported from West and East Africa. Single cases have been reported from Brazil and Indonesia.

2. Life Cycle and Morphology

Normally the adult worms are located in the large intestine. Morphologically they resemble hookworms. The eggs of *O. apiostomum* also resemble those of hookworms. In an appropriate environment and a temperature of about 26 °C, these eggs hatch and develop into the first- and second-stage larvae in about 10 days. The infective third-stage larvae are ingested by the final host, which is histotropic, and invade the submucosa of the end of the small or (usually) large intestine. Here the larvae develop to the fourth stage, then return to the lumen of the bowel and become mature worms. The prepatent period lasts about 5 weeks in the normal host. In man the infection probably occurs in the same way, but some authors suppose that percutaneous infections may be possible.

IX. *Strongyloides stercoralis*

Strongyloidiasis or anguilluliasis in man is normally caused by *Strongyloides stercoralis,* although human infections by *S. fülleborni,* a parasite of monkeys (chimpanzee and baboon), have been reported, especially in Africa (high prevalences in infants in Zaire and Zambia). *S. stercoralis* has also been reported in dogs and apes (CROVE 1980).

1. Geographical Distribution

Strongyloides stercoralis essentially is a cosmopolitan parasite. Since the larvae and free-living adults need a moist and warm soil for their development, the parasite is more abundant in the tropical and subtropical regions of Africa, Asia, and the western hemisphere. Its distribution corresponds largely with that of the hookworms. In patients with autoinfections, *S. stercoralis* can persist for decades outside the endemic regions.

Prevalences of strongyloidiasis are high in areas with low sanitary standards. All ages may be infected, although severe cases of disseminated strongyloidiasis occur only in patients with deficient immune responses.

Prevalences of 58% in Brazil (CHAIA 1980), 25%–40% in Surinam (ASIN and VAN THIEL 1963), 3% in mentally retarded children in New York (before control by chemotherapy 17%) (YOELI et al. 1972), and 27.5% in allied ex-prisoners of war in Southeast Asia (GROVE 1980) have been reported.

2. Epidemiology

The transmission of both *S. strongyloides* and the hookworms have many similarities. In all nematode infections which are transmitted by cutaneous penetration, fecal soil pollution as well as extensive contact of the human skin and the polluted soil are necessary for transmission. However, there are differences, and strongyloidiasis is not always coextensive with hookworm infections. In most areas the prevalence of *S. stercoralis* is lower than the prevalence of hookworm. The reasons for the differences have been insufficiently studied. On one hand the free-living generations increase the number of infective filariform larvae considerably and the parasitic females of *S. stercoralis* have a larger offspring. On the other hand the *S. stercoralis* infective larvae have a shorter longevity and the rhabiditiform larvae are more vulnerable than the hookworm eggs. They have little resistance to dry conditions and die within a few days at temperatures below 8 °C or above 40 °C.

It is impossible to make a reliable estimate of the worm load in strongyloidiasis because: (a) there are no methods for quantitative enumeration of *S. stercoralis* larvae in the feces and (b) in auto- and hyperinfections the number of larvae in the stool is not related to the worm load in the patient.

The population dynamics of the parasitic phase of *S. stercoralis* are strongly dependent on the immunological resistance of the host. In patients with suppressed or deficient immune responses, hyperinfections with extensive visceral invasions of *S. stercoralis* and an enormous increase in worm load are found.

Invasion of the intestinal mucosa by filariform *S. stercoralis* larvae may be stimulated by low motility of the intestine and stasis of the larvae. Therefore, diverticulosis of the gastrointestinal tract and ileus might predispose to autoinfection and overwhelming hyperinfections of *Strongyloides*.

3. Control

As in hookworm infection, control of strongyloidiasis depends mainly on: (a) the safe disposal of human feces by means of a combination of providing adequate sanitary facilities and health education and (b) chemotherapy.

A survey of the life cycle, morphology, clinical manifestations, and diagnosis can be found in Chap. 5.

X. *Ternidens deminutus*

Ternidens deminutus (*Triodontophorus deminutus*) is normally a parasite of monkeys in Africa and Asia. The infection in man is called "false hookworm infection."

1. Geographical Distribution

The first human infection was reported from an autopsy from the island of Mayotte. Later, human infections were reported from Zimbabwe (with locally very high prevalences of over 80%), Zambia, south Tanzania, South Africa, Zaire, and the Comoro Islands. Human infection is geographically more restricted than infection in the common hosts. No human cases have been reported from outside Africa. It is not known why human infections are restricted to Africa (GOLDSMID 1967; KILALA 1971; SANDGROUND 1931).

2. Life Cycle and Morphology

The adult worms inhabit the colon and occasionally the ileum. In size and appearance they resemble hookworms, but they are longer and may readily be distinguished by the presence of the corona radiata (a crown of cuticular bristles surrounding the mouth). The worms are also broader than the hookworms. The female worms measure 12–16 mm by 0.65–0.75 mm and the males 9.5 by 0.55 mm. The males have a characteristic caudal bursa. The eggs, which resemble hookworm eggs, may be differentiated by their greater mean size viz., 82 by 51 µm. When they pass out in the feces, they are normally in the eight-celled stage. In an appropriate environment they hatch and develop into the rhabditiform larvae in about 30 h, which feed on organic detritus and bacteria. After two molts and about 8 days later, the third-stage larvae are developed. Attempts to infect the final host with the third-stage larvae, either by the oral route or by skin penetration, have been unsuccessful.

XI. *Trichinella spiralis*

Trichinellosis, trichinosis, or trichinelliasis is a cosmopolitan parasitic disease of carnivorous animals. Heavy infections in man are followed by severe clinical symptoms and a high mortality (GOULD 1970).

1 Geographical Distribution

Trichinella spiralis is endemic in carnivorous animals throughout the world. Epidemics of human infections with severe morbidity and mortality have been reported from Germany, Eastern Europe, and Spain. In 1865 a severe epidemic caused 333 cases and 101 deaths in Hedersleben (Germany) and during the epidemic of 1883 in Madrid 763 cases and 173 deaths were reported. In most cases, however, the infections are mild with only light clinical symptoms. In the United States trichinellosis has been a widespread disease with a high prevalence. GOULD (1970) found a mean prevalence of 60% in the United States in the period between 1931 and 1942 and LINK (1952) estimated that in 1952 about 25 million people were infected in the United States. Most of these cases were mild, subclinical infections. After that, the prevalence rate in the United States diminished considerably and in 1968 it was estimated at 4.2% (ZIMMERMAN et al. 1973). Other important areas with human trichinellosis are Canada, Alaska (mainly amongst the Eskimos), Poland, the USSR, Latin America, the Pacific area, Indonesia, and Japan.

2. Life Cycle and Morphology

The adult female worms measure 2.5–3.5 × 0.06–0.07 mm and the males 1.0–1.5 × 0.03–0.035 mm. They taper toward the anterior end. The posterior part of the esophagus, which is typical for *Trichinella*, is relatively long and nonmuscular. It consists of cubical cells or stichocytes with a central intracellular canal. The female worms are ovoviviparous and the ova develop into larvae, which are discharged from the uterus. In a mature female worm the uterus is filled with larvae. The adult worms partly penetrate into the intestinal wall. Toward the end of the 1st week following the ingestion of infected food, the first larvae (80–120 × 5.6 μm) are deposited deep in the intestinal mucosa. During its lifetime of about 5 weeks, a female worm produces up to 2,000 larvae. These penetrate into the deep lymphatics and from there they enter the systemic blood circulation. They are capable of leaving the capillaries in many organs such as the myocardium, brain, retina, and liver, but the striated skeletal muscles are the sole site where they can develop into infective larvae. The diaphragm is the most frequently invaded muscle. After penetration into the muscle fibers they grow slowly. About 10 days after the invasion of the sarcolemma the larvae become U-shaped, and at about the 17th day of the infection they begin to coil and develop a spiral form. Soon after the invasion the typical cross striations of the sarcoplasma of the muscle fiber disappear and the fibers become more basophilic. Simultaneously the nuclei of the infected fiber show a marked proliferation, become spherical and increase numerically, as well as in size. The hypertrophic nuclei migrate to the axis of the fiber, but later they are again located beneath the sarcolemma. Four weeks after the invasion, the development of the larva is completed. It is supposed that the larva molts twice before it reachs the infective third stage. The tenfold growth in length of the larva and its spiraling cause the typical spindleform distension of the muscle fibers around the larvae. The swollen and edematous sarcoplasm forms the so-called basophilic halo of Nevinny surrounding the larva. The halo of Nevinny contains smooth membrane systems, mitochondria, altered nuclei, tubules of the endoplasmic reticulum, and an enlarged Golgi apparatus, which indicate that there is intensive metabolic activity of the altered sarcoplasm. In a later stage inflammatory reactions follow, with infiltrates of neutrophils, eosinophils, lymphocytes, and plasma cells; the edema then subsides. Gradually the larvae become encapsulated. The formation of the collagenous outer capsule is a complex process of tissue reactions in which the sarcolemma is involved. Inside the capsule, granulations and sarcoplasmic prolongations are found. Externally the capsule is surrounded by fibrillar connective tissue. After a few months the cyst walls gradually become calcified, but it may take a long time before the calcification becomes manifest. The encysted *Trichinella* larvae may stay alive for more than 20 years.

After ingestion of meat containing living larvae, the cyst wall is digested in the host's stomach and the larvae are liberated. They quickly pass to the duodenum and the anterior part of the small intestine. After two ecdyses, they are transformed into adult worms. After copulation the males die and the females penetrate into the mucosa.

3. Epidemiology

The main source of human infections in the temperate regions is provided by domestic pigs. Besides the "domestic" life cycle there are "sylvatic" or "feral" cycles of this zoonotic parasite, in which wild animals are the sources of infections. The trichinae involved in the sylvatic cycle have a low infectivity to domestic pigs and rats. Human infections by the strains of *Trichinella* with a sylvatic cycle are the result of the ingestion of undercooked or smoked meat of wild pigs and warthogs, or the meat of carnivorous animals such as polar bears, walruses, and dogs.

Some authors separate the *Trichinella* infections occurring in man into three separate species, viz., *T. spiralis,* with a domestic cycle; *T. nelsoni,* the etiological agent of sylvatic trichinellosis in East and South Africa, the USSR, Bulgaria, and Switzerland; and *T. nativa,* also having a sylvatic cycle and occurring in North America, Europe, and Asia. *Trichinella nelsoni* is common in wild foxes in Switzerland and occurs mainly in the southern part of the Old World up to a latitude of 48° north of the equator. Most researchers do not accept separation into three species, in spite of the distinct differences in infectivity to domestic pigs, in antigenic components, in pathogenesis, and in morphological differences of the cysts. In a recent outbreak of trichinellosis with two fatal cases among a tribe in Tanzania, a warthog (*Phacochoerus aethiopicus*) was the source of infection (BURA and WILLET 1977). The strain of *T. spiralis* was similar to that isolated in Kenya, where the infections resulted from eating meat of wild pigs.

In Africa the rodent *Mastomys natalensis,* which is a very susceptible host to *Trichinella,* can play a substantial role in the transmission of trichinellosis in a natural environment and is supposed to become an effective link between the domestic and sylvatic cycles. In the United States, both prevalences in the human population and the number of cysts in individual patients have diminished considerably over the past 2 decades. The average infection rate in pigs which are fed on garbage dropped from 11% in 1950 to 0.5% in 1966.

Small epidemics still occur in European countries. Recently a small epidemic was reported (GENTILINI et al. 1976) from the southern suburbs of Paris. Due to the difficulties of diagnosing mild infections, the real prevalences in man are not known. In northeast Iran the sylvatic strain of *Trichinella spiralis* is quite common. HAMIDI (1979) found 84% of the golden jackals, 30% of the red foxes, and 9% of the dogs infected. The main source of human infection in this area is the wild boar *Sus scrofa.*

In the Arctic regions seals probably become infected by ingesting marine amphipods (crustaceans). Experimental transmission via amphipods has been proven by FAY (1967). These amphipods may become infected by feeding on fragments of meat of dead infected mammals. The *Trichinella* cysts have a high resistance to low temperatures and putrefaction of the surrounding meat.

4. Immunity

In natural infections the host develops a strong and long-lasting immune protection. In experimental studies it has been demonstrated that antigenic fractions of the muscle larvae induce immunological responses in the host (DESPOMMIERS et al. 1977). After injection of the antigenic material, fewer muscle larvae developed in the muscles of the challenged hosts than in the controls. It has also been demonstrated that adult female *Trichinella* worms from immunized rats produce nearly 50% fewer newborn larvae. The protection of the host induced by antigens which are released by the pre-adult enteral stage of the parasite is as effective as the protection induced by natural infections.

Antibodies as well as specific subpopulations of lymphocytes are engaged in induction of the protective immune processes (CRUM et al. 1977).

Eosinophil-mediated destruction of newborn larva has been demonstrated in vitro (MACKENZIE et al. 1980).

The clinical manifestations and diagnosis are described in Chap. 5.

XII. *Trichostrongylus* spp.

Several species of *Trichostrongylus* which are normally parasites of ruminants are found as parasites in man. The species most commonly found in man is *T. orientalis, T. colubriformis, T. axei, T. brevis, T. instabilis, T. lerouxi, T. probolurus, T. skrajabini,* and *T. vitrinus* have also been reported as parasites in man (MARKELL 1968; MOTABAR and MONTAZEMI 1978).

1. Geographical Distribution

The prevalence of human infection with *Trichostrongylus* is related to the association between man and his domestic ruminants. The areas with the highest prevalences are those where there is a very close association between man and sheep. Prevalences of 27.6% have been reported in nomadic shepherds in Iran (MOTABAR and MONTAZEMI 1978). In southern Iran, infection rates of 87% have been observed. Other population groups with high prevalences have been found in Egypt, Ethiopia, Armenia, Turkey, Korea (one particular area with a prevalence of 80%), and Indonesia (MARKELL 1968; MÜLLER 1975).

2. Life Cycle and Morphology

The adult worms live in the duodenum and jejunum, where they are attached to the intestinal wall. They are small and thin, the females measuring 5–10 mm in length, while the males are somewhat smaller. There are three small lips around the mouth but no buccal capsule. The copulatory bursae of the males, particularly the spicules, are characteristic for the species. The worms penetrate with their head into the mucosa of the small intestine.

The eggs resemble those of hookworms, but are longer, narrower, and more pointed at one end. They measure 75–100 × 30–50 μm. When passed in the feces, the eggs are already embryonated to the morula stage. The eggs hatch under the appropriate conditions within about 24 h and reach the infective stage in about 3 days after two molts in the soil. The third-stage infective larvae are capable of penetrating the skin (as infective hookworm larvae), but in human infections the third-stage infective larvae are normally ingested with food. The worms reach maturity within 3–4 weeks.

3. Epidemiology

The embryonated eggs are very resistant to low temperatures, desiccation, and submersion in water. The infective larvae are susceptible to high temperatures and low humidity, but may survive long periods of cold weather; freezing kills them, however. In man the adult worms may survive for more than 8 years.

In man infections are generally light, but in the ruminant hosts the worm loads may be very high. The principal hosts constantly contaminate the soil; the peri-domiciliary soil is often heavily polluted especially when ruminants are kept in the backyards of houses or around houses. Human behavior resulting in a close association between man and ruminants may result in heavy infections.

4. Control and Prevention

Avoidance of the ingestion of infective larvae on raw vegetables or via fingers prevents human infection. Therefore, environmental sanitation and the provision of safe water and health education may be important measures of control. However, *Trichostrongylus* infections are common in people living in very poor sanitary conditions and in close association with ruminants. Sanitation and health education will not have much effect on transmission in populations with a low socio-economic level. Treatment of ruminants can also be applied as a control measure. In most situations the feasibility of these methods is low, such as in groups of nomadic shepherds.

Selective treatment of moderate and heavy infections is the most efficient method at present of controlling clinical trichostrongyliasis.

XIII. *Trichuris trichiura*

Trichuriasis, trichocephaliasis or whipworm infection is a widespread infection, particularly in children. The number of people infected with *Trichuris trichiura* (*Trichocephalus trichiurus*) is estimated at 750 million.

1. Geographical Distribution

Trichuris trichiura is a cosmopolitan parasite which is more common in the warm parts of the world with high rainfall. It is not as widespread as ascariasis and has a more patchy distribution. In some areas in tropical countries, prevalences of more than 90% have been found, but usually prevalences are between 30% and 60%. In most areas, prevalences of *Ascaris* infections are higher than those of *T. trichiura*, but this is not always the case. In Martinique (1980) prevalences of 37% for *T. trichiura* infections and 7% for *A. lumbricoides* were reported (CAREC SURVEILLANCE REPORT 1980). Prevalences of 75.6% for trichuriasis and 37.5% for ascariasis were found in pygmies in Zaire (1979) (PAMPIGLIONE et al. 1979), 84.3% and 96% in Brazil (1979) (ALMEIDA 1979), 83.8% and 64% in squatter areas in Kuala Lumpur (1978) (CHIA WEE 1978), 20.2% and 64.9% in Indonesia (1979) (LUBIS et al. 1979), 21% and 57% in Kar Kar Island, Papua (1976) (JONES 1976a), 19.8% and 55.5% in Dakka City (HUQ and SHAIKH 1976), 19.5% and 64.4% in Sri Lanka (FERNANDO and BALASURIYA 1976), and very few and 49% in East Timor (1976). Trichuriasis is not rare in the temperate zones (JONES 1976b).

2. Life Cycle and Morphology

The adult worms usually occur in the cecum, but may also be found throughout the colon, rectum, appendix vermiformis, and terminal ileum, particularly in heavy infections. The adult worms are whip shaped, having a narrow anterior portion and a much wider posterior portion (hence the name "whipworm"). They are pinkish-gray. The females measure 30–50 mm in length, and the males are slightly smaller, 30–45 mm, with a tightly coiled posterior end and a single spicule.

The anterior, narrow portion of the worms is partially embedded in the mucosa of the intestine and carries a simple mouth with a stylet which facilitates the penetration of the mucosa. Behind the mouth lies the simple nonmuscular esophagus. At the end of the anterior, narrow part of the body, the esophagus passes into the midgut. The anus is situated at the posterior end of the body. The worms obtain nutrition from the host tissue and from blood.

Estimates of the egg output by *T. trichiura* are very variable, viz., from 1,000 to 46,000/female per day, but the mean output is between 2,000 and 10,000 eggs/day. The characteristically barrel-shaped eggs have a mucoid, transparent polar prominence at each end. The eggs are yellowish-brown and measure 52×22 μm.

They have an inner and an outer shell. At oviposition, the eggs are unsegmented. After passing out in the feces, they take from 2 weeks to several months to embryonate in the soil, according to temperature, moisture, and protection against sunlight. They require a period of 4–6 months at 15 °C, 3–4 weeks at 26 °C, and 12 days at 35 °C to develop into the infective stage. The embryonated eggs which are ingested on contaminated hands or food, such as raw vegetables, hatch in the distal part of the small intestine. The first-stage larvae attach themselves to the villi or penetrate into the intestinal wall, where they lie coiled up. After a few days, the immature worms emerge, reenter the intestinal lumen, and migrate down to the cecum. They molt four times and reach the final predilection site at the time that they have achieved maturity. Eggs begin to appear 2–3 months after ingestion of the infective eggs. The longevity of the adult worms is not exactly known, but it is believed that they may live for between 3 and 8 years.

3. Epidemiology

The mode of infection of *T. trichiura* is similar to that of *A. lumbricoides,* and these two intestinal nematodes are commonly coextensive. However, *T. trichiura* infection is usually more common in areas with a high humidity and dense shade, whereas *A. lumbricoides* is more prevalent in drier and unshaded areas, because *T. trichiura* eggs have a lower resistance to cold, heat, and complete immersion in water. In temperate climates, the highest prevalences are found in institutes for mentally abnormal children and other institutionalized groups.

The same factors that increase the transmission of *Ascaris* also affect the transmission of trichuriasis, like pica (dirt eating), eating contaminated, unwashed fruit and vegetables, and indiscriminate defecation around the house. In their study of lettuces from markets in Penang, ANUAR and RAMACHANDRAN (1977) found 50% of the samples to be contaminated with *T. trichiura* eggs. The lettuce had been contaminated by night soil which had been used as manure.

4. Control and Prevention

Safe sanitary disposal of human feces, provision of safe household water, and health education are the main approaches for a lasting control of trichuriasis. However, environmental sanitation is not effective in a population which is not motivated to participate in the control and preventive measures. BONNEFOY and ISAUTIER (1978) evaluated the results of a decade of intensive efforts of environmental sanitation (sanitary disposal of feces, safe water supplies) and health education in the island of Réunion. The prevalences of trichuriasis had changed but little. In other intestinal helminthic infections, however, prevalences had diminished to about 50% of the previous level.

At short notice more benefit may be expected from mass treatment. The main objective of mass treatment programs is the reduction of the worm load in a community to below the level of clinical disease. Besides, mass treatment may reduce the contamination of the environment and thereby transmission of trichuriasis.

Complete eradication by chemotherapy is difficult. Nevertheless, good results of control by mass treatment, resulting in a drastical reduction of worm loads, have been reported from many countries.

The success of mass treatment programs of *T. trichiura* is improved by control of diarrhea before administration of anthelmintics and their use in higher doses or longer and/or repeated courses.

D. Trematodes

I. *Echinostoma* spp.

Echinostomiasis is caused by a number of echinostome flukes. Human infections have been occasionally reported. Dogs and rats are the main natural hosts of the species involved in human infections. A survey of echinostomiasis can also be found in Chap. 12.

1. Geographical Distribution

Echinostoma ilocanum, causing Garrison's fluke infection, has been reported as a human parasite from the Philippines. The normal definitive hosts are dogs and rats (TUBANGUI and PASCO 1933).

Echinostoma lindoense has been a common human parasite in the area around Lake Lindu in central Sulawesi. Prevalences of 25%–95% have been reported (BONNE et al. 1948). At present it is a rare parasite in man, as a result of changes in the eating habits of the population (CARNEY et al. 1980).

Echinostoma malayanum has been reported as a human parasite from Thailand and Malaya; it probably also occurs in north China (HARINASUTA 1969).

Human cases of *E. hortense* infection have been detected in the Akita prefecture in Japan. Metacercariae have been found in loach and it is supposed that human infection is caused by eating raw loach.

Other species that have been reported from man are *E. revolutum* and *E. melis*.

2. Life Cycle and Morphology

The adults are small flukes measuring 5–8 mm in length and 1–2 mm in width. The integument is scaly. They are characterized by a circumoral collar with spines. Each species has a characteristic arrangement of the spines. The ventral sucker is about four times larger than the oral sucker and lies near the anterior end of the body. The adult worms live in the small intestine of the host.

The eggs are similar to those of *Fasciola* or *Fasciolopsis,* but are slightly smaller and measure about 100×70 μm. Embryonation requires 1–2 weeks in fresh water with appropriate conditions. The miracidia penetrate the snail intermediate hosts (planorbid snails) and develop through a sporocyst and two redial stages to the cercarial stage. The cercariae penetrate the second intermediate snail hosts after a free-swimming period (particularly in *Indoplanorbis* and *Pila* spp.).

3. Epidemiology

Man acquires an infection by ingestion of raw edible second intermediate snail hosts, and human echinostomiasis occurs mainly in areas where these snails are eaten as delicacies. Dogs, rats, and other mammals are reservoir hosts.

CLARKE et al. (1974) and CARNEY et al. (1980) report that during the 1970s more than 30,000 stool specimens were examined from rural populations in Indonesia and that only occasionally were echinostome eggs found. In the Lake Lindu valley, central Sulawesi, high prevalences of *E. lindoense* were observed in 1937, 1940, and 1956, ranging from 24% to 96% (CARNEY et al. 1980). In 1971 and 1972 no echinostome eggs were found in the stools of the population in this area.

According to CARNEY et al. (1980), the population of the snail *Corbicula lindoensis,* which was the main source of human infections, has nearly disappeard from the Lindu valley. This decline of the snails may be the result of the introduction of the fish *Tilapia mozambica* in this area.

II. *Fasciolopsis buski*

Fasciolopsiasis, or giant fluke infection, is caused by *Fasciolopsis buski.* It is a common parasite of pig, man, and other mammals in Southeast Asia (MANNING and RATANARAT 1970; RAHMAN et al. 1981; SADUN and MAIPHOOM 1953). Information can also be found in Chap. 11.

1. Geographical Distribution

The most important endemic areas are central and south China, Taiwan, India (mainly in Assam and Bihar), Bangladesh, Thailand, Laos, and Cambodia. In China it occurs mainly in the Kwantung und Chekiang Provinces (CROSS 1969). The Yangtze valley is the northern limit of the endemic area. In Bangladesh a high infection rate has been reported from children in a rural area (36.2%) (MANNING and RATANARAT 1970).

2. Life Cycle and Morphology

The adults, which are situated in the small intestine, are large trematodes ranging in size from 25 to 75 mm in length and from 8 to 20 mm in width. In heavy infections the adults also occur in the stomach and colon of the host. They are fleshy, ovoid, pinkish-red worms with a cephalic cone. The tegument is covered by rows of small spines. The oval sucker has a diameter of about 0.5 mm, and the ventral sucker is about four times larger and is situated close to the oral sucker. The bulbous pharynx lies under the oral sucker. The unbranched ceca extend almost to the posterior end of the body. The highly branched testes lie behind each other in the posterior half of the body. The branched ovary occupies the middle of the body and the vitelline glands are situated in the areas lateral of the intestinal ceca. The uterus is packed with ova, which measure 130–140 × 80–85 μm.

The eggs look very much like *F. hepatica* eggs. The daily output per fluke is about 25,000 eggs. At oviposition, the eggs are not embryonated. They pass in the feces and need an aquatic environment for their development, which takes 3–7 weeks at a temperature of around 28°–30 °C. When the miracidia penetrate an appropriate snail intermediate host they develop through a sporocyst and two redial stages to the cercarial stage. Appropriate snails are the planorbids, such as *Polypylis* (= *Segmentina*) *hemisphaerula*, *Hippeutis cantori*, and *Trochocorbis trochoideus*. Development in the snail host takes 30–50 days. The cercariae emerge from the snail, swim in the water, and encyst on aquatic vegetation such as the water caltrop (*Trapa bicornis* and *T. natans*), water chestnut (*Eliocharis tuberosa*), and other freshwater plants. When the infested plants are ingested by a suitable host, the encysted metacercariae excyst and the young flukes attach themselves to the wall of the duodenum. Here they develop to maturity in 3–4 months. The life span of the adult worm in man is about 6 months.

3. Epidemiology

The miracidia are short lived and vulnerable. The encysted metacercariae are resistant to adverse environmental conditions, but are highly susceptible to desication.

High infection rates have been reported from some endemic areas, such as 85% in Chekiang and 70% in Maharashtral (Cross 1969). Worm loads may be very high in human infections, and cases of loads of several thousands of worms have been reported.

The prevalences of fasciolopsiasis are correlated to the feeding habits of the population. In villages where nightsoil is used as fertilizer for the water caltrop beds and where fresh seedpods are eaten raw, high prevalences may be expected. Since the water caltrop is grown in ponds with stagnant water, it is often the main source of infection. The infectivity of the metacercariae diminishes during transport due to desiccation. Therefore, infection rates are higher in the villages where the water caltrop is grown and where the cysts have not yet dried up. The seedpods of the water caltrop and the water chestnut bulbs may be covered by hundreds of metacercariae and consequently human infections may be very heavy.

In endemic areas where pigs are fed with water plants, they may be important reservoir hosts. Infection rates are much higher in pigs than in man.

III. *Gastrodiscoides hominis*

1. Geographical Distribution

Gastrodiscoides hominis is common in India, particularly in Assam, Bihar, and Orissa. Human infections have also been reported from Bangladesh, Vietnam, and the Philippines.

2. Life Cycle and Morphology (DUTT and SRIVASTAVA 1972)

The adult flukes occur in the cecum and ascending colon, where they are attached to the intestinal wall. They are reddish brown, piriform with a convex dorsal surface, and measure 5–8 × 3–5 mm. The oral sucker lies in the narrow anterior conical part of the body. The very large ventral sucker is situated close to the posterior extremity. The pharynx has a pair of lateral pouches arising just behind the oral sucker and bifurcates into the ceca, which extend to the middle of the disk-shaped part of the body. The large, lobate testes are situated at the anterior side of the discoid part of the body. The small ovary lies just behind the testes. The uterus opens on a genital cone which is situated near the posterior end of the pharynx. The eggs, which measure about 150 × 65 μm, are transparently greenish-gray in color and have a rhomboidal shape and a small operculum. They are unembryonated when they pass out in the feces and require a period of 9–14 days to develop to the miracidial stage in water at a temperature of 24°–30 °C. The natural snail intermediate host is not known, but *Helicorbis coenosus* could be infected experimentally. The first cercariae emerge 1 month after infection. The cercariae develop into metacercarial cysts on water plants.

3. Epidemiology

Man acquires an infection by ingesting the metacercariae on uncooked vegetables or in water. Man, pig, and some wild mammals are the normal hosts of this parasite. In some areas with high prevalences of human infections, man is probably the main host, as in Assam. In other areas, pigs are the natural host and man is only accidentally infected.

IV. *Heterophyes heterophyes*

Heterophyiasis (heterophyidiasis) or dwarf fluke infection is caused by the small trematode *Heterophyes heterophyes*.

1. Geographical Distribution

This fluke is common in Egypt (Nile delta) and the subtropical area in the Far East (southern China, Japan, the Philippines, Taiwan, South Korea). *H. heterophyes* has also been reported from Romania, Greece, Tunisia, and Israel (SHEIR and ABOUL-ENEIN 1970).

2. Life Cycle and Morphology

The adult flukes are small, measuring 1–2 mm in length and 0.3–0.7 mm in width. They occur in the jejunum and the upper ileum, where they are attached to the wall or lie in the crypts of Lieberkühn. The spinose body is elongate oval with a minute oral sucker 90 μm in diameter. Then ventral sucker, which is 2½ times as large as the oral sucker, is situated at two-thirds of the body length. The protrusible genital sucker lies near the posterior margin of the ventral sucker and is nearly two times as large as the oral sucker. The intestine consists of a narrow prepharynx, a small bulbous pharynx, an esophagus, and two intestinal ceca which nearly extend to the posterior end of the body. The ovoid testes occupy the posterior fifth of the body and the round ovary lies in the midline of the body at two-thirds of the body length. The long, coiled uterus is packed with eggs. The adult worms lie attached to the wall of the jejunum and upper ileum.

The brown, operculate, transparent eggs measure 30 × 15 μm and may have a small knob at the end, opposite to the operculum. They contain a fully developed miracidium when they are discharged in the feces and hatch when they are ingested by an appropriate water snail.

In Egypt, in the Nile delta, *Pirenella conica* and in China and Japan *Cerithidea cingulata microptera* are proven intermediate hosts. Within the snail, the parasite passes through a sporocyst and one or two redial stages before the cercarial stage is attained. Three to four weeks after infection, the first cercariae begin to emerge from the snail. They penetrate under the scales of various species of freshwater or brackish water fish, such as *Mugil cephalus* and *Tilapa nilotica* in Egypt and *Mugil japonicus* and *Acanthogobius* spp. in the Far East. They encyst in the fish muscles and develop into infective metacercariae in 2–3 weeks. The metacercariae measure about 160 μm. After ingestion of uncooked, infected fish, the metacercariae escape and mature in the small intestine of the final host.

3. Epidemiology

Man acquires an infection of *H. heterophyes* by eating raw, slightly pickled, marinated, or inadequately cooked fish. In Egypt, high prevalences have been recorded from communities as in Matazia near Port Said, where 88% of the school children have been found to discharge *H. heterophyes* eggs in their stools. In Egypt the main source of infection is pickled mullet, which is eaten traditionally at the feast of Sham-al-Nessim. The encysted metacerariae can survive at least a week in salted fish or in fish which is stored just above freezing point. The adult worms have a short life span and live for about 2 months. Heavy worm burdens of up to 4,000 worms have been recorded at autopsy.

Reservoir hosts, such as dogs, cats, and other fish-eating mammals, can maintain transmission even in the absence of man.

It should be noted that it is difficult to differentiate the eggs of *H. heterophyes* from those of *Metagonimus yokogawai*, but the former usually have a thinner shell.

4. Prevention and Control

The best preventive measure is adequate cooking of fish. However, this will not be easy in regions where raw or pickled fish is regarded as a delicacy. Anti-snail measures are not feasible and the control of promiscuous defecation by the infected people is impossible.

V. *Metagonimus yokogawai*

Metagonimiasis or Yokogawa's fluke infection is caused by *Metagonimus yokogawai,* a small fluke which is similar to *Heterophyes heterophyes*.

1. Geographical Distribution

This fluke is common in Japan, Korea, China, south Manchuria, Taiwan, and Siberia (Amur river). It has been demonstrated in Japan that snail intermediate hosts do not shed cercariae below a temperature of 18 °C and that consequently metagonimiasis is not endemic in areas where the summer temperature is lower.

2. Life Cycle and Morphology

Both the morphology and the life cycle of *M. yokogawai* are very similar to those of *H. heterophyes*. The principal morphological differences are that the ventral sucker is situated to the right of the median line and that there is no genital sucker.

The adult worms occur in the upper and middle parts of the jejunum, attached by the suckers to the mucosa. They are rarely found in the duodenum, ileum, and cecum.

The eggs measure 27 × 16 μm. The only proven intermediate snail host of *M. yokogawai* in China, Taiwan, Japan, and Korea is *Semisulcospira libertina,* but other species may be involved.

The second intermediate hosts are always freshwater fish, such as *Plecoglossus altivelis* ("sweet" fish), *Odontobuitis obscurus, Leuciscus hakuensis,* and *Mugil cephalus*. KIM (1980) reported that in the Geum river basin (Korea) 18 out of 22 species of fish which were examined were infected with metacercariae of *M. yokogawai* and that the prevalence rate in *Pseudogobio esocinus* was 90%.

In experimentally infected mice the development of the adult worms took 7 to 8 days and the passage of eggs began on the 10th day postinfection (HONG and SEO 1969).

3. Epidemiology

High prevalences have been reported locally. In the Hadong area in South Korea 42.4% of the population were passing eggs and prevalences were highest in adults, viz., 57.8% (YEO and SEO 1971). This agrees with the observations that the heaviest infections are found in the age group of between 30 and 50 years. In the river Takatsu area in Japan, a prevalence rate of 72% has been reported and in the Amur river area (Siberia) 15%. In the Tamjin river area in South Cholla Do in Korea it was found that 23.2% of the intermediate snail host *Semisulcospira* were infected, and that in 2 out of 20 of the second intermediate host, the trout *Plecoglossus altivelis,* metacercariae were observed, with a mean number/fish of 15,688. The prevalence rate in man was 26.4% and the mean eggs per gram output was 2,078 (CHAI et al. 1977). In another area in South Korea, the mean number of metacercariae was 3,851, with a maximum of 14,487. In the Province of Jeonra-Nam-Do no *M. yokogawai* infections were found in people living along the Yeongsan river, whereas 41.6% of the people living along the Seomyin river were infected with *M. yokogawai* (SOH et al. 1976).

The worm loads may be high in man. From a patient with chronic diarrhea for 6 months, 17,560 adult worms were recovered after treatment (SEO et al. 1971). The average egg output has been estimated at 1,505 eggs/worm per day. Several fish-eating mammals such as dogs and cats are reservoir hosts, and in some areas *Metagonimus* infections are common among animals, whereas human infections are rare.

More information on this infection can be found in CHAI et al. (1977), SEO et al. (1971), SOH et al. (1976), YEO and SEO (1971), and Chap. 12 in this volume.

E. Cestodes

I. *Diphyllobothrium latum*

Diphyllobothriasis or broad fish tapeworm infection is caused by the fish tapeworm *Diphyllobothrium latum*. Other *Diphyllobothrium* spp. have been reported as human parasites, i. e., *D. pacificum, D. dentriticum, D. ursi*, and *D. cordatum*.

The adult tapeworms live in the small intestine of fish-eating mammals and man. Further information can be found in VON BONSDORFF (1977) and in Chap. 14, this volume.

1. Geographical Distribution

The parasite mainly occurs in the subarctic and temperate lake areas of the northern hemisphere. The main focus in Europe is the Baltic region (Finland, Poland, USSR). Other endemic areas are the Great Lake areas in northern Italy and western Switzerland, the Danube Basin, and Romania. In Asia *D. latum* is endemic in Siberia, Japan, Korea, and China. The worm was introduced by Baltic immigrants into the Great Lakes region of the United States and Canada (VON BONSDORFF 1977).

Small endemic foci probably exist in Chile, Argentina, and Peru. *D. pacificum* infections have been reported in Chile.

In 1973, the number of carriers in the world was estimated at 9 million (VON BONSDORFF 1977).

2. Life Cycle and Morphology

The adult worm inhabits the small intestine. The length of the worm ranges from 3 to 10 m, but longer specimens have been reported. They may have up to 3,000–4,000 proglottids. The worm is attached to the mucosa by the scolex, which is ovoid and measures 1.5–2.5 mm in length and 0.5–1 mm in breadth. The scolex has no suckers, but is provided with dorsal and ventral sucking prooves or bothria. The scolex is connected to the strobila by a narrow "neck." The mature proglottids are usually broader than they are long and measure approximately 3 × 11 mm. However, the proglottids at the posterior fourth part may be square. They contain both male and female sexual organs. The testes consist of very small spherical bodies which occupy the dorsolateral fields. A bilobed ovary lies in the posterior half of the proglottid.

The long, coiled rosette-like uterus has a uterine or birth pore through which the eggs are discharged. The uterine pore is situated just behind the genital pore on the ventral surface of the proglottid.

The eggs are expelled in the intestinal lumen and pass out in the feces. The proglottids at the end of the strobila are wrinkled, with only a few eggs left and are finally sloughed off. Each worm may produce more than one million eggs daily. The yellowish-brown eggs are oval to ellipsoidal and are 55–70 µm long and 35–60 µm wide. They have an inconspicuous operculum and generally a small protuberance at the end opposite to the operculum. The egg is immature when discharged and around the ovum there are granular yolk cells. For its development it is necessary to reach freshwater. The development to the next stage, the coracidium, takes 12 days to several weeks, depending on the temperature of the water. The ciliated coracidium escapes from the egg when the operculum opens and can survive for 1 or 2 days after hatching. For further development it has to be eaten by a suitable copepod. Several species of copepod can serve as the first intermediate host, such as species belonging to the genera *Cyclops* and *Diaptomus*. After being ingested by the copepod, the coracidium discards the outer ciliated epithelium, migrates through the copepod's intestinal wall, and enters its hemal cavity, where the larva develops within 2–3 weeks to the next stage, the procercoid.

If the infected copepod is eaten by a plankton-eating fish, such as the perch, the procercoid penetrates the intestinal wall, passes into the abdominal cavity. and develops into a plerocercoid larva in the connective tissues or muscles of the second intermediate host. The white plerocercoid, with a maximal length of 5 cm, takes about 4 weeks to become infective. If the fish is eaten raw by a mammal, the larva is liberated by digestion in the small intestine from the surrounding fish tissue.

The larvae attach to the intestinal wall and develop into mature tapeworms within 3–4 weeks. When the small infected plankton-eating fish are eaten by larger predatory fish, the plerocercoids penetrate through the intestinal wall and stay alive in the new fish-intermediate host. In this way the number of plerocercoid larvae in the carnivorous fish may increase considerably, and these fish may cause heavy infections in man. The plerocercoids can live for years in the fish host.

3. Epidemiology

In areas where *D. latum* is a common parasite of man and of fish-eating mammals where raw, very slightly salted or smoked fish and raw roe of carnivorous fish are considered to be delicacies, the prevalences of infections may be very high. Shallow littorals with a vegetation which is favorable for copepods and fish are the best biotopes for the stages in the intermediate hosts. In Finland, the prevalence of the whole population was between 20% and 25% in 1926. In some areas, 100% of the population was infected. Since 1950 there has been a rapid decrease in prevalences and in 25 years the prevalence in the whole country has dropped from 20% to 1.8% (Von Bonsdorff 1977).

In some areas, pollution of rivers and lakes by sewage has considerably increased the prevalence rates in fish as well as in man, as in some of the Great

North American lakes and in Siberia. Finnish immigrants have imported *D. latum* infections to south Sweden. The construction of dams, power plants, and canals has caused the introduction and increase of *D. latum* infections, as in the Moscow region, where several foci arose after the construction of the Moscow canal.

The longevity of the adult worms is considerable and life spans of up to 25 years have been reported (VON BORNSDORFF 1977). The eggs are resistant to chemical reagents, but are destroyed by freezing and desication. The worm load is generally low, but occasionally high worm loads have been reported.

4. Clinical Manifestations

In the majority of cases the infections are asymptomatic. Many symptoms that have been attributed to *D. latum* are not related to its presence. In some patients, fatigue, vomiting, diarrhea, constipation, numbness of the extremities, and weight loss occur. The most important symptom is tapeworm pernicious anemia, which has occurred mainly in Finland. Locally, high prevalences of pernicious megaloblastic (macrocytic) tapeworm anemia have been observed, but generally the prevalence rate is low (VON BONSDORFF 1977).

The anemia results from a high uptake of vitamin B_{12} by the worms. *D. latum* has a great affinity for vitamin B_{12} and interferes with the absorption by the host of vitamin B_{12} from the intestine. When *D. latum* is located high up in the intestine, it affects the uptake of vitamin B_{12} by the host more than when the worm is located in the distal part of the ileum. In the proximal part of the there are few or no vitamin B_{12} receptors in the intestinal wall and here the young proglottids, which are metabolically very active, can take up large amounts of vitamin B_{12} before the host can absorb it. If the worm is located in a more distal part of the ileum, numerous receptors can absorb sufficient vitamin B_{12} before the worm has taken it up.

Other factors which contribute to the vitamin B_{12} deficiency of the host are: (a) the number of worms, (b) a reduced output of the intrinsic factor, and (c) the malabsorption of folates.

Partial vitamin B_{12} deficiency is common in *D. latum* carriers. However, serious tapeworm pernicious anemia occurs in cases of high *D. latum* location and a large amount of worms.

It is probable that a "releasing factor" produced by the worm can dissociate vitamin B_{12} from the intrinsic factor – vitamin B_{12} complex and interferes in this way with the absorption of this vitamin by the host. Degenerative changes in peripheral nerves and in the spinal cord occur with symptoms of nerve damage, such as optic neuropathy with scotoma, severe psychosis, paresthesiae, and disturbances in motility and coordination.

Cases of intestinal obstruction have been reported in patients with multiple infections of *D. latum*.

5. Diagnosis

In endemic areas the symptoms may be suggestive, such as a macrocytic anemia. A specific diagnosis depends on the demonstration of the characteristic eggs in the feces. The eggs must be differentiated from other operculated eggs by their form and size. Proglottids, with the characteristic rosette-shaped uterus, are seldom passed.

6. Prevention and Control

The plerocercoid larvae are killed if the fish is adequately cooked, thoroughly pickled, or stored at −10 °C for 2 days. In endemic areas, treatment of sewage in order to destroy the eggs may reduce prevalences, but many mammals are reservoir hosts, including bears, cats, and dogs.

Inhabitants of the endemic areas should be discouraged from eating raw fish or from feeding raw fish to cats and dogs.

II. *Dipylidium caninum*

Dipylidium caninum or the common dog tapeworm is a cosmopolitan parasite in dogs, cats, and wild carnivores.

1. Geographical Distribution

A few hundred cases of *D. caninum* infections in man have been reported from several parts of the world, mostly in children.

2. Life Cycle and Morphology

The adult worms which inhabit the small intestine measure from 10 to 70 cm and usually have 60–175 proglottids. The scolex is about 0.35 mm in diameter and has four acetabula and an ovoid, retractable rostellum with 30–150 thorn-shaped hooks in one to seven rows (usually three to four). The mature, elliptical proglottids are approximately 12 mm long and 3 mm wide. In the gravid proglottids, the uterus is divided into egg nests or capsules, which contain 8–20 eggs. The egg nests nearly fill all the available space in the gravid proglottid. The detached gravid proglottids migrate out of the intestine and are very active outside the host's body. The egg capsules are set free when the proglottid has left the body and are therefore seldom seen in the feces. The eggs measure from 25–40 μm in diameter and hatch when they are ingested by an appropriate arthropod intermediate host. These are the larval stages of ectoparasites, such as the dog flea (*Ctenocephalides canis*), the cat flea (*C. felis*), the human flea (*Pulex irritans*) and *Trichodectes* spp. from dog and cat.

The liberated oncospheres bore through the intestinal wall into the body cavity of the intermediate host and develop into tailed cysticercoid larvae in about 3 weeks. The definitive host is infected by swallowing an infected intermediate host. The cysticercoid larva is liberated by the digestion of the intermediate host and attaches itself to the mucosa of the small intestine.

3. Epidemiology

The eggs are very susceptible to unfavorable environmental factors, such as heat, freezing, desiccation, and sunlight. The worm burden in man is low and generally only one adult worm is found. The longevity of the worm is not known.

4. Clinical Manifestations

Generally human infections with *D. caninum* are asymptomatic or the symptoms are slight, such as intestinal discomfort with mild pain, anorexia, and pruritis.

5. Diagnosis

Diagnosis is by demonstration of the migrating gravid proglottids and of eggs or capsules in the feces.

6. Prevention

1. Control of ectoparasites of pet dogs and cats, particularly of the larval stages on carpets, rugs, and other sites where the pet animals lie
2. Treatment of dogs and cats infected with *D. caninum*

III. *Hymenolepis diminuta*

Hymenolepsis diminuta or the rat tapeworm is a common parasite of rats and mice, and occasionally a human parasite.

1. Geographical Distribution

It is a cosmopolitan parasite of rats, mice, and other rodents. Most cases of human infections have been reported from children and from various areas in the world. A prevalence of 1.9% has been observed in children in the New Guinea highlands (McMillan et al. 1971).

2. Life Cycle and Morphology

Hymenolepsis diminuta resembles *H. nana* morphologically, but there are some differences, i. e.:

1. *H. diminuta* is larger and normally measures between 20 and 60 cm in length and occasionally even over 80 cm.
2. The piriform scolex has four small suckers and a retractable rostellum, but lacks rostellar hooks. The strobila consists of 800–1,000 proglottids. The mature proglottids are about 0.75 mm in length and 2.5 mm in width. The reproductive organs resemble those of *H. nana*. The ovoid eggs are 60–80 µm in diameter and lack polar filaments.
3. An insect intermediate host is necessary for further development of the oncosphere larva. The most important insect intermediate hosts are: (a) flour beetles (*Tribolium* spp., *Tenebrio molitor*) and other beetles; (b) rat fleas (*Xenopsylla cheopis, Nosophyllus fasciatus*) and other fleas (*Pulex irritans, Ctenocephalides canis*); and (c) larvae of moths, larvae, and adults of cockroaches and earwigs.

When the oncosphere is ingested by the insect intermediate host, it hatches and penetrates through the intestinal wall. Then it develops into a tailed cysticercoid larva in the hemal cavity of the insect.

When the infected insect is eaten by a suitable definitive host (a rodent or a human being), the cysticercoids are liberated by the digestion of the host and attach to the intestinal mucosa by means of the scolex. They then mature within 18–20 days.

3. Epidemiology

The resistance of the eggs of *H. diminuta* to environmental factors is greater than that of *H. nana* eggs. However, they are also readily killed by heat and freezing. The worm load in man is small. Man acquires the infection by the ingestion of intermediate hosts when eating contaminated food. Another modus of infection has been reported from Southeast Asia, where live beetle are ingested as a drug. This practice occurs among Chinese and Malayan and originally the live beetles were used as an aphrodisiac, but the practice has been modified and now includes the treatment of a wide variety of diseases and ailments. Some of these beetles are able to serve as intermediate hosts for *H. diminuta*.

The direct mode of transmission of *H. diminuta* by means of eggs has not been observed. This is probably due to the chemical composition of the eggshell.

4. Clinical Manifestations

The clinical manifestations are very light, i.e., some diarrhea and abdominal pain.

5. Diagnosis

Diagnosis is as for *H. nana*.

6. Control and Prevention

1. Rodent control
2. Protection of the appropriate food from infestations with the insect intermediate hosts
3. Control of household insect pests

IV. *Hymenolepis nana*

The dwarf tapeworm infection or hymenolepiasis is caused by *Hymenolepsis nana*.

1. Geographical Distribution and Prevalence

Hymenolepis nana has a cosmopolitan distribution. Prevalences are higher in children than in adults. Dwarf tapeworm infections are common in South America (in some areas prevalences of up to 20% in children have been recorded), the Mediterranean countries, some areas in Asia (over 90% of children between 5 and 10 years in the Punjab), among aboriginal people in Western Australia (20.4%) (JONES 1980).

2. Life Cycle and Morphology

The adult worms inhabit the small intestine, mainly in the upper three-quarters of the ileum. They are attached by means of the scolex, which is embedded in the mucosa. The length generally ranges from 15 to 40 mm, but shorter and longer specimens have been found. The worm has approximately 200 proglottids. The scolex, measuring about 0.3 mm in diameter, is provided with four suckers and a retractable rostellum with a single row of 20–30 hooks. The scolex is connected to the strobila by a long, slender neck. The mature proglottids which are broader than long, measure 0.2 × 0.85 mm. There are three globular testes and a single globular ovary between them. The gravid proglottid is nearly completely filled by the broad uterus, containing 100–200 eggs.

The terminal gravid proglottids disintegrate inside the intestine and the free eggs are discharged in the feces.

The hyaline eggs measure 30–50 μm and are spherical or subspherical. They are enclosed in an outer and an inner transparent envelope. The inner membrane is lemon shaped and has two polar thickenings from which arise four to eight slender filaments, which lie between the inner und outer membrane.

The eggs are already infective when they are passed in the feces. When they are ingested by a host, they hatch in the small intestine and then the oncospheres penetrate the villi of the jejunum. Here the oncosphere loses its six hooklets and develops in about 4 days into a tailless cercocyst. The cercocyst reenters the lumen of the intestine and after the evagination of the scolex, it develops into a sexually mature adult tapeworm within 10 to 12 days. The complete cycle requires about 30 days and the first eggs are passed in the feces about 1 month after infection.

3. Epidemiology

The adult *H. nana* have a short life span and live for only a few months (MÜLLER 1975). Infections have been reported which continue in children who had left an endemic area several years previously. Probably, these long-lasting infections are the result of autoinfections. Freed oncospheres have been demonstrated in intestinal aspirates from infected children.

The eggs of *H. nana* are very sensitive to desiccation, heat, and cold. Their viability outside the host is limited to a maximum of 12 days.

The worm load may be very high and there may be thousands of adult worms. *H. nana* is probably the most common tapeworm infection of man. Infection is more common in children than in adults, and also more common in families and particularly in children in institutional groups. Hand to anus to mouth contact and food or water contaminated by feces of infected mice and rats are probably the principal sources of infection. In some areas, household rodents may be an important source of infection, whereas in other situations human fecal contamination is the principal source of infections. The role of rodents as a natural reservoir of human *H. nana* tapeworm is not clear. There is evidence that the morphologically identical rodent dwarf tapeworm, *H. nana* var. *fraterna,* is not well adapted to man and does not usually cause infection in man. The rodent variety often develops in insect intermediate hosts, such as fleas or beetles. The dwarf tapeworm was probably originally a murine parasite which has become adapted to man. In some areas the murine *H. nana* is of greater importance as a potential human parasite than in other areas.

Immunosuppression in experimental infections resulted in a considerable increase of the parasite in the intestine of the host. In a patient who was given immunosuppressive treatment, *H. nana* also multiplied strongly (LUCAS et al. 1980). Therefore it is recommended that *H. nana* infections are eliminated in patients before they are given immunosuppresive therapy.

4. Clinical Manifestations

Light infections are usually symptomless. Heavy infections may cause severe systemic toxemia, resulting in enteritis with abdominal pain, diarrhea, nausea, vomiting, headache, dizziness, and other nervous disorders. Mild eosinophilia (up to 16%) may occur.

5. Diagnosis

A specific diagnosis can be made by the identification of the characteristic eggs in the feces.

6. Control and Prevention

1. Improvement of sanitary conditions combined with health education in order to diminish ingestion of eggs
2. Destruction of rodents and avoidance of contact between rodents and food
3. Treatment of infected persons, especially infected children

V. *Taenia saginata*

The beef tapeworm infection or taeniasis saginata is caused by *Taenia saginata,* which is also named *Taeniarynchus saginatas* by some authors, since they consider it to be a separate genus from *Taenia,* because of the lack of hooks on the rostellum. In the past is has been confused with *T. solium* (PAWLOWSKI and SCHULTZ 1972).

1. Geographical Distribution

Taenia saginata is a cosmopolitan parasite which occurs in all countries where beef is eaten undercooked or raw. It is probable that there are more than 60 million cases in the world.

2. Life Cycle and Morphology

The adult worms are long, ranging in length from 4 to 10 m, but specimens as long as 25 m have been reported. Generally, they are about 6 m long and may have between 1,000 and 2,000 proglottids. The piriform scolex measures 1–2 mm in diameter and is provided with four prominent hemispherical suckers or acetabula, but has no rostellum or hooks. The scolex is connected to the strobila by a narrow neck which is several millimeters long. In the neck lies a proliferation zone where new proglottids are formed. A mature proglottid is about 9 mm long and 12 mm wide. Numerous spherical testes are scattered through the dorsal part of the proglottid, but are more numerous in the lateral fields. The bilobed ovary lies in the posterior part of the proglottid. The vitelline gland consists of numerous small bodies and lies in a band just behind the ovaries.

In the mature proglottids, the uterus extends forward from the ootype as a narrow cylindrical tube in the median line. The uterus has no opening to the exterior. The ripe or gravid proglottid measures approximately 18 mm in length and 6 mm in width. The gravid uterus is branched and filled with about 80,000 eggs. The number of the lateral branches is between 15 and 30 (usually 20–24) on each side.

The spherical eggs measure 40–30 μm in diameter and contain a larva or oncosphere which is surrounded by a thick radially striated embryophore. The eggs are originally enclosed in a hyaline membrane. The gravid proglottids come off the strobila and migrate actively outside the host's body by their movements. Some eggs may be found in the feces, but most eggs are pressed out through ruptured branches of the uterus when the proglottid is moving around after it has left its host's body. For further development the oncophere must be ingested by cattle. In the cow's duodenum, the embryophore is broken down by pancreatin and bile, and the hexacanth larva or oncosphere hatches. With the aid of the six hooklets and histolytic enzymes they enter the capillaries and mesenteric veins. They are carried embolically through the body and in the voluntary muscles they lose their hooks and develop into a *cysticercus bovis*.

The larva matures in 10–12 weeks into the infective cysticercus, which measures about 5×10 mm. It is a small white bladder and has an invaginated scolex with four acetabula. The outer layer has microvilli which probably have a trophoblastic function. When the infected muscles of the intermediate host are ingested by man, the larvae are liberated by digestion of the surrounding meat and the fibrotic cyst wall. In the duodenum, the cysticercus evaginates its scolex, attaches to the intestinal wall, and starts to produce proglottids. It develops into an adult worm in 6–8 weeks.

3. Epidemiology

Man becomes infected by eating raw, inadequately cooked, or underdone beef. In areas where beef is usually eaten undercooked, the infection prevalences are high, as in Ethiopia, where prevalences of up to 75% have been reported locally (Pawlowski and Schultz 1972). After World War II, prevalences increased in Europe. High infection rates have been recorded from the USSR, such as more than 40% in the Republic of Uzbekistan and 30% in the Republic of Azerbadjan.

The adult worms stay alive for several years and they may survive for as long as 25 years. The worm burden is light and man usually harbours not more than one *T. saginata*.

Eggs may stay alive in grassland for as long as 8 months and in sewage for 2 weeks. Adequate conditions for egg survival are a mild temperature and high humidity. They die rapidly when exposed to desiccation or low temperatures. In the USSR is has been demonstrated that eggs survived for 62 days at a temperature of −4 °C.

Cattle are usually infected at a young age. The sources of infection are: (a) proglottids on grassland and (b) pastures which have been polluted by inadequately treated sewage or by floods. Some cysticerci may remain viable throughout the life of the intermediate host, but others degenerate and calcify. Gulls feeding on sewage beds and flies may disseminate taenia eggs, but are not important sources of infection of cattle.

4. Clinical Manifestations

Usually *T. saginata* causes no distinct lesions in the intestinal wall and in most cases there are no clinical manifestations. The most frequent symptom (99%) is the active passing out of the gravid proglottids.

The patient often has an itching sensation for 5–10 min when the proglottids migrate through the rectum and pass out through the anus. In about 5% of cases it results in pruritis ani. There may be other symptoms, such as epigastric or umbilical pain (35%), nausea (34%), weakness (28%), loss of weight (21%), increase in appetite (17%), headache (17%), constipation (9%), vertigo (8%), and diarrhea (6%).

Occasionally, allergic manifestations such as urticaria and widespread pruritis occur. The systemic manifestations are probably caused by toxic products of the worm which are absorbed by the host.

Some complaints may be attributed to psychological reactions in patients who are well aware of the presence of the tapeworm, such as the "globus hystericus" reported from middle-aged women. The epigastric and umbilical pain decreases considerably after taking food.

One of the most severe clinical manifestations is intestinal obstruction, which may occur when the parasite becomes twisted. Cases of acute appendicitis due to obstruction of the lumen of the appendix by the tapeworm have been reported. Another acute situation may develop when part of the strobila is vomited and aspirated.

5. Diagnosis

Diagnosis depends on the examination of fresh gravid proglottids. The proglottid must be pressed between two slides and then the number of lateral branches of the uterus can be counted. *T. saginata* has between 15–30 branches on each side and *T. solium* only 7–12. The eggs of the *Taenia* species are morphologically identical and no differentiation between eggs of the two species is possible. Eggs can be recovered by the use of the adhesive cellophane swab.

If the scolex is recovered, the two species can easily be differentiated. However, the scolex is seldom seen after treatment with modern drugs.

Recently it has been demonstrated that by enzyme electrophoresis it is possible to differentiate between *T. saginata* and *T. solium*, since there is a consistent and reproducible difference in mobility of the isozymes.

6. Control and Prevention

The most important preventive measures are:

1. Meat inspection. The most heavily infected muscles should be examined on the presence of cysticerci. Six weeks after the infection the cyst can easily be recognized in the meat.
2. Adequate treatment of all beef before consumption. Meat should be cooked, baked, or grilled thoroughly and the temperature must have been at least 56 °C to kill the cysticerci. Freezing for 360 h at −5 °C, 216 h at −10 °C, or 144 h at −15 °C kills the cysticerci effectively.
3. Adequate treatment of sewage to prevent infection of cattle.
4. Prevention of promiscuous defecation by means of health education and provision of sanitary facilities.
5. Prevention of the use of night soil as a fertilizer.
6. Mass diagnosis of the population and treatment of all infected persons.

7. Immunity

The adult worm is only weakly immunogenic, but thy cysticercus induces a stronger immunological response in the invaded host. The immune responses are directed against the penetrating oncospheres in the small intestine and against the growing cysterci in the muscles.

In cattle a strong, lifelong resistance to reinfection develops. The lifespan of primary cysticerci in cattle can be diminished by secondary exposure.

It has been suggested that the presence of a *T. saginata* worm in the intestine induces a state of premunition and that in reinfections it becomes difficult for the worms to establish themselves.

VI. *Taenia solium*

The pork tapeworm infection or taeniasis solium has much in common with *T. saginata* infections, with regard to the adult worm. An important difference, with serious clinical consequences is that human infections with the cysticercus stage often occur.

1. Geographical Distribution

Taenia solium is a cosmopolitan parasite and infections occur in all countries where pork is eaten raw, very lightly salted, or undercooked. It is very common in Mexico, Chile, and other Central and South American countries, and also in east and central Europe, India, China, Papua New Guinea, and parts of Africa.

2. Life Cycle and Morphology

Morphologically *T. solium* closely resembles *T. saginata*, but there are some important differences:

1. The adult worm is shorter and is 2–10 m in length; the number of proglottids is generally less than 1,000, but may be up to 4,000.
2. The scolex is about 1 mm in diameter and is provided with a rostellum with a double row of 25–32 large (170-μm) and small (130-μm) hooks and four large suckers.

3. The proglottids are smaller than those of *T. saginata*; the gravid ones are about 10–12 mm long and 5–6 mm wide.
4. The gravid uterus has only 7–12 branches on each side.

The life cycle also resembles that of *T. saginata*, but the intermediate host is the pig. These become infected by ingesting either eggs or gravid proglottids when feeding on human feces. The eggs are identical to those of *T. saginata*. The larvae develop into *"cysticercus cellulosae"* in about 9–11 weeks. The living cysticerci measure about 5–8 mm and are found mainly in the heart muscles, diaphragma, tongue, and masseters ("measly pork"). Man acquires infections with adult *T. solium* by eating raw or underdone pork containing *cystercerci cellulosae*.

3. Epidemiology

The epidemiology is comparable to that of *T. saginata* except that beef meat is replaced by pork. Generally infection rates of *T. solium* are markedly lower than those of *T. saginata*.

4. Clinical Manifestations

The clinical manifestations caused by adult *T. solium* worms are very similar to those of taeniasis saginata. Patients infected with adult *T. solium* worms are a source of eggs which may be ingested by persons in their environment, causing cysticercosis cellulosae in man.

5. Control and Prevention

Preventive and control measures correspond principally with those of *T. saginata*.

VII. *Cysticercosis cellulosae*

Human infections with *T. solium* cysticerci are common in areas with taeniasis solium in the human population. The disease is called cysticercosis or cysticerciasis.

1. Epidemiology

Man acquires the infection by:

1. The accidental ingestion of eggs with contaminated food and water.
2. External reinfections. Most of the infections with cysticercosis are the result of anus to finger to mouth transfer of eggs.
3. Autoinfections following the regurgitation of gravid proglottids should not be excluded. The eggs must pass through the stomach and therefore regurgitation is a prerequisite for hatching. About 25% of patients with cysticercosis still harbour adult *T. solium* worms.

The introduction of *T. solium* into areas where much undercooked pork is eaten can cause serious public health problems. GAJDUSEK (1978) reported that in Papua New Guinea, where the pig is the main domestic animal, *T. solium* has been introduced recently. A few years after the introduction of pigs from other parts of Indonesia into the Enarotali region in the Central Highlands, cysticerci in pork and subcutaneous cysticerci in man were noted by the inhabitants of this area (1972). In 1973 it appeared that 9% of the patients in Enarotali hospital were excreting proglottids. In 1974 an epidemic of severe burns which were associated with epilepsy caused by cysticercosis was reported. In the mean-time, *T. solium* has been spread into neighboring areas. It is interesting that the epileptic attacks coincided with initial infections of the central nervous system, before the cysts died and calcified, although it has often been suggested that these symptoms occur after death and calcification of the cysts. One autopsy has been carried out and over 2,000 cysticerci were observed in the brain, which were nearly all alive and without surrounding tissue reactions.

2. Clinical Manifestations

All organs and tissues may be invaded by cysticerci. The clinical manifestations depend on the localization of the cysticerci and also on their number.

The most common sites in man are the muscles and the subcutaneous tissues. The subcutaneous nodules are usually painless, but are important for the diagnosis (see "Diagnosis").

The most serious pathological effects are caused by cysticerci which are localized in the brain. As long as the cysticerci are alive, they cause no serious reactions in the surrounding tissues. Following the death of the cysticerci, intense inflammatory reactions set in.

Initially the reaction is composed mainly of neutrophils, followed by foreign body giant cells and a small number of eosinophils. Small arteries near the parasite show endarteritis and may become occluded.

There are three forms of cysticercosis of the central nervous system: parenchymatous, meningeal, and ventricular cysticercosis. Mixed forms also occur. The cysticerci may cause epileptiform seizures, hydrocephaly with headache, vomiting, nausea, and various focal symptoms, such as paresthesia, localized anesthesia, visual symptoms, aphasia, and neural deterioration.

In most cases, the hydrocephaly is due to a basal meningitis causing a block in the absorption of the cerebrospinal fluid. Cysticerci in the ventricular system may cause obstruction hydrocephaly. In ocular cysticercosis the parasite may be found in the orbit, conjunctiva, anterior chamber, retina, or vitreous humor. They may cause iridocyclitis, cloudiness of the vitreous humor, inflammatory reactions, and atrophy in the retina and ablatio retinae.

3. Diagnosis

Biopsy of the palpable subcutaneous nodules may confirm the clinical diagnosis; however, these may be absent in some patients. X-ray examination may detect calcified cysticerci. Serological diagnosis can also be reliable.

References

Aketagawa H (1938) Some experimental contributions on oral and cutaneous infection of hookworms. Jap J Exp Med 16:85–107

Almeida IS (1979) Acão terapêutica do mebendazole em população infantil com polienteroparasitose no bairro de N.S. de Fátima em Planaltina – DF – 1978. Rev Inst Med Trop Sao Paulo 21:339–343

Anuar AK, Ramachandran CP (1977) A study on the prevalence of soil-transmitted helminths among lettuce leaves sold in local markets in Penang, Malaysia. Med J. Malaysia 31:262–265

Arfaa F, Sahba GH, Farahmandian I, Jalai H (1977) Evaluation of the effect of different methods of control of soil-transmitted helminths in Khuzestan, southwest Iran. Am J Trop Med Hyg 26:230–233

Asin HGR, Thiel PH van (1963) On the distribution of intestinal helminths in the urban and bushland population in Surinam. Trop Geogr Med 15:257–267

Banzon TC, Singson CN, Cross JH (1976) Mebendazole treatment for intestinal nematodes in a Philippine barrio. J Phillip Med Assoc 52:239–243

Beaver PC (1955) Observations on *Necator* infections resulting from exposure to three larvae. Rev Iber Parasitol [Suppl]:1–9

Beaver PC (1961) Control of soil-transmitted helminths. WHO Public Health Papers 10. WHO, Geneva

Berland B (1961) Sarsia 2:21

Bloch M, Rivera H (1977) La enfermedad ancylostomiasica: una lacre de Latinoamerica. Rev Inst Invest Med 6:105–184

Bonne C, Bras G, Lie Kian Joe (1948) Five human echinostomes in the Malayan Archipelago. Med Maandb 23:456–465

Bonnefoy C, Isautier H (1978) Variation de l'incidence des helminthiases à la Réunion en fonction de différents paramètres. Bull Soc Pathol Exot Filiales 71:70–78

Bradley DJ (1972) Regulation of parasite populations. A general theory of the epidemiology and control of parasite infections. Trans R Soc Trop Med Hyg 66:697–708

Bradley DJ (1974) Stability in host-parasite systems. In: Usher MB, Williamson MH (eds) Ecological stability. Halsted, New York

Bradley DJ, May RM (1978) Consequences of helminth aggregation for the dynamics of schistosomiasis. Trans R Soc Trop Med Hyg 72:262–273

Briscoe J (1976) Public health in rural India. Research Paper No 12. Thesis. Center for population studies. Harvard University

Bura MWT, Willett WC (1977) An outbreak of trichinosis in Tanzania. East Afr Med J 54:185–193

Capron A, Auriault C, Mazingue C, Capron M. Torpier G (1980) Schistosome mechanisms of evasion. In: Van den Bossche H (ed) The host-invader interplay. Elsevier/North Holland Biomedical, Amsterdam, pp 217–225

Carec Surveillance Report (1980) Parasitic survey in Martinique Port of Spain

Carney WP, Sudomo M, Purnomo (1980) Echinostomiasis: a disease that disappeared. Trop Geogr Med 32:101–105

Chabaud AG (1972) Description de *Stefankostrongylus dubosti* n.sp., parasite du potomagale et assai de classification des nématodes Angiostrongylinae. Ann Parasitol Hum Comp 47:735–744

Chai JY, Cho SY, Seo BS (1977) Study of *Metagonimus yokogawai* (Katsurada 1912) in Korea. IV. An epidemiological investigation along the Tamjin River Basin, South Cholla Do, Korea. Korean J Parasitol 15:115–120

Chaia G (1980) Human nematodes on the South American continent. R Soc Med Int Congr Symp Ser 24:103–108

Chandler AS (1954) A comparison of helminthic and protozoan infections in two Egyptian villages two years after the introduction of sanitary improvements in one of them. Am J Trop Med Hyg 3:59–73

Chatterji A, Chowdhury AB (1969) Bull Calcutta School Trop Med 17:3

Chen ER (1971) Recent studies on endemic ascariasis in Taiwan. Formosan Science 25:27–50

Chia Wee Yan (1978) The problem of soil-transmitted helminths in squatter areas around Kuala Lumpur. Med J Malaysia 33:34–43

Chobanov RE, Salekhov AA (1979) Prevalence of enterobiasis among the urban and rural population of the Azerbaijan SSR (in Russian with English summary) Med Parazitol (Mosk) 5:79–83

Chowdhury AB (1980) The importance of nematodes on the Indian continent. In: Wood C, Rue Y (eds) Health policies in developing countries. Proceedings of an international symposium held by the Janssen Research Foundation at Beerse. April 20–21, 1979. R Soc Med Int Congr Symp Ser 24:97–102

Clark MD, Carney WP, Cross JH, Hadidjaja P, Oemijati S, Joesoef A (1974) Schistosomiasis and other human parasitoses of Lake Lindu in Central Sulawesi (Celebes), Indonesia. Am J Trop Med Hyg 23:385–392

Crofton HDA (1971) A quantitative approach to parasitism. Parasitology 62:179–193

Cross JH (1969) Fasciolopsiasis in Southeast Asia and the Far East: a review. 4th South East Asian seminar on parasitoloy and tropical medicine, Bangkok

Cross JH, Banzon TC, Singson CN (1978) Further studies in *Capillaria philippinensis*: development of the parasite in the Mongolian gerbil. J Parasitol 69:208–213

Cross JH, Sinson CN, Battad S, Basaca-Sevilla V (1980) Intestinal capillariasis: epidemiology, parasitology, and treatment. In: Wood C, Rue Y (eds) Health policies in developing countries. Proceedings of an international symposium held by the Janssen Research Foundation at Beerse. April 20–21, 1979. R Soc Med Int Congr Symp Ser 24:81–87

Crum ED, Despommier DD, McGregor DD (1977) Immunity to *Trichinella spiralis*. I. Transfer of resistance by two classes of lymphocytes. Immunology 3:707–795

Daengsvang S (1968) Further observations on the experimental transmission of *Gnathostoma spinigerum*. Ann Trop Med Parasitol 62:88–94

Daengsvang S (1980) A monograph on the genus *Gnathostoma* and gnathostomiasis in Thailand. SEAMIC Publication (Tokyo) 21:9, 118

Davis A (1976) Epidemiology and control of intestinal dwelling nematodes. In: Cruickshank R, Standard KL, Russel HBL, Cruicksank EK (eds) Epidemiology and community health in warm climate countries. Churchill Livingstone, Edinburgh, pp 317–330

Despommier DD, Campbell WC, Blair LS (1977) The in vivo and in vitro analysis of immunity to *Trichinella spiralis* in mice and rats. Parasitology 74:109–119

Dutt SC, Srivastava HD (1972) The life history of *Gastrodiscoides hominis* (Lewis and McConnell 1876) Leiper, 1913 – the amphistome parasite of man and pig. J Helminthol 46:35–46

Eyles DE, Jones FE, Smith CS (1953) A study of *Entamoeba histolytica* and other intestinal parasites in a rural West-Tennessee community. Am J Trop Med Hyg 2:173–190

Fay FH (1967) Experimental transmission of *Trichinella spiralis* via marine amphipods. Can J Zool 46:597–599

Fernando MA, Balasuriya S (1976) Prevalence of soil-transmitted helminths in the Hindagala community health project area. Ceylon Med J 21:177–183

Fülleborn E (1926) Über das Verhalten der Hakenwurmlarven bei der Infektion *per os*. Arch Schiffs- u. Tropenhyg 30:638–653

Gajdusek DC (1978) Introduction of *Taenia solium* into West New Guinea with a note on an epidemic of burns from cysticercus epilepsy in the Ekari people of the Wissel Lake area. Papua New Guinea Med J 21:329–342

Gelpi AP, Mustafa A (1967) Seasonal pneumonitis with eosinophilia. Am J Trop Med Hyg 16:646–657

Gentilini M, Vernes A, Gentilini JL, Richard-Lenoble D, Bourée P, Wattez A (1976) Étude enzymatique et sérologique de la trichinose humaine. A propos d'une récente épidémie de la banliewe sud de Paris. Bull Soc Pathol Exot Filiales 69:525–531

Ghadirian E, Arfaa F, Arvanaghi A (1974) Prevalence of intestinal helminthiasis among settled nomads and those with moving habits in southern Iran. Iranian J Public Health 3:147–153

Gilles HM et al. (1964) Hookworm infection and anaemia. An epidemiological, clinical and laboratory study. QJ Med 33:1–24

Goldsmid JM (1967) *Ternidens deminutus* Raillet and Henry (Nematoda). Cent Afr J Med 13:54

Goulart EG, Jourdan MC, Brazil RP, Brazil BG, Cosendey AE, Bar M, DoCarmo EC, Gilbert B (1977) Ecological control of hookworm and strongyloidiasis. J Helminthol 51:131–132

Gould SE (1970) Trichinosis in man and animals. Thomas, Springfield

Grove DI (1980) Strongyloidiasis in allied ex-prisoners of war in southeast Asia. Br Med J 280:598–601

Haaf E, Soest AH Van (1964) Oesophagostomiasis in man in North Ghana. Trop Geogr Med 16:49–53

Hairston NG (1965) On the mathematical analysis of schistosome populations. Bull WHO 33:45–62

Hamidi AN (1979) Trichiniasis among the animals in north eastern Iran, 1969, 1971, 1977. Bull Soc Pathol Exot Filiales 72:254–257

Harinasuta C (ed) (1969) 4th Southeast Asian seminar on parasitology and tropical medicine, schistosomiasis and other snail-transmitted helminthiasis. Bangkok

Hong NT, Seo BS (1969) Study on *Metagonimus yokogawai* (Katsurada 1912) in Korea. I. On the metacercaria, its distribution in the second intermediate host and the development in the final host. Korean J Parasitol 7:129–142

Hsieh HC (1971) Combining MTFL and Stoll dilution egg counting for species analysis of hookworm in man. Chin J Microbiol 4:25–39

Huq MN, Shaikh AA (1976) Incidence of intestinal parasites in children of different socio-economic populations of Dacca city. Bangladesh Med Res Counc Bull 2:1–7

Jones HI (1976a) A study of human intestinal helminthiasis on Kar Kar Island, Madang Province. Papua New Guinea Med J 19:165–172

Jones HI (1976b) Human intestinal helminthiasis in East Timor. Southeast Asian J Trop Med Public Health 7:523–529

Jones HI (1980) Intestinal parasite infections in Western Australian aboriginies. Med J Aust 2:375–380

Kaminsky RG, Ndinya-Achola JO (1977) *Oesophagostomum* sp. from Kenya. Identification through tissue sections. East Afr Med J 54:296–297

Khalil M (1926) The relation between sanitation and parasitic infection in the tropics. JR Sanit Inst 47:210–215

Kilala CP (1971) *Ternidens deminutus* infecting man in southern Tanzania. East Afr Med J 48:636–645

Kim CH (1980) Study on the *Metagonimus* sp. in Geum River basin, Chung-cheung-nam Do, Korea. (English summary) Korean J Parasitol 18:215–228

Kleevens JWC (1966) Re-housing and infections by soil-transmitted helminths in Singapore. Singapore Med J 7:12–29

Kobayashi A et al. (1966) Jpn J Parasitol 15:340

Koike A (1960) The mode of infection of hookworms: experimental studies on oral infection of the infective larvae to the human host. Chiba Igakkai Zasshi 36:1133–1149

Koshy A, Raina V, Sharma MP, Mithal S, Tandon BN (1978) An unusual outbreak of hookworm disease in North India. Am J Trop Med Hyg 27:42–45

Latham L, Latham M, Basta SS (1977) The nutritional and economic implications of *Ascaris* infection in Kenya. World Bank Staff Working Paper 271:1–86

Link VB (1952) Trichinosis: a national problem. Proceedings 1st national conference on trichinosis, Chicago, pp 3–7

Loría-Cortés R, Lobo-Sanahuja JF (1980) Clinical abdominal angiostrongylosis. A study of 116 children with intestinal eosinophilic granuloma caused by *Angiostrongylus costaricensis*. Am J Trop Med Hyg 29(4):538–544

Lubis CP, Siregar H, Siregar A, Lubis RM (1979) Measuring malnutrition and intestinal helminthiasis in tobacco plantation workers' children. Paediatr Indones 19:84–90

Lucas SB, Hassounah O, Muller R, Doenhoff MJ (1980) Abnormal development of *Hymenolepsis nana* larvae in immunosuppressed mice. J Helminthol 54:75–82

MacDonald G (1965) The dynamics of helminth infections, with special reference to schistosomiasis. Trans R Soc Trop Med Hyg 59:489–506

MacKenzie CD, Jungery M, Taylor PM, Ogilvie BM (1980) Activation of complement, the induction of antibodies to the surface of nematodes and the effect of these factors and cells on worm survival *in vitro*. Eur J Immunol 10:594–601

Manning GS, Ratanarat C (1970) *Fasciolopsis buski* in Central Thailand. Am J Trop Med Hyg 19:613–619

Markell EK (1968) Pseudohookworm infection – trichostrongyliasis. New Engl J Med 278:831

Matsusaki G (1966) Hookworm disease and prevention. In: Morishita K, Komiya Y, Matsubayashi H (eds) Progress of medical parasitology in Japan, vol 3. Meguro Parasitological Museum, Tokyo, pp 187–251

Mayers CP, Purvis RJ (1970) Manifestations of pinworms. Can Med Assoc J 103:489–491

McDonald GSA, Hourihane DOB (1972) Ectopic *Enterobius vermicularis*. Gut 13:621–626

McMillan B, Kelly A, Walker JC (1971) Prevalence of Hymenolepsis diminuta infection in the New Guinea highlands. Trop Geogr Med 23:390

Mello DA (1974) A note on egg production of Ascaris lumbricoides. J Parasitol 60:380–381

Miyazaki I (1960) On the genus *Gnathostoma* and human gnathostomiasis, with special reference to Japan. Exp Parasitol 9:338–370

Miyazaki I (1966) *Gnathostoma* and gnathostomiasis in Japan. In: Morishita K, Komiya Y, Matsubayashi H (eds) Progress of medical parasitology in Japan. Meguro Parasitological Museum, Tokyo

Moore HA, Delacruz E, Vargas-Mendez O (1965) Diarrhoeal disease studies in Costa Rica. IV. Influence of sanitation upon the prevalence of intestinal infection and diarrhoeal disease. Am J Epidemiol 82:162–184

Morera P (1973) Life history and redescription of *Angiostrongylus costaricensis* Morera and Céspedes. Am J Trop Med Hyg 22(5):613–621

Morera P, Céspedes R (1971) Angiostrongylosis abdominal. Una nueva parasitosis humana. Acta Med Costarric 14:159–173

Motabar M, Montazemi K (1978) The prevalence of intestinal helminthiasis among the Qashqai tribe of southern Iran. Pahlavi Med J 9:200–207

Müller R (1975) Worms and disease. Heinemann, London

Nagalingam I, Lee EL, Robinson MJ, Dissanaike AS (1976) Mebendazole in treatment of severe *Trichuris trichiura* infection in Malaysian children. Am J Trop Med Hyg 25:568–572

Nawalinski T, Schad GA, Chowdhury AB (1978a) Population biology of hookworms in children in rural West Bengal. I. General parasitological observations. Am J Trop Med Hyg 27:1152–1161

Nawalinski T, Schad GA, Chowdhury AB (1978b) Population biology of hookworms in children in rural West Bengal. II. Acquisition and loss of hookworms. Am J Trop Med Hyg 27:1162–1173

Oshima T (1972) Anisakiasis (in Japanese). Prog Med Parasitol 4:301–305

Palmer ED (1955) Course of egg output over a 15-year period in a case of experimentally induced necatoriasis americanus in the absence of hyperinfection. Am J Trop Med Hyg 4:756–757

Pampiglione S, Nájera E, Ricciardi ML, Junginger L (1979) Parasitological survey on pygmies in Central Africa. III. Bambut group (Zaire). Riv Parassitol 40:187–234

Pawlowski Z, Schultz MG (1972) Taeniasis and cysticercocis (*T. saginata*). Adv Parasitol 10:269–343

Polak MF (1965) Ned Tijdschr Geneeskd 109:1004

Rahman KM, Idris M, Azad Khan AK (1981) A study of fasciolopsiasis in Bangladesh. J Trop Med Hyg 84:81–86

Ruitenberg EJ (1970) Anisakiasis: pathogenesis, serodiagnosis and prevention. Thesis, University of Utrecht

Sadun EH, Maiphoom C (1953) Studies on the epidemiology of the human intestinal fluke, *Fasciolopsis buski* (Lankester), in central Thailand. Am J Top Med Hyg 2:1070–1084

Sandground JH (1931) Studies on the life-history of *Ternidens deminutus*, a nematode parasite of man, with observations on its incidence in certain regions of southern Africa. Ann Trop Med Parasitol 25:147–184
Sakurai K (1960) An experimental study to confirm hookworm infection through the mouth. Nippon Ikadaigaku Zasshi 27:528–534
Sasa M, Hayashi S, Tanaka H, Shirasaka R (1958) Application of test-tube cultivation method on the survey of hookworm and related human nematodes infections. Jpn J Exp Med 28:129–137
Schad GA, Chowdhury AB, Dean CG, Kochar VK, Nawalinski TA, Thomas J, Jonascia JA (1973) Arrested development in human hookworm infections: an adaption to a seasonally unfavorable external environment. Science 180:502–504
Schliessmann DJ, Atchley FO, Wilcomb MJ, Welch SF (1958) Relation of environmental factors to the occurrence of enteric diseases in areas of eastern Kentucky. Public Health Monograph 54
Scragg JN, Proctor EM (1978) Further experience with mebendazole in the treatment of symptomatic trichuriasis in children. Am J Trop Med Hyg 27:255–257
Seo BS, Rim HJ, Lee SH, Cho SY, Kwack CW, Lee WJ, Yeo TH (1971) Two cases of metagonimiasis with special reference to the egg laying capacity in the human host. Seoul J Med 12:234–241
Sheir ZM, Aboul-Enein MS (1970) Demographic, clinical and therapeutic appraisal of heterophyiasis. J Trop Med Hyg 73:148–152
Shirai M (1926) Experimentelle Studien über die perorale Infektion von *Anchylostoma duodenale* mit besonderer Berücksichtigung des Durchwanderungsweges im Wirtskörper. Trans Jpn Pathol Soc 16:90–99
Soh CT (1973) Control of soil-transmitted helminths in Korea. Yonsei Rep Trop Med 4:102–105
Soh CT, Lee KT, Cho KM (1976) Prevalences of clonorchiasis and metagonimiasis along rivers in Jeonra-Nam-Do, Korea. Yonsei Rep Trop Med 7:3–16
Stephenson LS (1980) The contribution of *Ascaris lumbricoides* to malnutrition in children. Parasitology 81:221–233
Stoll NR (1947) This wormy world. J Parasitol 33:1–18
Takata J (1951) Experimental infection of man with *Ascaris* from man and the pig. Kitasato Arch Exp Med 23:49
Tripathy K, González F, Lotero H, Bolanos O (1971) Effects of *Ascaris* infection on human nutrition. Am J Trop Med Hyg 20:212–218
Tubangui MA, Pasco AM (1933) The life history of the human intestinal fluke, *Euparyphium ilocanum* (Garrison 1908). Philipp J Sci 51:581–606
Van Thiel PH (1976) The present state of anisakiasis and its causative worms. Trop Geogr Med 28:75–85
Van Thiel PH, Kuipers FC, Roskam RT (1960) A nematode parasitic to herring, causing acute abdominal syndromes in man. Trop Geogr Med 12:97–113
Venkatachalam PS, Patwardhan VN (1953) The role of *Ascaris lumbricoides* in the nutrition of the host. Effect of ascariasis on the digestion of proteins. Trans R Soc Trop Med Hyg 47:169–175
Von Bonsdorff B (1977) Diphyllobothriasis in man. Academic, London, pp xii–189
World Health Organisation (1964) Soil-transmitted helminths. WHO Tech Rep Ser 277
World Health Organization (1965) Bibliography of hookworm disease (*Ancylostomiasis*) 1920–1962. Geneva
World Health Organization (1967) Control of ascariasis. WHO Tech Rep Ser 379
World Health Organization (1979) Parasitic zoonoses. Report of a WHO Expert Committee. WHO Tech Rep Ser 637
World Health Organization (1981) Intestinal protozoan and helminthic infections. Report of a WHO Expert Committee. WHO Tech Rep Ser 666
Yanagisawa R, Mizuno T (1963) On the infection mode of hookworm. Med Cult 5:112–118
Yeo TO, Seo BS (1971) Study of *Metagonimus yokogawai* (Katsurada 1912) in Korea. III. Epidemiological observations of human Metagonimus infection in Hadong area, South Kyongsang-Do. Seoul J Med 12:259–267

Yoeli M, Most H, Hammond J, Scheinesson GP (1972) Parasitic infections in a closed communitiy. Trans R Soc Trop Med Hyg 66:764–776
Yokogawa S (1926) On the oral infection by the hookworm. Arch Schiffs Tropenhyg 30:663–679
Yoshikawa TT (1980) Antiparasitic drugs. Am Fam Physician 21:132–138
Zimmerman WJ, Steele JH, Kagan IG (1973) Trichiniasis in the U.S. population, 1966–1970. Public Health Serv Rep 88:606–623

CHAPTER 3

Epidemiology and Control of Gastrointestinal Helminths in Domestic Animals

J. F. MICHEL

A. Introduction

A chapter on the epidemiology of helminth infections has a place in a book devoted to anthelmintics only in so far as knowledge is sufficient to provide a rational basis for their use. In the case of the great majority of helminth infections, epidemiological knowledge is not sufficient. Inevitably therefore attention will be focused here on the gastrointestinal nematodes of sheep and cattle, only occasional references being made to other groups.

It is proposed to suggest answers to two questions which, because they are of fundamental importance, are rarely asked. Firstly, what is it necessary to know if helminths are to be controlled? Secondly and at a later stage, how is the knowledge to be effectively applied?

Animal management exerts a crucial effect on helminth infections; therefore it is both possible and necessary to consider their epidemiology within the context of particular systems of management and to design control measures specific to the particular farm enterprise. If control measures are to find application in the field, their design must recognise that the control of helminths is only one consideration among many in influencing management decisions. Control plans must make both agricultural and economic sense: worms are controlled for economic rather than aesthetic reasons.

It is necessary to understand the processes step-by-step that determine helminth populations in the host but in far too few countries is this seen as a fit objective of helminthological research. A majority of practical helminthologists when asked, "how does this infection work in your area?" have little conception of what kind of information is required. The issues were discussed in some detail by MICHEL (1971), who saw a life cycle as a series alternately of populations and processes. Each population was regulated by two processes, respectively adding and removing individuals. An understanding of each process could be gained by monitoring the populations that it connects. The populations to be monitored, and hence the complexity of the processes to be studied could be selected at will. In the first instance, it is necessary to establish, in broad outline, which are the important processes and it is those that are the most variable rather than those occasioning the greater loss that are of significance.

Progress has dependend on the realisation, firstly, that it is preferable to study and analyse the whole rather than to attempt to synthesise a picture of the whole from a knowledge of the parts and, secondly, that the direct observation of real situations is essential. All assumptions on which the indirect measurement of populations or the observation of artificially created situations is based are misleading and dangerous. In many parts both of the developed and the developing world there is still a crying need for simple observations in the field. This approach is too obvious to appeal to those who believe that nothing is worthy of the attention of highly educated scientists short of the exploration of the very frontiers of human knowledge. It is not suggested that some detailed work is not needed to supplement and illuminate the results of field observation, but if resources are scanty and a choice must be made between suitable observations in the field and detailed laboratory experimentation of limited scope, it is the field observations that should be undertaken.

The essential feature in which nematodes of the gastrointestinal tract differ from viruses, bacteria and protozoa is that the course of infections in the host does not conform to a standard pattern. Populations cannot increase in the host alone; each individual must undergo development outside the host before it can parasitise the host. The situation is commonly summarised by saying that every worm in the host has been picked up from the pasture as an infective larva, while every infective larva on the pasture has developed from an egg passed in the faeces of the host. The consequence, which cannot be sufficiently stressed, is that the course and magnitude of worm populations are infinitely variable and determined not only by the host response, but also by climate and, in the case of domesticated animals, by management. Indeed, the species that are common in any particular area may be assumed to be present in nearly every host. Very frequently, however, they are not in sufficient numbers to cause clinical signs though they may impair production.

I. Effect of Worm Infection on Production

It has long been accepted that most loss due to helminthiasis is attributable to impaired production rather than to death. The question whether and to what extent asymptomatic infections are the cause of biological or economic loss has been and continues to be actively debated and there is a growing literature on what is termed "subclinical parasitism." It may be argued that an infection that damages the host cannot be regarded as subclinical but what appears to be intended is that animals which appear normal to the casual observer may nonetheless be growing or producing less well than the uninfected animal. The issue has become confused because the accepted standard of normality has changed. Forty or fifty years ago severely worm affected animals were regarded as the norm and it was a novel idea that the normal animal was suffering from helminthiasis and that the worm-free and to that extent abnormal animal would grow a great deal faster.

Figure 1 contains evidence, if such were needed, that wormy stock was once regarded as normal. The print, which represents the birthplace of T. S. Cooper and is plainly intended to honour his memory, also shows two stirks severely stunted by the effects of ostertagiasis. It is highly significant that T. S. Cooper was a fashionable painter of cattle.

The discussion on the effects of "subclinical parasitism" must be seen against this background. Experimenters such as SYKES (1978) administer large numbers of infective larvae to their animals and measure the effects of the far from mod-

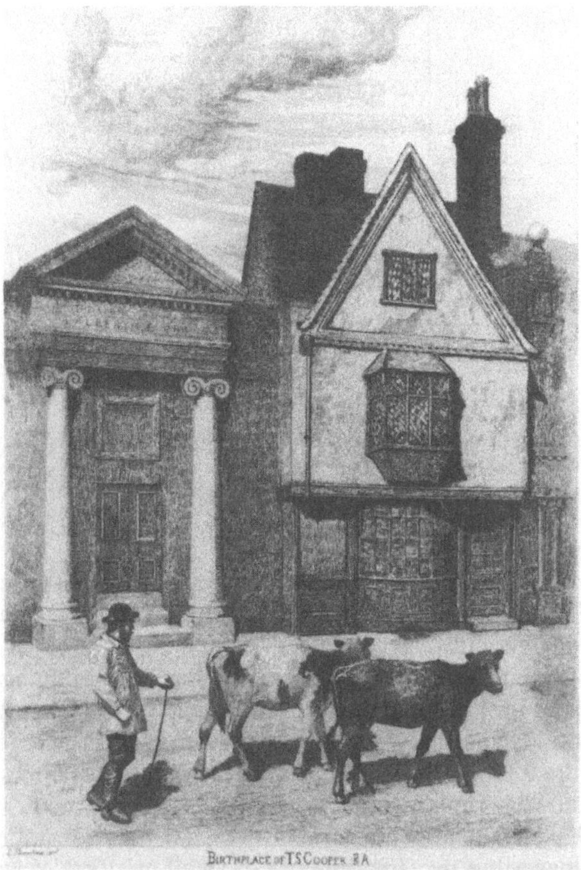

Fig. 1. The birthplace of T. S. Cooper

erate worm burdens that result. If they report these effects as being due to subclinical parasitism they are using a standard of normality which is out of date and no longer valid. There is a very real danger that their conclusions will be applied to animals seen as normal by today's standard. The idea is in fact widely current that no matter how thrifty an animal, there is always an increment of growth that could be achieved were its worm burden eliminated. To some extent this line of thought derived from the results of Spedding and Brown (1957), who studied the effects of different levels of worm infection in lambs and at the same time demonstrated means by which lambs could be kept virtually worm free on pasture. They discussed the concept of a tolerated level of worm burden but nonetheless their work was commonly and mistakenly taken to show that at all levels worm numbers and the resulting damage were proportional. On this basis it was possible to argue that worms should be controlled at levels such that the cost of control was just less than the cost of the damage. Meanwhile, working along a parallel line parasitologists in New Zealand were trying to establish a relationship be-

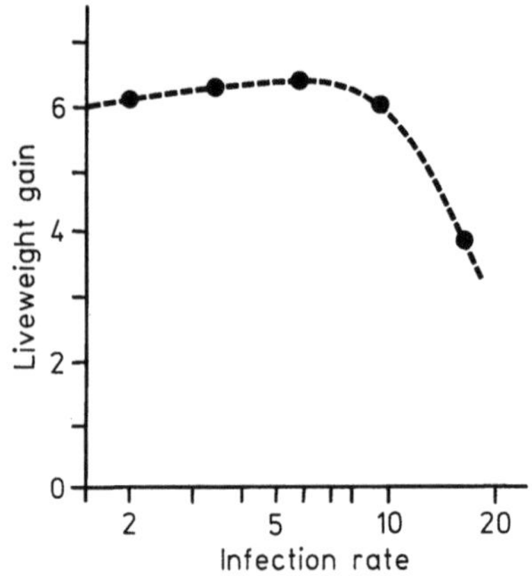

Fig. 2. The relationship between infection with *Ostertagia ostertagi* and the liveweight gain of calves

tween the number of routine anthelmintic treatments and the resulting production increase. These ideas still underlie much thinking on the economic effects of helminthiasis and its control.

It has been evident for some time, however, that worm numbers and the resulting loss are not proportional at all levels. The idea of a tolerated burden envisaged by SPEDDING and BROWN (1957) below which no production loss occurs is a reality. Figure 2 shows the relationship between the level of *Ostertagia ostertagi* infections in calves and liveweight gain. It is very clear that burdens below a certain level have no adverse effect on growth. There is not sufficient evidence to sustain the suggestion that the presence of small numbers of worms actually stimulates liveweight increase but the idea need not be dismissed out of hand. There are rather firmer grounds for believing that the tolerated level is affected by the nutritional status of the host (GORDON 1964; STEWART and GORDON 1953).

To measure production losses due to helminth infection is no easy matter. The production of experimentally infected animals can indeed be compared with that of worm-free controls but it is not readily possible to relate such experimental infections to naturally acquired infections in the field, the size of which cannot reliably be measured and which have in any case arisen in a very different way. The alternative is to compare naturally infected animals which are given frequent and regular anthelmintic treatment with comparable animals that are not treated. The difficulty here is that there is likely to be a marked difference between the production of exposed and dosed animals, and that of animals that are not exposed to infection. Moreover, most anthelmintics have potentially relevant effects other than their ability to remove worms.

A discussion of whether the production of animals judged normal by the standard of today is impaired by helminth infection is likely to arouse controversy because of the very small effects necessarily involved and the difficulties of measurement. A topical example is provided by the claim advanced by a number of workers that subclinical helminthiasis reduces the yield of healthy dairy cows (literature summarised by BAKER 1979). It is not in dispute that in certain circumstances large worm burdens can occur in milking cows, give rise to clinical disease and seriously depress milk yield. But in general, dairy cows carry only very small numbers of worms. The question is whether these small burdens are tolerated or whether they affect production.

Only an indirect answer can be provided to this question, namely whether anthelmintic treatment increased yield. If there was no response this might mean only that the effect of the worms persisted after their removal. If there was, it would be necessary to demonstrate that it was not due to the non-anthelmintic properties of the drugs used. Most important perhaps is the fact that because of the great natural variation in milk yield, the number of animals needed in each experimental group to reveal a small difference is very great indeed.

II. Economic Effects

If the assessment of biological loss due to helminth infection is difficult, translating this into economic loss is no simpler. The UNITED STATES DEPARTMENT OF AGRICULTURE (1942) assessed production losses by comparing actual with potential production, regarding an animal kept in less than optimal conditions as sustaining a production loss. This approach suffers from the fundamental defect that the objective of agriculture is maximising not output, but profit, and utilising existing resources to greatest advantage. The farmer lives on the margin between production cost and market return and it is notorious that this relationship is not the same at all levels of output.

The difficulties of assessment are not great where, as in the case of milk, the potential effect is on current yield. Estimating the economic effect of a retardation of growth is much less simple.

It is customary to do this by measuring the difference between anthelmintic-treated and control animals when this is at its greatest and then multiplying the difference by the unit price of the end product. This procedure can be very misleading because a considerable time may elapse before the animal comes to profit and compensatory growth during this interval may greatly decrease the difference.

This is one reason why the economic effect of a retardation of growth depends largely on the circumstances. The yearling heifers depicted in Fig. 1 will have sustained a reduction in liveweight gain of at least 30 kg but this will have occasioned no measurable economic loss. These animals will not have been expected to calve until 3 years old. They will have needed to grow at a very modest rate and in their second and third grazing seasons will have had great opportunities for compensatory growth. In contrast, the more intensively managed dairy heifer today which calves at the age of 24 months must grow consistently at a rapid rate. Even a small reduction in growth rate may have serious economic consequences. If her weight at calving is too low, this will reduce her yield; if bulling is postponed and she calves later, this may affect the market value of her lifetime yield. If service is delayed by a year, rearing cost is greatly increased.

A further important factor is that both market prices and production cost fluctuate. In Britain the successful fat lamb is ready for slaughter before it is exposed to damaging worm infection. It may not be advantageous too effectively to control helminthiasis in those lambs that have not been got away fat by early July for they would either be fit for slaughter when prices are at their lowest or overweight when prices rise again.

As a rule, the economic loss is greatest when the loss in production is unexpected and results in contingencies for which no provision has been made as, for example, in the case of beef cattle which should have been sold fat out of the yards but have failed to reach the required finish and must be sold as stores becauses no suitable pasture is available and stocks of winter feed are exhausted.

It follows from the fact that a particular loss is associated with the unexpected, that in an established agricultural system even a gross and obvious biological loss may be absorbed by production methods and marketing arrangements and consequently occasion little economic loss. Conversely, there is a tendency, in traditional systems, for considerable economic loss to be attributable to parasitisms which do not occur. This is because the system may contain uneconomic means of avoiding parasitism, the effects of which cannot be absorbed. The real economic significance of helminthiasis is that it is an obstacle, one of many, to change towards more efficient or more intensive production methods.

The commonly enunciated proposition that intensification increases the hazard of helminthiasis is misleading. It would be truer to say that the economic significances of such helminthiasis as does occur is greater in more intensive systems.

B. Spontaneous Regulation of Worm Burdens in the Host

As has been shown above, it is worm burdens above a tolerated level that cause a loss of growth or production and the object of control measures is to keep worm burdens within the host below that level. Control is a question of manipulating populations and demands a knowledge of the factors and processes by which the size of populations are regulated in the host in the absence of anthelmintic medication.

The mammalian host responds to invasion by parasitic nematodes by mechanisms having a variety of effects on the worms. Some workers take the view that a single mechanism produces a variety of effects. Others, of whom the present writer is one, think it preferable to consider different effects as springing from quite separate causes. They justify this by pointing to the fact that some manifestations of resistance may occur without others and that in different host/parasite systems they are not of the same relative importance and do not make their appearance in a constant order. Most hosts react to the presence of nematode parasites by an immune response, both humoral and cellular antibodies being formed (review by SINCLAIR 1970). It has proved difficult, however, to relate the manifestations of resistance to these antibodies. Moreover, in nearly every case the same effects can be demonstrated to be produced by causes other than an acquired immunity. Thus, most may appear as a result of an innate resistance of the host depending on breed, age, or condition. It is not essential to the present argument to consider the essential nature of immunity to helminths (reviews by OGILVIE and JONES 1971, 1973; JARRETT 1973; LARSH and RACE 1975), but it is necessary to discuss its effects.

The following are among the manifestations of host resistance to nematodes that have been described:

1. A resistance to the establishement of new infection
2. The sudden expulsion of almost the entire worm burden. For the present purpose this may be distinguished from:
3. A protracted form of worm loss
4. Depression of ovulation
5. A stunting of worms which fail to grow to their normal size
6. Morphological effects, the development of certain structures being prematurely terminated
7. Arrest of development at a precise early stage which is characteristic of the species

I. Self-cure and Protection

STOLL (1929) observed that when lambs were exposed to infection with *Haemonchus contortus* on pasture, the number of worm eggs in their facces rose and then fell spontaneously and rather abruptly after a few weeks. Thereafter, attempts experimentally to reinfect the lambs failed. STOLL called the termination of infection "self-cure" and the refractory state which appeared to follow "protection."

This simple observation profoundly influenced thinking on resistance to helminths. The notion became deeply entrenched that the development of an acquired resistance to gastrointestinal nematodes was always marked by the expulsion of worms followed by a refractory state.

Of almost equal influence was the observation by GORDON (1948) in Australia that when a period of dry weather was terminated by rain and fresh herbage growth resulted, burdens of *H. contortus* in sheep were abruptly terminated. Speculations about the anthelmintic properties of fresh grass were set aside by the work of STEWART (1950), who suggested that the elimination of worms was caused by massive reinfection with the infective larvae carried by the fresh grass. He demonstrated that the experimental administration of infective larvae speedily resulted in the elimination of the existing burden. Moreover, all the signs were that an allergic response was involved. The phenomenon was marked by a local oedema and could be prevented by means of antihistaminic drugs (STEWART 1953). This phenomenon, to which the term "self-cure" was now exclusively applied, was thought to be of a central importance in the epidemiology of gastrointestinal nematode infections. It was regarded as quite distinct from the spontaneous termination of primary infections.

Views on the nature and importance of the phenomenon studied by STEWART have changed. ALLONBY and URQUHART (1973) in East Africa showed that as visualised by GORDON (1948) a spontaneous expulsion of worms can occur on worm-free pasture. MICHEL (1952), working with *Trichostrogylus retortaeformis* in rabbits, concluded that, in this system at least, the spontaneous termination of an infection could not justifiably be distinguished from an expulsion of worms prompted by reinfection. A rapid loss of worms could occur in both circumstances and whether it did, depended on the presence of a critical biomass of worms.

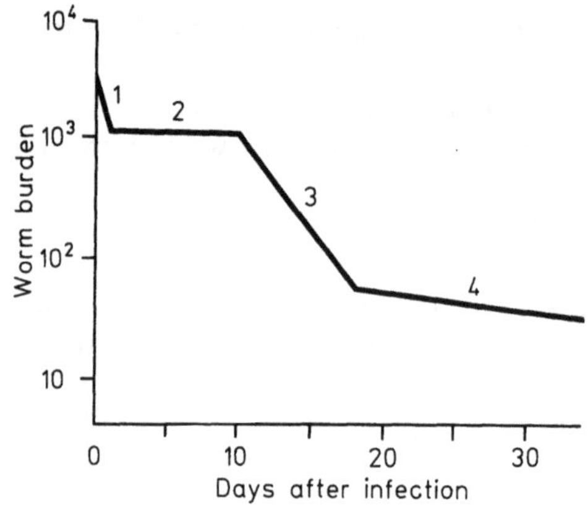

Fig. 3. The four phases of an infection of *Nippostrongylus brasiliensis* in the rat. (Based on data presented by JARRETT et al. 1968)

MULLIGAN et al. (1965), BARTH et al. (1968) and subsequently JARRETT et al. (1968) now investigated the spontaneous termination of experimental infections of *Nippostrongylus brasiliensis* in laboratory rats, describing this as self-cure. They described the course of an infection as consisting of four phases. First, an initial loss, i.e., the number of worms recovered very soon after infection was significantly less than the number of larvae administered; second, a plateau phase during which there was no drecrease in worm numbers; third, a logarithmic loss of worms which gave way to a fourth and final phase in which a small residue of worms was lost at a very much slower rate. This is shown in Fig. 3.

There are now grounds for questioning whether the more protracted loss of worms, which was once regarded as entirely distinct from self-cure, is not a phenomenon of a very similar kind. Before this can be considered, however, it is expedient first to discuss resistance to the establishment of worms, the phenomenon that STOLL (1929) called "protection."

II. Resistance to the Establishment of Worms

STEWART (1953) observed that when self-cure of a burden of *H. contortus* was elicited by reinfection, the new worms sometimes became established and sometimes failed to do so. MICHEL (1953) observed that in infections of *T. retortaeformis* in rabbits the appearance of "protection" could either precede or follow self-cure. The two phenomena must therefore be seen as entirely distinct.

As the term is commonly employed, an animal is regarded as immune to a parasite if new infection does not become established. There are, however, some difficulties of definition because it is not always easy to distinguish between the failure of worms to become established and the loss of worms subsequently to their establishment. This is not a mere matter of semantics as exemplified by the difference between those who choose to regard as an initial loss what others see as a failure of some of the worms administered to become established. It is rather

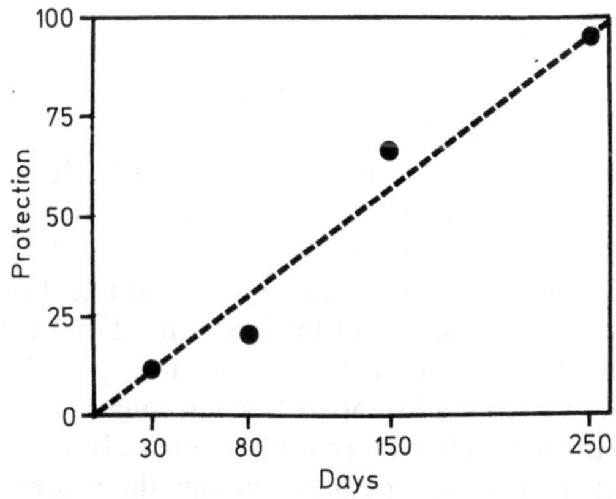

Fig. 4. The development of resistance to the establishment of *O. ostertagi* (protection) in calves infected daily with 1,000 infective larvae

a question of the stage to which the worms develop in the refractory host. An arbitrary definition proposed by the present writer, and which may or may not prove durable, was that a reaction of the host whereby worms were prevented from reaching the stage at which, characteristically, their development could be arrested, should be regarded as a resistance to establishment.

Except in circumstances to be discussed further below, most grazing animals, when adult, are highly resistant to reinfection with most gastrointestinal nematodes, a circumstance the importance of which is easily overlooked. The rate at which a resistance to the establishment of worms is acquired varies from one host/parasite system to another and this determines whether animals are susceptible to reinfection from pasture which they themselves have contaminated. Thus, calves develop a resistance to the establishment of *O. ostertagi* slowly but steadily (Fig. 4) over a period of several months, *Cooperia oncophora* and *T. colubriformis* engender an immunity rather more rapidly in cattle and sheep, respectively, calves are normally refractory to *Nematodirus helvetianus* 4 months after first exposure to infection on pasture and lambs can become resistant to the establishemnt of *N. battus* even more rapidly.

An innate resistance is not often expressed as a resistance to establishment, but animals that by virtue of breed, bodily condition or age are innately resistant, acquire a resistance to the establishment of worms more quickly. As demonstrated by MANTON et al. (1962) and URQUHART et al. (1966) lambs of a number of British breeds are incapable of acquiring this form of resistance to *H. contortus* before they are between 3 and 7 months old. Merinos do not appear to become refractory even when adult.

A resistance to the establishment of worms when once acquired is not necessarily permanent. In many systems it is largely in abeyance around parturition and in early lactation (CONNAN 1968; O'SULLIVAN and DONALD 1970). This and associated phenomena which have a crucial epidemiological significance are discussed further below.

III. The Loss of Worms

The time course of uniformly aged populations of *O. ostertagi* in cattle (a system which has been rather thoroughly studied) is similar in form to that of *Nippostrongylus brasiliensis* in the rat, but the time scale is rather longer. Only a proportion of the worms administered become established and there is then little or no decrease in worm numbers for a period which appears to be inversely related to the size of the inoculum. This is followed by a logarithmic decrease of which the slope is positively related to the size of the inoculum. Finally, there is a residual phase. This is shown for three levels of infection in Fig. 5. It is evident that the plateau phase for *O. ostertagi* is five or six times as long as that for *N. brasiliensis* and the half-life of the population is ten times as great. It is nonetheless tempting to speculate that in the two host parasite systems the process is essentially the same. Certainly, in both cases worm loss is an expression of host resistance.

In infections of *O. ostertagi* and a number of other species, the short mean life of the worms is the main factor by which worm burdens in the host are regulated. The importance of this has not long been fully recognised. TAYLOR (1943) considered the possibility but dismissed it because most parasites were known to be capable of living almost as long as their hosts. This is indeed true in the case of very small populations. TAYLOR was confusing what can happen with what does happen, a type of error from which helminthologists are not exempt.

If the life span of the worms is short relative to the period during which the host remains incapable of resisting their establishment, then it follows that during this period populations in the host are determined in just the same way as populations in free-living organisms. New individuals are added to the population, old ones are lost. The size of the population is the product of the number added per unit of time and their mean life expectancy. A change in either results in a proportional change in the population. Since the longevity of the worms does not vary very widely in normal circumstances, the worm burden of a grazing animal depends on the rate at which new infection is acquired.

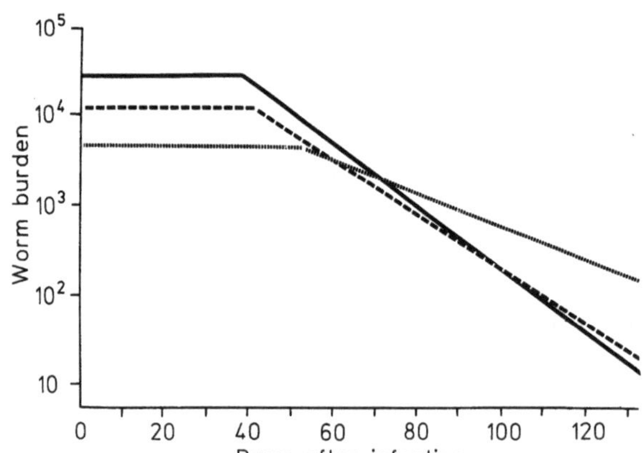

Fig. 5. The time course of populations of *O. ostertagi* in calves infected on day 0 with 8,3000 larvae (······), 25,000 larvae (–––––) and 75,000 larvae (———)

There are no adequate grounds for believing that populations of all species of gastrointestinal nematodes are regulated in this way and, certainly, it is possible to visualise a number of mechanisms. DINEEN (1963), for example, visualised the regulation of worm burdens as depending on the operation of immune mechanisms which were elicited when a threshold of worm numbers was exceeded, the worms being expelled or their development arrested. Subsequently a lower threshold operated.

Figure 6 shows a number of theoretically possible population curves in animals receiving infective larvae at a constant rate. Curve A represents the situation in which the life of the worms is long and resistance to their establishment develops slowly. Curve B might be expected if populations were regulated as visualised by DINEEN (1963). Increase is unrestrained whereupon worms are rapidly eliminated. Increase is then resumed and again abruptly declines from a lower peak. Curve C shows population changes where a resistance to the establishment of worms develops very quickly, where there is no violent synchronous expulsion of worms and the life expectancy of the worms is short. Curve D relates to a similar situation but in which the life of the worms is long. Curve E would be expected where the life of the worms is short and resistance to establishment develops slowly. It will be noted that curves D and E are of rather similar form.

Curves of populations of *O. ostertagi* in calves infected with the same number of larvae every day conform to this pattern. It is interpreted as indicating that worm burdens reach a level at which the number of new worms established is balanced by the worms lost. As the proportion of new larvae that become established

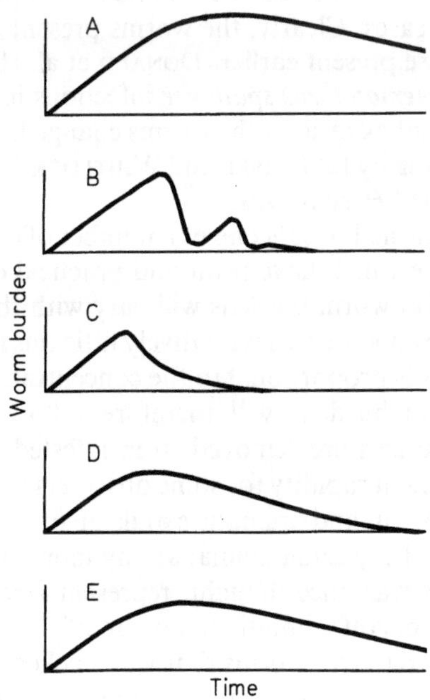

Fig. 6. Possible population curves (see text for explanation)

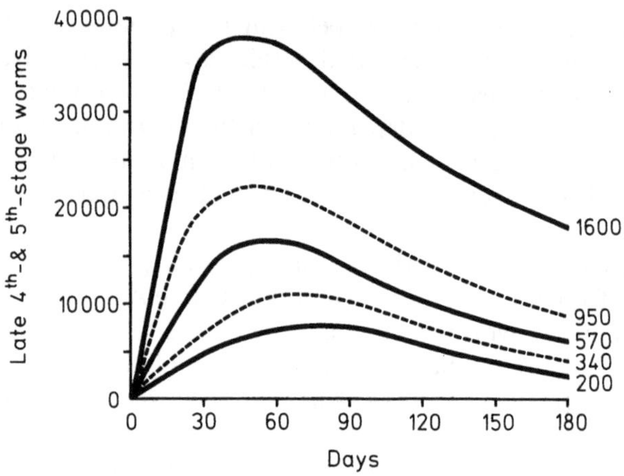

Fig. 7. The time course of burdens of developing and adult *O. ostertagi* in five groups of calves receiving infective larvae daily at different rates

decreases, so this equilibrium level also declines. Figure 7, which shows population curves of *O. ostertagi* in calves infected at five different rates, shows that the level at which the population is maintained is proportional to the infection rate. The deduction that, in this system at least, populations are regulated by a short mean life of the worms is reinforced by the circumstance that in animals constantly exposed to infection a turnover of worms can be demonstrated. With the passage of time, the worms present become smaller and the proportion with morphological abnormalities increases. Clearly, the worms present at one point in time are not identical with those present earlier. DONALD et al. (1964) made a similar deduction in the case of *Nematodirus spathiger* infections in lambs from the observation that with time the sex ratio of the worms changed. A similar interpretation is possible of the finding by LE JAMBRE and WHITLOCK (1968) of morphological changes in populations of *H. contortus*.

That populations are turned over is one of a number of consequences of regulation by a short mean life which have profound practical consequences. It has already been suggested that worm burdens will vary with the rate at which new infection is taken in. Since appetite varies relatively little this means that the worm burden of grazing animals is proportional to the concentration of larvae per unit weight of herbage. Worm burdens will therefore follow fluctuations in the herbage infestation. If animals are removed from infested pasture, their worm burdens decline with sufficient rapidity for some observers to interpret this as self-cure, i.e. the rapid synchronous and dramatic expulsion of worms.

The worms present in the grazing animal at any moment have been recently acquired. They do not, as was once thought, represent what has been accumulated over the whole season. Anthelmintic treatment of an animal that continues to be exposed to infection removes worms that were picked up recently and that will very quickly be replaced, the burden returning to its former level in 2 or 3 weeks.

IV. Arrested Development

In the previous section it was asserted that worms do not accumulate in the host over a long period and that their numbers are strictly dependent on the rate at which infective larvae are acquired. This is true only where the phenomenon of arrested development does not play a part.

Thirty years ago this phenomenon had been recognised in only very few host-parasite systems and was regarded as something of a curiosity. It was seen as a consequence of host resistance and it was assumed that the arrested worms did not subsequently develop. TAYLOR and MICHEL (1953) suggested that the arrested worms were capable of resuming their development and that this gave the phenomenon its significance as an adaptation permitting the parasite to survive through times when conditions were unfavourable. This interpretation is now accepted as broadly true. It is believed that nearly all species of nematodes are capable of interrupting their development, each species at a characteristic and usually early stage. Thus, *Toxocara* spp. are arrested at the second stage, *Trichostrongylus* spp. at the late third stage, *Ostertagia, Haemonchus*, and *Cooperia* at the early fourth stage and *Nematodirus* spp. at a more advanced point in the fourth stage.

This abilitiy to interrupt development appears chiefly to serve the purpose of synchronising the development of the worm with events in its environment. A number of different signals can cause arrest, even of one species, and it appears that the resumption of development can also be prompted by more than one cause.

Early workers often failed to distinguish between arrested development in which the worms are held at a precise stage, and retarded development in which the worms develop more slowly than normal. The real test of whether arrested worms are present is that the populations shows a bimodal size distribution of the kind shown in Fig. 8.

The causes of arrested development have been studied for many years. The original belief that the phenomenon is a consequence of host resistance can readi-

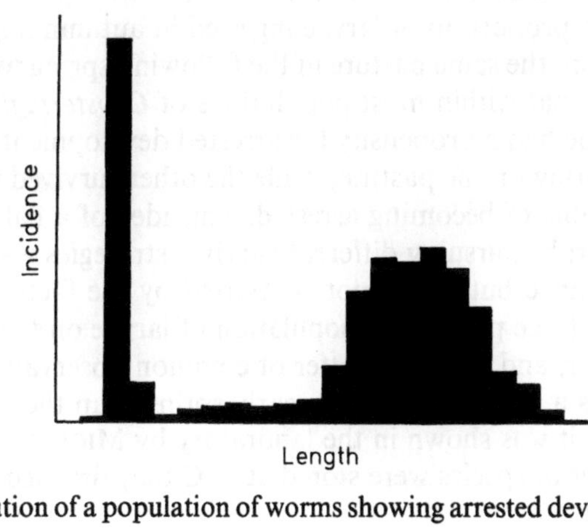

Fig. 8. Size distribution of a population of worms showing arrested development

ly be confirmed in a number of host/parasite systems. Closer re-examination of the evidence in some cases shows, however, that an alternative interpretation is possible, namely that an equal proportion of the worms initially established became arrested in both resistant and susceptible animals and that thereafter adult worms were more rapidly lost from the resistant animals while arrested worms were not lost. In consequence, a larger proportion of the worms, remaining in the resistant animals, was arrested. An explanation of this kind is not possible in every case, however. It is plain from observations by MICHEL (1952) with *T. retortaeformis* that arrested development can be the consequence of host resistance and more recently it has been shown that arrest of *O. ostertagi* in cattle can be caused by both acquired and innate resistance (MICHEL et al. 1979). The size of the inoculum can also play a part (DUNSMORE 1960; MARTIN et al. 1957).

By the mid-1960s it had become evident that the observed facts could not adequately be explained by the theory that host resistance was the only cause of arrested development. ANDERSON et al. (1966) in Scotland demonstrated that when susceptible calves were grazed for a short time on infested pasture in autumn or early winter, a larger proportion of the worms they acquired were arrested, but that this did not occur at other times of the year. It transpired that seasonal factors acting on the free-living stages caused changes in them which led to their parasitic development being interrupted and it was soon shown that low or decreasing temperature was the operative factor. FERNANDO et al. (1971) in Canada made very similar observations on infections of *Obeliscoides cuniculi* in rabbits and more recently a number of other species have been shown in regions of temperate climate to react in the same way.

It is a feature of the phenomenon in most species that only a proportion of the worms becomes arrested and, indeed, this proportion is used as an index of the intensity of arrest. ARMOUR et al. (1967) compared an isolate of *O. ostertagi* which had been maintained in the laboratory for 10 years with a new isolate and found that in the same conditions a very much greater proportion of the larvae of the fresh isolate became arrested. They deduced that *Ostertagia* larvae were of two kinds, respectively incapable of becoming arrested and readily induced to become arrested or "inhibition-prone."

ARMOUR (1970) and SOLLOD (1967) used this idea to explain the observation that, though a large proportion of larvae ingested in autumn might be arrested, larvae picked up from the same pasture in the following spring were not arrested at all. They argued that within most populations of *O. ostertagi* there were two morphs of which one had a propensity for arrested development but was unsuccessful in overwintering on the pasture, while the other survived well on the pasture but was incapable of becoming arrested. This idea of a balanced polymorphism with two morphs pursuing different survival strategies was attractive and not without importance but it was not supported by the facts. The theory demanded that a very large part of the population of larvae on the pasture should die during the winter, and it was a matter of common observation that herbage infestations were, as a rule, no smaller in early spring than they had been in the autumn. Moreover, it was shown in the laboratory by MICHEL et al. (1975) that if larvae of a number of species were stored at 4 °C they first acquired the ability

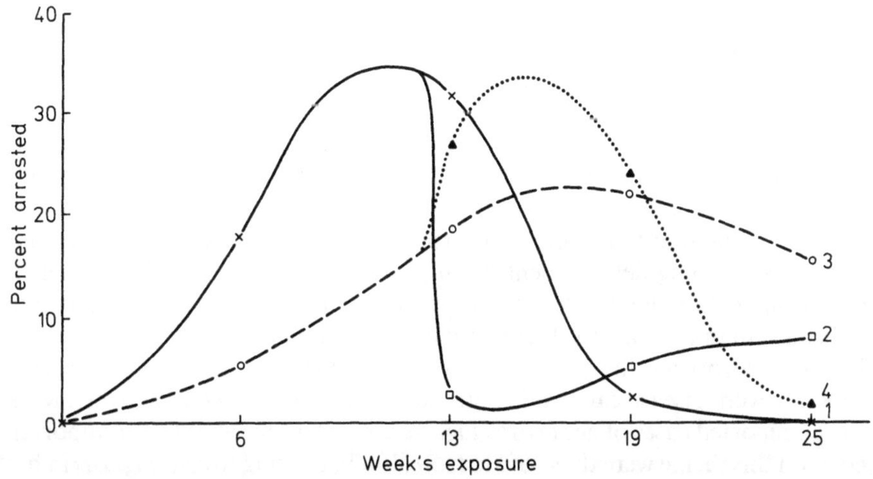

Fig. 9. The mean proportion of *O. ostertagi* that became arrested when infective larvae were administered to calves after storage for different periods at 4 °C (group 1,*X*) and 15 °C (group 3,*O*). Also shown is the effect of an increase in storage temperature after 12 weeks from 4 °C to 15 °C (group 2,□) and a decrease in temperature from 15 °C to 4 °C (group 4,▲). MICHEL et al. (1975)

to become arrested, the proportion doing so reaching a peak after 12 weeks, and then lost this ability until by the 24th week none could do so.

Meanwhile, mortality was negligible. In the jargon that grew up, the larvae were first conditioned and then deconditioned. It was also demonstrated that changes in temperature could expedite both conditioning and deconditioning. An abrupt fall in temperature greatly speeded up conditioning; a rise in temperature rapidly deconditioned the larvae (Fig. 9).

While exposure of free-living stages to low temperature is obviously an important cause of arrested development in temperate climates, other signals evidently operate in other regions. HOTSON (1967) had reported that in winter rainfall areas of Australia, *O. ostertagi* began to be arrested in the same calendar month as in Britain, i.e. in spring instead of in autumn. Since Australian *O. ostertagi* is almost certainly of British origin, it followed that, in response to different selection pressures, its reactions had changed. In Britain, the relevant factors are that the life of adult worms is short and that *O. ostertagi* eggs passed during late autumn and winter have a negligible chance of reaching the infective stage. In consequence, worms that grow to maturity in late autumn or winter leave virtually no progeny. In winter rainfall areas of Australia it is during the dry summer that the transmission of infection is prevented and worms that develop to maturity in summer are selected against. Reports of worms being arrested during the dry season are becoming more frequent. Examples are provided by the observation of OGUNSUSI and EYSKER (1979) in northern Nigeria and of MICHEL and HOOSHMAND-RAD (1978) in southern Iran.

SMEAL (1977) has investigated the factors that cause arrest in Australian *Ostertagia* populations and found that the larvae are not conditioned by high or rising temperatures. The operating signal is evidently of a different kind, possibly depending on photoperiod.

It must not be assumed that in all cases where worms are arrested in winter, low temperature is the relevant signal. In Britain, *H. contortus* which fails to survive on the pasture and overwinters in the host as an arrested larva begins to be arrested in late summer, from which it follows that the larvae were conditioned in the hottest part of the year (WALLER and THOMAS 1975).

There is little question today that arrested development should be seen as a means of postponing development during an unfavorable period. In spite of the obvious implication that the resumed development of the worms is of even greater significance than their arrest, this phase of the phenomenon has been little studied. This is surprising for if arrested worms resume their development in large numbers, severe disease can result. This has been known since 1957, when MARTIN et al. reported cases of acute *ostertagiasis* caused in this way. Other important reports on this theme were those of HOTSON (1967), relating to *ostertagiasis* in beef cows in Australia, and of GIBBS (1964), who reported an outbreak of *Haemonchus* in housed ewes in Canada.

ARMOUR and BRUCE (1974) on the basis of experiments on calves experimentally infected with cold-conditioned larvae of *O. ostertagi* concluded that all the arrested larvae resumed their development after a fixed interval of 16–18 weeks from infection or, as seems more probable, after a fixed interval of time from conditioning of the larvae. MICHEL et al. (1976a, b) were not able to draw the same conclusions from a number of series of observations both in experimentally and naturally infected cattle. They found that a constant 600–700 larvae resumed their development daily and their number was in no way influenced by whether many arrested worms were present initially or not. In spring, or earlier in certain circumstances, a very large proportion of the arrested worms that remained, developed over a short period.

These results suggested the operation of a rather more complex mechanism than that envisaged by ARMOUR and BRUCE (1974) and posed some conceptual difficulties. In animals carrying a large burden of arrested *O. ostertagi*, developing and adult worms are constantly present and their numbers are entirely consistent with the usual turnover of the population of adults. The same number of developing and adult worms begins to develop every day and survives thereafter for an average 28–30 days. The steady release from arrest of a fixed number of worms daily is very difficult to explain except in terms of a mechanism whereby the loss of adult worms allows an equal number of arrested larvae to resume their development. But since the number of adult worms lost daily, plainly depends on the number of arrested worms that resume their development, the argument becomes circular and implausible.

The possibility that the presence of adult worms plays a part in restraining the development of arrested larvae has been discussed for many years and may derive support from a series of observations described by GIBSON (1953) in which housed horses carrying burdens of *Trichonema* spp. were treated with phenothiazine, a drug without effect on arrested worms. Every time that the horses were dosed, adult worms were recovered from the faeces, the faecal egg count fell to zero, and, although accidental reinfection was prevented, counts gradually rose again to near their former level.

GIBSON concluded that it was the removal of adult worms that had stimulated the resumed development of arrested forms. An alternative explanation is possible, however. If small numbers from a large reservoir of arrested larvae developed constantly, a turnover of adult worms being fed from this source, events exactly as described by GIBSON would follow the removal of adults by anthelmintic treatment.

It has proved very difficult to obtain direct evidence that the resumed development of arrested worms is prompted by the removal of adult worms. An experiment by MICHEL (1970) using *O. ostertagi* in calves does provide some evidence but the extent of the phenomenon is small.

Although there is now no doubt that host resistance can be an effective cause of arrested development, it has not yet been very clearly demonstrated that development is resumed if there is a failure of immunity. Certainly, development of massive numbers of *Ostertagia* tends to occur earlier than normal in weak animals and there are indications that acute stress may have the same effect. On the other hand, working with another system, *H. contortus* in sheep, BLITZ and GIBBS (1971) failed to induce arrested worms prematurely to resume their development by transferring them from resistant to susceptible ewes. Development is not prompted by parturition or lactation of the host although at this time the proportion of newly acquired worms that become arrested can be shown to be greatly reduced.

The circumstance that there is more than one cause of arrest and that a variety of factors may be involved in resumed development has raised the problem, keenly debated, of whether arrested development should be seen as a simple mechanism with alternative causes or, as argued by ARMOUR (1980), as two or more entirely separate and distinct mechanisms, each with its own causes of arrest and of resumed development. This theory is illustrated in Fig. 10. The question is of more than theoretical interest for it would be of considerable practical use to know whether larvae arrested because of seasonal conditioning could be prompted to resume their development by changes in host resistance or whether seasonal signals would prompt the development of worms that were arrested because of the resistance of the host. Because of very considerable technical difficulties, the matter is still the subject of debate rather than experiment.

On the basis of the results of ARMOUR and BRUCE (1974), the massive development of arrested larvae that occurs in spring is attributed to the operation of a biological clock which measures time from either conditioning of the larvae or from infection. But development tends to occur over a rather shorter period than either conditioning of the larvae or their acquisition by the host and the possibility should not be neglected that a second mechanism may be involved to give added precision. A vernal signal might be transmitted by the host's endocrine system. Such endocrine signals do in fact appear to play an important part in a number of host-parasite systems.

A brief discussion of the life history of various species of ascarids, hookworms, and *Strongyloides* is indicated here not only for its intrinsic interest, but

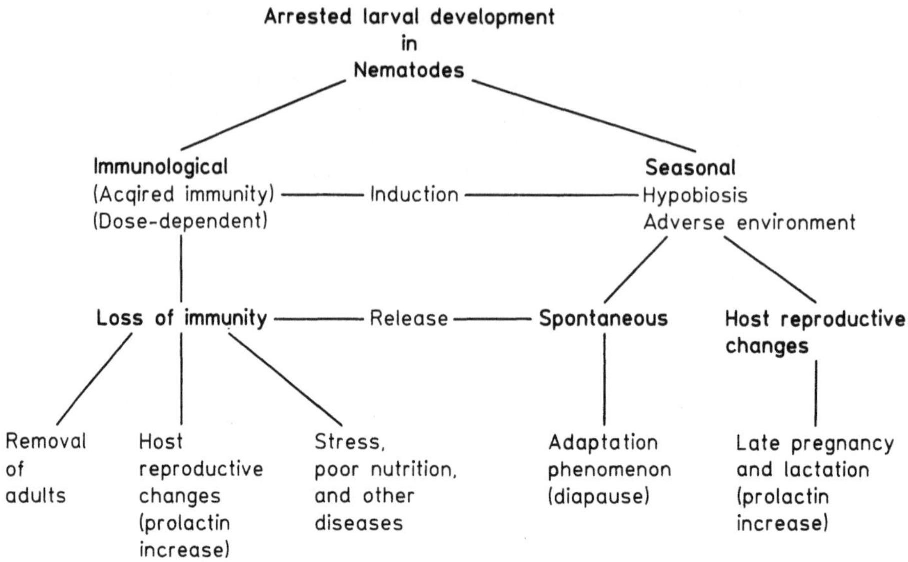

Fig. 10. Diagrammatic representation of the causes of arrested development and of resumed development according to the view of ARMOUR (1980)

because it may give a broader view of arrested development and its significance. The literature has been summarised by MICHEL (1974). *Toxocara canis* provides a good starting point, showing how the phenomenon plays an essential part in the transmission of infection between carnivorous hosts. If infective eggs of *Toxocara* are ingested by a young susceptible dog they perform what is termed a tracheal migration, passing into the circulation, breaking into the alveoli of the lung, being swept up the trachea and swallowed, and establishing themselves in the intestine. If the eggs are ingested by an unsuitable host, as for example a small rodent, then a rather different migration takes place. The larvae pass through the capillaries of the lung and into the systemic circulation, so reaching the somatic tissues, where they persist for long periods without growing. If now the small rodent, or larvae isolated from it, are ingested by a young dog, the larvae perform a tracheal migration and develop in the intestine. In other words, *Toxocara* can use small rodents or other unsuitable hosts as paratenic hosts.

Hosts may be "unsuitable" for *T. canis* for different reasons. Adult dogs, resistant on account of age or previous infection, may also be unsuitable in the sense that *Toxocara* larvae swallowed by them perform a somatic migration. Sex also plays a part and a somatic migration is more likely to occur in bitches than in dogs. It can be argued that the bitch also serves as a paratenic host of a specialised kind, for the larvae are mobilised in late pregnancy and infect the foetus via the placenta. Larvae also migrate to the mammary gland and appear in the colostrum. Of particular significance in the present context is the accuracy with which the reactivation of the larvae is synchronised with the stage of the pregnancy, the fetus being invaded very close to the 42nd day. Eggs appear in the faeces of the pup 21 days after birth, 9 days earlier than if pups are given infective eggs immediately after birth. It appears that when the arrested larvae in the bitch resume their activity they may also reach the gut and develop to maturity, eggs appearing in the faeces of the bitch at exactly the same time as in the pups. It is difficult to avoid the conclusion that the development of the worms, arrested because of the resistance of the host, is resumed in response to an endocrine signal associated with late pregnancy. Interestingly, if infective eggs are administered to a pregnant mouse, the larvae perform a tracheal migration.

A further interesting feature in this system is that only a proportion of the somatic larvae in the bitch are mobilised on any occasion. Even if withheld from new infection, a bitch can infect at least three successive litters prenatally or via the colostrum.

Prenatal infection was at one time believed to occur in a number of host-parasite systems, but it is now recognised that *T. canis* in the dog is the only well-documented instance. In all other cases the evidence consisted not of the demonstration of worms in the foetus or the neonate, but the appearance of eggs in the faeces earlier than could, on the basis of the normal prepatent period, be explained by infection after birth. Because larvae that appear in the colostrum have already undergone some development, this evidence is not valid. *Neoscaris vitulorum* (= *Toxocara vitulorum*), *Strongyloides* spp. and several species of hookworms can all be transmitted via the colostrum. In every case a tracheal migration occurs in the susceptible host and a somatic migration in the aged or resistant host, and the mobilisation of larvae from the tissues is accurately timed.

It is tempting to speculate that the advantage to the species of this device to ensure that the host is infected as early as possible is that immune tolerance results. As yet, however, there is no very striking evidence that infection in the neonate persists longer than infection in older hosts.

There are clearly sufficient similarities between these examples and cases of arrested development among the *Trichostrongylidae* to justify the view that this phenomenon may serve a variety of functions, that some form of synchronisation appears always to be involved and that different causes of arrest and different signals for resumed development may operate. Of particular interest is the finding by SCHAD et al. (1973) that a seasonally induced arrest occurs in infections of *Ancylostoma duodenale* in humans, a system in which the colostral transmission of infection also appears to occur.

V. Stunting and Morphological Effects

Arrested development as noted above must be distinguished from retarded development. In the resistant host, and in this context the term includes both innate and acquired resistance, worms tend to grow more slowly and to reach a smaller adult size. Effects on the morphology of the worm also occur, the best-documented example perhaps being provided by the vulval flap of *O. ostertagi*, which in the resistant host may stop growing at a number of points along the course of its normal development. Effects of a less specific kind are the smaller spicules reported by KEITH (1967) to occur in *Cooperia pectinata* from resistant hosts and the uteri of *O. ostertagi*, which in worms from a resistant host are smaller and therefore contain fewer eggs.

Because, in many infections all the worms present at any point in time have recently been acquired, these characters can be used to give an indication of the current state of resistance of the host. As long ago as 1935, TETLEY suggested that the number of eggs present in the uteri of *Nematodirus* spp. were a measure of "the pitch of the host-parasite relationship". TETLEY (1941) believed that the number of eggs contained in the uteri of the worm reflected the rate of ovulation. In fact, uterine capacity appears to be a more important factor.

VI. Regulation of Egg Output

It has long been recognised that in the resistant host the fecundity of the worms tends to be depressed. There have been very few detailed studies of this phenomenon and in the most thoroughly studied system, *O. ostertagi* in cattle, the mechanisms involved are of a singular nature which may not be typical. In this system, if more than a relatively small number of adult worms is present, total egg output is independent of worm numbers and runs a stereotyped course, rising quickly to a peak and then decreasing logarithmically. This pattern, which is shown in Fig. 11, occurs whether worm numbers are increasing or decreasing, whether the same worms are present throughout, or whether reinfection and a turnover of the population are occurring.

It is not easy to suggest of what kind the underlying mechanism might be. If cumulative egg output is plotted, a logistic curve results and it has been suggested that this should be seen as the normal pattern for the proliferation of cells, whether in a bacterial culture, the growth of an elephant, or the shedding of worm eggs. But the form of a normal growth curve is conditioned by feedback mechanisms and in the three examples cited, these are rather different in kind. Since egg output of a population of *O. ostertagi* takes the same course whether the population is turned over or not, it must follow that the limit to total egg output is determined by the host and not by the worms. Since it is the output of the whole

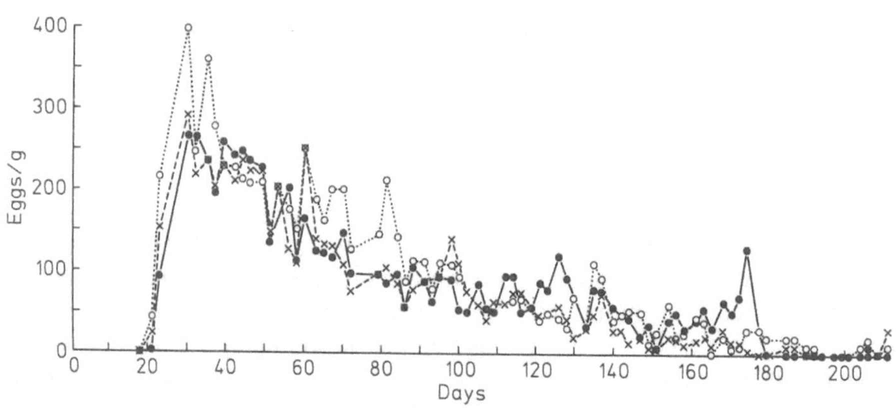

Fig. 11. Mean faecal egg counts of three groups of calves infected with different numbers of *O. ostertagi* larvae. Calves infected daily with 500 (●——●), 1,000 (×-----×) and 1,500 (o·········o) larvae. MICHEL (1967)

population that is subject to this limit, it appears probable that a rationing mechanism of some kind is involved. It is a feature of the logarithmic decrease that egg output at any point in time bears the same relation to egg output at a point earlier by a constant interval. This suggests a self-contained mechanism. One might visualise a situation in which egg output is limited by the availability of some factor of which a fixed quantum is required for the production of each egg, the supply of the rationed factor being determined by previous egg output. The limit to egg output may be raised or set aside altogether by the administration to the host of immunosuppressants. Equally, it may lapse if the animal becomes severely debilitated from any cause. It appears not unlikely therefore that if a rationing mechanism operates, the supply of the rationed factor is limited by an immune mechanism of some kind.

While egg output of a number of nematode parasites of cattle appears to be regulated in this way, and while there is some evidence that a similar mechanism controls the egg output of hookworms in dogs (KRUPP 1961), the relationship between egg output and worm burden is rather closer in many host-parasite systems. This may, however, be a difference of degree rather than of kind. Egg output from *O. ostertagi* populations is independent of worm number within a certain range of which the lower border is set by the number of worms which can just reach the limit if ovulating at the maximum rate of which, in the absence of any restraint, they are capable. The upper and less clearly defined border is where the number of worms is sufficient to cause clinical disease, severe debility and the suspension of the regulatory mechanism.

It seems not unlikely that in gastrointestinal nematode infections in sheep the range of worm burden within which such a mechanism operates is very much narrower. One may visualise that in susceptible sheep, infected with *O. circumcincta*, egg output and worm numbers are roughly proportional up to a fairly high level of worm numbers. Above this level egg output would be independent of worm numbers and at a higher level again great variation might be expected in the relationship, with some very high egg counts occurring. With continuous experience of

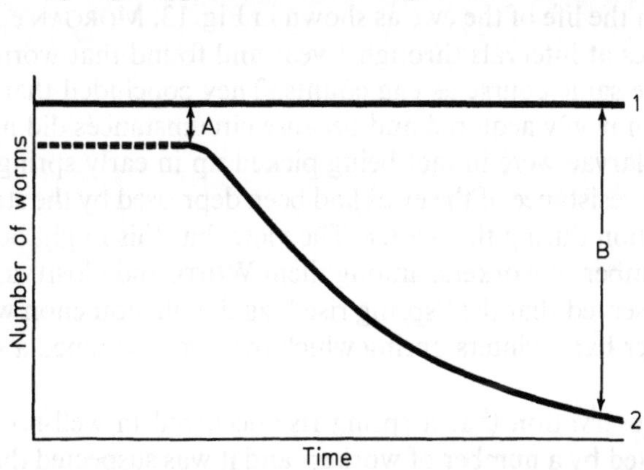

Fig. 12. Illustration of a theory on the regulation of egg output. Curve *2* represents the number of worms which when ovulating without restraint can just reach the limit to total egg output. Above the horizontal line *1* the regulatory mechanism fails. Egg output is not related to worm numbers over a much smaller range at *A* than at *B*

infection, the limit to egg output might be expected to fall and the range of worm burden within which regulation of egg output occurs to get wider. This is illustrated in Fig. 12. No systematic work has been done to verify this theory, but the results of GIBSON and EVERETT (1977) are not inconsistent with it.

It is clear that faecal egg counts are more likely to serve as a guide to worm numbers in some host-parasite systems than in others. In every case they are likely to be misleading in animals that have been exposed to infection for some time.

The use of faecal egg counts as a means of measuring worm burdens has led to great confusion in epidemiological studies. Faecal egg counts are, however, a direct and essential measure of the extent to which pasture is being contaminated. The manner in which egg output from *O. ostertagi* infections in calves is regulated has important epidemiological consequences, for there is a strong tendency for pasture contamination to be the same every year and in a wide range of circumstances. Meanwhile, this is not true in the case of *O. circumcincta* in lambs.

VII. Effect of Parturition and Lactation on Host Resistance

Without attempting to explain the phenomenon, ZAVADOWSKII and ZVIAGINTSEV (1933) reported the occurrence of a seasonal fluctuation in the faecal egg count of a camel in the Zoological Gardens of Moscow. Prompted by this report, TAYLOR (1935) examined monthly composite faeces samples from a group of housed ewes at Weybridge. He found that in spring, when the ewes lambed, there was a marked increase in their egg counts. Because these ewes had been kept in conditions calculated to prevent reinfection, TAYLOR concluded that there had been an increase in the rate of ovulation of the worms.

A very thorough study of the egg counts of sheep on Scottish hill farms by MORGAN et al. (1950) provided the next landmark. This revealed the same seasonal pattern, counts rising in spring and falling again in late summer and this continuing through the life of the ewe as shown in Fig. 13. MORGAN et al. (1951) now slaughtered ewes at intervals through 1 year and found that worm numbers followed much the same course as egg counts. They concluded that the additional worms had been newly acquired and because circumstances did not suggest that more infective larvae were in fact being picked up in early spring, they thought it probable that resistance of the ewes had been depressed by the stress of lambing and poor nutrition during the winter. The view that this might be the cause was shared by a number of workers, among them WHITE and CUSHNIE (1952). PAVER et al. (1955) observed that the "spring rise", as the phenomenon was now called, was greater after hard winters during which the ewes sustained a severe decrease in body weight.

TAYLOR'S observation that a spring rise occurred in well-nourished housed ewes was repeated by a number of workers and it was suspected that the methods used by MORGAN et al. (1951) had failed to reveal the presence of arrested worms during the winter. It soon came to be accepted that the worms involved in the spring rise were arrested worms that had resumed their development. Meanwhile, CROFTON (1954a) had published data suggesting a close connection between par-

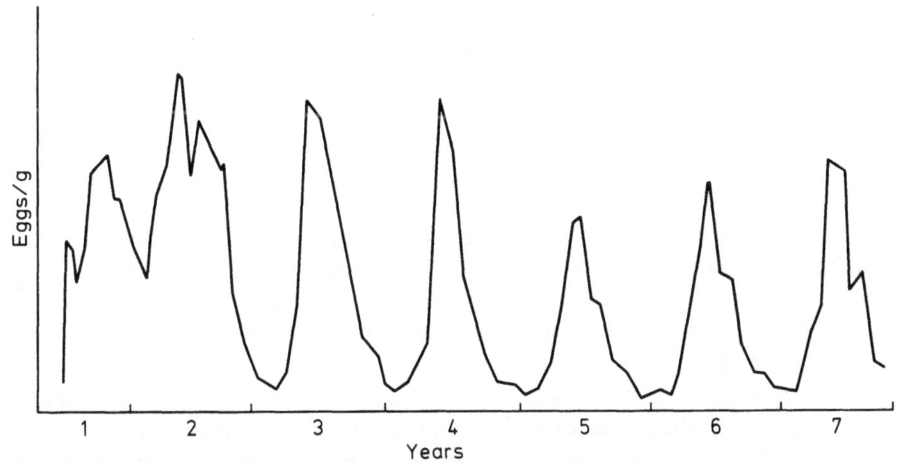

Fig. 13. The seasonal pattern of faecal egg counts of Scottish hill sheep. MORGAN et al. (1951)

turition and the rise in egg counts. He claimed that in individual ewes the peak egg count occurred between 6 and 8 weeks after lambing. In barren ewes and wethers a very much smaller rise was seen at about the same time. Although other workers failed to confirm that there was so close a temporal relationship between parturition and the rise, it was soon generally believed that the stress associated with parturition caused the development of arrested worms and the phenomenon was renamed the "postparturient rise." A similar postparturient increase in worm burden and in faecal egg count was described in many host-parasite systems. JACOBS (1966) and CONNAN (1967) found that the postparturient rise in sows due to *Oesophagostomum* spp. and *Hyostrongylus rubidus* could be abruptly terminated by prematurely weaning the piglets. This was also shown to occur in sheep. It was therefore assumed that the development of arrested worms was triggered by endocrine events associated with lactation.

This position was soon eroded. CVETKOVIĆ et al. (1971), working with *Haemonchus contortus* in ewes, provided evidence that the resumed development, of this species at least, occurs at a particular time of year and was not occasioned by parturition or lactation as such. The nearer the date of lambing was to the time that a small spring rise occurred in unmated ewes, i.e. March to May, the greater was the postparturition rise in the ewes that had lambed. Similar results had been obtained by BRUNSDON (1967) and SALISBURY and ARUNDEL (1970). CVETKOVIĆ et al. did, however, obtain a large postparturient rise in ewes lambing in the autumn, as had CROFTON (1958). The explanation of this apparent anomaly emerges from the work of CONNAN (1968) and of O'SULLIVAN, and DONALD (1970), who showed that the adult worms involved in the postparturient rise could be derived not only from arrested worms that had resumed their development, but also from larvae newly acquired from the pasture. There was also some evidence that the rate of ovulation of the worms increased. Therefore, while particularly in housed ewes the postparturient rise in spring lambing ewes depends on the development of arrested worms, in autumn lambing ewes it is due to worms newly acquired.

It was now suggested among others by KELLY (1973) that during lactation there was a total suspension of all expressions of host resistance, but MICHEL (1974) suggested that it was not necessary to assume this and that all the observed facts could be explained by postulating that the turnover of the population of adult worms ceased during early lactation. In experiments with *O. ostertagi* in heifers, however, MICHEL et al. (1979) found that the turnover rate was not affected by pregnancy, parturition or lactation, although resistance to the establishment of worms was greatly reduced. Meanwhile, DONALD et al. (1980) produced conclusive evidence that the susceptibility of ewes to the establishment of *Ostertagia* spp. was increased during lactation.

Although the literature devoted to the postparturient rise is very voluminous and still growing, the extent of truly useful knowledge is rather limited. In view of the crucial importance of the phenomenon in the epidemiology of parasitic gastroenteritis in sheep, this is surprising. As will appear in a later section, the worm eggs passed by ewes during the postparturient rise are an important source, sometimes the only source, of the herbage infestation that is the cause of disease in the lambs. The suppression of the postparturient rise is therefore an essential component of many procedures for controlling nematode infection and represents an important use or, as some would say, the most important single use of anthelmintics.

C. The Free-Living Stages

The objectives of much early work on the free-living phase of the life cycle of gastrointestinal nematodes were founded on concepts and assumptions which have, in the event, proved not to be entirely appropriate. Partly, this was because populations were seen in rather static terms.

Before the eggs of Trichostrongylid nematodes passed in the faeces of the host are capable of infecting another host, they must develop through three stages. In most cases, the first and second stages feed on coliform bacteria in the faeces; the third stage, which generally retains the cuticle of the second stage, does not feed and may be seen as a resting stage. It is more resistant than the other stages to extremes of temperature and desiccation. When ingested by a suitable host it casts the retained second-stage cuticle and begins its parasitic development. Some authors, notably ROGERS (1961), have attributed a central importance to the act of exsheathement which marks the transition from a free-living to a parasite way of life. It is not of significance to the present argument and will not therefore be mentioned further.

The ultimate purpose of studies on the free-living stages is to make it possible to predict when the host will be exposed to infection and how heavy that infection will be. Although the free-living phase is superficially very simple, the processes involved may be defined and investigated in a number of ways. Some researchers have taken the path of ultimate subdivision and analysis, studying every component in refined laboratory conditions in the hope of ultimately synthesising a composite picture from which practically useful deductions might be drawn. Others, notable among whom were LEVINE and ANDERSEN (1973), went to the opposite extreme and in studying the effects of climate factors on the free-living stages used a single parameter, the "transmission factor," to include the whole of free life. This was the area subtended by the curve of larval population following deposition of worm eggs onto pasture plots. This approach is attractive in its boldness, but it is now conceded that because conditions favouring development to the infective stage, on the one hand, and the persistence of infective larvae on the other are very different, some subdivision is essential. Another problem confronting these and a number of other workers was that the climate to which their larvae were exposed was the microclimate within the sward, and to relate the reactions of the free-living stages to the microclimate meant producing knowledge with little practical value because records of microclimate are not generally available.

A third group of workers, pre-eminent among whom were GIBSON and EVERETT (1967), adopted a more empirical approach. They contaminated plots of pasture with infected faeces every 2 weeks through the year and monitored the resulting infestation on the herbage. From the resulting family of curves a seasonal pattern of herbage infestation appropriate to any pattern of pasture contamination could be calculated. There is, however, a danger that artefacts will be introduced by the slightly artificial conditions of such experiments and considerable resources are required to maintain a supply of infective material. Therefore a fourth group of workers, who are now in the majority, prefer to study the entirely natural situation in which pastures are contaminated by grazing animals. This form of experimentation has proved the key to progress, but this is not to say that more detailed experiments are not essential to the interpretation of its results.

It is now customary to divide the free-living phase into two processes, "translation," which includes all steps from the freshly passed egg to the infective larva on the pasture, and survival of the infective larvae. But it could be argued that this division, which was conceived by ROSE and MICHEL (1957) with *Dictyocaulus viviparus* in mind, is inadequate in the case of gastrointestinal nematodes. Here it is necessary to separate development to the infective stage from the translocation of the larvae from the faeces to the herbage. Conditions that favour development are not identical with those that are best for emergence of the larvae from the faeces and survival is most successful in conditions in which development does not occur.

When considering populations of free-living stages, a number of basic phenomena must be recognised. Firstly, the size of any population depends on the rate at which individuals are recruited to it and the rate at which they are lost from it. Secondly, if the speed of a process increases over a period of time then individuals entering the process over that period will complete it over a shorter period and a large increase in the terminal population may occur. Conversely, if the speed of a process decreases, individuals entering it over a short period will complete it over a longer period, resulting potentially in a decrease in the terminal population. Third are what may be called "reservoir effects." A reservoir in which individuals can be stored can postpone an event or process without changing its rate, it can turn a sustained input at a low rate into a high output over a short period or it can turn a large input over a short period into an output at a low rate over a long period.

It will be realised that these basic phenomena may be seen in populations within the host as well as in populations of the free-living stages on the pasture.

I. Development

In its development from egg to infective larva, trichostrongylid nematodes require moisture, oxygen and a sufficiently high temperature. The last of these, being easiest to measure, has been most extensively studied. Surprisingly, most attention has been devoted to the lowest temperature at which development, or in some cases only the hatching of eggs, can proceed. Critical temperatures in the region of 5°–10 °C have been worked out for most trichostrongylids, but as CROFTON et al. (1965) have shown populations in warmer regions may have a higher critical temperature than populations in cooler regions; critical temperature for development is not a fixed character of the species.

In practice, the lowest temperature at which development can occur is not of great interest, nor for that matter is the highest temperature or the shortest time in which development can be completed. At the extremes the yield of larvae tends to be very small. The optimum temperature for development, i.e. the temperature at which the greatest number of infective larvae is produced, is of rather greater interest. Some determinations by CROFTON (1963) are shown in Fig. 14. This difference between the minimum and the optimum temperature probably underlies the disparity which at one time existed between different assessments of the critical temperature for development of *H. contortus*, which was estimated by DINABURG (1944) at 18 °C, while all other workers since RANSOM (1906) had determined it to lie between 4 °C and 8 °C. The matter became somewhat confused because GORDON (1948) used DINABURG's figure with conspicuous success in predicting the geographical and seasonal incidence of clinical haemonchiasis.

With the exception of the larvated egg (the egg shortly before the first-stage larva hatches from it) and the infective larva, the free-living stages are susceptible to desiccation. The availability to the larva of moisture is greatly modified by the character of the faeces. Large aggregates of faeces, as those of cattle or of ewes on fresh pasture, dry out sufficiently slowly for the development of most larvae to be completed before humidity declines to a lethal level. As against this, oxygen tension in the centre of a large mass of faeces may be insufficient for development. The faecal pellets produced by lambs or by ewes on dry feed can dry out very much more quickly and eggs may even fail to reach the relatively protected larvated egg stage before desiccation has progressed too far. Because of differences between the conditions in different parts of one faecal aggregate and the great variation in their size and location on the pasture, there tends to be considerable variation in the time taken by development from egg to infective larva.

The free-living development of *Nematodirus* spp. differs from that of other trichostrongylids in that it is completed within the eggshell. Because the infective larvae cannot migrate and become available to the grazing animal until they have hatched from the egg, hatching and the factors by which it is prompted has been the subject of some study especially in the case of *Nematodirus battus*. In this species hatching of most of the eggs tends to be greatly delayed and to occur in the spring, many months after development has been completed. As first suggested

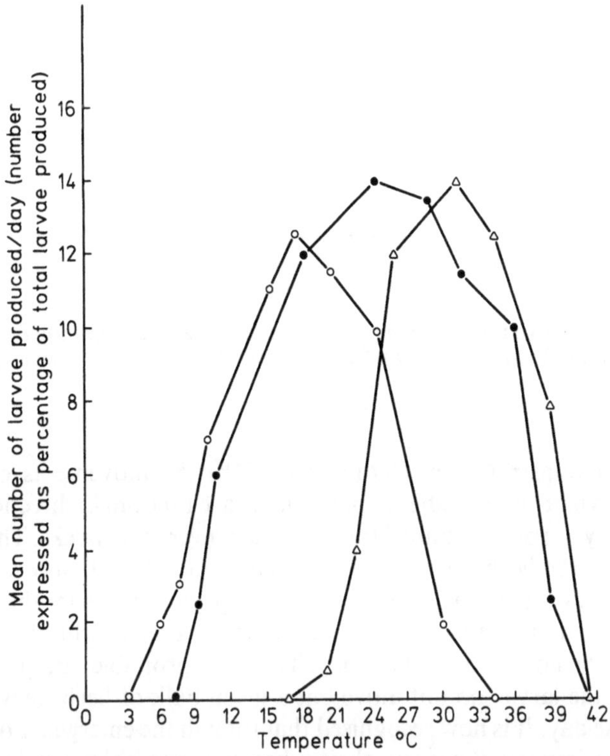

Fig. 14. Optimum temperature for development of the free-living stages of *Haemonchus contortus*, (●), *Ostertagia circumcincta*, (○), and *Cooperia curticei*, (△). CROFTON (1963)

by CHRISTIE (1962), the eggs must experience a period of exposure to cold before a rise in temperature to 10 °C will prompt them to hatch. In other species of *Nematodirus* such cold-conditioning does not appear to be necessary.

II. Migration

If infective larvae are to be accessible to the grazing animal, they must be transferred from the faeces to the herbage. When infected faeces are incubated in a glass jar, infective larvae can, after a time, be seen streaming in narrow and branching bands up the walls of the jar. On this observation, early helminthologists based the belief that larvae migrated up the herbage in a purposive manner. It was thought that the larvae showed either a negative geotaxis or a positive phototaxis. Since movement of the larvae seemed to demand the presence of a continuous film of moisture, it was further believed that larvae were present on the herbage only in the early morning and the evening, performing a regular twice daily movement up and down the grass. It could be, however, that the particular piece of folk wisdom which seemed to support this belief, namely that pasture was not safe when there was dew on the herbage, derived from the fact that in most years in Britain the dew never dries off the herbage after St. Swithuns day.

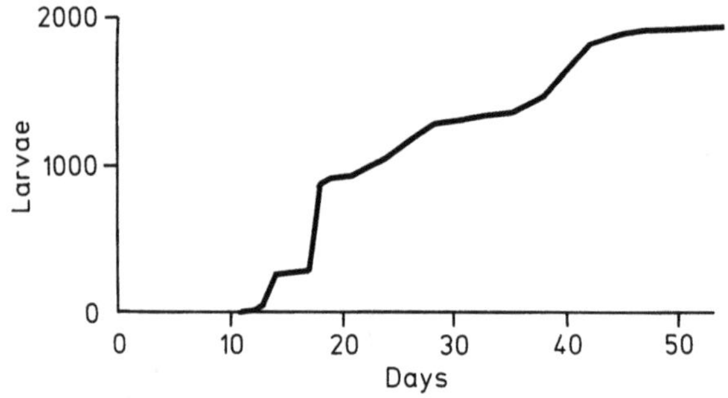

Fig. 15. The cumulative total of *Haemonchus contortus* larvae migrating from 11 pellets of sheep faeces cultured at 11 °C (Drawn from data of SILVERMAN and CAMPBELL 1958)

In fact, as demonstrated by CROFTON (1954b) the movements of the larvae, though more vigorous at higher temperatures, are random in direction. More significantly, they are not continued for more than a very few weeks. The notion that infestations on the herbage are greater at dawn and at dusk may safely be abandoned. CROFTON (1949), who examined herbage samples from the same area at 2-h intervals, found that the number of larvae per unit weight of herbage was at its highest in the hottest part of the day. The most propable interpretation of this result is that the larvae do not move but a given bulk of herbage weighs least in the heat of the day. It is now recognised that though the emergence of larvae from the faeces is an important process, their subsequent vertical migrations are of little interest.

The time that elapses from the completion of development to the emergence of the infective larva from the faeces is very variable and, consequently, as shown by the observations of SILVERMAN and CAMPBELL (1958) on *H. contortus*, larvae may continue to migrate from a pellet of sheep faeces over a period of several weeks (Fig. 15). Where the faecal mass is larger the process of emergence can take many months. The faeces on a pasture may act as a reservoir of infection, a very important factor in determining the seasonal course of herbage infestations. Wet weather favours the transference of larvae from faeces to herbage both by facilitating the movement of larvae and by speeding the disintegration of the dung. Conversely, dry conditions delay emergence and where faecal masses are large enough for larvae to reach the infective stage before the faeces dry out, wet weather after a prolonged dry spell can result in the rapid appearance on the herbage of very large numbers of larvae.

III. Survival

The infective third-stage larva is the resistant resting stage and considerable attention has been devoted to its longevity. Again, most workers have been preoccupied with maxima instead of with modal values and have regarded maximum longevity as a fixed characteristic of the species. Maximum longevity is of course extremely difficult to determine even if an arbitrarily defined end point is used.

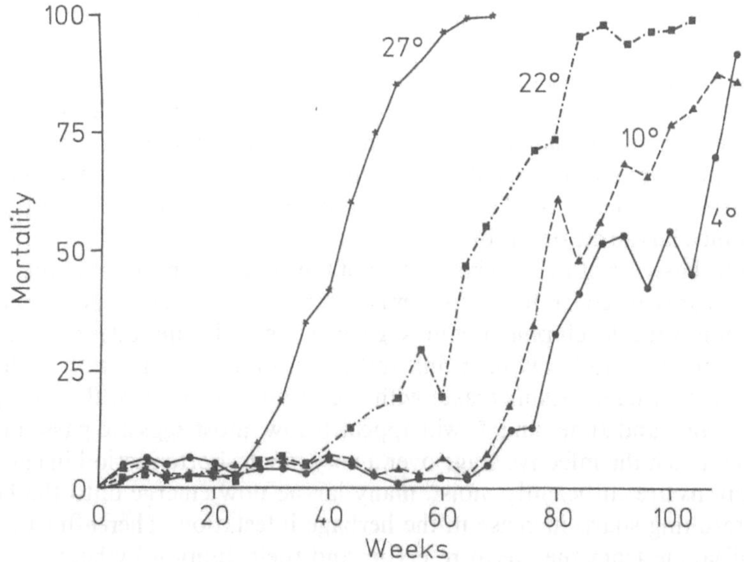

Fig. 16. The effect of temperature on the mortality of thirdstage larvae of *Oesophagostomum dentatum* (Drawn from data made available by Dr. J. H. Rose, Central Veterinary Laboratory, Weybridge)

Figure 16 shows a family of curves, drawn from data kindly made available by Dr. J. H. Rose, of the mortality of *Oesophagostomum dentatum* larvae maintained at different temperatures in otherwise uniform and favourable conditions. With increasing temperature the time before a significant mortality begins gets longer and the death rate during the ensuing period becomes greater. At higher temperatures the larvae are more active and their food reserves are exhausted more rapidly. In the field, of course, temperature and humidity fluctuate and vary widely in different parts of the environment. In consequence, as the population declines, the rate of decline will decrease, and a very small number of larvae will persist for a very long time. There are therefore considerable technical difficulties in determining maximum longevity in the field. The question which is so frequently asked, how long larvae of this or that species survive on the pasture, is probably based on the false analogy of the three score years and ten that are the alloted span of human existence. The form of population curves on the pasture depends, as will be shown in the next section, on factors other than a natural life span.

IV. Herbage Infestations

Infestations on the herbage are measured to give an indication of the infectivity of the pasture. As the appetite of any class of grazing animal varies relatively little, it is rational and convenient to measure them as a concentration, a number of larvae per unit weight of herbage. It follows that herbage infestations are influenced by changes not only in the number of larvae but also in the quantity of herbage.

Grass growth will tend to decrease the herbage infestation whether the herbage is removed or not.

Conditions that favour herbage growth also tend to favour development and emergence from the faeces. Therefore the course of herbage infestation may very readily be seen as a dynamic process. The size of a population of larvae on the herbage (measured as a concentration) is determined by the rate at which larvae emerge from the faeces, on the one hand, and the rate of herbage growth and the rate at which larvae die on the other.

On this basis a picture may be built up of how seasonal patterns in the herbage infestation are caused. In Britain and much of northwestern Europe, temperature severely limits the development of most gastrointestinal nematodes of bovines. As temperatures rise gradually in spring and early summer, so the rate of development of free-living stages increases with the result that most of the eggs passed in April, May, and June (and as will appear below, most eggs are passed in May and June) reach the infective stage over a very much shorter period in early July. If conditions are sufficiently moist, many larvae now emerge onto the herbage with a resulting sharp increase in the herbage infestation. Thereafter the emergence of larvae from the faecal reservoir and their dilution by herbage growth tend to remain roughly in balance, whether or not the reservoir is replenished by further contamination of the pasture. In the second half of the grazing season, conditions become increasingly unfavourable for the development of larvae and, in England at least, eggs reaching the pasture after the end of September have a very small chance indeed of completing their development. By the beginning of winter the faecal reservoir normally contains relatively few larvae and the rate of emergence is therefore reduced. But herbage growth has also virtually ceased and therefore there is no reduction in the herbage infestation. The final disintegration of the faeces during the winter and the release of the remaining larvae are not balanced by herbage growth and commonly the infestation rises to its highest level. In spring, the faecal reservoir being exhausted, and the herbage beginning to grow, the herbage infestation rapidly declines, the process being speeded by the death of aged larvae as temperature rise.

This seasonal pattern of events may be used as a standard with which others may be compared. In very wet summers herbage infestations will initially be very high but because of early depletion of the reservoir, levels will tend to be low in autumn and winter. In very dry summers there will be little or no release of larvae which will persist and even accumulate in the reservoir. When wet weather returns in the autumn, virtually all the larvae that have developed throughout the season will emerge and very high herbage infestations result. There will be a tendency, therefore, for this to be reflected in correspondingly higher levels in spring. Cold winters with prolonged snow cover retard the disintegration of faeces and the release of larvae. Therefore, if the faeces still contained appreciable numbers of larvae in the autumn, these may be released in spring and large infestations may persist for longer than normal.

The seasonal pattern of infestations on the herbage of larvae of the gastrointestinal nematodes of sheep is broadly similar to that described above, differences being due to the smaller size of the faecal aggregate and consequently more rapid emergence of larvae. Thus, the midsummer increase in the infestation tends to be

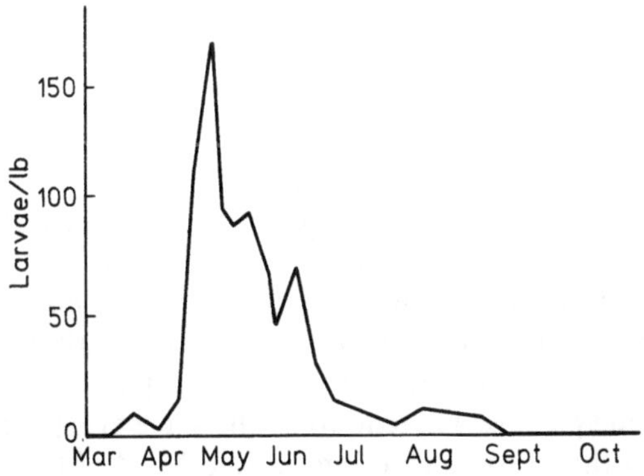

Fig. 17. Seasonal pattern of infestation on pasture herbage of *Nematodirus battus* larvae. THOMAS and STEVENS (1956)

earlier than for cattle worms, and because the capacity of the reservoir is less, infestations decline more rapidly. This is seen most clearly in infestations of *Nematodirus battus* larvae. Here there is no reservoir effect, the faeces having long since disintegrated when the eggs hatch. In consequence, as shown in Fig. 17, the infestation rises rapidly to a peak and as rapidly declines. In contrast infestations of *Nematodirus* species which hatch in autumn follow much the same course as infestations of trichostrongylids of other genera.

If the summer is long and very dry so that in mid-summer the faeces dry out too quickly for development of the larvae to be completed, the infestation that appears on the herbage in autumn when wet weather returns will be derived partly from eggs passed in spring or early summer and partly from eggs passed in autumn.

Where winters are long and the growing season short and cool, development may not be completed until the autumn and little emergence of larvae from the faeces may occur until the following spring.

It will be evident from this brief account of some factors influencing the course of herbage infestations that such questions as "how long does free-living development take?" or "how long do infective larvae survive on the pasture?" are without meaning unless the context is precisely defined.

In Britain it is possible to say that herbage infestations of most trichostrongylid nematodes other than *N. battus* and *N. filicollis* may be assumed to have fallen by the end of April to a level at which the growth of susceptible hosts will not be affected. By the middle of June they will have fallen to a level at which worm-free animals grazing the pasture will not become a sufficient source of contamination, in their turn to build up a potentially dangerous infestation. When the last larva disappears from the pasture, a question that is meaningful only in a discussion of the eradication of nematodes, demands an arbitrarily defined end point related to the probability of the introduction of infection from outside.

Arbitrarily defined degrees of cleanliness of pastures are an important ingredient in the design of control measures and are discussed below.

D. Epidemiology of Gastrointestinal Nematode Infections

I. Cattle

Perhaps the simplest system, and certainly the first to be studied comprehensively, is ostertagiasis and cooperiasis in hand-reared calves in Britain and northwest Europe. If such calves are turned out in late April onto a pasture similarly grazed in the previous year, they will encounter an overwintered infestation which is by this time small and decreasing rapidly. Their growth will not be affected but they will contaminate the pasture. Unless the overwintered herbage infestation is very small, their egg output will follow the stereotyped pattern so that the resulting contamination of the pasture will tend to be the same every year and will not depend on the size of the overwintered infestation. Most of the eggs passed by the calves will be put out in late May, June, and early July and for reasons already discussed the herbage infestation will rise steeply in July or later. In Britain this increase occurs typically between mid-July and early August but if the summer is abnormally dry it may be delayed until the autumn. The level reached by the herbage infestation as a result of what has come to be called the "mid-season rise" is variable and influenced by the weather, but commonly it is sufficient to retard the growth of the calves; not infrequently it is the cause of clinical disease and can be fatal. The herbage infestation tends to remain at a high level until the following spring whether or not the pasture is contaminated in the second half of the grazing season; contamination of the pasture at this time is far less effective in creating an infestation on the herbage than is contamination in the first half. Further, even though the worm burdens of the calves are often large in late summer and autumn, this is not necessarily reflected in greater faecal egg output, although a proportion of clinically affected calves may show high counts.

Ostertagia and *Cooperia* in cattle in Britain therefore behave as annuals. Little more than one generation is completed each year. Eggs that are the progeny of the new generation of worms do indeed make some contribution to the overwintering herbage infestation, which may not, however, be very great. The results of an observation on this point by PACENOWSKY et al. (1971) in Holland suggests that half the overwintered infestation is of the second generation.

The resistance of the calves to the establishment of worms increases gradually through the grazing season, but in the autumn they are still receptive to new infection. If they continue to graze on infested pasture, a proportion of the worms established will be arrested in their development. While worms that develop normally have a short mean life so that their number is directly related to the rate at which new infection is acquired, arrested worms accumulate in the host and their number depends not only on the rate of infection but also on the length of time for which it continues. A moderate herbage infestation, if cattle are exposed to it for a long time, can result in large burdens of arrested worms. It is a common finding that the number of arrested *Ostertagia* present in members of a group of outwintered cattle is extremely variable but the reasons for this are obscure.

There is some development of arrested worms through the winter with the result that numbers of adult and developing worms tend to remain constant while the number of arrested worms shows a linear decrease. In weak or debilitated animals a large number of arrested worms may develop during the winter to cause disease but, more commonly, it is not until the spring that a large proportion of the worms develops over a shorter or longer space of time. If many arrested worms remain and they develop over a short time, acute ostertagiasis occurs. The term "ostertagias type II" is often used for outbreaks of this kind, but the objection is sometimes raised that this implies that type II disease differs from type I in something other than the circumstances in which a large burden of developing and adult worms arises. Moreover, the related term "pre-type II ostertagiasis" is objectionable because it implies that the presence of large burdens of arrested worms in the winter inevitably means that type II disease will occur in the spring. Indeed the idea has taken hold that an animal which is carrying large numbers of arrested *Ostertagia* is in fact suffering from type II ostertagiasis. The rather older term "winter ostertagiasis" also has defects, not so much because outbreaks occur in spring (a shift of season is not uncommon in agricultural terminology in Britain, where an autumn-born calf may be born in summer and a spring-born calf in winter) but because in regions where *Ostertagia* is arrested during the summer, disease due to the resumed development of arrested forms occurs in the autumn.

In Britain, while ostertagiasis occurring in summer and autumn usually affects almost every animal in the group, winter ostertagiasis is often confined to a relatively small proportion. This must be related to the observation, already referred to, that there is very great variation in burdens of arrested worms among animals grazing together.

In its second grazing year, the young beast is only a very moderate source of pasture contamination. Even if many arrested worms develop in the spring, egg counts are not high and the adult worms do not persist for very long. Further, cattle in their 2nd grazing year are not very susceptible to the establishment of new infection. These two factors together mean that this age group is not usually at risk. Nor indeed is it likely either to give rise to herbage infestations that are directly harmful to calves or to be damaged themselves if they graze pasture that has been contaminated by calves.

In Britain it is unusual for cattle at the end of their 2nd year to acquire large numbers of arrested worms, but though rare, it is not impossible and very occasionally incidents diagnosed as due to ostertagiasis occur in spring calving heifers. In Australia such incidents are not uncommon in recently calved beef cows.

Reference has been made to the effect of the weather on the course of herbage infestations. Clearly both these and the management of the animals will affect the pattern outlined above. Thus if the calves are turned out very early in the spring they may encounter the overwintering infestation when this is still at a high level and clinical disease may result. The hazard of this is greater if the preceding summer was very dry and the overwintered infestation may remain at a dangerous level later than normal after a hard winter. Parasitic gastroenteritis in summer will be more severe and will tend to occur early if the early summer was very wet. In a very dry summer, outbreaks will not occur until the autumn and will then be very severe. The longer the cattle are kept out after the beginning of October on pasture that they have contaminated during the summer, the greater will be the hazard of winter (or type II) ostertagiasis in the following spring. The hazard is further increased after very dry summers.

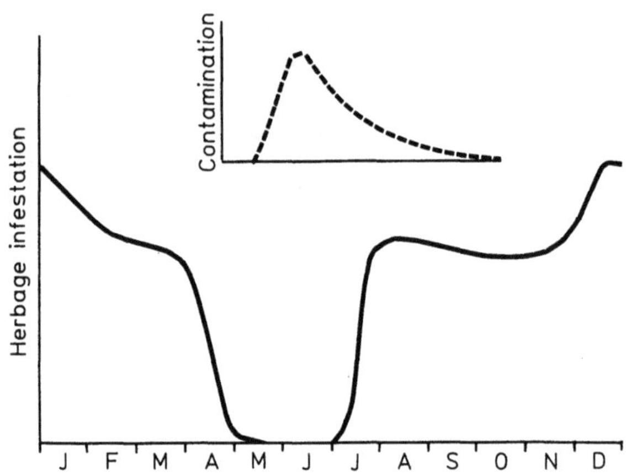

Fig. 18. The seasonal pattern of infestation on the herbage of larvae of *O. ostertagi* and *C. oncophora* on a pasture grazed every year by calves. Egg output by the calves is also shown

The picture presented above and illustrated in Fig. 18 of the epidemiology of ostertagiasis and cooperiasis in hand-reared calves in Britain is commonly used as the standard in relation to which patterns seen with other systems and in other regions are discussed. For example, the new generation of *N. helvetianus* appears on the pasture in Britain rather later than *Ostertagia* and *Cooperia*, i.e. in August rather than in July, and by the time it does, the calves are no longer susceptible to reinfection. Therefore clinical nematodiriasis is likely to occur in calves only where these are turned out exceptionally early and encounter a large overwintered infestation or where spring-born calves are turned out late in the season on pasture contaminated earlier by autumn-born calves.

In northern Europe and presumably also in Siberia and northern Canada, it is the overwintered infestation that is the cause of disease. There is only one generation. The calves are turned out at the end of May or in June, become heavily infected and contaminate the pasture mainly in July and August. The original overwintered infestation declines during the summer. The new generation of larvae does not appear on the herbage to any significant extent before the end of the grazing season. Arrested development does not appear to play an important part.

The beef herd in Britain presents a slightly more complex picture than that for the hand-reared calf, the pattern depending largely on the time of year that the calves are born. The cows are resistant to infection and pass very few worm eggs. Although a periparturient rise does occur it is of very modest proportions and transient. Meanwhile, the egg output of the calves follows the normal stereotyped pattern. Because the cows pass several times as much faeces as the calves, the mean worm egg content of all the faeces passed is low and consequently herbage infestations also tend to remain low.

At this point a brief discussion is appropriate of the related topics of mixed grazing and density of stocking in relation of the hazard of helminth infection. These subjects are often the cause of difficulty. It is generally asserted that a high stocking rate inevitably leads to greater worm burdens in the stock. Indeed, TAY-

LOR (1930) argued that infection rates must vary as the square of the stocking density. Closer examination of the question, however, shows that stocking density, as such, need not enter into the matter. In conditions of agriculture, as opposed to ranching, an increase in stocking rate implies an increase in herbage production and whether the herbage to feed a given number of animals is grown on a larger or small area is not, of itself, relevant. Indirect effects, of course, there will be. In particular at a higher stocking rate a greater proportion of the herbage will, as the season advances, be in close proximity to faeces, and the stock will be forced to graze less selectively.

Difficulties also arise over the effect of grazing helminthologically inert stock together with susceptible animals. It is often argued that because the resistant animals destroy the larvae that they ingest they tend to clean the pasture. In its extreme form, the so-called vacuum cleaner fallacy, this argument claims that an infested pasture can rapidly be rendered safe by grazing resistant stock on it. But the resistant stock do not lick the larvae off the herbage, nor do they selectively take the most heavily infested tufts of grass. In fact, the opposite is the case and the short-term effect of grazing an infected pasture with resistant stock is to render it more rather than less infective, and the long-term effect is negligible. The real effect of grazing inert and susceptible stock together occurs in the contamination phase. In effect, the animals grazing a pasture may be seen as converting a flow of herbage into a flow of faeces which, in turn, contaminates the flow of herbage. If, in the mixed stocking situation, only a proportion of the herbage processed is turned into infected faeces, then the resulting contamination of the pasture will be correspondingly reduced.

In Britain the suckler herd may calve at any time of year and the hazard of parasitic gastroenteritis in the calves depends on the date of calving. While cows and calves graze together, dangerous herbage infestations are not likely to arise, but if the calves are weaned in summer and graze together, they can create a dangerous herbage infestation. Therefore, the autumn-born calf which is weaned at this time is at risk, either being affected in autumn or, if outwintered, acquiring large burdens of arrested worms which can result in disease in the spring. The spring-born calf, on the other hand, which is not weaned until late autumn or winter, is not at risk. The herd calving in summer is of some interest for the calves are born after the overwintered pasture infestation has died out. Therefore it is only the very small periparturient rise in the egg output of the cows that carries on the infection from year to year.

II. Sheep

The epidemiology of gastrointestinal nematode infections in sheep is dominated by the postparturient rise in the ewe, which is a most important source of pasture contamination. The view of early workers, pre-eminent among whom was CROFTON (1958), was that the postparturient rise provided an initial infection which was then built up by the lambs through several generations. It is now accepted, however, that the eggs passed by the ewes in the course of the postparturient rise do not appear as larvae on the herbage until the end of June or later, and that this first new generation of larvae is the cause of disease in the lambs. If there is

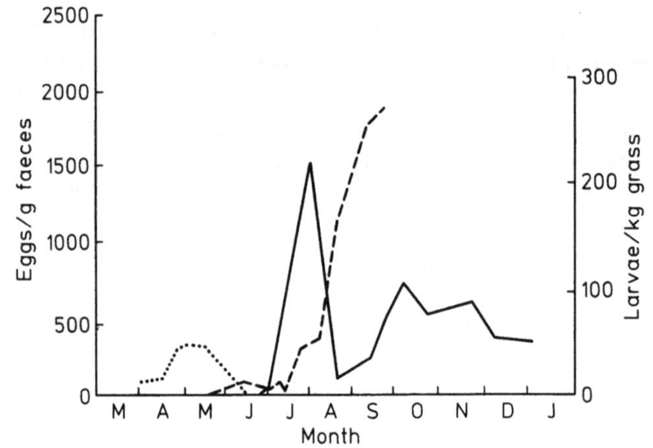

Fig. 19. The pattern of egg output by ewes and lambs and of herbage infestation on a pasture initially carrying no overwintered infestation. ········, ewe egg output; -----, lamb egg output; ———, pasture larval level. BOAG and THOMAS (1971)

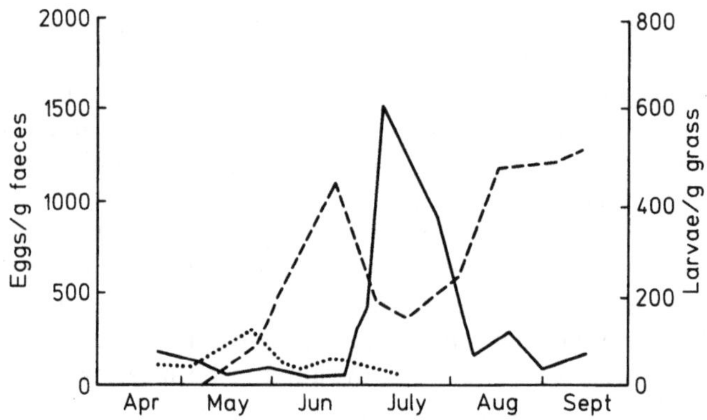

Fig. 20. The pattern of egg output by ewes and lambs and of herbage infestation on a pasture on which, initially, there was an overwintered infestation. ······, ewe egg output; -----, lamb egg output; ———, pasture larval level. THOMAS and BOAG (1972)

no overwintered infestation on the pasture, the eggs passed by the ewe are virtually the sole source of this dangerous infestation. If there is an overwintered infestation the lambs, becoming infected from it, will also make a contribution and infective larvae derived from eggs passed by ewes and by lambs will make their appearance on the herbage about the same time. Because of their importance, the classical graphs published by BOAG and THOMAS (1971)and THOMAS and BOAG (1972) are reproduced in Figs. 19 and 20. These relate to flocks in northeast England lambing in April. Figure 19 shows the sequence of events when ewes and their newborn lambs are put on a pasture carrying no overwintered infestation. The postparturient rise in egg output by the ewes produces a sharp rise in the herbage infestation which, in turn, gives rise to large worm burdens in the lambs. A second peak in the herbage infestation in autumn is thought to be due to eggs passed by the lambs and this seems probable, although it could be due to delayed emergence of larvae from the faeces of the ewes. It has been suggested that the lambs are the chief source of the overwintered infestation. What happens when there is an overwintered infestation on the herbage is shown in Fig. 20. Here the eggs put out by the ewes are still of great importance. The graph shows the number of eggs passed per unit weight of faeces and since the weight of faeces passed by the ewes is very much greater than that passed by young lambs, total contamination from the ewes is as great or greater than that due to the lambs. It will be noticed that the egg output of the lambs attributable to the worms picked up in July is not very great, and underestimates the worm burden. This is due to suppression or regulation of egg output.

A further difference between these situations must be appreciated. On pasture carrying no overwintered larvae, the postparturient rise is derived entirely from arrested worms that have developed. Where an overwintered infestation is present, it is derived both from such worms and from worms newly acquired from the pasture. When and in what circumstances burdens of arrested worms accumulate in the ewes has not been worked out in detail, although a series of observations by REID and ARMOUR (1975) in Scottish hill ewes suggests that they are picked up in October.

There have also been no detailed studies of the effect of the date of lambing. It is evident that the early lamb is likely to have been sold for slaughter before the end of June when the new generation of larvae is liable to appear on the herbage. On the other hand the early lamb, in so far as it grazes in early spring, could encounter an overwintered infestation but it is a subject of speculation whether this would be at a dangerous level.

The helminthological effects of late lambing are also the subject of complex speculation and until the necessary observations have been made comment is difficult. The overwintered infestation would have fallen to a low level and it is possible that the postparturient egg output of the ewes would be small. Hence, herbage infestations might not reach high levels.

The case of the autumn lambing flock has also not been adequately studied. CROFTON (1958) found that a postparturient rise occurred and it is more than likely that this was due to worms currently acquired. Since the lamb would be sold during the winter and the herbage infestation attributable to the postparturient rise would not persist beyond May, it is difficult to see how there could be a sufficiently elevated infestation when the ewes lamb again.

Clinical infections of *H. contortus* are now relatively rare in Britain, chiefly, it is assumed, because of its great susceptibility to commonly used anthelmintics, but it occurs occasionally in sheep of any age. The larvae do not survive readily through the winter on the pasture and, as shown by WALLER and THOMAS (1975) survival is almost entirely as arrested larvae in the ewe. These larvae develop in the spring (there appears to be no development during the winter) and contamination of the pasture by the ewe in the course of the postparturient rise leads to the appearance of a new herbage infestation in July. It is this infestation that may be the cause of disease. As early as August, however, a large proportion of the larvae ingested, whether by ewes or lambs, becomes arrested. It is not inevitable, however, that the pattern must be of this form. For example, CONNAN (1979, personal communication) observed that on one farm where very through anthelmintic treatment of ewes had been undertaken every winter for a number of years, *Haemonchus* was successfully overwintering on the pasture.

The essential features of the epidemiology of *N. battus* infections were worked out in the early fifties by workers in northeast England and in Scotland. Because lambs become resistant to reinfection quickly (age alone confers some resistance to the effects of infection), the infection is transmitted from one crop of lambs to the next and, because hatching is delayed until the spring, the first contact of the lambs is with a potentially dangerous infestation. Whether and when this infestation will reach a high level varies from year to year. Meanwhile, the lambs are at risk from the time they ingest significant quantities of grass until they are too old to be vulnerable, a period that will be rather longer for twins than for singletons, but is of the same order of magnitude as the variation in the date when the peak herbage infestation occurs. Therefore there is variation from year to year not only in whether outbreaks occur but also in which lambs, in relation to the date when they were born, are at risk.

Besides northwest Europe and New Zealand, it is only in Australia that the epidemiology of the nematode infections of grazing animals has been studied in any detail. The results are summarised in what is familiarly termed *The Golden Book* (DONALD et al. 1978), to which the reader is referred.

In northwest Europe, also in northern Europe and other areas having long winters and a short growing season, it is almost entirely temperature that determines seasonal patterns. The availability of moisture plays a significant part only in very dry years. In Australia both temperature and moisture play an important part. In winter rainfall areas *Ostertagia* predominates, in summer rainfall areas, *Haemonchus*. Each has its own epidemiological pattern wherever it occurs. The postparturient rise is an important source of contamination of the pasture with *Haemonchus*. Where the ewes lamb in early spring, this contamination occurs in the spring and results in the appearance of large numbers of infective larvae on the herbage about mid-summer, shortly after the lambs are weaned. The herbage infestation declines during the autumn but larvae ingested at this time accumulate as arrested larvae and are the chief source of the postparturient rise. The seasonal pattern for *Ostertagia* infections in winter rainfall areas is rather different. Pasture contamination due to the postparturient rise of spring lambing ewes raises the herbage infestation rather quickly and the lambs are already heavily infected by the time they are weaned in early summer. During the dry summer the herbage infestation falls to low levels. Contamination of the pasture by the lambs in late spring and early summer and again at the end of summer and in early autumn leads to a rise in the herbage infestation as soon as wet weather returns. It is larvae picked up from the pasture in late spring and early summer that become arrested.

III. Intraspecific Variation

The tendency, where the transmission of infection is prevented by arid conditions in summer, for nematodes to be arrested during this period, has already been discussed. An important feature is that species which are arrested in winter in one environment are arrested in summer in another. Recognition that the characteristics of nematodes are labile and change rapidly in response to new selection pressures is recent and its far-reaching consequences have not yet been thought through. This realisation was brought about by the cumulative influence of a number of findings, none of which alone would have attracted very great notice. DRUDGE et al. (1954) reported having found a population of *H. contortus* resistant to phenothiazine. CROFTON and WHITLOCK (1965) observed that eggs of this nematode from Bristol hatched at a significantly lower temperature than eggs from Ithaca in upstate New York. HOTSON (1967) found that Australian *O. ostertagi* although descended from British ancestors became arrested in spring instead of in winter, ARMOUR et al. (1967) noted with some surprise that worms of a culture of *O. ostertagi* that had been maintained in the laboratory for some years did not become arrested in response to cold-conditioning while a recent isolate did. It was soon realised how the so-called Weybridge strain had lost its aptitude for seasonally induced arrest. The worms had been passaged between twice and three times annually. This had meant that the larvae were stored at 4 °C for about 3 months before being administered to calves. Larvae were then cultured when egg counts were at a high level. Clearly, this had effectively selected against larvae that become arrested in response to cold-conditioning. Attempts to avoid similar changes in another isolate are of interest. Larvae were cold-conditioned before being administered to calves. When the faecal egg count had risen, the adult worms were removed by anthelmintic treatment and larvae were cultured when the egg count rose again. This procedure threatened to produce a strain remarkable for the promptitude with which arrested worms resumed their development. Accordingly, isolates were passaged as infrequently as possible but this had the effect of markedly increasing the longevity of the larvae. It is now widely recognised that experimental helminthologists cannot be sure that they are using material identical with that of colleagues in other laboratories, nor that their own material is not changing.

Similar changes can also occur in the field. MICHEL et al. (1972) observed that the progeny of worms that had overwintered as arrested larvae in the host had a greater aptitude for arrested development than the progeny of worms that had overwintered on the pasture. SMEAL (1977) made similar and more striking observations of the same kind. It follows that differences in animal management can exert a selection pressure and populations of worms on adjacent farms could have different characteristics.

Two important consequences flow from the fact that nematodes respond readily to selection pressures. The first is that worms of different species occurring in one environment will show a large measure of convergence. At one time, possibly because most helminthologists were taxonomists, it was believed that every species had its own fixed characteristics, its own epidemiology, and its own susceptibility to anthelmintics. It has become evident that this is only partly true. In any one environment, worms of different taxa tend to be similar; worms of the same species in different environments may be very different. Where populations of hosts and of their parasites have remained in the same environment for many years, it should be possible to deduce from climate, landscape and animal management how nematode infections work. Where animals are periodically introduced or where there is an active livestock trade between regions, the picture is clearly more complicated.

The second consequence is that control measures of any kind may be expected to have a finite period of usefulness. The use of anthelmintics obviously selects against worms susceptible to the anthelmintic and, depending on how vigorous is the selection, will sooner or later lead to the creation of resistant populations. Control procedures depending on an annual alternation of sheep and cattle on different blocks of pasture will, in time, lead to populations of reduced host specificity. Since host specificity of the gastrointestinal worms of sheep and cattle is not absolute and since selection in this situation is rather rigorous it is not impossible that such procedures may prove not to have a very long useful life. Control procedures that are based on seasonal patterns of herbage infestation may be expected, in time, to select worms having different reactions to temperature or able in some other way to give rise to herbage infestations at atypical times of year. It was for this reason that a report by BAIRDEN et al. (1978) attracted attention. These authors suggested that infective larvae of *O. ostertagi* can survive in the soil for long periods and appear on the herbage in quantity when not expected. As yet, this is an isolated observation which in no way invalidates the position that for the foreseeable future the control of gastrointestinal nematodes must be based on certain fixed points in their epidemiology. There should, however, be an awareness that all control procedures must exert their own selective pressures.

The renewed interest in efforts to select strains of sheep that are resistant to nematode infections may be seen in this context for it could be argued that, in time, maintaining flocks of such sheep separately may result in the selection of worms more successful in parasitising resistant sheep.

Hosts may avoid the effects of worm infection in two distinct ways. They may be inherently resistant, i.e. particularly efficient in recognising the presence of nematodes and mounting an immune response against them. Alternatively they may be inefficient in recognising the presence of the worms and, since an immune response is an important component of the pathological process, tolerant of infection. There are a number of well-documented cases in which a nematode parasites two different species of host of which one may be regarded as resistant and the other as tolerant. The first to be reported (WETZEL and ENIGK 1938) concerned *Dictyocaulus arnfieldi* in the horse and in the donkey. The reaction of the horse to infection with this parasite is fairly violent, relatively small infections result in clinical disease but they are short lived and pasture contamination is limited. In the donkey, even large infections do not produce symptoms of disease but the worms persist for a very long time and the pasture is heavily contaminated. In consequence, *D. arnfieldi* infection is not a major problem where the two species of host graze separately but very troublesome if they graze together (ENIGK and WEINGÄRTNER 1973). *Elaephora schneideri* provides another example (HIBLER et al. 1968). It is almost without pathogenicity to mule deer or to white-tailed deer, but highly pathogenic to the American elk. Severe disease is seen in elk only where its grazing overlaps with that of the deer.

A difference in response may also occur between different breeds of the same host species. For example, sheep of the Wiltshire Horn breed appear to be tolerant to lungworms and if grazed together with Clun Forest sheep, which are not, are the cause of lungworm disease in these. It is highly probable that within a single breed some individuals will be more resistant and some more tolerant and it may be that the severity of nematode infections may be aggravated by the fact that most flocks contain a mixture of them. It should be possible either to select inherently resistant sheep, on the basis of their immunological responsiveness, as practised by DINEEN and WINDON (1980), or to select tolerant sheep, by separating out those that are thrifty in spite of carrying large worm burdens. If these characters were intensified by selective breeding, sheep of both kinds should perform well if grazed alone, but the consequence of mixing them might be serious.

E. The Control of Gastrointestinal Nematode Infections of Sheep and Cattle

As was shown in an earlier section of this chapter, worm burdens above a tolerated level impair production and this, in some but not all circumstances, has adverse economic effects. In most cases, the presence of large worm burdens is the consequence of exposing susceptible animals to heavily infested grazing. The objective of control measures should therefore be to whithhold susceptible animals from such grazing.

I. Eradication

From time to time, discussion of the possibility of eradicating gastrointestinal nematodes becomes fashionable. To be eradicable, an infection must either be quickly recognised or, provided it spreads only slowly through the flock or herd, its presence must be reliably identified by means of some simple test, and it must not persist outside the host. Gastrointestinal nematodes do not satisfy these requirements. They can be present in a flock or herd for many years without their presence becoming clinically evident. Laboratory tests are notoriously incapable of demonstrating the absence of helminth infection, whole groups of animals are nearly always infected at once and a large part of the worm population may be outside the host at any one time. To these difficulties must be added the practical problem of preventing the introduction of infection from outside, which may occur on the wheels of vehicles, on the feet of animals or by the agency of paratenic hosts (JACOBS et al. 1971). Larvae may also be transported in running water or wrapped around the legs of psychodid flies (TOD et al. 1971). It is hardly surprising that SPEDDING (1969), after long experience of conducting grazing experiments under worm-free conditions, concluded that the nematode parasites of grazing animals could not be eradicated.

II. Suppressive Dosing

A point of view that is still not uncommon, especially among those who think of themselves as practical men, is that the epidemiology of helminth infections is too complex and unpredictable to be the basis for control measures and that farmers are incapable of conducting their grazing management to a prearranged plan.

Therefore, so it is argued, suppressive anthelmintic treatment is the only possible course. In Australia, JOHNSTONE et al. (1976) advocated regular 3-weekly treatment, a total of 17 doses per year, and were able to demonstrate that at the prices of anthelmintics, labour and sheepmeat then prevailing, this practice was marginally more profitable than giving no treatment at all. This is not to say that other means of control might not be economically much more advantageous. Dosing at 3-weekly intervals throughout the year does prevent the contamination of pasture almost entirely. While it achieves the objectives of control, it is an expensive way of doing so.

Less frequent treatment does not prevent, though it may reduce, pasture contamination. Its function is pre-emptive rather than suppressive and it may fail to give an adequate measure of control.

III. Monitoring and Forecasting

While many veterinary helminthologists now believe that an understanding of the epidemiology of gastrointestinal nematode infections can provide a basis for their control, there is a fundamental difference of opinion between those who think in terms of routine procedures of management and medication founded on a supposedly constant seasonal pattern of events and those who stress the effects of climatic variation and believe that farmers are unwilling to employ any procedure routinely. Advocates of the second view consider that control should depend on the timely publication of warnings, information and advice based on the techniques of forecasting, monitoring or both. Proposals for monitoring numbers of worm eggs in faeces samples as a means of determining when anthelmintic treatment should be given merit only brief mention. NEUMANN and KIRSCH (1968) operated a scheme of this kind in Schleswig-Holstein to advise when calves should be treated against *O. ostertagi* and *C. oncophora*. In view of the stereotyped pattern of egg output, this is likely to have resulted in the treatment of calves when their worm burdens were at a harmlessly low level and before they encountered any significant challenge. The proposal of ROSS and WOODLEY (1968) to use faecal egg counts to determine when lambs should be dosed against nematodiriasis can be criticised on the grounds that *Nematodirus* spp. exert a pathogenic effect before eggs appear in the faeces and that dangerous herbage infestations tend to arise very suddenly.

There has been considerable progress in recent years in the development of techniques for forecasting the likely incidence, the severity and the timing of outbreaks of a number of parasitic infections (review by GETTINBY and GARDINER 1981). The present discussion concerns not the accuracy of these forecasts but their use. For example, means are being developed for predicting the date in summer when the new generation of gastrointestinal nematode larvae appears on the herbage. The correct response when this is about to happen is to move susceptible animals to safe pasture. If this is to be possible, such alternative grazing must have been provided. If it is available, it must be grazed when it is ready. The grazing plan must make such a pasture available at the earliest date that it may be needed and the forecast therefore becomes largely irrelevant.

The same argument applies with less force to a forecast of those years in which the overwintered pasture infestation is likely to remain at a dangerous level longer than normal. Here it could be argued that farmers could readily react by turning the calves out later or onto a safer pasture. It could equally be argued, however, that if a less heavily infested pasture were available and its use a viable option, then it should be used routinely and as a matter of course. This is an extreme view, however. The safest pasture may be unsuitable for other reasons and its use might not be contemplated in the absence of compelling reasons.

In Britain a forecast of the likely severity and timing of outbreaks of nematodiriasis in lambs is issued annually. The most effective means of controlling this infection is by ensuring that young lambs do not graze pastures contaminated by lambs in the previous year. Where this is not possible, the forecast allows an adequate measure of control to be achieved by means of one, or at most two, anthelmintic treatments instead of the five that might otherwise be needed.

At present the basic assumption underlying the monitoring/forecasting approach is that the practices of farmers are immutable and take no account of the needs of helminth control. This is untrue. It is the position of a growing number of helminthologists, of whom the present writer is one, that the only viable policy in preventing economic losses from gastrointestinal nematode infections is to foster the routine use of systems of management and of anthelmintic medication that are based on fixed points in the epidemiological pattern. Forecasts derived from meteorological data can serve as a valuable adjunct to this approach and may have a wider role to play during a transitional period. What may be termed "scientifically guided opportunism" has no long-term future in helminth control.

IV. Control Strategies

The aim of withholding susceptible animals from excessively infested grazing may be achieved by the use of one of three basic strategies. To explain the operation of these, a brief consideration is first needed of what constitutes a clean pasture because the term is very loosely used. A distinction must be made between pastures that are safe in that they will not directly damage susceptible animals grazing on them, and pastures that are CLEAN and will not turn animals grazing on them into a source of contamination that could render pastures unsafe.

The account that follows relates to gastrointestinal nematodes under British conditions. Whether or not a pasture is safe at the beginning of the grazing season depends both on its grazing history in the previous year and on the date. Thus a pasture grazed by calves in the previous year will not be regarded as safe for calves until the last week in April, one grazed by yearling cattle in the previous year may be regarded as safe for calves a little earlier and a pasture grazed by cows in the previous year may safely be grazed by calves as early in the spring as desired. In the second half of the season, i.e. from 15 July onwards, safe pastures are those that were not grazed by young cattle in the first half of the grazing season. It is important to realise that, even if contaminated, a pasture that was safe at the beginning of the grazing season will remain safe until the middle of the season. In contrast, a pasture that was safe in the middle of the season, if then contaminated, may not remain safe for very long.

For lambs, a pasture grazed by lambs in the previous year is not safe until mid-June or, if the hazard of nematodiriasis can be disregarded, until late April. A pasture grazed only by dry adult sheep in the previous year can safely be grazed by lambs as early as desired. In the second half of the season, i.e. from the end of June onwards, safe pastures for lambs are those that were not grazed by lambs earlier in the same season. Normally these will be aftermaths, provided they were not grazed by ewes and lambs before being shut up.

CLEAN pasture for calves will, in the first half of the grazing season, be pasture not grazed by cattle of any kind in the previous year. In the second half, it will be pasture not grazed previously in the same year by cattle. But if a pasture that was CLEAN at the beginning of the season is then grazed only by hand-reared calves straight out of the buildings, it may be expected to remain safe for the rest of the season. For lambs, CLEAN pasture at the beginning of the season will be pasture not grazed by sheep of any kind in the previous year. In the second half of the season it will be pasture not grazed by sheep in the same year. But if a pasture that was CLEAN at the beginning of the grazing season is then grazed only by dosed ewes and their lambs, it may be regarded as safe for the rest of the season. In practice, CLEAN pastures at the beginning of the season will either be new leys after an arable crop or pastures grazed by another species in the previous year.

The three distinct strategies that may be used in the control of gastrointestinal nematodes are described, respectively, as preventive, evasive and diluting.

Preventive procedures aim to avoid the creation of a large herbage infestation quite simply by preventing the contamination of pasture. Commonly this implies putting uninfected animals only on a CLEAN pasture and excluding any other source of contamination such as potentially infected older animals or unprocessed dung or slurry. Where, as in the case of ewes and lambs, it is not possible to exclude older animals, these must be rendered virtually worm free by anthelmintic treatment. It is particularly in the context of a preventive control strategy that the postparturient rise and its suppression by anthelmintic treatment are of crucial importance. The anthelmintic used must be highly effective against both arrested and developing worms and the ewes must not be exposed to infection between being dosed and turned out onto the CLEAN pasture. The requirements of a preventive strategy are, in some respects, rather exacting; in others, they allow for greater freedom in management, permitting animals to be turned out sooner and lambs to be weaned later than might otherwise be prudent.

Evasive procedures make no effort to prevent the contamination of pasture but remove the animals before the contaminated pasture becomes infective. In practice this means that the animals are turned out on a safe pasture and moved in the middle of the season to another safe pasture, usually an aftermath. Either a second move is undertaken a month later or else anthelmintic treatment is given when the animals are moved in mid-season with the aim of preventing or reducing contamination of the aftermath. Evasive procedures are applicable to many enterprises but they impose some limitations. Early turning out may well not be possible, in difficult years hay aftermaths may not be available in time and the safe utilisation of the infective pasture in the second half of the season may pose difficulties. Moreover, in the case of sheep the lambs must, in practice, be weaned when they are moved to safe pasture, and for late lambs this may be earlier than desirable.

Diluting procedures depend on reducing pasture contamination by grazing helminthologically inert animals together with the susceptible animals. Reference has already been made to the application of this principle in the case of the single-suckled calf. Another example is the Ruakura system in which calves graze rotationally ahead of the dairy herd. In a more recent variant of this, the so-called leader-follower system of managing dairy followers, the calves graze ahead of an equal number of heifers. The dilution in this case is considerably less and the system is not successful in all circumstances.

The choice of an appropriate strategy for any particular enterprise and its successfull implementation demands design and advisory skills which are still imperfectly developed. Management techniques are involved as well as anthelmintic medication, and any change in management is likely to have repercussions throughout the enterprise. In any management decision, the needs of helminth control are only one consideration of many. What is proposed must make sense agriculturally and economically and take account of the farmer's objectives as well as of existing resources in capital, labour, skills and installations. Some enterprises afford great freedom of manoeuvre in the design of helminth control plans, many options being available. At the other extreme are cases in which some change is needed in the structure of the enterprise before rational control measures can be devised.

V. Dairy Followers

The control of gastrointestinal nematodes in dairy followers can often be undertaken by more than one strategy. Which is the most eligible depends on the size of the herd, whether the followers are kept on the same holding as the milking cows and how much of the land can only be grazed by dry stock.

In Britain, because of seasonal fluctuations in the price of milk, the aim in most dairy herds is to calve the cows in autumn. In self-contained herds therefore, the calves are born in autumn and must in their turn calve in autumn. Therefore they should calve when 24 or 36 months old. There are compelling economic reasons for choosing the 24 months option but this demands steady and rapid growth throughout the rearing period and helminth infections must be effectively controlled. In many herds the interval between calvings is greater than 365 days and therefore cows tend to calve later in the year as they grow older. The aim is therefore that the heifers should calve in August. As a rule, calves born before the end of November are managed to calve when 24 months old or less. Calves born after the end of November are either disposed of or, especially on larger farms, are reared to calve in August when 2½ years old or more.

If the followers are reared on the farm where the dairy herd is kept, an evasive strategy is usually the most suitable. The calves are turned out on any suitable pasture, preference being given to those not grazed by calves in the previous year. Where grass is conserved as hay, the calves are moved to aftermath grazing in mid-July (i.e. just before the new generation of larvae appears on the herbage). If they are to remain on the same aftermath until the end of the grazing season, they are given anthelmintic treatment when they are moved to reduce or postpone contamination of the aftermath. Alternatively, a second move should be undertaken in the middle of August. Because of the seasonal pattern of herbage growth over much of Britain, the area of pasture required during the first half of the grazing season is substantially smaller than that needed in the second half. The pasture contaminated during the first half of the season will of course remain potentially dangerous to calves for the rest of the season and beyond; and the calves must not return to it. It can, however, become part of the grazing area of either heifers or cows and in some cases it can be conserved. It is common, at the end of their first grazing season, to keep heifers that are to calve in autumn at pasture until Christmas so that a bull may conveniently be run with them. Clearly this introduces the risk that they will acquire large burdens of arrested worms and therefore the pasture to be used for this purpose must be carefully chosen.

Because of the high capital cost involved, few dairy farmers are equipped to make both hay and silage. On farms where grass is conserved as silage, the first aftermaths are ready in June. Further aftermaths, after two cuts of silage, are available at the end of July or in August. The most convenient procedure is to move the calves to a first-cut aftermath and then to a second-cut aftermath, the pasture that they vacate being conserved. On some intensively managed farms, three cuts of silage are taken and this permits the use of a preventive strategy for it is possible to turn out the calves onto a pasture not grazed at all in the previous year. In this case the grazing area is enlarged, as the season goes on, by the addition of aftermaths and no anthelmintic medication should be needed.

If the rearing of dairy followers is undertaken on a separate holding, then the choice of strategy depends on what area of grass is conserved. On intensively managed rearing units, the leader-follower system is attractive. The calves graze rotationally just ahead of the heifers and are therefore provided with ample unsoiled herbage. The presence of the heifers which pass relatively few worm eggs dilutes pasture contamination and the fact that the calves can graze selectively also assists in reducing the numbers of larvae that they pick up. The system is successful for autumn-born calves but tends to fail when used for spring-born calves. This is due partly to the greater age of the autumn-born animals in their first grazing season and, more importantly, to the fact that while in the case of the autumn-born animals the grazing pressure is reduced in the second half of the season as the heifers join the dairy herd, in the spring-born situation the grazing pressure increases throughout the season.

Helminth control in the leader-follower system can be improved by suppressing the egg output of the calves while the overwintered herbage infestation is declining. Two treatments are given, respectively 3 and 6 weeks after turnout. Meanwhile, contamination due to the second-year animals is not great and does not in any case affect the herbage infestation until the second half of the grazing season.

The size of the herd may influence the procedures used. Very large milking herds must graze all the pasture within walking distance of the milking parlour; therefore conservation is almost entirely outside this radius and few aftermaths are grazed by the cows. They can be grazed by the followers and evasive procedures can very easily be used. In smaller herds, aftermaths are not infrequently reserved for the milking herd. Here an evasive procedure may nonetheless be used, the calves being moved in mid-season to pastures previously grazed by the cows.

On many dairy farms a parcel of pasture which, by virtue of its situation, is unsuitable for the dairy herd and which, because of its configuration, must be grazed, is used for the followers. If it is not too big, it should be reserved for heifers in their second grazing year and the calves kept nearer home. If it is large enough to satisfy the requirements of both calves and heifers and if no part of it can be mown, then consideration might be given to moving the calves in mid-July to pasture previously grazed by heifers while incorporating the pasture that they have vacated in the grazing area of the heifers.

Clearly, where there is a second enterprise, where arable crops are grown, or where sheep are kept, the opportunities for devising control plans are greatly increased as both can provide CLEAN pasture and permit the use of a preventive strategy.

VI. Beef

The single-suckled calf presents few problems. In general, it is only the autumn-born calf that is at risk, and this only after it is weaned. The calves are usually weaned onto an aftermath and should be given anthelmintic treatment when they are moved. Alternatively they may be moved a second time after a month. Often, a second aftermath is not available but pasture previously grazed by cows or by cows and calves together may be used until the beginning of October.

Semi-intensive beef production on permanent pasture using calves from the dairy herd can pose serious helminth control problems. Autumn-born calves are preferred and these have only one season at grass, being finished in their second winter when 18 months old. On permanent pasture an evasive strategy cannot readily be employed. The cattle require three times the area of pasture in the second half of the grazing season as in the first. Therefore they graze one-third of the pasture in the first half of the season while the remaining two-thirds are conserved.

In the second half of the season, the entire area is grazed. This arrangement provides enough conserved forage for the two winters. The problem is how, during the second half of the season, to utilise the pasture that the calves contaminated during the first half and to which they must not return. Grazing one-quarter of the whole area while three-quarters are conserved and then grazing the aftermaths while the quarter that was grazed in the first half of the season is conserved, is rarely a viable option because it produces an excess of hay or silage.

The problem is a little less acute where the cattle are less intensively fed during their second winter and are finished after 3 months of a second grazing season. In this situation, an evasive procedure can be used. In the second half of the grazing season, the calves graze partly on aftermaths and partly on pastures previously grazed by the 2nd-year animals. Meanwhile the pasture that was grazed by calves in the first half of the season is conserved.

Spring-born calves can be finished off grass in their second grazing season only if they grow rapidly during their 1st year. An evasive strategy can be used, the calves being moved to aftermaths while the pasture that they grazed in the first half of the season is added to the area grazed by the 2nd-year animals.

Clearly, where they can be used, preventive procedures are more appropriate to semi-intensive beef production. On arable farms it is not uncommon to grow 1-year leys as a break between white-strawed crops and to graze these with semi-intensively managed beef cattle. Three-year leys may be used with equal advantage. In this case, the new ley should be grazed in the first half of the season while the 2nd- and 3rd-year grass is conserved. In the second half of the season 1st-, 2nd-, and 3rd-year grasss is grazed. The only precaution that must be observed is that if the new ley is grazed by cattle in the autumn of the year in which it was sown, these cattle should be given anthelmintic treatment before they are put on. A preventive strategy may be employed on permanent pasture by the integration of sheep and cattle grazing. This will be discussed further, below.

VII. Sheep

The principal problem in the design of grazing plans for the control of gastronintestinal nematodes in fat lamb production is that little conservation is needed, one-third of the total area being considered sufficient. Moreover, since most flockmasters make hay rather than silage, aftermaths are not commonly available by the beginning of July when, for the purposes of an evasive strategy, they would be required. The need to control nematodiriasis is a further complicating factor.

Increasingly, early lambs, i.e. those born from December to February, are housed, in many cases until they are sold. Early lambs that are reared on pasture are likely to be at risk from *Nematodirus* and from the overwintered infestation of other trichostrongylids. Since the lambs will have been disposed of before the new generation of larvae appears on the herbage, no danger need be apprehended from this source and there are no adequate grounds for attempting to suppress the postparturient egg output of the ewes. On permanent pasture it is not possible to design entirely satisfactory procedures for the early lamb. One-third of the pasture will have been conserved in the previous year and grazed by dry ewes thereafter. From this pasture, *Nematodirus* larvae will virtually be absent and the overwintering infestation of other trichostrongylids will be very small. Accordingly, this pasture should be reserved for ewes with twins.

Integration with some other enterprise is essential if effective worm control is to be possible for the entire flock. Where 3-year leys are used, the following is the most satisfactory plan.

Stubble	Dosed ewes
Year 1	Ewes and twin lambs; subsequently ewes
Year 2	Conservation; aftermath grazed by dosed lambs
Year 3	Ewes and single lambs

By the time lambs born after the beginning of March graze to a significant extent, the overwintered infestation of trichostrongylids other than *Nematodirus* is not likely to be at a dangerous level. There is, however, a danger that a large infestation of *N. battus* will appear. If management is good, a significant proportion of the lambs will have been sold fat before July. Those that remain are likely to encounter the new generation of larvae of "other trichostrongylids." Where silage rather than hay is made, an evasive strategy can be employed. Aftermath grazing should be ready at this time and its area, usually one-third of the total, should be sufficient to finish the remaining lambs. In practice, moving the lambs means weaning them and for lambs born near the end of April implies weaning at 9 weeks. If an evasive procedure of this kind is used, the control of nematodiriasis must depend on pre-emptive anthelmintic treatment. The use of five doses, as envisaged by GIBSON (1963), is not regarded as practicable, but in Britain the Ministry of Agriculture, Fisheries and Food issues an annual forecast of the expected severity of nematodiriasis and indicates when anthelmintic treatment should be given.

Special measures against nematodiriasis are not needed if a preventive strategy is employed. Where the flock is kept on a predominantly arable farm and 1-year leys are grown as a break crop, this can readily be arranged. The ewes are given anthelmintic treatment after lambing but just before being turned out on the new ley in order to suppress the postparturient rise. No further change of pasture or anthelmintic medication is needed. Where the ley is sown under spring corn, it normally provides some grazing in the stubble and it is common practice to use this to flush the ewes. Where this is done it is of course necessary to dose the ewes before they are put on. The present tendency is for the area of spring corn to decrease and for leys to be sown direct after winter corn. It is less likely, therefore that the leys are grazed that autumn.

Two-year leys are also less commonly grown. Three-year leys do not furnish sufficient clean pasture to permit the design of a preventive procedure for the flock lambing in March or April. A hybrid system can, however, be devised. Ewes with twins are dosed and turned out on the 1st-year ley. Their lambs need not be dosed and can be weaned whenever is considered desirable. The 2nd-year ley is conserved. Ewes with singletons are put on the 3rd-year ley. They need not be dosed. The single lambs are weaned at the beginning of July and moved to the aftermath. They are dosed when moved in order to limit the infestation of both *Nematodirus* and other trichostrongylids in the following spring.

VIII. Integration of Sheep and Cattle Grazing

Where both sheep and cattle are kept on the same farm, advantage can be taken of the fact that gastrointestinal nematodes of the two hosts do not overlap to an important degree. In Britain, *Trichostrongylus axei, Cooperia oncophora* and *Ostertagia leptospicularis* do indeed parasitise sheep and cattle with almost equal success and a number of species including *Haemonchus contortus, Nematodirus battus, N. spathiger, N. filicollis,* and *N. helvetianus* are not entirely species specific. For practical purposes, however, this does not appear to be of great importance.

At one time it was suggested that mixed grazing of sheep and cattle was an advantageous way of exploiting the presence of the two host species for the purpose of helminth control, but the extent of the dilution achieved is not sufficient. For many years the annual alternation of sheep and cattle grazing has been advocated by a number of writers but it is only relatively recently that it has been taken up in practice. A system devised by J. Rutter in southeast Scotland (ANON 1974) takes the form of a three-course rotation of pasture use, namely, cattle-sheep-conservation, the changeover taking place when the ewes have lambed. They are then dosed and moved to the clean pasture. Lambs and calves graze on the aftermath. This system, in which the cattle are usually represented by an autumn-calving suckler herd, has been shown to result in rapid growth of lambs running at unprecedentedly high stocking rates. It does, however, suffer from one or two limitations. It can be operated only where there are equal numbers of sheep and cattle livestock units and where all the pasture can be mown. Moreover, the system is designed expressly to cater for the needs of the lambs. The cattle do not start on clean pasture. Each year they graze where calves grazed in the second half of the previous grazing season. This means that unless they are given anthelmintic treatment when they are weaned, they will contaminate the aftermath and could create a dangerous infestation on it.

According to a more flexible and more commonly used system, the pastures are divided into two blocks, cattle and sheep alternating between them annually. Conservation is taken from both blocks. This means that calves do not graze pasture that was contaminated as an aftermath in the previous year so that the system can be used for cattle enterprises more intensive and more profitable than the suckler herd. It can also be used where not all the pasture can be mown and where there are unequal numbers of livestock units of the two species, a greater or smaller proportion of one block or the other being taken for conservation. This system is finding increasing acceptance in northern England and southern Scotland and since set stocking is the rule, it can be introduced gradually onto a farm, only two fields and a small proportion of the stock being involved in the first instance. The chief difficulty is a practical one. To avoid mis-mothering, especially when trough food is given, shepherds like ewes and lambs to run in small groups for the first 3 or 4 weeks after lambing. For this reason and because grass is short at this time, sheep tend to graze every pasture on the farm in the month after lambing. Therefore, half the ewes, when in early lactation and therefore susceptible, are exposed to the overwintered pasture infestation and, unless dosed, which they very rarely are, when moved back to the pastures reserved for sheep could create a damaging infestation there.

This outline of the control of gastrointestinal nematodes of sheep and cattle in Britain has sought to show how intimately agricultural and helminthological factors are associated. This owes much to the fact that on British lowland farms every phase of production is tightly controlled. The pastures, the animals, the very landscape are all man-made.

In contrast, Australian thinking on helminth control has been conditioned by a background in which, generally speaking, the opportunities for the detailed control of grazing are small. Traditionally, therefore, regular routine anthelmintic treatment has been the rule and most thought has been devoted to putting the timing of anthelmintic treatments on a more rational basis. GORDON (1948) introduced the idea that it should be adjusted to take account of seasonal fluctuations in worm burdens. He distinguished between "strategic" treatments, which were given routinely, and "tactical" treatments, which were given in response to some meteorological event. It has been suggested, however, that in its practical application this approach differed little from the six or seven evenly spaced routine doses that were commonly given each year.

Newer epidemiological knowledge led to attempts to exploit the fact that in winter rainfall areas the infectivity of pastures is low in summer and that it is chiefly pasture contamination at the beginning and end of the dry season that is the source of the herbage infestations that arise when wet weather returns. ANDERSON (1972, 1973) therefore advocated two "critical" anthelmintic treatments given at the beginning and end of the dry season, and demonstrated that they were as effective as a considerably greater number of routine doses. A similar approach has been used in other parts of Australia.

Particularly in summer rainfall areas, there has been considerable interest in simple systems of grazing management. BARGER and SOUTHCOTT (1975, 1978) have investigated alternate grazing either annually or 6-monthly by sheep and cattle and there has been interest in alternately grazing ewes and lambs and adult wethers (DASH et al. 1975).

F. Conclusions

An attempt has been made in this chapter to show what constitutes a working knowledge of the epidemiology of a single group of helminth infections in a single climatic zone. This picture has been built up through successive levels of complexity. At the lowest level were the basic components, the reaction of the host to infection and the biological properties of the free-living stages. How these basic phenomena affected the course of worm burdens in the host and infestations on the pasture, respectively, constituted the next level. At the third level, infestations on the pasture and worm burdens in the host were put together in a consideration of the relationships between worm burden and pasture contamination, between pasture contamination and infestations on the herbage and between infestations on the herbage and worm burdens. At the fourth level of complexity, the effect of operations of husbandry was taken into account and control measures considered.

In Britain it has taken a quarter of a century and the efforts of a number of major laboratories to reach the present position but much remains to be done before existing knowledge can effectively be put to use. The underlying problem, the great diversity of livestock enterprises, appears in particularly acute form in Britain and efforts are under way to create a capability of formulating advice for the individual enterprise.

A working knowledge of the epidemiology and control of the important nematode parasites of sheep and cattle exists in very few countries. The question arises, if this is to be rectified, how extensive a research effort would be needed and of what kind it should be.

If, as was formerly believed, all species of nematodes had their own fixed characteristics, then it would be possible from a knowledge of climate and animal husbandry to predict what species were of importance in any particular area and what form seasonal patterns would take. But, as has been shown, the relevant characteristics of any given species of nematode are far from constant. It has therefore been urged that it is a relatively easy matter, in any area, to work out the bold outlines of epidemiology by the direct and simple observation of reality.

As a minimum, worm burdens, pasture contamination and herbage infestations would be monitored. A class of barefoot helminthologists would be needed.

It is tempting to speculate, however, whether, by considering the selection pressures acting on the worms, it might not be possible to deduce from climate, landscape and animal management what the characteristics of indigenous helminth populations might be and whether it might not therefore be possible, after all, to work out epidemiology by dead reckoning. In situations that had not been disturbed for some centuries, this might well be possible but over large parts of North and South America and in Australasia, exotic breeds of livestock have been introduced, and their parasites with them, and there have subsequently been frequent or even regular movements of livestock from one area to another. Nematode populations may, in these circumstances, be in a state of transition and their characteristics largely unpredictable. The conclusion is inescapable that observational work is essential although its planning and interpretation will be assisted if due regard is paid to the selection pressures likely to be operating.

There is an entirely deplorable tendency, in many countries, to devote scarce resources to laboratory experiments either of a simple but irrelevant kind or, worse still, of a more esoteric and supposedly prestigious order. The distinction between "fundamental" and "applied" science is an artificial one. Work may be classified according to its relevance to practical problems but there is no connection between this and its complexity or difficulty.

That so-called fundamental science and its practitioners are excessively esteemed, while work relevant to practical problems and those involved in it are seriously undervalued, is an important reason why it is still not possible to write a coherent account of the epidemiology of any group of helminth infections except, perhaps, that which is the main subject of this chapter.

References

Allonby EW, Urquhart GM (1973) Self-cure of *Haemonchus contortus* infections under field conditions. Parasitology 66:43–53

Anderson N (1972) Trichostrongylid infections of sheep in a winter rainfall region. I. Epizootiological studies in the Western District of Victoria. 1966–1967. Aust J Agricult Res 23:1113–1128

Anderson N (1973) Trichostrongylid infections of sheep in a winter rainfall region. II. Epizootiological studies in the Western District of Victoria. 1967–1968. Aust J Agricult Res 24:599

Anderson N, Armour J, Jennings FW, Ritchie DS (1966) In: Corradetti A (ed) Clinical bovine ostertagiasis. Proceedings of the first international congress of parasitology, Rome 1964, vol 2. Pergamon, Rome

Anon (1974) Worms in sheep. Publication No 2. The Scottish Agricultural College

Armour J (1970) Bovine ostertagiasis: a review. Vet Rec 86:184–190

Armour J (1980) The epidemiology of helminth disease in farm animals. Vet Parasitol 6:7–466

Armour J, Bruce RG (1974) Inhibited development in *Ostertagia ostertagi* infections – a diapause phenomenon in a nematode. Parasitology 69:161–174

Armour J, Jennings FW, Urquhart, GM (1967) The possible existence of two strains of *Ostertagia ostertagi*. Vet Rec 80:208

Bairden K, Parkins JJ, Armour J (1979) Bovine ostertagiasis: a changing epidemiological pattern? Vet Rec 105:33–35

Baker NF (1979) Economic impact and control of parasitism in dairy cattle. Bovine Practitioner 14:42–49

Barger IA, Southcott WH (1975) Control of nematode parasites by grazing management I. Decontamination of cattle pasture by grazing with sheep. Int J Parasitol 5:39–44

Barger IA, Southcott WH (1978) Parasitism and production in weaner sheep grazing alternatively with cattle. Aust J Exp Agric Anim Husbandry 18:340–346

Barth, EEE., Jarrett WFH, Urquhart GM (1965) Studies on the mechanism of the self-cure reaction in rats infected with *Nippostrongylus brasiliensis* Immunology 10:459–464

Blitz NM, Gibbs HC (1971) An observation on the maturation of arrested *Haemonchus contortus* larvae in sheep. Can J Comp Med 35:178–180

Boag B, Thomas RJ (1971) Epidemiological studies on gastro-intestinal nematode parasites of sheep. I. Infection patterns on clean and autumn contaminated pasture. Res Vet Sci 12:132–139

Brunsdon RV (1967) The spring-rise phenomenon: the relationship between the time of lambing and the commencement of the rise in faecal worm egg counts. NZ Vet J 15:35–40

Christie MG (1962) On the hatching of *Nematodirus battus*, with some remarks on *N. filicollis*. Parasitology 52:297–313

Connan RM (1967) Observations on the epidemiology of parasitic gastroenteritis due to *Oesophagostomum* spp. and *Hyostrongylus rubidus* in the pig. Vet Rec 80:424–429

Connan RM (1968) Studies on the worm populations in the alimentary tract of breeding ewes. J Helminthol 42:9–28

Crofton HD (1949) The ecology of immature phases of trichostrongyle nematodes III. Larval populations on hill pastures. Parasitology 39:274–280

Crofton HD (1954a) Nematode parasite populations in sheep on lowland farms. 1. Worm egg counts in ewes. Parasitology 44:465–477

Crofton HD (1954b) The vertical migration of infective larvae of strongyloid nematodes. J Helminthol 28:35–52

Crofton HD (1958) Nematode parasite populations in sheep on lowland farms. V. Further observations on the post-parturient rise and a discussion of its significance. Parasitology 48:243–250

Crofton HD (1963) Nematode parasite populations in sheep and on pasture. Technical Communication, vol 35. Commonwealth Bureau of Helminthology, St Albans

Crofton HD, Whitlock JK, Glazer RA (1965) Ecological and biological plasticity of sheep nematodes. II. Genetic and environmental plasticity in *Haemonchus contortus* (Rud. 1803) Cornell Veterinarian 55:251–258

Cvetkovic L, Gološin R, Kosanović M (1971) Seasonal fluctuations in the trichostrongylid worm egg counts in the faeces of unmated ewes and ewes which lambed in different months of the year. Acta Vet (Beograd) 21:77–88

Dash KM, Southcott WH, Le Jambre LF, Barger A (1975) Evaluation of management options in simulated whole farm systems for the control of helminth infections in sheep. CSIRO Division of Animal Health, Annual Report, pp 73–75

Dinaburg AG (1944) Development and survival under outdoor conditions of eggs and larvae of the common ruminant stomach worm, *Haemonchus contortus*. J Agric Res 69:421–433

Dineen JK (1963) Immunological aspects of parasitism. Nature (Lond) 197:471–472

Dineen JK, Windon RG (1980) The effect of site selection on the response of lambs to vaccination with irradiated *Trichonstrongylus colubriformis* larvae. Int J Parasitol 10:189–196

Donald AD, Dineen JK, Turner JH, Wagland BM (1964) The dynamics of the host-parasite relationship. 1. *Nematodirus spathiger* infection in sheep. Parasitology 54:527–544

Donald AD, Southcott WH, Dineen JK (eds) (1978) The epidemiology and control of gastrointestinal parasites of sheep in Australia. Commonwealth Scientific and Industrial Research Organisation, Australia

Donald AD, Waller PS, Dobson RJ (1980) Regulation of *Ostertagia* populations in ewes. Australian Society for Parasitology Meeting May 19–21, 1980. Australian Society for Parasitology, Adelaide, p 29

Drudge JH, Leland SE, Wyant ZN, Elam GW (1954) Observations on the effectiveness of phenothiazine in control of gastrointestinal nematodes of sheep. 67th Annual Report of the Director, Kentucky Agricultural Experiment Station, p 56
Dunsmore JD (1960) Retarded development of *Ostertagia* species in sheep. Nature (Lond) 186:986–987
Eingk K, Weingärtner E (1973) Zur Verbreitung und Behandlung der Dictyocaulose der Einhufer. Dtsch tierärztl Wochenschr 80:145–148
Fernando MA, Stockdale PHG, Ashton GE (1971) Factors contributing to the retardation of development of *Obeliscoides cuniculi* in rabbits. Parasitology 63:21–29
Gettinby G, Gardiner WP (1980) Disease incidence forecasts by means of climatic data. Int J Biometeorology 24 [2]:87–103
Gibbs HC (1964) Observations on an outbreak of clinical parasitism in ewes during the winter months. Can Vet J 5:8–11
Gibson TE (1953) The effect of repeated anthelmintic treatment with phenothiazine on the faecal egg counts of housed horses with some observations on the life cycle of *Trichonema* spp. in the horse. J Helminthol 27:29–40
Gibson TE (1963) The control of nematodiriasis by strategic anthelmintic medication. Res Vet Sci 4:480–490
Gibson TE, Everett G (1967) The ecology of the free-living stages of *Trichostrongylus colubriformis*. Parasitology 57:533–547
Gibson TE, Everett G (1977) The effect of different levels of larval intake on the output of eggs by *Ostertagia circumcinta* in lambs. Br Vet J 133:360–364
Gordon HMcL (1948) The epidemiology of parasitic diseases with special reference to studies with nematode parasites of sheep. Aust Vet J 24:17–45
Gordon HMcL (1964) Studies on resistance to *Trichostrongylus colubriformis* in sheep. Influence of a quantitative reduction in the ration. Aust Vet J 40:55–61
Hibler CPAD, Cock JL, Abdelbaki TZ (1968) Elaephorosis in deer and elk in Gila Forest, New Mexico. Bull Wildlife Dis Assoc 5:27–30
Hotson IK (1967) Ostertagiasis in cattle. Aust Vet J 43:383–387
Jacobs DE (1966) The periparturient egg-rise of the sow. Vet Rec 79:272–273
Jacobs DE, Dunn AM, Walker J (1971) Mechanisms for the dispersal of parasitic nematode larvae. 2. Rats as potential paratenic hosts for *Oesophagostomum* (Stongyloidea). J Helminthol 45:139–144
Jarrett EEE (1973) Reaginic antibodies and helminth infection. Vet Rec 93:480–483
Jarrett EEE, Jarett WFH, Urquhart GM (1968) Quantitative studies on the kinetics of establishment and expulsion of intestinal nematode populations in susceptible and immune hosts. *Nippostrongylus brasiliensis* in the rat. Parasitology 58:625–639
Johnstone IL, Bowen FL, Smart KE (1976) Production in merino weaners following anthelmintic therapy. N South Wales Vet Proc 12:31
Keith RK (1967) Studies on *Cooperia pectinata*. Vet Rec 81:209–210
Kelly JD (1973) Mechanisms of immunity to intestinal helminths. Aust Vet J 49:91–97
Krupp IM (1961) Effects of crowding and of superinfection on habitat selection and egg production in *Ancylostoma caninum*. J Parasitol 47:957–961
Larsh JE, Race GJ (1975) Allergic inflammation as a hypothesis for the expulsion of worms from tissues: a review. Exp Parasitol 37:251–266
Le Jambre LF, Whitlock JH (1968) Seasonal fluctuation in linguiform morphs of *Haemonchus contortus cayugensis*. J Parasitol 54:827–830
Levine ND, Andersen FL (1973) Development and survival of *Trichostrongylus colubriformis* on pasture. J Parasitol 59:147–165
Manton VJA, Peacock R, Poynter D, Silverman PH, Terry RJ (1962) The influence of age on naturally acquired resistance to *Haemonchus contortus* in lambs. Res Vet Sci 3:308–314
Martin WB, Thomas BAC, Urquhart GM (1957) Chronic diarrhoea in housed cattle due to atypical parasitic gastritis. Vet Rec 69:736–739
Michel JF (1952) Self-cure in infections of *Trichostrongylus retortaeformis* and its causation. Nature (Lond) 169:881

Michel JF (1953) Phenomenon of protection in infections of *Trichostrongylus retortaeformis*. Nature (Lond) 172:312
Michel JF (1970) Adult worms as a factor in the inhibition of development of *Ostertagia ostertagi*. Int J Parasitol 1:31–36
Michel JF (1971) Some reflections on the study of epidemiological problems in veterinary helminthology. In: Centraal Diergeneeskundig Instituut. Facts and reflections: a symposium. The Institute, Lelystad, pp 19–29
Michel JF (1974) Arrested development of nematodes and some related phenomena. Adv Parasitol 12:279–366
Michel JF, Hooshmand-Rad P (1978) Arrested development of nematodes in sheep in Southern Iran. Parasitology 77:XVIII
Michel JF, Lancaster MB, Hong C (1972) The inhibition of development; variation within a population of *Ostertagia ostertagi*. J Comp Pathol 83:351–356
Michel JF, Lancaster MB, Hong C (1975) Arrested development of *Ostertagia ostertagi* and *Cooperia oncophora*. The effect of temperature at the free-living third stage. J Comp Pathol 85:133–138
Michel JF, Lancaster MB, Hong C (1976a) Observations on the resumed development of arrested *Ostertagia ostertagi* in naturally infected yearling cattle. J Comp Pathol 86:73
Michel JF, Lancaster MB, Hong C (1976b) The resumed development of arrested *Ostertagia ostertagi* in experimentally infected calves. J Comp Pathol 86:615–619
Michel JF, Lancaster MB, Hong C (1979) The effect of age pregnancy and lactation on some reactions of cattle to infection with *Ostertagia ostertagi*. Parasitology 79:157–168
Morgan DO, Parnell IW, Rayski C (1950) Further observations on the seasonal variation in worm egg output in Scottish hill sheep. J Helminthol 24:101–122
Morgan DO, Parnell IW, Rayski C (1951) The seasonal variations in the worm burden of Scottish hill sheep. J Helminthol 25:177–212
Mulligan W, Urquhart M, Jennings FW, Neilson JTM (1965) Immunological studies on *Nippostrongylus brasilensis* infection in the rat: the "self-cure" phenomenon. Exp Parasitol 16:341–347
Neumann HJ, Kirsch H (1968) Großflächige Parasitenbekämpfung unter kontrollierten Bedingungen in Schleswig-Holstein. Tierärztl Umschau 23:565–571
Ogilvie BM, Jones VE (1971) *Nippostrongylus brasiliensis*: a review of immunity and the host parasite relationship in the rat. Exp Parasitol 29:138–177
Ogilvie BM, Jones VE (1973) Immunity in the parasitic relationship between helminths and hosts. Progr Allergy 17:93–144
Ogunsusi RA, Eysker M (1979) Inhibited development of trichostrongylids of sheep in Northern Nigeria. Res Vet Sci 26:108–110
O'Sullivan BM, Donald AD (1970) A field study of nematode parasite populations in the lactating ewe. Parasitology 61:301–315
Pacenowsky J, Kloosterman A, Antonisse HW (1971) Observations on the translation process of trichostrongylid nematodes. Netherlands J Agric Sci 19:114–122
Paver H, Parnell IW, Morgan DO (1955) Some factors influencing the seasonal variation in worm egg counts in Scottish hill sheep. J Comp Pathol 65:220–235
Ransom BH (1906) The life history of the twisted wire worm (*Haemonchus contortus*) of sheep and other ruminants. Preliminary report. Bureau of Animal Industry USDA No. 93, 7pp
Reid JFS, Armour J (1975) Seasonal variations in gastro-intestinal nematode populations of Scottish hill sheep. Res Vet Sci 18:307–313
Rogers WP (1961) The nature of parasition: the relationship of some metazoan parasites to their hosts. Academic, New York, pp 287
Rose JH, Michel JF (1957) Quantitative studies on the contamination of pasture herbage with husk worm larvae. J Comp Path 67:57–68
Ross JG, Woodley K (1968) Parasitic disease forecasts: experiences in Northern Ireland. Record of Agriculture Research, Ministry of Agriculture, Northern Ireland 17:23–29
Salisbury JR, Arundel JH (1970) The relationships between lactation and post-parturient rise in faecal nematode egg counts of ewes. Aust Vet J 46:267–271

Schad GA, Chowdhury AB, Dean CG, Kochar VK, Nawalinski TA, Thomas J, Tonascia JA (1973) Arrested development in human hookworm infections. An adapation to a seasonally unfavourable external environment. Science 180:502–504

Silverman PH, Campbell JA (1958) Studies on parasitic worms of sheep in Scotland. 1. Embryonic and larval development of *Haemonchus contortus* at constant conditions. Parasitology 49:23–37

Sinclair IJ (1970) The relationship between circulating antibodies and immunity to helminthic infections. Adv Parasitol 8:97–138

Smeal MG (1977) Studies on inhibited developments of nematode parasites in cattle. PhD Thesis, University of Sydney

Sollod AE (1967) The possible existence of two stains of *Ostertagia ostertagi*. Vet Rec 81:547–548

Spedding CRW (1969) The eradication of parasitic disease. Vet Rec 84:625

Spedding CRW, Brown TH (1957) A study of subclinical worm infestation in sheep. 1. The effect of level of infestation on the growth of the lamb. J Agric Sci 48:286–293

Stewart DF (1950) Studies in resistance of sheep to infestation with *Haemonchus contortus* and *Trichostrongylus* spp. and on the immunological reactions of sheep exposed to infestation. II. The antibody response to infestation with *H. contortus*. Aust J Agric Res 1:301–321

Stewart DF (1953) Studies in the resistance of sheep to infestation with *Haemonchus contortus* and *Trichostrongylus* spp. and on the immunlogical reactions of sheep exposed to infestation. V. The nature of the "self cure" phenomenon. Aust J Agric Res 4:100–117

Stewart DF, Gordon HMcL (1953) Studies on resistance of sheep to infestation with *Haemonchus contortus* and *Trichostrongylus* spp. and on the immunological reactions of sheep exposed to infestation. VI. The influence of age and nutrition on resistance to *Trichostrongylus colubriformis*. Aust J Agric Res 4:340–348

Stoll NR (1929) Studies with the strongyloid nematode *Haemonchus contortus*. I. Acquired resistance of hosts under natural reinfection conditions out of doors. Am J Hyg 10:384–418

Sykes AR (1978) The effect of sub clinical parasitism in sheep. Vet Rec 102:32–34

Taylor EL (1930) Some factors concerning the occurrence of disease due to strongyloid worms in grazing animals – verminous gastritis, hoose and equine strongylidosis. Vet Rec 10:602–605

Taylor EL (1935) Seasonal fluctuation in the number of eggs of trichostrongylid worms in the faeces of ewes. J Parasitol 21:175–179

Taylor EL (1943) The interaction of nutrition and parasitism with special reference to parasitic gastritis. Vet Rec 55:117–118

Taylor EL, Michel JF (1953) The parasitological and pathological significance of arrested development in nematodes. J Helminthol 27:199–205

Tetley JH (1941) The egg-laying function of a nematode as shown by study of *Nematodirus* eggs in utero. J Parasitol 27:481–491

Thomas RJ, Boag B (1972) Epidemiological studies on gastro-intestinal nematode parasites of sheep. Infection patterns on clean and summer contaminated pasture. Res Vet Sci 13:61–69

Thomas RJ, Stevens AJ (1956) Some observations on *Nematodirus* disease in Northumberland and Durham. Vet Rec 68:471–476

Tod ME, Jacobs DE, Dunn AM (1971) Mechanisms for the dispersal of parasitic nematode larvae. 1. Psychodid flies as transport hosts. J Helminthol 45:133–137

United States Department of Agriculture (1942) Keeping livestock healthy. Yearbook of Agriculture 1942. Government Printers Office, Washington, 14, 127 pp

Urquhart GM, Jarrett WFH, Jennings FW, McIntyre WM, Mulligan W (1966) Immunity to *Haemonchus contortus* infection. II. Relationship between age and successful vaccination with irradiated larvae. Am J Vet Res 27:1645–1648

Waller PJ, Thomas RJ (1975) Field studies on inhibition of *Haemonchus contortus* in sheep. Parasitology 71:285–291

Wetzel R, Enigk K (1938) Zur Biologie von *Dictyocaulus arnfieldi* dem Lungenwurm der Einhufer. II. Mitteilung. Arch Wissenschaftl Prakt Tierheilkd 73:106–114
White EG, Cushnie GH (1952) Nutrition and gastro-intestinal helminths in sheep on hill grazing: the effect of a dietary supplement on faecal worm egg counts, worm burden, body weight and wool production. Br J Nutr 6:376–386
Zavadovskii MM, Zviagintsev SN (1933) The seasonal fluctuations in the number of eggs of *Nematodirus* spp. in faeces. J Parasitol 19:269–279

CHAPTER 4

Pharmacology of Anthelmintics

H. VANDEN BOSSCHE

A. Introduction

As noted in the different chapters of this volume, most infections due to worms living in the gastrointestinal tract can now be cured by anthelmintics. In general these drugs can be divided into four classes: herbal preparations, inorganic and metallorganic compounds, "antibiotics," and synthetic organic compounds.

The chemotherapy of helminthiasis was reviewed comprehensively by DE CARNERI; CAVIER; and CAVIER and ERHARDT in CAVIER and HAWKING'S book *Chemotherapy of Helminthiasis* (1973). Properties of some herbal preparations of the natural anthelmintics and of metallorganic and inorganic compounds can be found in VANDEN BOSSCHE (1980a).

The present chapter gives a few data on the older anthelmintics and will be limited to the "antibiotics" avermectins and paromomycin, and to synthetic organic compounds. Information on arecoline, di-*n*-butyl tin dilaurate, bunamidine, and nitroscanate can be found in the chapter in this volume on the chemotherapy of tapeworm infections in animals (Chap. 13).

B. Albendazole

Albendazole is the generic name for methyl[5-(propylthio)-1-*H*-benzimidazol-2-yl]carbamate, a product synthesized at the Smith-Kline-Beckman Corporation. The chemical structures of albendazole and of two of its metabolites are shown in Fig. 1. It is almost insoluble in water and only slightly soluble in most organic solvents (THEODORIDES et al. 1976).

I. Pharmacokinetics

Ring-labeled [^{14}C]albendazole was administered to calves at a single oral dose of 20 mg/kg body weight. Peak plasma levels of 5.5 µg/ml albendazole and/or metabolites were achieved 15 h after the administration of the drug; 46% of the administered dose was recovered in the urine within 72 h. Total radioactivity in muscle and fat depleted to less than 0.1 ppm within 5 days. However, total radioactive residues in the liver and kidney remained 30 days after treatment at 0.4 and 0.3 ppm (DICUOLLO et al. 1977).

In sheep peak plasma levels of 3.7 µg/ml of albendazole and/or metabolites were found 15 h after the oral administration of 16 mg/kg; 51% of the admin-

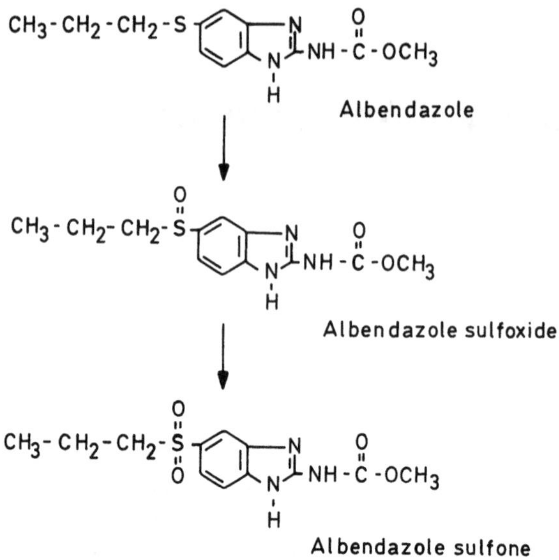

Fig. 1. Chemical structures of albendazole and its metabolites

istered dose was recovered in the urine within 120 h. Total radioactive residues in all tissues including liver and kidney decreased to below 0.1 ppm within a period of 10 days (DICUOLLO et al. 1977).

In these studies no distinction was made between the parent drug and metabolic products. More recently MARRINER and BOGAN (1980) described the pharmacokinetics of albendazole and its major metabolites (the sulfoxide and sulfone) in plasma, ruminal fluid, and abomasal fluid of sheep. Surprisingly, the concentrations of unchanged albendazole in plasma were at all times lower than 0.05 μg/ml even when albendazole was administered orally at a dose rate of 10 mg/kg.

Peak concentrations of 6.2 μg/ml albendazole were reached in the abomasal fluid within 8 h and persisted up to 16 h after drug administration.

Albendazole sulfoxide, the anthelmintic active metabolite, was detectable in plasma and in abomasal fluid at mean peak concentrations of 3.2 and 26.2 μg/ml 20 h after administration (MARRINER and BOGAN 1980). Both sulfoxide and sulfone were not detectable in ruminal fluid at detection limits of 0.3 and 0.05 μg/ml respectively. The results obtained by MARRINER and BOGAN (1980) demonstrate that albendazole is rapidly metabolized to the sulfoxide and sulfone. The authors suggest that the activity of albendazole against lungworm and liver fluke may be due to these metabolites.

The dissolved concentrations of albendazole in the rumen are small and persist for 3–4 days, indicating that, because of the relatively insoluble nature of albendazole, the rumen may serve as a "reservoir" of undissolved drug, which will lead to a markedly enhanced plasma bioavailability. MARRINER and BOGAN (1980) conclude that for improved activity in ruminant animals, the divided dose intervals should be at least 24 h and possibly 48 h. It is of interest to note that they mention a divided-dose regimen as a necessity for good activity in monogastric animals.

II. Toxicology

The oral LD_{50} in rats was about 2.4 g albendazole/kg body weight (THEODORIDES et al. 1976). No untoward effects were observed in sheep drenched with 26.5 and 37.5 mg albendazole/kg body weight (JOHNS and PHILIP 1977). In a reproductive safety study no abnormalities were found in any of the lambs born to ewes dosed with albendazole doses up to 15 mg/kg on days 21, 24, and 28 after service. Skeletal abnormalites were found in 3 of 44 lambs born to ewes dosed 17 days after service with 15 mg/kg and in 4 of 44 lambs born to ewes dosed with 11 mg/kg (JOHNS and PHILIP 1977).

III. Mode of Action

The mode of action of all benzimidazole carbamates seems to be identical to that of mebendazole and will therefore be dealt with in the section of mebendazole. In summary: benzimidazole carbamates cause degenerative changes in the intestinal and tegumental cells of helminths, an effect attributed to interaction with cytoplasmic microtubules. IRELAND et al. (1979) compared the sensitivity of mammalian brain microtubules to a range of benzimidazoles with their efficacy in vivo and found some correlation between the antimicrotubular activity and anthelmintic efficacy in mice infected with *Nematospiroides dubius* for albendazole.

Another possible biochemical mode of action of albendazole has been proposed by MCCRACKEN et al. (1982). They studied the effects of this and other benzimidazoles (thiabendazole, cambendazole, oxibendazole) on the electrical resistance of planar bimolecular lipid membranes and found that all compounds lowered membrane resistance at concentrations down to 0.1 μM and were better transmembrane proton conductors than 2,4-dinitrophenol. They conclude that the anthelmintic activity of these benzimidazoles is due to bioenergetic disruptions resulting from transmembrane proton discharge.

C. Amoscanate

Amoscanate, an anthelmintic from CIBA-GEIGY, with activity against intestinal nematodes, some filariae, and schistosomes, is an isothiocyanate compound. This 4-isothiocyanato-4′-nitro-diphenylamine (C9333-GO/CGP 4540), of which the chemical structure is shown in Fig. 2, is a yellow crystalline substance which is insoluble in water and most organic solvents (STRIEBEL 1976).

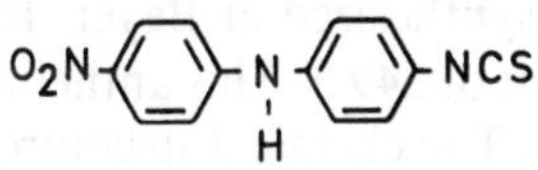

Fig. 2. Amoscanate

I. Pharmacokinetics

Pharmacokinetic studies in animals revealed poor absorption of the compound after oral administration. Preliminary human pharmacokinetic studies showed a total urinary excretion (72 h) of 1%–6%. Drug elimination via urine plus feces seems to be complete 48 h after oral drug administration (RAJAGOPALAN, results cited in VAKIL et al. 1977).

II. Toxicology

Amoscanate is well tolerated in acute toxicity tests; it has an extremely high margin of safety. The oral LD_{50} is certainly higher than 5 g/kg in rats, mice, dogs, cats, and rhesus monkeys. For this study the micronized form (median particle size, 4.23 μm; specific surface, 1.94 m^2/g) was used (STRIEBEL 1976).

The isothiocyanate derivative, of which the average particle size was approximately 0.5 μm, failed to exhibit any detectable mutagenic activity when tested in the absence or presence of liver microsome preparations with two *Salmonella* tester strains TA-98 and TA-100 (BUEDING et al. 1976). Following the oral administration of amoscanate to mice, one of several urinary metabolites was found to be mutagenic for *Salmonella* strain TA-100; none was mutagenic for strain TA-98. This mutagenic effect of amoscanate can be eliminated by the simultaneous oral administration of succinylsulfathiazole, suggesting a role of intestinal bacteria in the formation of a mutagenic compound from amoscanate (BUEDING et al. 1976).

III. Mode of Action

The mode of action of this isothiocyanate is not known. In an interesting study MIKO and CHANCE (1975) described isothiocyanate derivatives as potent uncouplers affecting the respiration of tumor cells and isolated mitochondria. These isothiocyanates are similar to known uncouplers (e.g., 2,4-dinitrophenol) in that they: stimulate respiration of state four mitochondria; stimulate mitochondrial ATPase activity; release the inhibition of mitochondrial respiration by oligomycin; and inhibit both mitochondrial respiration and mitochondrial ATPase activity at higher molar concentrations.

It should be of interest to study the effects of amoscanate on energy-forming systems.

D. Amidantel

Amidantel is the generic name for *N*-[4-[[(1-dimethylamino)ethylidene]amino] phenyl]-2 metoxyacetamide, synthesized at Bayer. It is a white crystalline compound with a molecular weight of 249.3. This anthelmintic is soluble in water and ethanol but insoluble in ether. The chemical structure is shown in Fig. 3 (THOMAS 1979; WOLLWEBER et al. 1979).

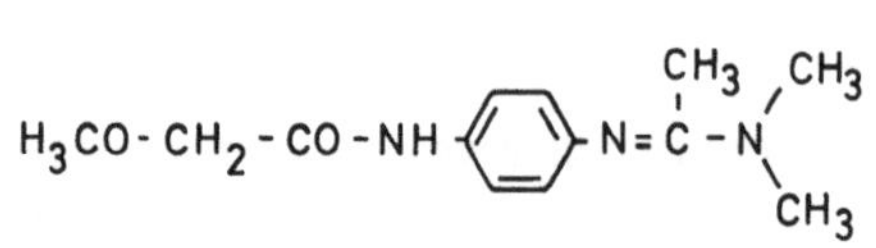

Fig. 3. Amidantel

Toxicology

Amidantel seems to be well tolerated. The LD_{50} values were assessed for several animal species (WOLLWEBER et al. 1979). For example, when the compound was given to mice p.o. or s.c., LD_{50} values of 1,207 and 569 mg/kg were found respectively. Oral treatment of other animals gave the following LD_{50} values (in mg/kg): rat, 4,693–5,968; rabbit, 500–1,000; cat, 750; and dog, 500–1,000.

Daily oral doses of 30 and 100 mg/kg for 28 days to dogs were tolerated without any or with only minor clinical symptoms such as salivation. Amidantel did not show teratogenic effects in rats treated orally with 300 mg/kg/day from the 6th to 15 th day of pregnancy (WOLLWEBER et al. 1979).

E. Avermectins

The avermectins are a family of closely related macrocyclic lactones produced by an actinomycete, *Streptomyces avermitilis* MA-4680 (NRRL8165), which was isolated at the Kitasato Institute, Japan, from a soil sample (BURG et al. 1979). There are eight major avermectins and their structures are shown in Fig. 4. The

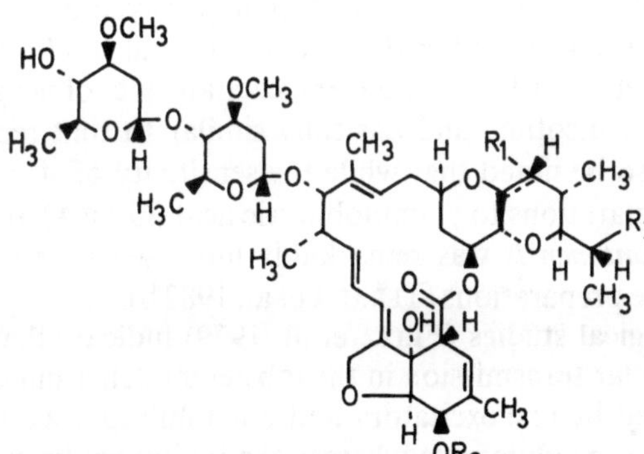

Avermectin nos.	R_1*	R_2	R_3
A_1a	—	C_2H_5	CH_3
A_1b	—	CH_3	CH_3
A_2a	OH	C_2H_5	CH_3
A_2b	OH	CH_3	CH_3
B_1a	—	C_2H_5	H
B_1b	—	CH_3	H
B_2a	OH	C_2H_5	H
B_2b	OH	CH_3	H

* Where R_1 is absent, ≕ is present

Fig. 4. Structures of major avermectins. BURG et al. (1979)

22,23-dihydroavermectin B_1 or ivermectin has been chosen for commercial development (Merck, Sharp, and Dohme). Ivermectin contains at least 80% 22,23-dihydroavermectin B_{1a} and not more than 20% 22,23-dihydroavermectin B_{1b} (MERCK 1981). Ivermectin is an α-L-oleandrosyl-α-L-oleandroside macrolytic lactone with broad-spectrum anthelmintic and insecticidal activity (EGERTON et al. 1979). The generic name of this new family of compounds was derived from the anthelmintic ("*a*nti-*verm*es") activity and from the activity against *ect*oparasites (CAMPBELL 1981). No grossly observable toxic reactions were noted in cattle, sheep, dogs, and chickens with the efficacious levels of this natural product (EGERTON et al. 1979).

For a survey article see CAMPBELL (1981).

Mode of Action

Avermectin B_{1a} quickly immobilizes parasitic nematodes at low doses, indicating an effect on the nematode nervous system. In fact, using an isotonic transducer, avermectin B_{1a} at concentration $\geqq 3.6 \times 10^{-18}$ *M* caused a sustained paralysis in *Angiostrongylus cantonensis* (SANO et al. 1981). The time required to cause complete paralysis varied from about 100 min at 3.6×10^{-18} *M* to about 10 min at 3.6×10^{-10} *M*. The concentration of avermectin paralyzing 50% of *Caenorhabditis elegans* in 30 min was $0.4–1.0 \times 10^{-6}$ *M* (PONG et al. 1980). It is of interest to note that TERADA et al. (1982a) found the excitatory cholinergic mechanism in *A. cantonensis* to be nicotinic and basically similar to that reported in *Ascaris suum*. It should also be noted that while the sensitivity of *A. cantonensis* and of *Ascaris* muscle preparations to γ-aminobutyric acid (GABA) and piperazine was not different, *A. cantonensis* was remarkably more sensitive to avermectin B_{1a} than *Ascaris* muscle preparations (TERADA et al. 1982b).

Neurophysiological studies (FRITZ et al. 1979) indicate that avermectin B_{1a} blocks neuromuscular transmission in the lobster stretcher muscle. The stretcher muscle is innervated by one excitatory and one inhibitory axon. The excitatory transmitter seems to be glutamate whereas the inhibitory transmitter is GABA. Studies by FRITZ et al. (1979) indicate that avermectin B_{1a} irreversibly blocks the inhibitory postsynaptic potentials and reduces the excitatory postsynaptic potentials in this muscle. These authors hypothesize that the reduction in excitatory postsynaptic potentials after avermectin B_{1a} treatment is caused solely by reduction in membrane resistance. The resistance change appears to be the result of increased Cl^- conductance and this action is reversed by picrotoxin, a well-known GABA antagonist. The authors argued that avermectin might either act as a GABA agonist or cause an increase in tonic GABA release from lobster nerve terminals.

Further studies on the mechanism of action of avermectin B_{1a} (PONG et al. 1980) revealed that this macrocyclic lactone causes a marked and sustained increase of GABA release from rat brain synaptosomes.

An action of avermectin on GABA neurons is further supported by binding experiments using radiolabeled drug (study cited by PONG and WANG 1980). Maximum level of binding to the synaptosomes of whole dog brain was estimated as 1.5 pmol [^{3}H]avermectin B_{1a}/mg protein. The specific binding sites were concentrated in the cerebellum, where GABA nerves are most abundant. The studies by PONG and WANG (1979, 1980) suggest that the binding sites are on the presynaptic end of GABA nerves. Interesting is that the EC_{50} value (effective concentration for 50% maximal stimulation) of avermectin B_{1a} for stimulating synaptosomal GABA release (2–3 μ*M*) and that for paralyzing the free-living *C. elegans* (0.4–1 μ*M*) are within the same order of magnitude (PONG et al. 1980). However, it is premature to conclude from these studies that the stimulation of GABA release may be the basis of the antiparasitic action of avermectin B_{1a}. Studies carried out by FRITZ et al. (1979) indicate that the GABA-induced relaxation of *Ascaris* muscle strips is not blocked by picrotoxin, suggesting that the GABA system in *Ascaris* is pharmacologically distinct from that in, e.g., lobster. The action of avermectin B_{1a} on *A. cantonensis* was also not antagonized by the treatment with picrotoxin (3×10^{-5} *M*) or by the activator of the acetylcholine release, *N*-methylcytisine (1.2×10^{-4} *M*). However, the combination of both compounds did antagonize the action of avermectin (SANO et al. 1981).

According to KASS et al. (1980), avermectin B_{1a} paralyzes nematodes without causing hypercontraction or flaccid paralysis. Using selective stimulation techniques they showed that this macrocyclic compound blocks transmission between interneuron(s) and excitatory motoneurons in the ventral nerve cord of *A. suum*. This disruption of the signaling between interneurons and motoneurons would lead to paralysis of the worm (KASS et al. 1980). It is of interest to note that avermectin B_{1a} immobilizes both the wild strain and a mutant of *C. elegans* (E 107e) which is resistant to levamisole. These data suggest that the mode of action of avermectin B_{1a} is not related to that of levamisole (KASS et al. 1980). As will be discussed later levamisole acts as a ganglion-stimulation compound, after which it induces a neuromuscular inhibition of the depolarizing type (VAN NUETEN 1972; COLES et al. 1975).

CAMPBELL (1981) summarizes the mode of action as follows: avermectins seem to stimulate the presynaptic release of GABA and enhance its binding to the postsynaptic receptors. The function of the inhibitory neurotransmitter, GABA, is to open the chloride channels on the postsynaptic side, allowing Cl^- ions to flow in and to induce the "resting" condition. In the presence of avermectins the chloride channels are open when they should be shut. Cl^- ions flow in even when Na^+ ions alone should be entering. The motorneuron remains negatively charged and so both inhibitory and excitatory signals are not registered by the recipient muscle cell. Thus the muscle cell does not function and the result will be paralysis.

The lower susceptibility of cestodes and trematodes to avermectins may be attributed to a lack of the GABA mechanism in those parasites (CAMPBELL 1981; TERADA et al. 1982c).

F. Bephenium Hydroxynaphthoate

Bephenium hydroxynaphthoate (Fig. 5) or benzyldimethyl(2-phenoxyethyl) ammonium 3-hydroxy-2 naphthoate is a light-yellow, bitter-tasting crystalline substance (Wellcome). It is weakly soluble in water (0.02%) and has a molecular weight of 427.

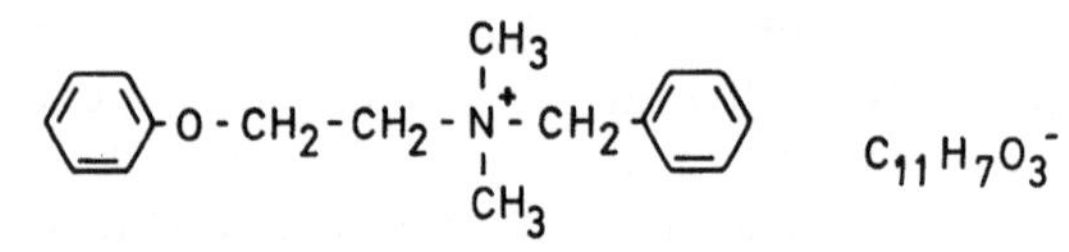

Fig. 5. Chemical structure of bephenium hydroxynaphthoate

I. Pharmacokinetics

The excretion in the urine of bephenium and its metabolites in man is low. In fact after the administration of 1 g bephenium base, given as hydroxynaphthoate, 0.52% of the dose was recovered in the urine collected in 24 h (ROGERS 1958).

II. Toxicology

The compound is normally well tolerated. The oral LD_{50} value in mice is 5–7 g/kg (CAVIER 1973). Monkeys given 300 mg/kg bephenium base, given as hydroxynaphthoate daily for 3 months, showed no histological abnormality (DAVIS 1973).

III. Mode of Action

Bephenium produces contraction of *Ascaridia galli* muscle preparations. This contraction can be blocked by piperazine and the bephenium-treated preparation fails to respond to acethylcholine even after repeated washings (KAUSHIK et al. 1974). This compound also produces a spastic paralysis of *A. suum* muscle that may be counteracted by adding *d*-tubocurarine and piperazine (BROOME 1962; DEL CASTILLO 1969).

Bephenium also lowers the histamine content of *A. suum* (PHILLIPS et al. 1976). This may be the result of a stimulated metabolism or of a decreased uptake of histamine rather than by an inhibition of its synthesis.

G. Bithionol

Bithionol or 2,2′-thiobis(4,6-dichlorophenol) is practically insoluble in water (0.0004%); it is soluble in acetone (15 g/100 ml), propylene glycol (0.5 g/100 ml), corn oil (1 g/100 ml), and ethanol (0.3 g/100 ml). Its chemical structure is given in Fig. 6.

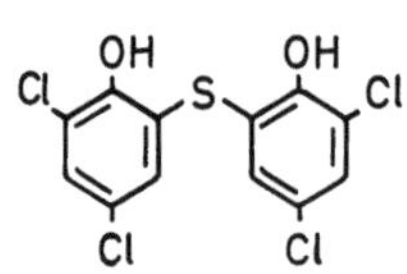

Fig. 6. Bithionol

I. Toxicology

After oral administration, the LD_{50} of bithionol in mice is 1.43 and in rats 5.77 g/kg. No side effects could be shown in studies on subacute toxicity in which mice and rats were treated with 70 mg bithionol/kg/day for 5–8 days (UENO et al. 1959, 1960).

II. Mode of Action

Many phenols and their derivatives are known uncouplers of oxidative phosphorylation. In worms bithionol has been shown to inhibit ATP synthesis (VANDEN BOSSCHE 1976a). HAMAJIMA (1973) carried out detailed studies on the action of bithionol on glycolytic and oxidative metabolism of the adult lung fluke, *Paragonimus westermani*. He suggested that the mode of action of bithionol may be due to the phenolic OH groups which act by interfering with glycolysis, the tricaboxylic acid cycle, and the oxidation-reduction system similar to the action of 2,6-dichlorophenol.

H. Bitoscanate

Bitoscanate or 1,4-diisothiocyanatobenzene (Hoechst) is a yellow-white crystalline powder. This phenylene 1,4-diisothiocyanate (Fig. 7) has a molecular weight of 192.2; it is almost insoluble in water but dissolves in methanol, ethanol, and chloroform.

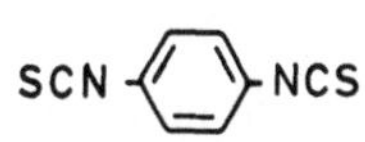

Fig. 7. Bitoscanate (phenylene-1,4-diisothiocyanate)

I. Pharmacokinetics

Bitoscanate is slowly resorbed. In dogs maximum serum concentration is reached only after 16–24 h. In dogs as well as in man, elimination from the blood proceeds very slowly. The half-value periods are respectively 26 and 12 days (DAVIS 1973).

II. Toxicology

The oral LD_{50} s for mice and rats are respectively 230 and 495 mg/kg body weight. Bitoscanate is not a carcinogen in mice nor a teratogen in mice and rabbits (DAVIS 1973).

I. Bromoxanide

Bromoxanide or *N*-[4-bromo-2-(trifluoromethyl)phenyl]-3-*tert*-butyl-2-hydroxy-6-methyl-5-nitrobenzamide (Fig. 8) is a salicylanilide active against *Fasciola hepatica* and *Haemonchus contortus* in sheep (THEODORIDES et al. 1974). A single oral dose of 20 mg/kg had no adverse effects; 30 mg/kg was found to be the maximum

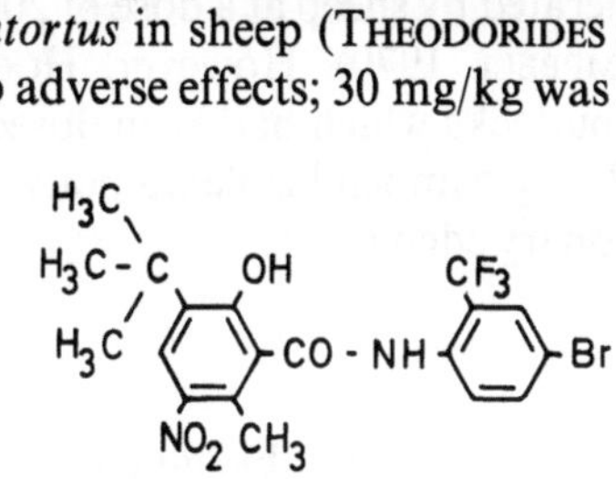

Fig. 8. Structural formula of bromoxanide

tolerated dose by sheep. Details of the mode of action of salicylanilides are given in the section on closantel.

J. Brotianide

The substituted anilide of thiosalicylic acid, brotianide (3,4′-dibromo-5-chlorothiosalicyl-anilide acetate ester), is an antifluke agent (ROSEBY and BORAY 1970) available in combination with thiophanate. Its molecular weight is 463.41. The chemical structure is given in Fig. 9 [information available in PROUS et al. (1982)].

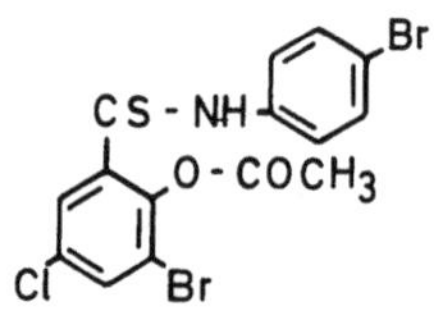

Fig. 9. Brotianide

K. Cambendazole

Cambendazole (Fig. 10) is the generic name for 2-(4-thiazolyl-5-isopropoxycarbonyl-aminobenzimidazole, a tiabendazole derivative from Merck, Sharp, and Dohme (HOFF et al. 1970; EGERTON and CAMPBELL 1970). It is a white crystalline solid with a molecular weight of 302.35. Cambendazole is soluble in alcohol, dimethylformamide, very slightly soluble in 0.1 *M* HCl, and practically insoluble in water (0.02 mg/ml).

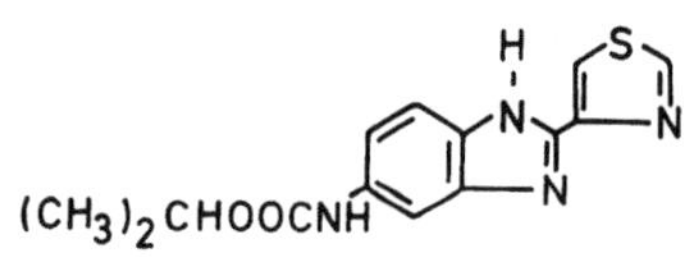

Fig. 10. Cambendazole

I. Pharmacokinetics

According to POUPLARD (1976) most of the cambendazole administered orally is absorbed in the intestinal tract. Residues have been found in milk and according to the same author this excludes the use of this benzimidazole derivative in dairy cows.

II. Toxicology

This anthelmintic is well tolerated by sheep at a dose of 200 mg/kg, but not at 300 mg/kg (EGERTON and CAMPBELL 1970). However, HOGG (1978) reported the death of two 7-month-old bullocks which had been dosed twice by the farmer at the recommended rate of 25 mg cambendazole/kg body weight. Gross postmortem features included pulmonary edema.

III. Mode of Action

Cambendazole inhibits aerobic and anaerobic glucose uptake and increases glycogen utilization in the anterior portion of *Moniezia expansa*. Anaerobically it reduces succinate production by inhibiting phosphoenolpyruvate carboxykinase and fumarate reductase. Cambendazole also increases lactate production. The benzimidazole derivative diminishes ATP synthesis in *Moniezia* within 30 min of incubation under both aerobic and anaerobic conditions, an effect also observed in *M. expansa* collected from sheep treated orally with 20 mg/kg and killed after 8 h (RAHMAN and BRYANT 1977; BRYANT et al. 1976).

It is interesting to note that cambendazole, like other benzimidazole derivatives, affects the polymerization of sheep (IRELAND et al. 1979) and bovine (FRIEDMAN and PLATZER 1980a) brain microtubules in vitro. Further details are given in the section on mebendazole.

L. Ciclobendazole

Ciclobendazole is the generic name for methyl-[5-(cyclopropylcarbonyl)-1*H*-benzimidazol-2yl]carbamate (Janssen Pharmaceutica). It is almost insoluble in water and most organic solvents (DEGREMONT and STAHEL 1978). The molecular weight of this mebendazole analogue is 259.26 (Fig. 11).

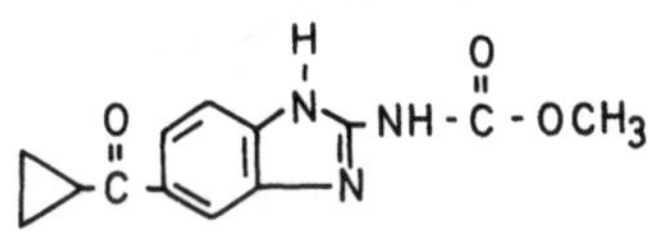

Fig. 11. Ciclobendazole

I. Pharmacokinetics

(BRODIE et al. 1977; DEGREMONT and STAHEL 1978)

After a single oral dose of 4 mg [^{14}C]ciclobendazole/kg body weight to rats most of the radioactivity was excreted during the first 48 h. In the first 24 h, 52% and 22% of the administered radioactivity was excreted in the feces and urine respectively. Experiments with biliary cannulated rats showed that 70%–80% of an oral dose of [^{14}C]ciclobendazole was eliminated in the bile. The radioactivity eliminated in urine and bile and retained in the carcass indicates that a mean of 91% of the administered dose was absorbed.

After an oral dose at a level of 4 mg/kg to rats, the peak mean plasma concentration of radioactivity (0.073% dose/ml) occurred at 15 min. Thereafter the concentration declined with a half-life of approximately 22 h. Plasma levels of radioactivity were low at all times after oral administration of [^{14}C]ciclobendazole (4 mg/kg) to dogs. The peak (0.0005% dose/ml) occurred at 30 min.

After a single oral dose of 4 mg [^{14}C]ciclobendazole/kg to dogs about 80% and 10% were excreted in the feces and urine within 48 h. Bile duct-cannulated dogs in the first 24 h excreted between 26% and 35% of an oral dose in the bile and 14.5% in the urine, 44.2% remaining in the tissues and gastrointestinal tract.

In man treated with ciclobendazole, 45% and 12% of the administered radioactivity was excreted during the first 48 h in the feces and urine respectively. During the 5 days posttreatment 72% of the dose was found in the feces and 14% in the urine.

II. Toxicology

The oral LD_{50} values found were: mice, 1.03 g/kg; rats, 2.46 g/kg; and rabbits, 183.3 mg/kg. In dogs treated with 1.2 g/kg, apart from anorexia no adverse reactions were observed.

Ciclobendazole administered to mice, rats, and rabbits produced no teratological effects (DEGREMONT and STAHEL 1978).

M. Closantel

Closantel or *N*-[5-chloro-4-[(4-chlorophenyl)cyanomethyl]-2-methylphenyl]-2-hydroxy-3,5-diiodobenzamide (Janssen Pharmaceutica) is a salicylanilide derivative. Its structure is shown in Fig. 12. It has a molecular weight of 663.08.

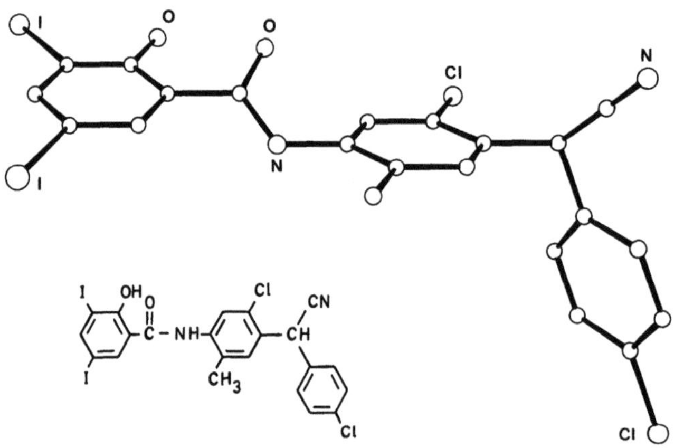

Fig. 12. Chemical structure of closantel and three-dimensional structure of closantel as derived by TOLLENAERE et al. (1979) from crystallographic data

I. Pharmacokinetics

Closantel was administered orally and intramuscularly to sheep at dose rates of 10 and 5 mg/kg respectively. Maximal plasma levels of nearly 55 µg/ml plasma were reached 8–24 h after dosing. Closantel was eliminated from the plasma with a half-life of about 15 days (MICHIELS et al. 1977a). Maximum concentrations of closantel in plasma were reached 24–48 h after subcutaneous or intramuscular injection of dairy cows at a dose of 5 mg/kg. Mean peak levels of 44 µg/ml and 29 µg/ml were found after subcutaneous and intramuscular administration (MICHIELS et al. 1978).

II. Toxicology

The acute toxicity of closantel (R 31 520) has been studied in mice and rats after oral and intramuscular administration. The LD_{50}s are given in Table 1.

Table 1. LD_{50}s of closantel in mice and rats (NIEMEGEERS 1976)

Species	Sex	Route of administration	LD_{50} (mg/kg)
Mice	♂	i.m.	56.8
	♀	i.m.	56.8
	♂	Oral	331.0
	♀	Oral	453.0
Rats	♂	i.m.	35.9
	♀	i.m.	28.4
	♂	Oral	342.0
	♀	Oral	262.0

III. Mode of Action

The salicylanilide derivative, closantel, affects in vitro the mitochondrial phosphorylation system in *Fasciola hepatica, Ascaris suum* muscle, and rat liver (VANDEN BOSSCHE et al. 1979; VANDEN BOSSCHE and VERHOEVEN 1982). In vivo *Ascaris* seems to be insensitive to closantel; however, in vitro 50% inhibition of the mitochondrial (muscle) malate-induced ^{32}Pi incorporation into ATP was obtained at 3×10^{-7} *M* closantel. In *Fasciola* mitochondria this inhibition was achieved at 2×10^{-6} *M*. The same concentration gives an almost equal inhibition of the ATP-^{32}Pi: exchange reaction. The mitochondrial ATPase of *Fasciola* is stimulated by 5×10^{-7} *M* and inhibited by higher concentrations; 50% inhibition is reached at 10^{-4} *M*. An increase in cytochemically demonstrable mitochondrial ATPase activity in several fluke tissues after host treatment was demonstrated by VERHEYEN et al. (1979).

Twelve hours after i.m. treatment of the sheep host with 5 mg closantel/kg body weight the ATP content of the liver flukes was decreased by more than 60% and the adenylate energy charge was 0.53 instead of the 0.84 found in liver flukes from control sheep (VANDEN BOSSCHE and VERHOEVEN 1982). KANE et al. (1980) also found a diminished ATP synthesis in fluke recovered from sheep drenched intraruminally with 5% w/v formulated closantel at 5 mg/kg body weight. A study of the ultrastructural changes in the liver fluke after intramuscular treatment of the sheep host with 5 mg/kg also revealed that the most common change after closantel administration concerned the mitochondria (VERHEYEN et al. 1980).

No effect on the oxidative phosphorylation was found in mitochondria isolated from livers of uninfected rats and from hearts of rats infected and uninfected with *Fasciola* 4 and 16 h after i.m. injection with 5 mg closantel/kg. Liver mitochondria from control rats infected with *Fasciola* were uncoupled (VANDEN BOSSCHE et al. 1980). Elimination of the parasites from the bile duct by closantel resulted in a normalization of the mitochondrial activity (VANDEN BOSSCHE and VERHOEVEN 1982).

In conclusion: all the experimental evidence obtained thus far indicates that closantel in vivo selectively disturbs phosphorylation in *Fasciola* mitochondria.

Studies are needed to evaluate the effect of closantel on blood-sucking nematodes, e.g., *H. contortus*.

N. Dichlorophen

Dichlorophen(e) (2,2′-methylenebis[4-chlorophenol]) is practically insoluble in water. One gram dissolves in 1 g 95% ethanol. Molecular weight is 269.12. The chemical structure is shown in Fig. 13.

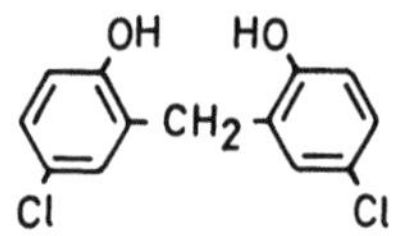

Fig. 13. Dichlorophene

I. Toxicology

The oral LD_{50} in rats is 2.63 g/kg; in mice it was found to be 1.2 g/kg.

II. Mode of Action

High concentrations of dichlorophen have been found to inhibit phosphorylation in *Ascaris* mitochondria; 48% inhibition was found at 5×10^{-5} *M* (SAZ 1972). Dichlorophen reduces the incorporation of ^{32}Pi into ATP by intact *Hymenolepis diminuta* in vitro and by isolated mitochondria from this rat tapeworm (SCHEIBEL et al. 1968). It can act as an uncoupler of electron-transport-linked phosphorylation in isolated mitochondria of *H. diminuta* (YORKE and TURTON 1974) and of rat liver (STRUFE and GÖNNERT 1967). The low toxicity of dichlorophen can be ascribed to the fact that little is absorbed from the gastrointestinal tract (BUEDING 1969).

O. Diphetarsone

The arsenic compound diphetarsone (Fig. 14) or [1,2-ethanediylbis(Imino-4,1-phenylene)]bis[arsenic acid]disodium salt (molecular weight, 504.1) has already been known for quite some time as a contact-amebicide (WHO 1974). In 1965 JUNOD described its activity against *Trichuris trichiura*.

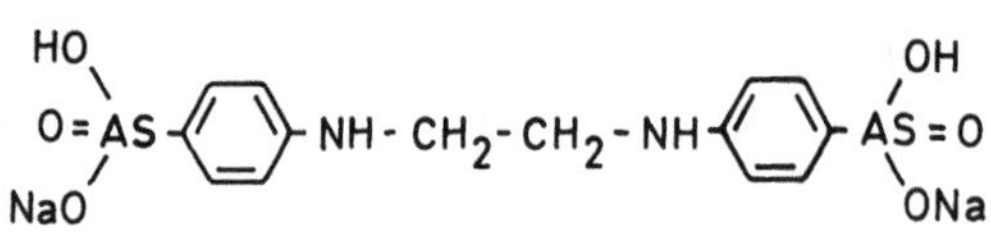

Fig. 14. Diphetarsone

The decahydrate (molecular weight: 684.1) is freely soluble in water and practically insoluble in acetone, chlorofrom, and absolute ethanol.

P. Disophenol

Disophenol or 2,6-diodo-4-nitrophenol (Fig. 15) is a drug used in veterinary medicine for the treatment of dogs infested with *Ancylostoma caninum, A. braziliense,* and *Uncinaria stenocephala.* Disophenol is very sparingly soluble in water; π (log partition coefficient between octanol and water of disophenol divided by that of phenol) = 2.88; $pK_a = 3.6$. It is freely soluble in alcohol. Its molecular weight is 390.9 (available as Ancylol, Iodophene, Syngamix).

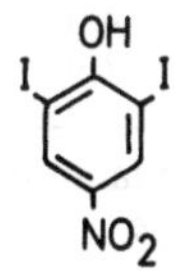

Fig. 15. Structural formula of disophenol

I. Toxicology

The pharmacology of disophenol in dogs is considered similar to that of the uncoupler of oxidative phosphorylation, 2,4-dinitrophenol (KAISER 1964). In fact qualitatively the two compounds produced similar toxicological signs in laboratory animals (mice, rats, dogs): increase in respiration, heart rate, and body temperature and an extremely quick rigor mortis. Quantitatively 2,4-dinitrophenol and 2,6-diodo-4-nitrophenol differed significantly. Although on a molecular weight basis the acute toxicity in mice and rats was nearly equal; following repeated administration disophenol appeared to be the more toxic compound. LD_{50} values for disophenol are 170 and 212 mg/kg when administered orally to rats and mice respectively (KAISER 1964).

Perfusion of isolated rat hearts with disophenol caused significant alterations in spontaneous heart rate, coronary flow, isometric systolic tension, metabolite levels, and electrical activity (ARONSON and SERLICK 1977). Phosphorylase *a* levels decreased significantly at 1,000 ng/ml. At the same dose, spontaneous heart rate, coronary flow, and isometric systolic tension were depressed. Diastolic tension increased more than threefold after 60 min of perfusion with 1,000 ng/ml. Disophenol at concentrations $\geqq 100$ ng/ml decreased tissue glycogen, ATP, total adenine nucleotides, and creatine phosphate levels whereas it increased lactate levels (ARONSON and SERLICK 1977).

CAMPBELL and MONTAGUE (1981) determined the safety indices for disophenol used in the treatment of both mature (12 weeks after infection) or immature (6 weeks after infection) liver flukes in Merino crossbred sheep and compared them with those obtained for other "uncouplers" (Table 2).

II. Mode of Action

The effects of disophenol observed in laboratory animals are reflections of its uncoupling properties. Disophenol is a potent uncoupler of rat liver mitochondria (TOLLENAERE et al. 1976; CAMPBELL and MONTAGUE 1981) and an inhibitor of mitochondrial phosphorylation in *Ascaris* mitochondria (VANDEN BOSSCHE 1972b;

Table 2. Safety index of "uncouplers"[a] (CAMPBELL and MONTAGUE 1981)

Compound[b]	Safety index	
	Mature *F. hepatica*	Immature *F. hepatica*
Disophenol	2.7	1.2
Hexachlorophene	2.0	1.5
Oxyclozanide	4.0	1.5
Rafoxanide	8.9	3.0

[a] Safety index = maximum tolerated dose/therapeutic dose
[b] Oxyclozanide: 3,3′,5,5′,6-pentachloro-2′-hydroxysalicylanilide; rafoxanide: 3′-chloro-4′-(*p*-chlorophenoxy)-3,5-diiodosalicylanilide

TOLLENAERE et al. 1976). For example, maximal stimulation of the mitochondrial ATPase from rat liver is obtained at 9×10^{-7} *M* and 50% inhibition of the malate-induced phosphorylation in *Ascaris* muscle mitochondria is obtained at 5×10^{-6} *M*.

PRICHARD (1973) showed that at higher doses (1.5×10^{-4} *M*) disophenol also inhibits the fumarate reductase system in both tiabendazole-susceptible and -tolerant strains of *Haemonchus contortus*.

It is surprising that many of the available anthelmintics are uncouplers of oxidative phosphorylation in mammalian mitochondria and inhibitors of mitochondrial phosphorylation in helminths. Some examples are given in Table 2; others are bithionol, bromophenophos, desaspidin, dichlorophen, niclofolan, niclosamide, and resorantel (VANDEN BOSSCHE 1976a).

Q. Febantel

Febantel (Fig. 16) is the generic name of dimethyl {[2-(2-methoxy-acetamido)-4-phenyl-thiophenyl]imido-carbonyl} dicarbamate (Bayer). It is a white crystalline solid which is only slightly soluble in most organic solvents and has a molecular weight of 446.48 (CASTAÑER 1978; WOLLWEBER et al. 1978).

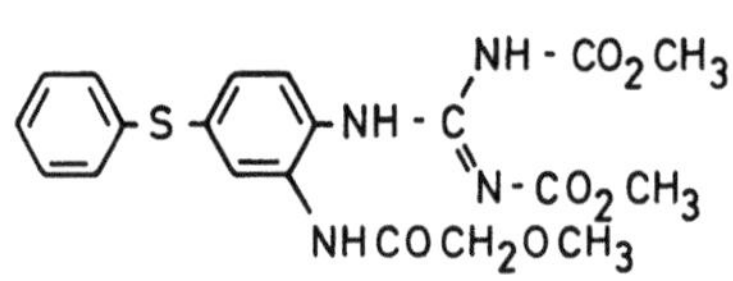

Fig. 16. Febantel

I. Pharmacokinetics

Febantel is absorbed from the intestinal tract, metabolized in the liver, and eliminated – up to 70% – by the bile at a half-life of 9 h in rats (DÜWEL et al. 1981). Febantel is quickly metabolized to fenbendazole (ŠPALDONOVA 1981).

II. Toxicology (WOLLWEBER et al. 1978)

In acute toxicity studies febantel was well tolerated. The oral LD_{50}s in g/kg were: >10, 10.6, 1.25, and >10 for mouse, rat, rabbit, and dog respectively. In sheep, 200 mg/kg was well tolerated.

III. Mode of Action (ZINTZ and FRANK 1982)

The effects of febantel on *Heterakis spumosa* were investigated by means of electron microscopy. Mice infected with *H. spumosa* were treated with 200 mg/kg febantel and the mice were killed 6, 12, 18, 24, 28, 36, 48, or 72 h later. Changes were only seen in the intestinal cells. Microtubules disappeared and the number and size of autophagic vacuoles increased. Seventy-two hours after treatment the parasites isolated from the gut showed only sluggish movements and they were rolled up like small springs. The authors suggest that febantel may have some neurotoxic effects and these may help to expel the damaged worms by the intestinal peristalsis of the host.

R. Fenbendazole

Fenbendazole (DÜWEL et al. 1975; DÜWEL 1979) or methyl[5-(phenylthio)-2-benzimidazole carbamate (Hoechst) is a crystalline powder insoluble in water and insoluble or only slightly soluble in most organic solvents. It is soluble in dimethylsulfoxide. Its molecular weight is 299.35 and its chemical structure is shown in Fig. 17.

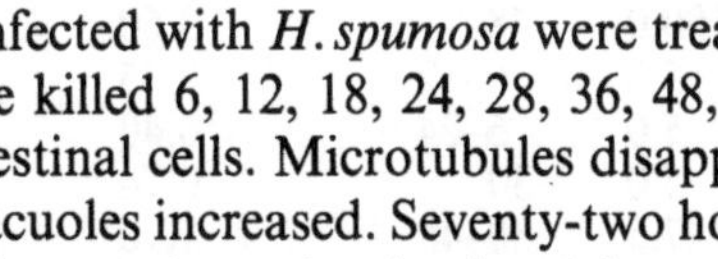

Fig. 17. Fenbendazole

I. Pharmacokinetics

Following oral administration of 10 mg [^{14}C]fenbendazole/kg to rats and dogs and of 5 mg/kg to farm animals, the radioactivity was mostly excreted in the feces and only one-tenth in the urine. In experiments using rabbits one-fifth of the administered dose was found in the urine.

Serum levels of fenbendazole found in different animals are summarized in Table 3. Following an oral dose of 7.5 mg/kg to cattle a maximum concentration of 0.30 µg fenbendazole/ml milk was found after 28 h (DÜWEL 1977).

It is of interest to note that plasma radioactivity after [^{14}C]fenbendazole administration to rats was higher in iron- and protein-deficient rats than in rats with sufficient iron and protein. However, the uptake of radioactivity by *Nippostrongylus brasiliensis* in iron and protein-deficient rats was significantly less than in worms from diet-sufficient rats (PRICHARD et al. 1981 a). In an earlier study PRICHARD et al. (1978 b) compared the incorporation of radiolabel from fenbendazole in benzimidazole-susceptible with that in benzimidazole-resistant *Haemonchus contortus* and *Trichostrongylus colubriformis*. Incorporation of

Table 3. Serum levels of fenbendazole (DÜWEL et al. 1975; DÜWEL 1977, 1979)

Species	Oral dose (mg/kg)	Time to reach maximum level (h)	Peak level (μg/ml)	Half-life in serum (h)
Rat	10.0	5– 7	0.19	6
Dog	10.0	6–24	0.04–0.40	15
Rabbit	50.0	30	2.60	15
	100.0	48	3.60	21
Pig	5.0	6–12	0.45	10
Sheep	5.0	6–24	0.40	26
Cattle	5.0	30	0.74	27
	7.5	30–48	1.10	13
	10.0	24–30	1.60	14

radioactivity was significantly greater in the susceptible than in resistant worms. The same authors also found that the rate of absorption was markedly greater if fenbendazole was administered directly into the abomasum instead of the rumen. They suggest that in sheep the rumen may act as a reservoir of anthelmintic, prolonging the period of high anthelmintic concentration in the host.

PRICHARD et al. (1981 b) also studied the gastrointestinal absorption and pharmacokinetic behavior of fenbendazole (5 mg/kg) administered intrarumenally to cattle. This study shows that slower rates of absorption and urinary excretion and extensive recycling of absorbed drug back to the gastrointestinal tract may contribute to the anthelmintic potency (e.g., against arrested *Ostertagia ostertagi* larvae) of fenbendazole in cattle.

Results of residue studies with nonradioactive fenbendazole in sheep, cattle, and pigs showed that, in most tissues, residues after 2 days are low and approach the limit of detection (0.05 mg/kg) after 5 days. Seven days after treatment the liver of cattle, pig, and sheep contained about 0.3, 0.3, and 0.9 mg/kg respectively. After 14 days these livers contained <0.1, 0.1, and 0.2 mg/kg (DÜWEL 1977).

The principal metabolite in sheep and bovine urine results from hydroxylation at the para- place of the phenyl ring. A 2-amino derivative was also found (CHRIST et al. 1974; DÜWEL 1977). An important route of metabolism of fenbendazole, as for the other sulfide benzimidazole, albendazole, was found to be via the sulfoxide to the sulfone. Mean peak concentrations in plasma of fenbendazole, oxfendazole, and sulfone of 0.15, 0.29, and 0.17 μg/ml occurred 24, 30, and 36 h after oral administration of 10 mg fenbendazole/kg body weight to sheep. Mean peak concentrations in abomasal fluid were 1.86, 0.66, and 0.07 μg/ml occurring at 30, 48, and 72 h respectively (MARRINER and BOGAN 1980, 1981). It is of interest to note that AVERKIN et al. (1975) in a comparative study in mice found the sulfoxide metabolite of fenbendazole (oxfendazole) more active than the parent compound. This was further proven in sheep by HALL et al. (1978). Much of the anthelmintic activity may be due to the oxfendazole metabolite (MARRINER and BOGAN 1981). More details are given in the section on oxfendazole.

II. Toxicology (DELATOUR and BURGAT-SACAZE 1981)

Fenbendazole is like the other benzimidazole carbamates well tolerated. The oral LD_{50} is >10 g/kg in rats and mice. Apart from transient increases of transaminases in a few members of each group of domestic animals the following high doses were well tolerated: cattle, >2 g/kg; dogs >0.5 g/kg; and pigs and sheep, >5 g/kg. Repeated administrations of several times the therapeutic dose were also well tolerated, e.g., sheep, 30 × 34 mg/kg; rat, 90 × 1.6 mg/kg; and dog, 90 × 125 mg/kg.

No evidence of teratogenic effects in rats, sheep, and cattle has been found.

III. Mode of Action

In *Fasciola hepatica* fenbendazole seems to disturb the synthesis or breakdown of serotonin and the metabolism of amino acids (METZGER and DÜWEL 1974). In nematodes, this benzimidazole carbamate was found to interfere with the absorption of glucose and with the "incorporation" of glucose into glycogen (DÜWEL 1977). According to DÜWEL and SCHLEICH (1978) fenbendazole is neurotoxic for *Hymenolepis diminuta*.

Fenbendazole shares with the other benzimidazole carbamates the property to interact with cytoplasmic microtubules, causing degenerative changes in the intestinal or tegumental cells of nematodes and cestodes respectively. More details will be given in the section on mebendazole. However, it is of interest to note here that FRIEDMAN and PLATZER (1980b) determined the inhibition constants (K_i) of fenbendazole for bovine brain tubulin and *A. suum* embryonic tubulin polymerization. The K_i of fenbendazole for *A. suum* embryonic tubulin was 262 times smaller than the K_i for bovine brain tubulin.

S. Flubendazole

Flubendazole (Fig. 18) is the generic name of methyl [5-(4-fluoro-benzoyl)-1*H*-benzimidazol-2yl] carbamate and is the *p*-fluoroderivative of mebendazole (Janssen Pharmaceutica). Flubendazole is insoluble in water and inorganic acids. It is

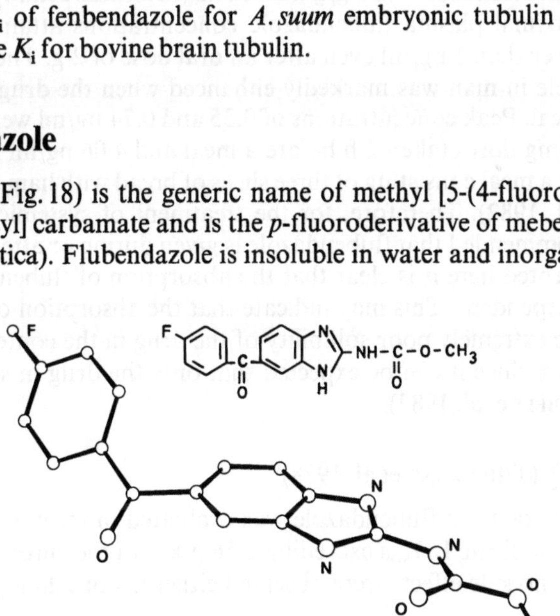

Fig. 18. Chemical structure of flubendazole and perspective drawing as derived by TOLLENAERE et al. (1979) from crystallographic data

slightly soluble in organic acids (e.g., 34.05 g per 100 ml formic acid) and solvents. Its molecular weight is 313.29.

I. Pharmacokinetics

After oral treatment of rats, dogs, pigs, and man only small quantities of flubendazole are resorbed. Plasma levels of flubendazole determined with a radioimmunoassay 4 h after oral administration of 40 mg/kg were 81.4 ng/ml in Wistar rats and 17 ng/ml in multimammate rats (*Mastomys natalensis*). Peak flubendazole plasma levels of 8.4 and 7.4 ng/ml were found 8 h after subcutaneous administration of 40 mg flubendazole/kg to Wistar and multimammate rats (MICHIELS et al. 1982).

Beagle dogs were injected intramuscularly with a microsuspension of flubendazole either once or for five consecutive days at a dose level of 2.5 or 25 mg/kg. After a single dose plasma peak levels amounted to about 0.5 ng/ml at 3–5 days for the 2.5-mg/kg dose and to 2 ng/ml at 5–7 days for the 25-mg/kg dose. Intramuscular flubendazole in dogs for five consecutive days produced sustained fairly high plasma levels for at least 6 weeks after the last dose. Plasma levels were maximal 3–4 days after the last dose, representing peak concentrations of 2.4 and 13 ng/ml for the low- and high-dose levels respectively (MICHIELS et al. 1982).

Pigs treated orally with a single dose of 5 mg flubendazole/kg were slaughtered 24, 48, and 72 h after treatment. Plasma concentrations determined with a high-pressure liquid chromatography (HPLC) method were 20, 30, and <10 ng/ml. Tissue levels in the liver, kidney, and muscle were about 10 ng/g tissue up to 72 h after treatment. In fat 60–70 ng/g was found (MICHIELS et al. 1977 b).

In man, maximal plasma flubendazole concentrations attained 1–4 h after dosing were lower than 5 ng/ml even after an oral dose of 2 g. The absorption of oral flubendazole in man was markedly enhanced when the drug was taken together with a meal. Peak concentrations of 0.35 and 0.74 ng/ml were obtained for 100- and 2,000-mg doses taken 2 h before a meal and 4.06 ng/ml for a 2,000-mg dose taken after a meal consisting of three slices of bread with ham, eggs, and milk (MICHIELS et al. 1982). Therefore, for the treatment of systemic localized helminths it is recommended that flubendazole is given during or after a meal. From the results presented here it is clear that the absorption of flubendazole is completely dose independent. This may indicate that the absorption of flubendazole is limited by the extremely poor solubility of the drug in the contents of the gastrointestinal tract since it can be expected that only the drug in solution can be absorbed (MICHIELS et al. 1982).

II. Toxicology (THIENPONT et al. 1978)

The acute oral toxicity of flubendazole was evaluated in mice, rats, and guinea pigs. The results indicate LD_{50}s exceeding 2.56 g/kg. In the chronic toxicity tests in rats and dogs no side effects were observed either histopathologically or clinically.

Doses up to 40 mg/100 g food (approximately 40 mg/kg body weight) given to rats from day 6 through day 15 of pregnancy produced no teratogenic effects. Flubendazole also had no effect on either male or female fertility. No differences were observed between the control and the dosed (up to 40 mg/kg) female rats with regard to mortality, pregnancy, weight, and food consumption. Litter size, weight at birth, weight gain during a 3-week postnatal period, and survival rate were considered to be normal in all groups even in those that were treated with 40 mg/kg/ day from day 16 of gestation through a 3-week lactation period. No teratogenic effects were observed in rabbits treated orally by gavage at doses of 10 and 40 mg/kg from day 6 through day 18 of pregnancy.

III. Mode of Action

Since the mode of action of flubendazole is identical to that of mebendazole it will be discussed in the section on mebendazole.

T. Levamisole and Tetramisole

Levamisole (RAEYMAEKERS et al. 1967) is the levorotatory enantiomer of tetramisole or (±)-2,3,5,6-tetrahydro-6-phenylimidazo[2,1-b]thiazole monohydrochloride (molecular weight, 204.29+36.46; Janssen Pharmaceutica). Most of the anthelmintic activity of the racemate resides in levamisole, which is several times more potent but not more toxic than dexamisole, the dextrorotatory isomer. Both isomers are highly soluble and quite stable in acid aqueous media. In alkaline solutions, hydrolysis opens the thiazoline ring to produce the insoluble OMPI [(−)-2-oxo-3-(2-mercapto-ethyl)-5-phenylimidazolidine]. The chemical structures are given in Fig. 19. The three-dimensional structure of levamisole is given in Fig. 20. One milligram of levamisole hydrochloride corresponds to 0.848 mg base. It is a stable white crystalline solid. For survey articles see JANSSEN (1976) and SYMOENS et al. (1979).

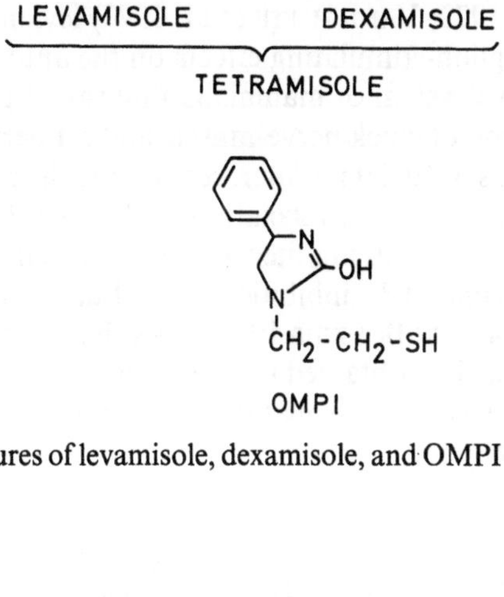

Fig. 19. Chemical structures of levamisole, dexamisole, and OMPI

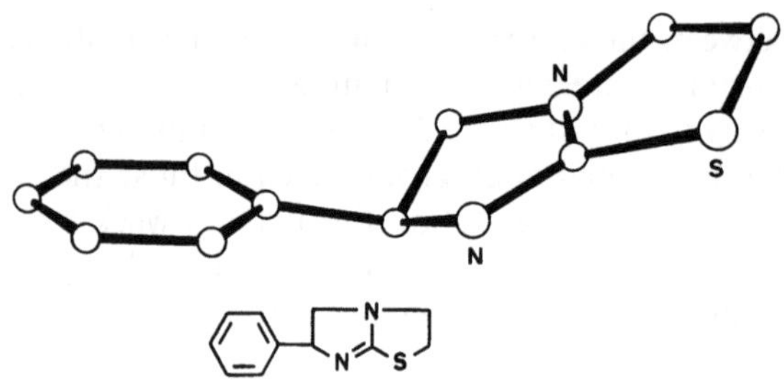

Fig. 20. Chemical structure of tetramisole and perspective drawing based on X-ray crystallography. TOLLENAERE et al. (1979)

I. Pharmacokinetics

Levamisole is rapidly absorbed from the gastrointestinal tract, from the intact skin, and from the injection site. In man peak plasma levels of about 0.7 μg/ml are reached within 1–2 h after oral administration of one single dose of 150 mg (GRAZIANI and DE MARTIN 1977b). In man the drug has a plasma half-life of about 4 h and is eliminated from the body in about 2 days.

In animals, intramuscular doses can elicit plasma concentrations of up to 10 μg/ml. With the same dose, peak plasma levels are about twice as high after intramuscular injection as after oral administration (GRAZIANI and DE MARTIN 1977a). A gas chromatographic method is now available to determine levamisole levels as low as 4 ng (ROUSSEAU et al. 1981).

The metabolism of levamisole has been studied in rats; four initial reactions seem to occur: (a) oxidation of the imidazoline moiety, (b, c) oxidation and hydrolysis of the thiazolidine group, and (d) para hydroxylation of the phenyl ring (BOYD et al. 1969).

One of the major metabolites of levamisole is OMPI. α-Ketoaldehydes, especially glyoxal and methylglyoxal, are very specific catalysts for the hydrolysis of levamisole into the thiol derivative OMPI. The reaction proceeds rapidly at ambient temperature and a slightly alkaline pH (VAN BELLE and JANSSEN 1979).

II. Pharmacology

1. In Vitro Experiments

In vitro (VAN NUETEN 1972; VANHOUTTE et al. 1977) levamisole and tetramisole produce reversible ganglion-stimulating effects on the autonomous as well as on the sympathetic nervous system of mammalian intestinal tissues. They produce neuromuscular inhibition of chick nerve-muscle and rat nerve-diaphragm preparations at concentrations of 10–30 mg/liter, resembling the activity of nicotine.

Levamisole induces a reversible relaxation of the KCl-depolarized guinea pig ileum at concentrations of 2.5–40 mg/liter. It also inhibits the acetylcholinesterase of erythrocytes and serum; 50% inhibition was obtained at $10^{-4}\,M$ and $2.5\times10^{-4}\,M$ respectively (VANDEN BOSSCHE 1976b). As the reversible ganglion-stimulating activity of levamisole is obtained between 2.6×10^{-6} and $4.1\times10^{-5}\,M$, the inhibition of the cholinesterases is probably not directly connected with the effects on the neuromuscular system.

An interesting property of levamisole is its ability to inhibit at 10^{-6} *M* alkaline phosphatases of most mammalian tissues. The intestinal and human placental isoenzymes are exceptions. The inhibition is of the uncompetitive type. It is of interest to note that dexamisole is inactive (VAN BELLE 1972, 1976; BORGERS and THONE 1976).

2. In Vivo Experiments

Therapeutic doses of tetramisole, levamisole, and dexamisole are devoid of measurable effects on the autonomous nervous system, thermoregulation, reflexes, and gross behavior in mice and rats. At subtoxic and toxic dose levels tetramisole and its enantiomers act as convulsants (SYMOENS et al. 1979).

III. Toxicology

The acute toxicity of levamisole has been evaluated in different animal species. In Table 4, some LD_{50}s are given.

Table 4. LD_{50} values after a single dose of levamisole (SYMOENS et al. 1979)

Species	Route of administration	LD_{50} (mg/kg)
Albino mouse	i.v.	22
	s.c.	84
	Oral	210
Wistar rat	i.v.	24
	s.c.	130
	Oral	480
Rabbit	Oral	700

Chronic toxicity tests in rats at oral doses up to 80 mg/kg did not produce a drug-related mortality. Analysis of blood and urine showed normal values except for a lower creatinine content at the highest dose.

The subacute 1-month and 3-month toxicity studies in dogs also revealed no drug-related effects. However, daily administration of a toxic dose of 20 mg/kg to beagle dogs for 2 months produced reversible hemolytic anemia. This effect was not observed in Labrador dogs, Wistar rats, or Suffolk sheep. This could indicate that the erythrocytes of the beagle dog are abnormally sensitive to levamisole (SYMOENS et al. 1979).

Levamisole did not affect the fertility of male and female rats when they were dosed for 60 and 14 days before mating. Nor could any embryotoxic or teratogenic effect be shown in rabbits and rats treated with 100 and 75 mg/kg respectively (information from Imperial Chemical Industries).

IV. Mode of Action

In vitro, levamisole is immediately and almost completely absorbed by *A. suum* via a transcuticular mechanism (VERHOEVEN et al. 1976). This is consistent with the rapid occurrence of a levamisole- and tetramisole-induced spastic contraction of the *Ascaris* muscle (VAN NUETEN 1972). In incubated larval and adult nematodes the presence of levamisole causes a contraction followed by tonic paralysis (VANDEN BOSSCHE 1976a). Whether this effect is reversible depends on the worm species, the stage in the life cycle, the concentration, and the incubation circumstances (VAN NUETEN 1972; VANDEN BOSSCHE 1976a). Pharmacological experiments have demonstrated that levamisole acts as a ganglion-stimulating compound and that afterwards it induces a neuromuscular inhibition of the depolarizing type (COLES et al. 1975; COLES 1977). By using *Ascaris* muscle preparation it could be shown that levamisole alters the rest potential from −30 mV to −15 mV (XHONNEUX, unpublished results).

Levamisole and tetramisole also interfere with the fumarate reduction system in mitochondria of nematodes and of *F. hepatica* (for review articles see VANDEN BOSSCHE 1976a, 1978, 1980b). In various parasitic worms, this fumarate reductase system plays a key role in the mitochondrial energy production. Although it is certain that levamisole primarily influences the neuromuscular system of nematodes, it is possible that in some helminths the inhibition of the fumarate reductase system contributes to the anthelmintic efficacy of levamisole (VANDEN BOSSCHE 1976a; BEHM and BRYANT 1979).

U. Mebendazole

Mebendazole (Fig. 21) or methyl [5-(benzoyl)-1*H*-benzimidazol-2yl] carbamate (Janssen Pharmaceutica) is almost insoluble in water and most organic solvents. In dimethyl sulfoxide (DMSO) its solubility is 2.4 g/100 ml. The log P value, i.e., the logarithm of the partition coefficient of the substance between octanol and water is 3.10. Molecular weight is 295.3.

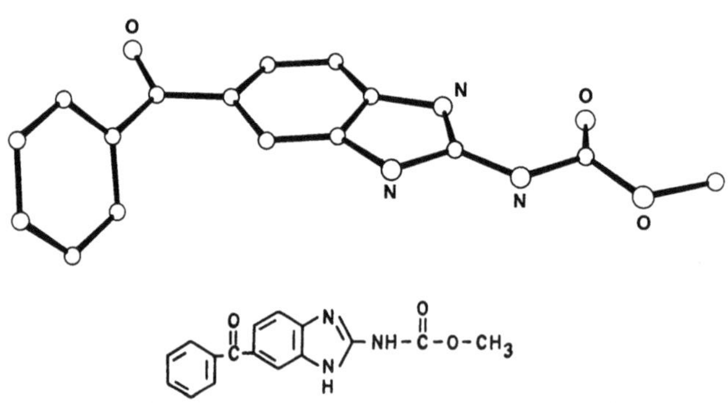

Fig. 21. Chemical structure of mebendazole and its three-dimensional structure. TOLLENAERE et al. (1979)

I. Pharmacokinetics

The survey in Table 5 shows the excretion via the urine is only 1% in dogs, whereas in pigs 32%–48% of the administered dose is found.

In rats mebendazole is excreted almost unaltered via the feces; the only metabolite found is (2-amino-1*H*-benzimidazol-5yl) phenylmethanone, which has no anthelmintic activity. This metabolite represents 14.8% of the total radioactivity found in the urine; 7% is mebendazole and 18% methyl[5-(α-hydroxy-α-phenyl-methyl-1*H*-benzimidazol-2yl)] carbamate formed by reduction of the ketone group of mebendazole (MEULDERMANS et al. 1977).

In Wistar rats and multimammate rats (*Mastomys natalensis*), treated orally with 40 mg/kg, plasma levels (radioimmune assay method) reached 400 ng/ml and 130 ng/ml, respectively, at 4 h after drug administration. At 8 h, plasma levels remained near peak levels in the Wistar rat (349 ng/ml) but decreased to 37.8 ng/ml in the multimammate rats. By 24 h, mebendazole in the Wistar group had almost disappeared from the plasma (5.3 ng/ml).

After subcutaneous injection, mebendazole was absorbed more gradually, reaching peak plasma levels of about 60–70 ng/ml for both strains within 4–8 h after administration (MICHIELS et al. 1982).

In jirds infected with *Echinococcus multilocularis* that were treated with 100–1,000 ppm mebendazole in their food, plasma concentrations varied between 118 and 1,062 ng/ml (measured with an HPLC method). In infected animals drug plasma levels of >73.7 ng/ml were associated with a significant decrease in parasitic weights (SCHANTZ et al. 1982).

When turkeys were treated with 63 ppm mebendazole in their food for 48 h, 6.7 ng/ml mebendazole and/or metabolites were found per *Syngamus trachea* worm pair. Even samller amounts of mebendazole reached *Syphacia muris*. Twenty-four hours after oral treatment of the rat host with a single dose of 2.5 mg/kg, 60 pg mebendazole was found (VANDEN BOSSCHE and JANSSEN 1983).

The distribution of mebendazole and/or metabolites was studied (VANDEN BOSSCHE and DE NOLLIN 1973; VANDEN BOSSCHE et al. 1975) in the different organs and pseudocoelomic fluid of *Ascaris suum* after 24 h of incubation in the presence of ^{14}C-labeled mebendazole. Highest specific activity was encountered in the alimentary system. However, highest total activity was found in the pseu-

Table 5. Excretion of mebendazole plus metabolites (Department of drug metabolism, Janssen Pharmaceutica, unpublished data)

Species	Oral dose (mg/kg)	Collection time (hours)	Excretion (% of dose)		
			Feces	Urine	Total
Rat	2.5	0→24	82.7	5.1	87.8
		0→96	85.6	5.8	91.4
	10.0	0→96	92.1	12.6	104.7
Dog	10.0	0→96	90.5	0.9	91.4
Pig	1.0	0→96	45–64	32–48	93–96

docoelomic fluid (37.5%) and muscle plus cuticle (31.3%). Almost similar figures have been published by KÖHLER and BACHMANN (1981). It is of interest to note that after 1 h of incubation the highest specific activity and the highest percentage of total radioactivity in the worm was found in the cuticle plus muscle (VANDEN BOSSCHE et al. 1975). This may indicate a partial transport of mebendazole through the cuticle.

In the intestinal cells mebendazole (and metabolites?) were found to bind partly to soluble high molecular weight proteins (about 100,000 and 50,000–60,000). A similar binding occurred when a soluble cell extract (the supernatant of a 1-h centrifugation at 235,000 g) was incubated in the presence of mebendazole (VAN DEN BOSSCHE et al. 1975).

Ascaris has a limited capacity for metabolizing mebendazole within a 24-h incubation period. Accoring to KÖHLER and BACHMANN (1981) this pharmacodynamic behavior may allow the drug to increase steadily under chemotherapeutic conditions within the parasite tissues and result in concentrations of the drug high enough to inhibit microtubule assembly (see Sect. U.III).

The two metabolites formed in *A. suum* tissues (KÖHLER and BACHMANN 1981) are also among the major metabolites of mebendazole in mammals (HEYKANTS 1972) and liver tissues (MEULDERMANS et al. 1976), i.e., methyl [5-(α-hydroxy-α-phenylmethyl-1*H*-benzimidazol-2yl)] carbamate and 2-amino-benzimidazol-5-yl phenylmethanone. Both are without anthelmintic activity (MEULDERMANS et al. 1976).

In man, after receiving 200 mg/day orally for 3 days, plasma levels never exceeded 30 ng/ml of the parent compound and 90 ng/ml of the amino derivative (DEMOEN et al. 1973). After oral administration of 1.5 g mebendazole to fasting volunteers, plasma concentrations $\leqq 5$ ng/ml were found. However, plasma concentrations of 5–39.5 ng/ml were found if mebendazole tablets were swallowed during a meal. In a patient with cholestasis a plasma concentration of 112 ng/ml was found (MÜNST et al. 1980).

From 24 observations made in seven patients during treatment with 40–60 mg/kg/day, serum levels, 1–3 h after administration, remained below 90 ng/ml. By contrast, concentrations exceeded this value on 14 occasions when determined from four patients during treatment with 200 mg/kg/day (BRYCESON et al. 1982).

II. Toxicology (JANSSEN PHARMACEUTICA 1972; MARSBOOM 1973; VANDEN BOSSCHE et al. 1982)

Pharmacologically, mebendazole is almost an inert substance. It has no effect on the central nervous system and it has no analgesic, anticonvulsive, and hypnotic effects.

The acute oral toxicity was evaluated in different species: the LD_{50} was higher than 640 mg/kg in rabbits, dogs, and cats and higher than 1.28 g/kg in mice, rats, and guinea pigs.

No clinical abnormalities were seen in sheep treated with 320 mg/kg. The temperature and the cardiac and respiratory rhythm of horses remained normal. Only after treatment with 400 mg/kg was diarrhea observed. Transient softening of the feces and diarrhea was also seen in some pigs.

Dogs tolerated daily doses of 40 mg/kg body weight for 104 weeks with no hematological or clinical changes. After daily treatment of horses with a standard dose of 5 g mebendazole for 19–74 days the intake of food, weight, physical appearance, and blood analysis were normal.

When mebendazole is given to dogs, sheep, and horses during organogenesis, no teratogenic or embryotoxic effects were observed. In rats when 40 mg mebendazole/kg body weight was given on the 7th or 10th day of gestation, some skeleton abnormalities were seen. Mebendazole does not affect the fertility of rats when a dose of 40 mg/kg is given to male and female rats for 14 and 60 days respectively prior to mating and to female rats again throughout gestation. When the same dose was given to rats from the 16th day of gestation throughout a 3-week lactation period, no effect on mortality, pregnancy, weight, and intake of food could be shown. The number of the offspring, their weight at birth, and weight increase were also not affected.

III. Mode of Action (VANDEN BOSSCHE et al. 1982)

Mebendazole shares with other benzimidazole derivatives the ability to bind to tubulin, the dimeric subunit protein of microtubules, and to inhibit the assembly of these microtubules (HOEBEKE et al. 1976; FRIEDMAN and PLATZER 1978; IRELAND et al. 1979; KÖHLER and BACHMANN 1980, 1981). FRIEDMAN and PLATZER (1980a, b) presented evidence of differential binding affinities of mebendazole for *A. suum* embryonic tubulin and mammalian brain tubulin, *A. suum* embryonic tubulin being 384 times more sensitive to the drug than bovine brain tubulin. KÖHLER and BACHMANN (1980, 1981) described the partial purification of *Ascaris* intestinal tubulin and the interaction of mebendazole with this tubulin and that of pig brain. The results indicate that mebendazole could bind about twice as tightly to *Ascaris* tubulin. Therefore it is doubtful that this small differential affinity of parasite and host tubulin could be responsible for the apparently selective interaction of the drug with the cytoplasmic microtubule of the *Ascaris* intestine (BORGERS et al. 1975a). However, it would be of interest to compare the affinity to *Ascaris* intestinal tubulin with that to mammalian intestinal tubulin.

Increasing evidence has accumulated which supports the assumption that tubulin is the primary target of the anthelmintic action of mebendazole (BORGERS et al. 1975a, b, c; BORGERS and DE NOLLIN 1975), flubendazole (VERHEYEN et al. 1976) and other mebendazole analogues (IRELAND et al. 1979). This interaction induces the disappearance of cytoplasmic microtubules of the tegumental or intestinal cells of cestodes or nematodes causing degenerative changes in these cells. This may also lead to impaired coating of the membranes, followed by a decreased digestion and absorption of nutrients. Mebendazole affects in vitro and in vivo the glucose uptake by helminths (VANDEN BOSSCHE 1972a, 1976a; VANDEN BOSSCHE and DE NOLLIN 1973; DE NOLLIN and VANDEN BOSSCHE 1973; RAHMAN and BRYANT 1977). This decreased glucose uptake is followed by an enhanced utilization of endogenous glycogen and/or decreased synthesis of this reserve polysaccharide (VANDEN BOSSCHE 1972a, 1976a; RAHMAN and BRYANT 1977; BEHM and BRYANT 1979). The drug also diminished ATP synthesis and/or turnover of adenine nucleotides. In *Moniezia expansa* these effects became apparent within 30 min of exposure to mebendazole in vitro (RAHMAN and BRYANT 1977). A similar effect has been observed in vivo (RAHMAN et al. 1977). It is therefore probable that an early effect of mebendazole is on the phosphorylation of ADP.

V. Metrifonate

Metrifonate (Trichlorfon) (Fig. 22, Bilarcil, Bayer) is the pharmaceutical grade of the agricultural chemicals Trichlorfon, Dipterex, Dylox, and Clorofos (ALDRIDGE and HOLMSTEDT 1981). Metrifonate or *O,O*-dimethyl-(1-hydroxy-2,2,2-trichloroethyl)-phosphonate is a white crystalline solid, soluble in water (15.4 g/100 ml) and most organic solvents. Its molecular weight is 257.45. There is a spontaneous breakdown of metrifonate to dichlorvos (Fig. 22). The half-life of metrifonate in aqueous solution is, at pH 7 and 37.5 °C, 6.4 h (METCALF et al. 1959; ALDRIDGE and HOLMSTEDT 1981). Dichlorvos is a colorless liquid. It is slightly soluble in water (about 1 g/100 ml) and most organic solvents. A survey of the chemistry of metrifonate and dichlorvos was presented at the symposium: "Metrifonate and Dichlorvos: Theoretical and Practical Aspects," Stockholm, 3–4 November, 1980, of which the proceedings are published in Acta Pharmacol Toxicol (ALDRIDGE and HOLMSTEDT 1981).

It should be noted that Neguvon A also contains metrifonate and, as a minor ingredient, the other organophosphorus compound, coumafos.

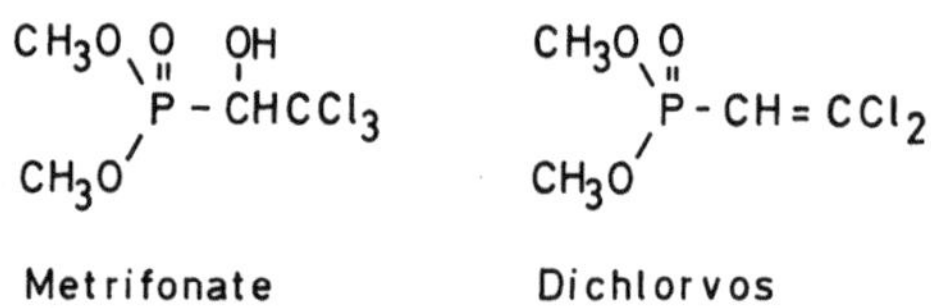

Fig. 22. Structural formulae of metrifonate and dichlorvos

I. Pharmacokinetics

A method is available for the simultaneous quantitation of metrifonate and dichlorvos (2,2-dichlorovinyl dimethyl phosphate, DDVP) in human blood. This method is based upon labeling of the compounds with deuterium ($[^2H_6]$metrifonate and $[^2H_4]$DDVP) and gas-phase analysis using the mass spectrometer as a selective detector (NORDGREN et al. 1981). The amount of DDVP in plasma of man is about 1% of the amount of metrifonate. In erythrocytes the corresponding amount of DDVP is 0.5% or less of metrifonate (NORDGREN et al. 1981). If, as seems likely, the conversions of metrifonate to dichlorvos in vivo and in vitro are the same, then dichlorvos must be destroyed very rapidly in vivo. According to ALDRIDGE and HOLMSTEDT (1981) the half-life of DDVP ist 1–2 min. Both compounds reach peak levels in blood within 2 h after oral dosing and are detectable for at least 8 h. Clearance of metrifonate occurs primarily via DDVP.

NORDGREN et al. (1981) also relates levels of both metrifonate and DDVP in plasma and erythrocytes in man to cholinesterase activity. After administration of metrifonate at 10 mg/kg, cholinesterase activity in plasma reaches zero levels within 15 min, and remains inhibited for more than 8 h, recovering slowly after the first day. Red blood cell cholinesterase is inhibited by 60%–80% and recovered more slowly than the activity in plasma.

It is of interest to note that metrifonate does not seem to react with cholinesterases, while dichlorvos is a potent inhibitor (REINER 1981).

II. Toxicology

The tolerable dose for oral treatment depends on the species: rabbits, 150 mg/kg; dogs, 50–75 mg/kg; cats, 40 mg/kg (CAVIER 1973).

Experiments in animals showed metrifonate not to be mutagenic, teratogenic, or carcinogenic (DAVIS 1975).

The toxicological profile of trichlorfon has been reviewed by MACHEMER (1981). In rats cholinesterase activity was depressed in serum at dietary levels of 500 ppm and also in erythrocytes at a dietary concentration of 1,000 ppm. In dogs, cholinesterase activity of erythrocytes and serum was inhibited at 200 ppm. In rhesus monkeys plasma cholinesterase activity was reduced significantly at 5 mg/kg; that of the erythrocytes was already reduced at 0.2 mg/kg.

Although the described inhibition of acetylcholinesterase results in accumulation of acetylcholine at nerve synapses, according to DAVIS (1975) there is no evidence of a relationship between depressed blood cholinesterase activity and the occurrence of organ malfunction.

III. Mode of Action

The mechanism of action is not known. Studies on the effects of metrifonate and dichlorvos on esterases revealed no basic differences between esterases in *Schistosoma mansoni* and *S. haematobium*, nor between mammalian enzymes and enzymes from parasitic helminths such as *Metastrongylus apri* and *A. suum* (REINER 1981). Thus the differences in the chemotherapeutic activities of metrifonate in man infected with *S. haematobium*, on the one hand, and with *S. mansoni* on the other, cannot be explained from the reactions of metrifonate and dichlorvos with cholinesterase (EC 3.1.1.7, EC 3.1.1.8) and arylesterases (EC 3.1.1.2) (BUEDING et al. 1972; REINER 1981).

W. Morantel

Morantel tartrate (Pfizer) is the 3-methyl derivative of pyrantel tartrate. The molecular weight of 1,4,5,6-tetrahydro-1-methyl-2-[2-(3-methyl-2-thienyl)ethenyl] pyrimidine is 220.3 (Fig. 23).

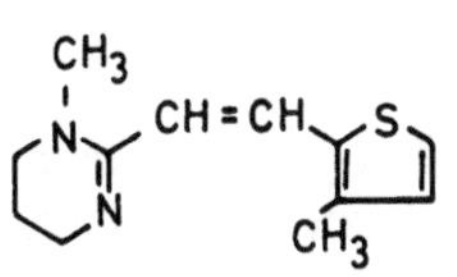

Fig. 23. Morantel

I. Pharmacokinetics (O'BRIEN 1970)

In sheep this pyrimidine derivative is absorbed rapidly from the upper small intestine, and peak blood levels are reached 4–6 h after administration.

Seventeen percent of morantel is excreted as metabolites in the first 96 h. The rest is excreted in the feces.

II. Toxicology

The oral LD_{50} in mice is between 300 and 437 mg/kg; the intraperitoneal LD_{50} is 28 mg/kg. In rats an oral LD_{50} value of 927 mg/kg is found. Rats that died of acute toxicity showed convulsions, erection of the hair, and ataxia (O'BRIEN 1970).

III. Mode of Action

It is believed that the mode of action of morantel is similar to that of its hydrogen analogue, pyrantel. It is of interest to note that the fumarate reductase system of *Haemonchus contortus* is sensitive to high concentrations (2.5×10^{-3} *M*) of morantel tartrate (PRICHARD 1973).

X. Niclosamide

Niclosamide (Fig. 24) is 2′,5-dichloro-4′-nitrosalicylanilide (Bayer) and is a crystalline powder which is practically insoluble in water and only moderately soluble in ethanol, chloroform, and ether. Its molecular weight is 327.1.

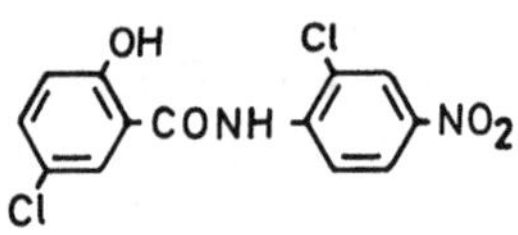

Fig. 24. Chemical structure of niclosamide

I. Pharmacokinetics

The antitapeworm drug, niclosamide, is almost not absorbed through the intestinal wall of the host (HECHT and GLOXHUBER 1960; GÖNNERT et al. 1963). The small part absorbed is metabolized into aminoclosamide, which is about 80 times better tolerated and inactive as an anthelmintic (STRUFE and GÖNNERT 1967).

In vivo, *Hymenolepis diminuta* absorbs a significant amount of niclosamide. After oral treatment of the host rats with 50 or 100 mg/kg up to 90 mg/100 g of dry weight was found in this cestode (STRUFE and GÖNNERT 1960).

II. Toxicology

Experiments in rats, rabbits, and dogs have shown that niclosamide, when administered orally, is well tolerated (HECHT and GLOXHUBER 1960). Rats and rabbits even survived a single oral dose of 5 g/kg. Intraperitoneal treatment of rats yielded an LD_{50} value of 0.75 g/kg. However, niclosamide is a toxic compound when given intravenously to mice (LD_{50}, 7.5 mg/kg). The low oral and intraperitoneal toxicity may be due to the inability of niclosamide to penetrate the host tissues.

III. Mode of Action

A number of studies have shown that niclosamide, like other salicylanilides, inhibits the formation of mitochondrial energy. A few examples to illustrate this: the anaerobic incorporation of ^{32}Pi into ATP by *H. diminuta* and the ^{32}Pi-ATP exchange in the mitochondria of this tapeworm are inhibited by niclosamide (SCHEIBEL et al. 1968). Low concentrations (2×10^{-7} *M*) of this compound stimulate oxygen utilization by *H. diminuta* mitochondria (YORKE and TURTON 1974). This salicylanilide has the same inhibitory effect upon the ^{32}Pi-ATP exchange reaction in *A. suum* mitochondria as demonstrated in *H. diminuta* mitochondria (SAZ and LESCURE 1968). Niclosamide also inhibits the malate-induced ^{32}Pi incorporation into ATP by *Ascaris* mitochondria (SAZ 1972a; VANDEN BOSSCHE 1972b), indicating that *Ascaris* and *H. diminuta* mitochondria are almost similar. The failure of niclosamide to affect intact nematodes may be due to differences in uptake and distribution (SAZ 1972b). The inability to penetrate the host tissues may also be at the origin of niclosamide's low toxicity. In fact, in vitro niclosamide also uncouples, e.g., rat liver (GÖNNERT et al. 1963; WILLIAMSON and METCALF 1967; STRUFE and GÖNNERT 1967). It also affects house fly muscle mitochondria (WILLIAMSON and METCALF 1967).

Niclosamide causes spastic and/or paralytic actions on various preparations of parasitic helminths, e.g., *Dipylidium canium, Paragonimus westermani, Fasciola hepatica,* and *Angiostrongylus cantonensis* (SANO et al. 1982). The latter investigators suggest that the spastic and/or paralytic action is via a neuropharmacological mechanism including acetylcholine and 5-hydroxytryptamine. These neuropharmacological effects may be elicited through the action of niclosamide on the energy production needed to release the neurotransmitter (SANO et al. 1982).

Y. Oxantel

Oxantel pamoate or 1-methyl-1,4,5,6-tetrahydro-2-(3-hydroxystyryl) pyrimidine pamoate (Fig. 25; molecular weight, 604.67) is a light yellow crystalline salt, practically insoluble in water (DRUGS OF TODAY 1981; BOTERO 1978). After oral ad-

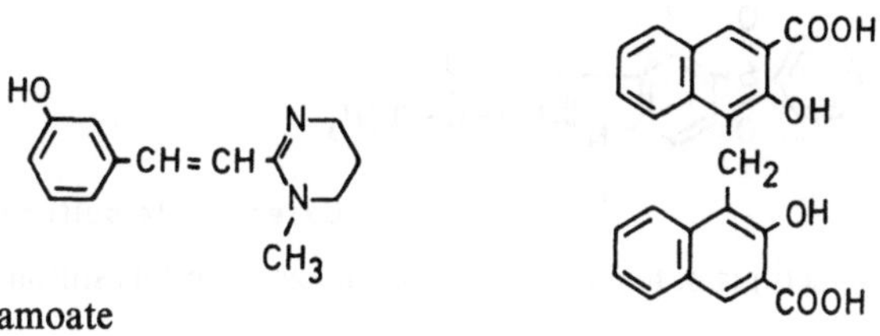

Fig. 25. Oxantel pamoate

ministration oxantel pamoate is poorly absorbed so that high concentrations are reached in the cecum and colon (GARCIA 1976).

Z. Oxfendazole

Oxfendazole is a member of the benzimidazole group of anthelmintics (AVERKIN et al. 1975). It is the generic name of methyl-5(6)phenylsulfinyl)-2-benzimidazole carbamate (Syntex Research).

I. Pharmacokinetics

PRICHARD et al. (1978a) determined the plasma levels of fenbendazole plus metabolites (using [^{14}C]fenbendazole) and of oxfendazole (Fig. 26) (using a radioimmunoassay) in sheep infected with *Haemonchus contortus* and *Trichostrongylus colubriformis*, both resistant to benzimidazoles. Sheep were treated orally with 5 mg/kg. Almost 3 µg oxfendazole/ml plasma was found against 0.5 µg/ml for fenbendazole plus metabolites. The plasma half-decay time was 22 h for fenbendazole and 28 h for oxfendazole.

Direct intra-abomasal oxfendazole administration of 5 mg/kg to sheep artificially infected with *T. colubriformis* and *H. contortus* resulted in a peak plasma oxfendazole concentration of 1.25 µg/ml after 65 h. A peak plasma level of 1.15 µg/ml was reached after 26 h when the same dose of oxfendazole was given intraruminally (PRICHARD and HENNESY 1981).

MARRINER and BOGAN (1981) also carried out pharmacokinetic studies of oxfendazole and its sulfone metabolite (Fig. 26) in sheep. They found a peak plasma

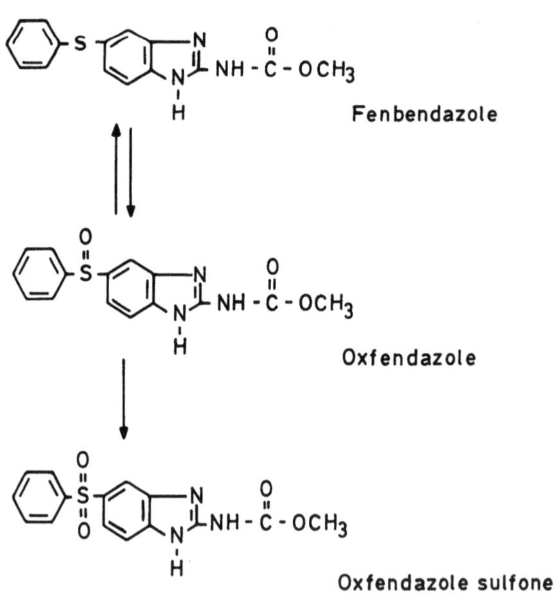

Fig. 26. Chemical structures of fenbendazole, oxfendazole, and its sulfone. MARRINER and BOGAN (1981)

oxfendazole concentration of 0.76 μg/ml at 30 h after oral administration of 10 mg/kg body weight and concentrations of 0.07 μg/ml were detectable 7 days after administration. Mean peak abomasal concentrations of 3.55 μg/ml occurred 20 h after administration and were detectable up to 9 days. In a number of plasma samples, fenbendazole (Fig. 26) was also measured. In all cases, concentrations of fenbendazole were 0%–20% of those of oxfendazole. Mean peak plasma oxfendazole sulfone concentrations of 0.24 μg/ml were found 48 h after oral administration of oxfendazole. Mean peak abomasal oxfendazole sulfone concentrations of 0.27 μg/ml occurred after 36 h.

Oxfendazole is known to be more potent than its sulfone (AVERKIN et al. 1975) and since fenbendazole is present at much lower concentrations in the plasma as compared with oxfendazole it is reasonable to consider that the anthelmintic activity is mainly due to oxfendazole and not to fenbendazole or oxfendazole sulfone (MARRINER and BOGAN 1981).

II. Toxicology

Acute toxicity studies indicated an LD_{50} for beagle dogs of more than 1.6 g/kg and over 6.4 g/kg in rats and mice (AVERKIN et al. 1975).

DELATOUR et al. (1977) studied the potential embryotoxicity and showed that the dose recommended for sheep must be strictly respected for the ewe at the onset of the gestation period. A dose 4.5 times the therapeutic dose is teratogenic and embryotoxic when given on the 17th day of gestation. They also found oxfendazole to be embryotoxic in rats treated daily with 15.75 and 21 mg/kg from the 15th day of the gestation period.

III. Mode of Action

The limited solubility of oxfendazole precluded accurate measurements of the concentrations needed to obtain 50% inhibition of the brain microtubule assembly (IRELAND et al. 1979). However, all benzimidazole carbamates studied have in common the property to bind to tubulin so that a similar mode of action may be proposed.

PRICHARD et al. (1978a) found that 5×10^{-5} *M* oxfendazole inhibited completely the fumarate-stimulated oxidation of NADH (fumarate reductase). However, as with mebendazole, further studies are needed to determine the involvement of this interference with energy metabolism in the anthelmintic activity of oxfendazole.

AA. Oxibendazole

Oxibendazole is the generic name of methyl[5-(*n*-propoxy)1*H*-benzimidazole-2yl]carbamate (Smith Kline Corporation). It is slightly soluble in most organic

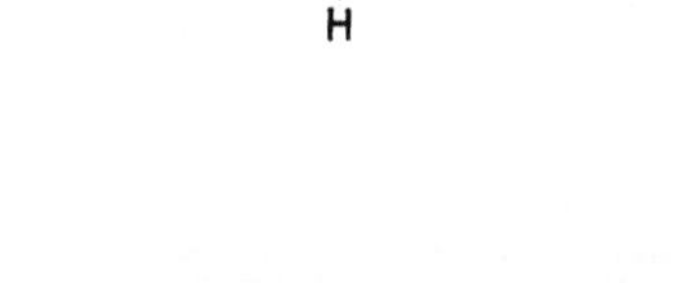

Fig. 27. Oxibendazole

solvents and insoluble in water (THEODORIDES et al. 1973). The chemical structure of this parbendazole derivative is given in Fig. 27.

I. Pharmacokinetics

Oral administration of oxibendazole at 53 mg/kg to sheep resulted in peak plasma levels of 2.43 μg/ml after 6 h. Approximately 34% of the dose was recovered in the urine in 24 h (THEODORIDES et al. 1973).

II. Toxicology

Oxibendazole administered orally to mated Long Evans rats from day 6 through day 15 of gestation at dose levels of 1, 3, 10, and 30 mg/kg did not affect pregnancy rate, implantation efficiency, and fetal size mortality, and did not induce malformations (THEODORIDES et al. 1973).

DELATOUR et al. (1976b) found therapeutic doses of oxibendazole devoid of teratogenic activity in rat and sheep. At doses four times the therapeutic dose oxibendazole was found embryotoxic in both species.

III. Mode of Action

Oxibendazole, like the other benzimidazole carbamate derivatives, is a potent inhibitor of brain microtubule polymerization (FRIEDMAN and PLATZER 1978).

BB. Parbendazole

Parbendazole (Fig. 28) is the generic name of methyl-5(6)-butyl-2-benzimidazole carbamate (ACTOR et al. 1967). It is practically insoluble in water. Its molecular weight is 247.3.

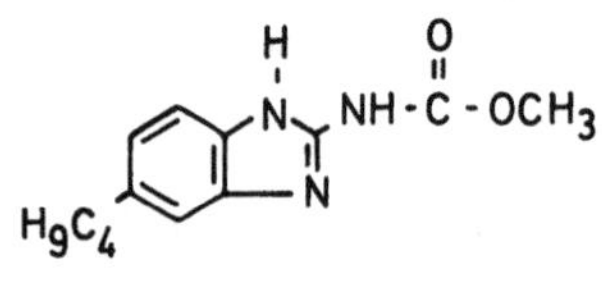

Fig. 28. Chemical structure of parbendazole

I. Pharmacokinetics

In sheep, residues in bile, fat, heart, kidney, liver, muscle, plasma, and skin were less than 0.1 ppm 16 days after administration of an oral dose of 45 mg [^{14}C]parbendazole/kg body weight (ACTOR et al. 1967).

Oral administration of [^{14}C]parbendazole to pigs resulted in a peak plasma concentration after 6 h. In 24 h 11% of the administered radioactivity was detected in the urine. Tissue residues were less than 0.1 ppm 21 days after oral administration of 50 mg [^{14}C]parbendazole/kg (ACTOR et al. 1976).

DUNN et al. (1973) determined the structures of seven metabolites isolated from sheep and cattle. The two major metabolites were methyl-5(6)-(3-carboxypropyl)-2 benzimidazole carbamate and methyl-*threo*-5(6)-(1,2-dihydroxybutyl)-2-benzimidazole carbamate. The first metabolite was also found in the fungus *Cunnighamella bainieri* (ATCC No. 9244).

II. Toxicology

The oral LD_{50}s for rats and mice exceed 4 g/kg body weight (ACTOR et al. 1976).

In subacute experiments in sheep, 75 mg/kg/day and 250 mg/kg/day (i.e., 3.75 and 12.5 times the normal dose) were administered for six consecutive days. None of the animals died, though animals showed anorexia, weight loss, and a slight reduction in the bromosulfalein clearance time. At autopsy irritation of the omasum and reticulum and abnormal liquid ruminal contents were found (O'BRIEN 1970).

DELATOUR et al. (1974, 1976a) found parbendazole to be teratogenic and embryotoxic in rats. Congenital abnormalities in lambs from ewes treated with parbendazole between the 9th and 21st day of gestation were reported (LAPRAS et al. 1973).

III. Mode of Action

Parbendazole, like the other benzimidazole carbamates, can bind to bovine brain tubulin and prevent the polymerization process (FRIEDMAN and PLATZER 1978). Parbendazole inhibits the monoamine oxidases of *Hymenolepis diminuta* and rat liver (MORENO and BARRETT 1979). However, it is doubtful that this effect is part of the anthelminthic activity of parbendazole. In fact doses too high (5×10^{-3} *M*) are needed to obtain a rather small inhibition (30%–49%).

CC. Paromomycin

Paromomycin, or *O*-,2,6-diamino-2,6-dideoxy-*β*-L-idopyranosyl-(1→3)-*O*-*β*-D-ribofuranosyl-(1→5)-*O*-[2-amino-2-deoxy-*α*-D-glucopyranosyl-(1→4)]-2-deoxystreptamine, is an oligosaccharide-type antibiotic related to streptomycin and iso-

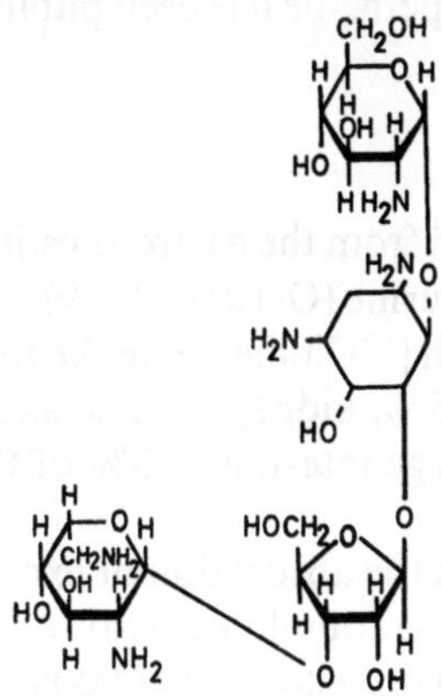

Fig. 29. Paromomycin

lated from various *Streptomyces*, e.g., *Streptomyces rimosus forma paromomycinus*. The chemical structure is given in Fig. 29. Its molecular weight is 615.6. This antibiotic is soluble in water and sparingly soluble in absolute alcohol. Paromomycin is very slightly absorbed from the intestine (BOTERO 1978).

The LD_{50} values in rats are: >1.625 g/kg orally >0.65 g/kg subcutaneously; and 156 mg/kg i.v. (The MERCK INDEX 1983).

The mode of action is unknown. It has been suggested that the action against *Taenia* may be by changing the ultrastructure of the tegumental membrane. This would make the parasite susceptible to the host's digestive mechanisms (GARIN et al. 1970).

DD. Piperazine

The diethylenediamine piperazine (Fig. 30), or hexahydropyrazine, is an alkaline crystalline compound which has been used against gout since 1891 (OELKERS 1959). Piperazine (molecular weight, 86.1) is available as a hexahydrate (containing 44.34% anhydrous piperazine; molecular weight, 194.1), as an adipate [calcium edetate (ethylenedinitrolo)-tetraacetic acid; molecular weight, 232.3), a citrate (molecular weight, 642.68), a phosphate (molecular weight, 184), and a tartrate (molecular weight, 236.2). The adipate, citrate, and phosphate contain 37.1%, 13.4%, and 46.8% piperazine respectively. The tartrate is formed from 1 mol piperazine and 1 mol tartaric acid (HEFFERREN et al. 1955).

Fig. 30. Piperazine

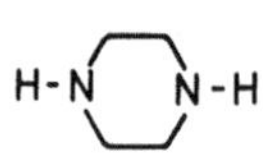

Piperazine and its hexahydrate; calcium edetate; and citrate are freely soluble in water. The phosphate is very slightly soluble in water. The solubilities in water of the adipate and tartrate are respectively 5.53 g/100 ml (at 20 °C) and 26 g/100 ml (at 25 °C) (MERCK INDEX 1976).

Piperazine and its salts have been discussed in several excellent survey articles (see, for example, OELKERS 1959; CAVIER 1973; DAVIS 1973). An interesting paper on the intriguing history of piperazine has been published by GOODWIN 1980).

I. Pharmacokinetics

Piperazine is readily absorbed from the gastrointestinal tract; in 24 h, 33.2±8.3% of the dose is excreted via the urine (OELKERS 1959).

After injection of rats with [^{14}C]piperazine the total content (5–15 min) in the muscles was 27.5%; liver, 8.5%; kidneys, 7.8%; skeleton, 7.1%; small intestine, 12%; stomach, 3.9%; and large intestine, 3.3% of the dose administered (SAVIN et al. 1977).

No essential differences in the absorption or excretion patterns of the adipate, citrate, or phosphate have been found but great individual differences have been observed in the rates of piperazine excretion (DAVIS 1973).

In rats fed with piperazine and nitrite, nitrosation of piperazine was observed in the stomach (SANDER et al. 1975). Nitrosation also occurs under simulated gastric conditions (MIRVISH 1975).

N,N-Dinitrosopiperazine and *N*-mononitrosopiperazine can be formed; both are animal carcinogens, *N,N*-dinitrosopiperazine being the most potent (DRUCKREY et al. 1967; GARCIA et al. 1970). It should be noted that lung adenomas can be induced in mice by long-term administration of nitrite in the drinking water plus piperazine in the food (MIRVISH 1975). In man mononitrosation occurs (BELLANDER et al. 1981).

When piperazine syrup (480 mg total dose) was given to fasting, healthy, nonsmoking, male volunteers considerably amounts of *N*-mononitrosopiperazine were found in the gastric juice. Thirty minutes after treatment 0.36–0.59 μg/ml was found. *N*-Mononitrosopiperazine was also excreted in the urine. The peak was reached within 2 h. In one subject even 2.14 μg/ml was found. *N*-Mononitrosopiperazine was not found in the blood within the 45 min studied; *N,N*-dinitrosopiperazine was not found in any of fluids examined (BELLANDER et al. 1981).

II. Toxicology

Orally, piperazine seems to be without pharmacodynamic activity (DAVIS 1973). Oral LD_{50}s for piperazine adipate in mice and rats are respectively 11.4 g/kg (i.e., 4.2 g piperazine) and 7.9 g/kg (CAVIER 1973).

Oral treatment of rats with 300 mg piperazine adipate/kg/day for 8 weeks or treatment of rabbits subcutaneously with 250 mg/kg/day (five times/week) for 5 weeks showed no pathological changes, apart from local necrosis at injection sites (CROSS et al. 1954).

III. Mode of Action

In *Ascaris* piperazine induces a reversible paralysis by directly affecting the neuromuscular system (NORTON and DE BEER 1957; OSTEUX et al. 1971). These paralyzed worms lose their ability to retain their position against the peristalsis of the small intestine, are carried down the gastrointestinal tract, and are voided with the feces (for survey articles see, e.g., DEL CASTILLO 1969; VANDEN BOSSCHE 1976a).

The effects of piperazine on the electrophysiological activity of the muscle cells of *Ascaris* have been studied, especially by DEL CASTILLO (1969). In summary: piperazine (10^{-5} up to 10^{-3} *M*) changes the rest potential of the *Ascaris* muscle cells from −30 to −45 mV. As the rhythmic action potentials disappear when the rest potential is −40 mV and since these action potentials are the basis of the muscular contractions, the hyperpolarizing effect is concomitant with paralysis. Further studies by DEL CASTILLO (1969) have shown that an increased permeability of the muscle membranes to chloride ions may cause hyperpolarization.

It should be noted that the incubation of *Ascaris lumbricoides* in the presence of piperazine (2 mg/ml) results in a decrease in the total phospholipid level. This may result from a stimulation of phopholipase C (a catabolic enzyme) and inhibition of choline kinase (an anabolic enzyme) (SASI and RAJ 1975).

EE. Praziquantel

Praziquantel or 2-(cyclohexylcarbonyl)-1,2,3,6,7,11b,hexahydro-4*H*-pyrazino [2,1-*a*]isoquinolin-4-one (molecular weight, 312.2) has been developed by E. Merck (Darmstadt) (SEUBERT et al. 1977) and Bayer. It dissolves very well in chloroform and dimethylsulfoxide. In ethanol its solubility is 9.7 g/100 ml whereas in water this pyrazino isoquinolone derivative is almost insoluble (GÖNNERT and ANDREWS 1977). The chemical structure is given in Fig. 31. It is available for schistosomiasis (Bayer) and against cestodes (Merck). For a survey article see ANDREWS and THOMAS (1983).

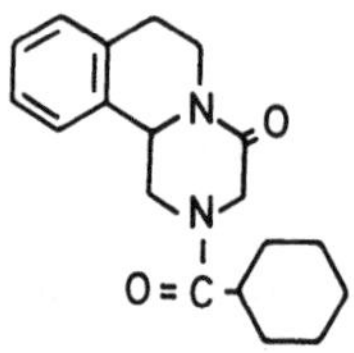

Fig. 31. Chemical structure of praziquantel

I. Pharmacokinetics

In man, more than 80% of the radioactivity coming from [^{14}C]praziquantel is found in the urine during the first 24 h after oral treatment (BÜHRING et al. 1978). STEINER et al. (1976) found similar results in Wistar rats, beagle dogs, and rhesus monkeys. When examining the urine, it was shown that only 0.1% of the dose is excreted as praziquantel (DIEKMANN and BÜHRING 1976), which indicates that the latter is rapidly metabolized. As soon as 4 h after oral treatment – the time of maximum serum-radioactivity – the amount of unchanged drug is less than 5% of the total radioactivity in the serum (BÜHRING et al. 1978). The major metabolites in serum and urine of man were, according to their mass spectra, predominantly hydroxylation products of praziquantel. In all metabolites with two or three hydroxy groups at least one hydroxy group is located in the cyclohexane ring (ring D). The other hydroxy groups are preferably located in ring B. The metabolism in man appeared to be independent of sex and dose and the metabolic pathway seems to be similar in man and rhesus monkey. In vitro studies with rat liver homogenates showed that the metabolism of praziquantel can be induced by phenobarbital (BÜHRING et al. 1978).

[^{14}C]Praziquantel is rapidly taken up by *Schistosoma mansoni* and not transformed metabolically (ANDREWS 1981). The binding of praziquantel in the tissues of *S. mansoni* appears to be easily reversible. Praziquantel is also rapidly taken up by *F. hepatica* and *H. diminuta* (ANDREWS 1981).

II. Toxicology

Praziquantel's acute toxicity tested in rats, mice, and rabbits is very low. The acute toxicity of praziquantel in female mice infected with *S. mansoni* was in the same range. The acute toxicity for dogs could not be evaluated owing to the emetic effect of higher doses (>200 mg/kg) of the compound in this species

(FROHBERG and SCHENCKING 1981). Rats tolerated daily oral doses of up to 1 g/kg for 4 weeks and dogs up to 180 mg/kg for 13 weeks without any organ damage.

Oral treatment of *S. mansoni*-infected mice with 1 × 250 mg praziquantel/kg resulted in a temporary elevation of plasma L-alanine: 2-oxoglutarate aminotransferase (GOT)- and L-aspartate: 2-oxoglutarate aminotransferase (GTP) activities on day 1 after treatment (ANDREWS et al. 1980). Values had returned to normal on day 5. Treatment also resulted in a slight but prolonged elevation of alkaline phosphatase activities, a high leukocyte count on day 5 after treatment and a normalization of the underweight and anemic state of the infected mice. ANDREWS et al. (1980) conclude that the changes observed can be regarded as secondary, reflecting host responses to damaged parasites and healing processes.

CHUBB et al. (1978) studied the effects of praziquantel on the isolated rat atria. Praziquantel produced a dose-dependent positive inotropic effect at concentrations between 10^{-6} and 5×10^{-4} *M*, with a maximum response occurring at 10^{-4} *M*. The inotropic action seems to result from alterations in calcium flux which is mediated by a mechanism other than adrenergic stimulation, Na^+, K^+ -adenosine triphosphatase inhibition, or cation ionophore translocation.

In daily oral doses up to 300 mg/kg, praziquantel had no effect on: male and female fertility, parturition and the newborn, lactation, weaning, postnatal development of the offspring, reproductive ability of the F_1 generation, and development of the F_2 generation in rats. Results so far give no indication of cancerogenic effects (FROHBERG and SCHENCKING 1981). Investigations on mutagenic potential revealed no mutagenic activity (reviewed by DAVIS et al. 1981).

III. Mode of Action

The primary point of attack seems to be the neuromuscular system (for review see ANDREWS 1981; VANDEN BOSSCHE et al. 1981). According to ANDREWS (1981) addition of 10^{-6} *M* praziquantel to *S. mansoni* caused instantaneous contraction of the parasite. It is interesting to note that the concentrations of praziquantel in the serum of animals and man receiving therapeutic doses are above the threshold of about 0.3 μg/ml plasma, which causes almost instantaneous contraction and paralysis of the parasites (ANDREWS 1981). According to PAX et al. (1978) and FETTERER et al. (1980a, b) the praziquantel-induced contracture of SCHISTOSOMA muscle is due to the ability of the drug to increase, nonspecifically, the permeability of the schistosome cells to Na^+ and Ca^{2+} ions. This increase in permeability results in an accumulation of Ca^{2+} within these cells, which triggers the cells to contract. COLES (1979) also suggested that in *S. mansoni* praziquantel opens pores in the membrane and permits a rapid influx of Ca^{2+} either directly or indirectly through an effect on the influx of Na^+.

In *Schistosoma*, the contraction is very rapid; half-maximal contraction was reached 11.2 s after the application of praziquantel at a concentration of 0.3 μg/ml (9.6×10^{-7} *M*) (ANDREWS 1981).

TERADA et al. (1982d) studied the in vitro effects of praziquantel on the motility of various cestodes, trematodes, and nematodes. In the presence of praziquantel the muscle system was paralyzed spastically at 10^{-8} *M* in *Taenia pisiformis;* at 10^{-7} *M* in *Dipylidium caninum* and *Paragonimus westermani;* and at

10^{-6} *M* in *Diplogonoporus grandis*, *Metagonimus yokogawai*, and *S. japonicum*. At much higher concentrations (10^{-4} *M*) *F. hepatica*, *Ancylostoma caninum*, and the isolated mouse ileum were also paralyzed. To affect the motility of *Angiostrongylus cantonensis* and *Trichuris vulpis* 2×10^{-4} and 3×10^{-4} *M* were needed.

The spastic paralysis must certainly be regarded as a "primary" effect of praziquantel. However, another "primary" effect of the pyrazino isoquinolone derivative has been discovered by ultrastructural investigations. In light and electron microscopic studies it was shown that the drug initiates a sudden vacuolization (within 5 min) of the tegument of *S. mansoni* (MEHLHORN et al. 1981). This vacuolization led to extensive lesions and finally to the complete destruction of the tegument of the parasites. The effects of praziquantel on the ultrastructure of trematodes pathogenic to man in Asia were also investigated (MEHLHORN et al. 1983). *Clonorchis sinensis*, *Opisthorchis viverrini*, and *S. japonicum* reacted with severe tegumental vacuolization within 5 min after exposure to 1 μg praziquantel/ml. In *M. yokogawai* the same degree of vacuolization was observed with 100 μg praziquantel/ml. *P. westermani* was the least sensitive: only very few vacuoles were formed after incubation in 100 μg/ml for 60 min. The authors assume that the thick tegument is responsible for the relative refractoriness to praziquantel in vitro. Another species against which the drug has no effect in vitro is *F. hepatica*, which possesses an equally thick tegument (MEHLHORN et al. 1983).

There is some evidence that vacuolization and contraction may be related phenomena. For example the time courses are similar: 11.2 s for half-maximal contraction and 10–20 s for vacuoles to appear. However, both processes are not identical. Vacuolization can be inhibited by media containing high Mg^{2+} but not by media free of Ca^{2+}. The initiation of contraction can be inhibited by both high Mg^{2+} content and media lacking Ca^{2+} (MEHLHORN et al. 1983).

The effects on the neuromuscular system and the induced tegumental lesions may be instrumental in the parasite's death. As soon as 4 h after treatment of mice, host cells of the defense system (eosinophilic granulocytes) are found attached to damaged regions of the schistosomal tegument; 24 h after treatment these cells have invaded the schistosomes in great number. It is hypothesized that vacuolization and the subsequent partial erosion of the tegument deprives schistosomes of their immunological escape mechanism and thus renders them susceptible to attack by host defense mechanisms (MEHLHORN et al. 1983).

FF. Pyrantel

Pyrantel (Fig. 32), 1,4,5,6-tetrahydro-1-methyl-2-[2-(2-thienyl)vinyl pyrimidine ($C_{11}H_{14}N_2S$; molecular weight, 206.3) is available as a pamoate salt ($C_{34}H_{30}N_2O_6S$; molecular weight, 594.69; Pfizer). It is a tasteless, yellow crystalline powder which is almost insoluble in water. It is also available as a tartrate ($C_{18}H_{20}N_2O_6S$; molecular weight, 392; Pfizer), which is soluble in water (180

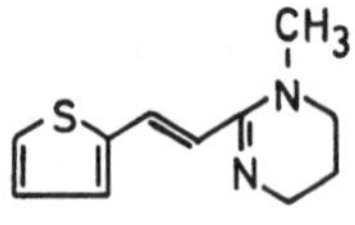

Fig. 32. Pyrantel

mg/ml). Pyrantel pamoate was synthesized in order to provide an anthelmintic that is poorly absorbed from the gut. Some 50%–70% of the ingested dose is excreted in the feces, and blood levels are not higher than 1 μg/ml (Davis 1973).

I. Pharmacology

Aubry et al. (1970) and Eyre (1970) studied the pharmacological properties of pyrantel tartrate.

Pyrantel showed activity characteristic of depolarizing neuromuscular-blocking agents on the rat phrenic nerve diaphragm preparation, chick semispinalis, and toad rectus abdominis muscles. The drug produced contraction of the guinea pig ileum, which was abolished by atropine, showing that muscarinic receptors were stimulated either directly or indirectly to induce contraction. It potentiated acetylcholine. Hexamethonium abolished the responses due to pyrantel, which suggests that pyrantel is acting by stimulating nicotinic receptors of the ganglionic synapses of the ileum.

High concentrations of pyrantel inhibit the acetylcholinesterase of sheep erythrocytes. It was a weaker inhibitor of the butylcholinesterase of horse plasma.

II. Toxicology

The oral LD_{50} in mice is 175 mg/kg and in rats 170 mg/kg. Daily administration of 20 mg/kg/day to dogs for 90 days produced no changes attributable to the drug. Dogs receiving daily doses of 50–75 mg/kg for 90 days showed sporadic symptoms including prostration, retching, and depressed respiration. One animal that died showed acute enteritis, fecal hemorrhage, and central nervous disturbance (O'Brien 1970).

The maximum tolerated oral dose of pyrantel tartrate in sheep is 175 mg/kg (Austin et al. 1966). The toxicity in adult sheep varies according to the method of administration of a solution of pyrantel tartrate in water (Cornwell 1966). Oral drenching with a 15% solution resulted in deaths at 200 mg/kg. Using a 5% solution, drenching with an esophageal tube gun, deaths occurred at 500 mg/kg but not at 400 mg/kg. With copper sulfate premedication to stimulate the closure of the esophageal groove, doses of 100 mg/kg were tolerated. A group of six sheep were given daily doses of 50 mg/kg every day for 1 week without ill effect. The drug is safe to use in pregnant ewes (Cornwell 1966).

III. Mode of Action (Aubry et al. 1970)

Pyrantel is, like levamisole, an anthelmintic that paralyzes nematodes. Pyrantel causes a slowly developing contracture of *Ascaris*-muscle preparations. It is more than 100 times more active than acetylcholine in this respect. Piperazine and (+)-tubocurarine block the responses to pyrantel. This antagonizing effect was not observed with *Ascaris*-muscle preparations treated with levamisole (Coles 1977). Pyrantel caused depolarization and increased spike discharge frequency in single muscle cells of *Ascaris*, an effect antagonized by piperazine (Aubry et al. 1970).

GG. Pyrvinium Pamoate

Pyrvinium pamoate (Fig. 33), or bis [6-(dimethylamino)-2-[2-(2,5-dimethyl-1-phenylpyrrol-3yl)vinyl]-1-methyl-quinolinium]4,4′-methylene bis (3-hydroxy-2-naphthoate), is a red tasteless powder which is practically insoluble in water (Park & Davis). Its molecular weight is 1151.4. Pyrvinium is almost not absorbed from the intestine (BUCHANAN et al. 1974; SMITH et al. 1976).

The activity of pyrvinium pamoate against *Enterobius vermicularis* is said to be due to inhibition of carbohydrate uptake (DAVIS 1973; BOTERO 1978).

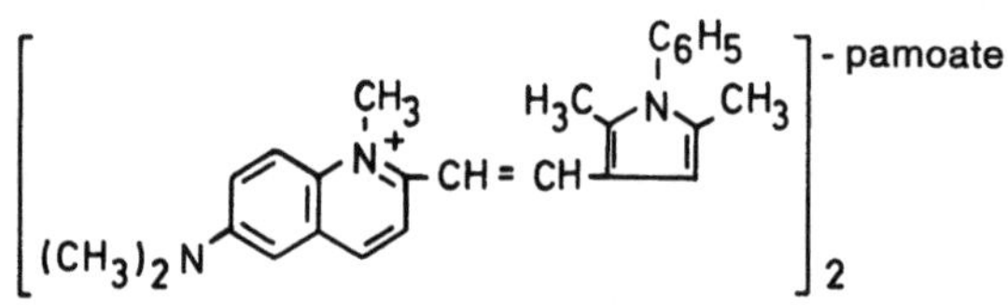

Fig. 33. Pyrvinium pamoate

HH. Rafoxanide

Rafoxanide (Flukanide) is the generic name for 3,5 diiodo 3′-chloro-4′-(*p*-chlorophenoxy)-salicylanilide (Fig. 34; Merck, Sharp, and Dohme). It is a colorless crystalline solid, moderately soluble in acetone and acetonitrile and insoluble in water (MROZIK et al. 1969). Its molecular weight is 626.01.

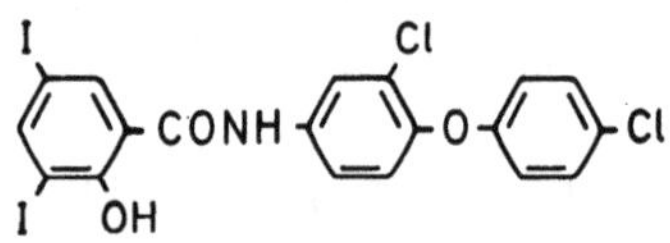

Fig. 34. Chemical structure of rafoxanide

I. Toxicology

Sheep suffering from liver fluke infection are less tolerant to drugs than are noninfected sheep. No deaths occurred among noninfected sheep given rafoxanide at a dose of 200 mg/kg. In infected sheep death occurred in some animals given 200 mg/kg but in none of those given 100 or 150 mg/kg. Some of the noninfected animals treated with 200 mg/kg and some of the infected animals treated with 100 mg/kg or more showed signs of ocular toxicity.

Calves naturally infected with liver fluke have tolerated dosages of 150 mg/kg repeated three times at monthly intervals with no signs of toxicity (MROZIK et al. 1969).

II. Mode of Action

Rafoxanide affects in vitro and in vivo, like the other salicylanilides (see, for example, closantel), mitochondrial phosphorylation in *F. hepatica* (CORNISH and

BRYANT 1976; CORNISH et al. 1977; PRICHARD 1978) and in vitro also that in *Ascaris* muscle (VANDEN BOSSCHE 1972 b).

The safety index is given in Table 2. More details on the effects of uncouplers on helminth metabolism are given in the chapters on, e.g., closantel, disophenol, and niclosamide.

II. Tetrachloroethylene

Tetrachloroethylene (C_2Cl_4) is an unsaturated halogenated hydrocarbon. It is a colorless nonflammable, volatile liquid, almost insoluble in water. It is decomposed slowly by light and various metals in the presence of moisture and forms phosgene (CCl_2O). Its molecular weight is 165.85.

The oral LD_{50} in mice in 8.85 g/kg. In the absence of alcohol or lipids and in a normal gastrointestinal system absorption is minimal. An elaborate survey can be found in DAVIS (1973) and CAVIER (1973).

JJ. Tiabendazole

Tiabendazole (thiabendazole) (Merck) or 2-(4-thiazolyl)-1*H*-benzimidazole (Fig. 35) was the first so-called broad-spectrum anthelmintic. The three-dimensional structure of tiabendazole is given in Fig. 36. It has a molecular weight of 201.26, is soluble in dimethylformamide, but it is only slightly soluble in alcohols, esters, and chlorinated hydrocarbons. Its maximal solubility in water at pH 2.2 is 3.8%. Tiabendazole is a chelating agent and forms stable complexes with a number of metals including iron. However, it does not bind calcium (ROBINSON et al. 1965).

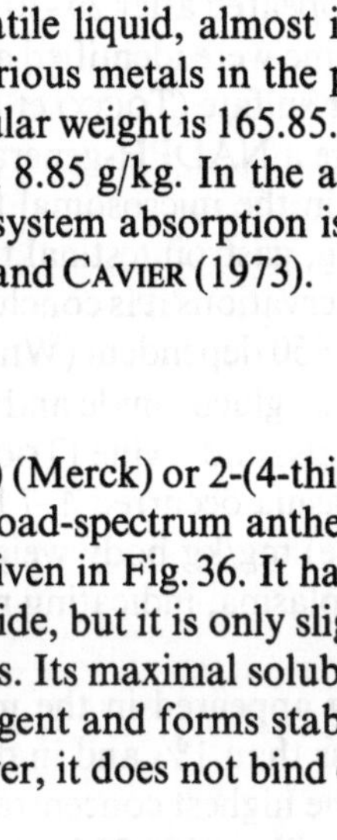

Fig. 35. Tiabendazole and 5-hydroxy tiabendazole

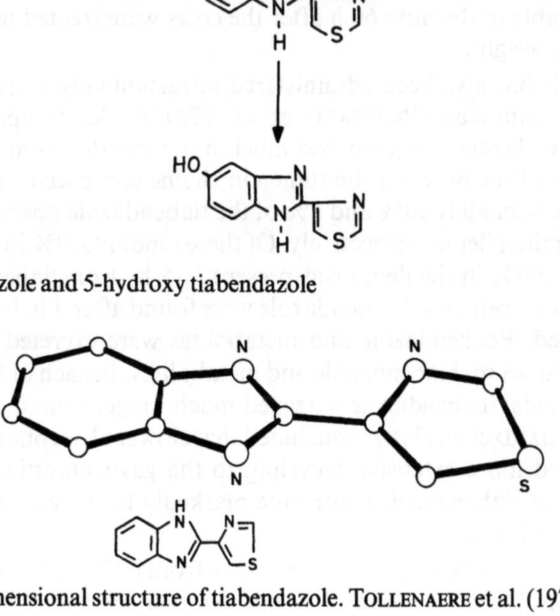

Fig. 36. Three-dimensional structure of tiabendazole. TOLLENAERE et al. (1979)

I. Pharmacokinetics

TOCCO et al. (1964) studied the absorption, excretion, metabolic transformation, tissue distribution, and retention of tiabendazole following oral administration of this anthelmintic at 50 mg/kg body weight to sheep. Peak plasma levels were found about 4 h after drug administration. Sheep excreted approximately 75% of the dose in the urine and 14% in the feces in 96 h. Tissue residues of radioactivity in eight lambs receiving 50 mg tiabendazole (^{14}C- or ^{35}S-labeled)/kg body weight were found to be extremely low in lambs killed 5, 8, or 16 days after dosing. No detectable residue in tissue appeared after 20–30 days.

Metabolites isolated from urine were identified as free 5-hydroxytiabendazole (Fig. 35) or as its glucuronide or sulfate (TOCCO et al. 1964). Tiabendazole 5-hydroxylation was found to require a NADPH-generating system and oxygen, was inhibited by CO, and occurred in the microsomal fraction of both rat liver and kidney but not in the heart, lung, gastrointestinal tract, or serum (WILSON et al. 1973). From these and other observations it is concluded that the 5-hydroxylation of tiabendazole is cytochrome P-450 dependent (WILSON et al. 1973).

5-Hydroxytiabendazole and its glucuronide and sulfate ester are also the only known metabolites in cattle, goats, and swine (TOCCO et al. 1965). In goats and cattle peak concentrations in plasma occurred 4–7 h after treatment with 50 and 100 (goats) or 50 and 200 (cattle) mg/kg body weight. Unchanged tiabendazole was essentially absent from the plasma, indicating rapid metabolism of the compound.

Small quantities of the drug appeared in the milk of dairy cows and goats (TOCCO et al. 1965). In goats less than 1% and in dairy cows about 0.1% of the dose was secreted in the milk. The highest concentration of tiabendazole and metabolites (90%) appeared in the milk within 24 h and residues were not detectable in milk 4 days after the goats were treated with 150 mg/kg. Tiabendazole residues were not detectable in the milk 60 h after the cows were treated with doses up to 220 mg/kg body weight.

Tiabendazole has also been administered intraruminally to cattle fitted with gastrointestinal cannulae (PRICHARD et al. 1981 b). As compared with fenbendazole, tiabendazole was absorbed much more rapidly from the rumen and only about 12% of the dose left the rumen in chyme compared with 30% of fenbendazole. Approximately 10% and 8% of the tiabendazole dose appeared at the pylorus and terminal ileum, respectively. Of these amounts, 9% in the abomasum and practically 100% in the ileum was present as 5-hydroxytiabendazole. Maximal plasma concentrations of tiabendazole were found after 4 h; for fenbendazole 24 h were needed. Fenbendazole and metabolites were excreted in urine much more rapidly than were thiabendazole and metabolites. In each of the gastrointestinal compartments, fenbendazole persisted much longer than did tiabendazole. Therefore, PRICHARD et al. (1981) concluded that slower absorption and excretion and the observed more extensive recycling to the gastrointestinal tract of fenbendazole than of tiabendazole contribute markedly to the greater anthelmintic potency of fenbendazole.

Incorporation of tiabendazole radioactivity from [^{3}H]tiabendazole into benzimidazole-susceptible or -resistant *Haemonchus contortus* and *Trichostrongylus colubriformis* was not significantly different when the drug was administered into the abomasum of sheep artificially infected with the nematodes (PRICHARD et al. 1978).

In vitro, *Nippostrongylus brasiliensis, F. hepatica,* and *Hymenolepis diminuta* concentrate tiabendazole 60, 2.8, and 2.4 times respectively (COLES 1977). The high concentration of tiabendazole found in *N. brasiliensis* may reflect its high sensitivity to this benzimidazole derivative.

II. Toxicology (ROBINSON et al. 1965)

Studies on the acute toxicity in mice, rats, and rabbits have shown that oral treatment with tiabendazole is well tolerated. The LD_{50}s were 3.6, 3.1, and >3.8 g/kg respectively when tiabendazole was administered orally as a suspension.

Single oral doses of 200 mg/kg or more caused emesis in most dogs, and because of this effect the acute oral toxicity could not be determined in dogs. Intravenous injection of 25 mg/kg or more at a rate of 2.5 mg/kg/min caused vomiting and transient ataxia shortly after the injection was completed.

Except for a modest increase in the rate of weight gain noted in both male and female rats at 100 and 400 mg/kg dose levels fed by gavage for 30 days, there were no outward signs of toxicity. At 800 mg/kg there was a marked suppression of weight gain and a 30% mortality.

All rats treated by gavage with tiabendazole at dose levels ranging between 12.5 and 400 mg/kg for 180 days survived treatment. A daily dose of 200 mg/kg caused no depression in rate of weight gain in female rats and even at the 400-mg/kg level the difference in the weight curves between the controls and treated animals was not striking. In contrast, in male rats, dose levels of 200 mg/kg or more significantly affected the rate of weight gain. However, except for the foregoing effects on weight, there were no outward signs of toxicity in any of the treated rats.

None of the dogs treated orally with 20, 100, or 200 mg/kg tiabendazole daily, 7 days/week over a period of 2 years or more, died as a result of treatment. Except for an occasional episode of vomiting during the early phase of the study, there were no outward signs of toxicity.

In conclusion: acute, subacute, and chronic oral toxicity studies have proved tiabendazole to be well tolerated in rats and dogs.

III. Mode of Action

It has been shown that tiabendazole affects the fumarate reductase system in *Haemonchus contortus, F. hepatica,* and *Hymenolepis diminuta* (PRICHARD 1970, 1973, 1974; MALKIN and CAMACHO 1972; ROMANOWSKI et al. 1975; COLES 1977). The fumarate reductase system is an essential component of carbohydrate metabolism in many parasitic stages of helminths (for a review see BARRETT 1981). However, *N. brasiliensis,* being susceptible to tiabendazole, is an aerobic metabolizing organism (SAZ et al. 1971) in which until now no significant fumarate reductase activity has been found (COLES 1977). Therefore it appears unlikely that inhibition of the fumarate reductase system alone is at the origin of the anthelmintic activity of tiabendazole.

At high concentration, tiabendazole affects the polymerization of bovine brain tubulin. Fifty percent inhibition was achieved at 5.49×10^{-4} *M* (IRELAND et al. 1979). Tiabendazole also binds to fungal tubulin, a property common to the benzimidazole carbamate, nocodazole (DAVIDSE 1976, 1978).

The appearance of large numbers of autophagic vacuoles in the cytoplasm of the intestinal cells of *Aspiculuris tetraptera* after treatment of the mice host with both tiabendazole and mebendazole (COMLEY 1980) is similar to the formation of these vacuoles in the intestinal cell of *Ascaris suum* and *Syngamus trachea* observed after treatment of pig and turkey hosts with mebendazole (BORGERS and DE NOLLIN 1975; BORGERS et al. 1975a). The latter authors suggest that the formation of such autophagic vacuoles is the result of the intracellular release of hydrolytic enzymes from secretory granules accumulating in the cytoplasm as a result of the mebendazole-induced disappearance of cytoplasmic microtubules. Although further studies are needed, the binding to tubulin suggests that the anthelmintic activity of tiabendazole may originate from the same mechanism as described for mebendazole and other benzimidazole carbamate derivatives.

It is of interest to note that in the cambendazole-sensitive strain of *Haemonchus contortus* tiabendazole (5 m*M*) depressed ethanol, propanol, acetate, and propionate accumulation by 42%. However, in the cambendazole-resistant strain the accumulation of the end products of glucose catabolism increased by 50% when the worms were exposed to tiabendazole in vitro and 80% when exposed in vivo (REW et al. 1982). Thus resistance appeared to be associated with the ability to increase the carbon flow in the presence of tiabendazole (REW et al. 1982).

KK. Thiophanate

Thiophanate (May & Baker), or diethyl 4,4′-*O*-phenylene bis (3-thioallophanate) (Fig. 37), is a white crystalline solid that is virtually insoluble in water (molecular weight, 370.44) (EICHLER 1973). Both thiophanate and methylthiophanate [1,2 bis (3-methoxycarbonylthioureido)benzene] (Fig. 37) were introduced in 1970 for the control of fungal diseases in plants. Methylthiophanate is soluble in acetone, methanol, and chloroform. It is slightly soluble in other organic liquids and insoluble in water.

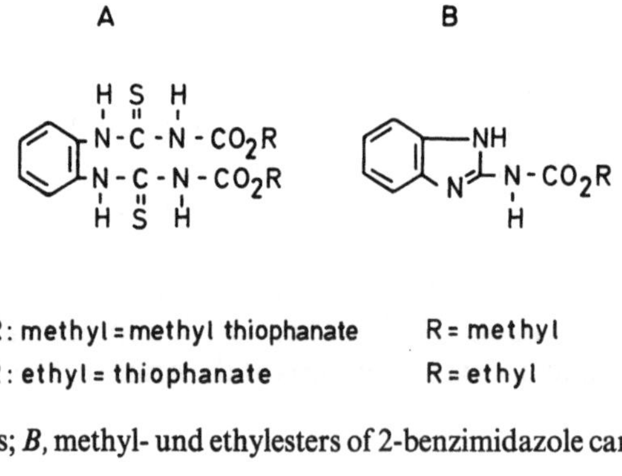

Fig. 37. *A*, thiophanates; *B*, methyl- und ethylesters of 2-benzimidazole carbamic acid

I. Pharmacokinetics

Thiophanate is a benzimidazole precursor. SELLING et al. (1970) found that methylthiophanate can be converted into the fungicide 2-benzimidazole carbamic acid methyl ester (BCM) and thiophanate is the ethyl analogue of BCM. BCM appears to be the only fungitoxic compound present in plants treated with benomyl (1[butylamino)carbonyl]-1*H*-[benzimidazole-2-yl] carbamic acid methyl ester).

The anthelmintic activity of thiophanate might be related to cyclization to the active moiety, 2-benzimidazole carbamic acid ethyl ester.

II. Toxicology

Oral LD_{50}s for thiophanate in mice and rats are > 15 g/kg (EICHLER 1973). When administered to cattle and sheep as a single dose of 1,000 mg/kg, which is 13–14 times the median standard dose (75 mg/kg), this compound was well tolerated. Death occurred among sheep dosed up to 2 g/kg; calves were not seriously affected at 5 g/kg (EICHLER 1974). Analyses of blood and urine and histopathological examination of the kidneys of sheep treated with five daily doses of 100 mg/kg thiophanate indicated transient dysfunction, but a single dose of 500 mg/kg produced no effect, probably due to a smaller proportion of thiophanate being absorbed when administered as a single dose. According to EICHLER (1974) renal failure was the most probable cause of death in sheep.

The oral LD_{50}s of methylthiophanate in female rats, mice, guinea pigs, and rabbits are 6.6, 3.4, 6.7, and 2.5 g/kg respectively. In dogs the minimal lethal dose (oral) is 4 g/kg (HASHIMOTO et al. 1972).

References

Actor P, Anderson EL, Dicuollo CJ, Ferlanto RJ, Hoover JRE, Pagano JF, Ravin LR, Scheidy SF, Stedman RJ, Theodorides VJ (1967) New broad spectrum anthelmintic, methyl 5(6)-butyl-2-benzimidazolecarbamate. Nature 215:321–322

Aldridge WN, Holmstedt B (1981) History and scope of the conference. Acta Pharmacol Toxicol [Suppl V] 49:3–6

Andrews P (1981) A summary of the efficacy of praziquantel against schistosomes in animal experiments and notes on its mode of action. Arzneimittelforsch 31:538–541

Andrews P, Thomas H (1983) Praziquantel. Medical Research Reviews 3:147–200

Andrews P, Dycka J, Frank G (1980) Effect of praziquantel on clinical-chemical parameters in healthy and schistosome-infected mice. Ann Trop Med Parasitol 74:167–177

Aronson CE, Serlick ER (1977) Effects of disophenol on the isolated perfused rat heart. Biochem Pharmacol 26:2297–2305

Aubry ML, Cowell P, Davey MJ, Shevde S (1970) Aspects of the pharmacology of a new anthelmintic: pyrantel. Br J Pharmacol 38:332–344

Austin WC, Courtney W, Danilewicz JC, Margan DH, Conover LH, Howes HL, Lynch JE, McFarland JW, Cornwell RL, Theodorides VJ (1966) Pyrantel tartrate, a new anthelmintic effective against infections of domestic animals. Nature 212:1273–1274

Averkin EA, Beard CC, Dvorak CA, Edwards JA, Fried JH, Kilan JG, Schiltz RA, Kistner TP, Drudge JH, Lyons ET, Sharp NL, Corwin RM (1975) Methyl 5(6)-phenylsulfinyl-2-benzimidazole carbamate. A new potent anthelmintic. J Med Chem 11:1164–1166

Barett J (1981) Biochemistry of parasitic helminths. Macmillan, London

Behm CA, Bryant C (1979) Anthelmintic action. A metabolic approach. Vet Parasitol 5:39–49

Bellander BTD, Hagmar LE, Österdahl BG (1981) Nitrosation of piperazine in the stomach. Lancet 2:372

Borgers M, Nollin S de (1975) Ultrastructural changes in *Ascaris suum* intestine after mebendazole treatment in vivo. J Parasitol 61:110–122
Borgers M, Thoné F (1976) Further characterization of phosphatase activities using non-specific substrates. Histochem J 8:301–317
Borgers M, Nollin S de, Verheyen A, Brabander M de, Thienpont D (1975a) Effects of new anthelmintics on the microtubular system of parasites. In: Borgers M, Brabander M de (eds) Microtubules and microtubule inhibitors. Elsevier, Amsterdam, pp 497–508
Borgers M, Nollin S de, Verheyen A, Vanparys O, Thienpont D (1975b) Morphological changes in cysticerci of *Taenia taeniaeformis* after mebendazole treatment. J Parasitol 61:830–843
Borgers M, Nollins S de, Brabander M de, Thienpont D (1975c) Influence of the anthelmintic mebendazole on microtubules and intracellular organelle movement in nematode intestinal cells. Am J Vet Res 36:1153–1166
Botero DR (1978) Chemotherapy of human intestinal parasitic diseases. Ann Rev Pharmacol Toxicol 18:1–15
Boyd JE, Bullock NW, Champagne DA, Gotterdam PE, Morici IJ, Plaisted PH, Spicer LD, Wayne RS, Zulalian J (1969) Metabolism of L-tetramisole in rats. In: 158th National meeting of the American Chemical Society, New York, 7–12 September
Brodie RR, Mayo BC, Chasseaud LF, Hawkings DR (1977) The disposition of radioactivity after administration of the anthelmintic methyl-14*C*-5-cyclopropylcarbonyl-2-benzimidazole carbamate (ciclobendazole) to rats and dogs. Arzneimittelforsch 27:593–598
Broome AWJ (1962) Mechanisms of anthelmintic action with particular reference to drugs affecting neuromuscular activity. In: Goodwin LG, Nimmo-Smith RM (eds) Drugs, parasites and hosts. Churchill, London, pp 43–61
Bryant C, Cornish RA, Rahman MS (1976) Adenine nucleotides as indicators of anthelmintic efficacy. In: Bossche H vanden (ed) Biochemistry of parasites and host-parasite relationships, Elsevier, Amsterdam, pp 599–604
Bryceson ADM, Woestenborghs R, Michiels M, Bossche H vanden (1982) Bioavailability and tolerability of mebendazole in patients with inoperable hydatid disease. Trans R Soc Trop Med Hyg 16:563–564
Buchanan RA, Barrow WB, Heffelfinger JC, Kinkel AW, Smith TC, Turner JC (1974) Pyrvinium pamoate. Clin Pharmacol Ther 16:716–719
Bueding E (1969) Some biochemical effects of anthelmintic drugs. Biochem Pharmacol 18:1541–1547
Bueding E, Liu CL, Rogers SH (1972) Inhibition by metrifonate and dichlorvos of cholinesterases in schistosomes. Br J Pharmacol 46:480–487
Bueding E, Batzinger R, Petterson G (1976) Antischistosomal and some toxicological properties of a nitrodiphenylaminoisothiocyanate (C 9330-GO/CGP 4540). Experientia 32:604–606
Bühring KU, Diekmann HW, Müller H, Garbe A, Nowak H (1978) Metabolism of praziquantel in man. Eur J Drug Metab Pharmacokinet 3:179–190
Burg RW, Miller BM, Baker EE, Birnbaum J, Currie SA, Hartman R, Kong YL, Monaghan RL, Olson G, Putter I, Tunac JB, Wallick H, Stapley EO, Oiwa R, Omura S (1979) Avermectins, new family of potent anthelmintic agents: producing organism and fermentation. Antimicrob Agents Chemother 15:361–367
Campbell AJ, Montague PE (1981) A comparison of the activity of uncouplers of oxidative phosphorylation against the common liver fluke *Fasciola hepatica*. Mol Biochem Parasitol 4:139–147
Campbell WC (1981) An introduction to the avermectins. NZ Vet J 29:174–178
Castañer J (1978) Febantel – veterinary anthelmintic. Drugs of the future 3:377–378
Cavier R (1973) Chemotherapy of intestinal nematodes. In: Cavier R, Hawking F (eds) Chemotherapy of helminthiasis, vol 1. Pergamon, Oxford, pp 215–436
Cavier R. Hawking F (eds) (1973) Chemotherapy of helminthiasis. Pergamon, Oxford
Christ O, Kellner H-M, Klöpffer G (1974) Studies on pharmacokinetics and metabolism with fenbendazole – a new anthelmintic. In: Proceedings 3rd international congress of parasitology, vol 3. Facta Publication, Vienna, pp 1448–1449

Chubb JM, Bennett JL, Akera T, Brody TM (1978) Effects of praziquantel, a new anthelmintic, on electromechanical properties of isolated rat atria. J Pharmacol Exp Ther 207:284–293

Coles GC (1977) The biochemical mode of action of some modern anthelmintics. Pestic Sci 8:536–543

Coles GC (1979) The effect of praziquantel on *Schistosoma mansoni*. J Helminthol 53:31–33

Coles GC, East JM, Jenkins SN (1975) The mechanism of action of the anthelmintic levamisole. Gen Pharmacol 6:309–313

Comley JCW (1980) Ultrastructure of the intestinal cells of *Aspiculuris tetraptera* after in vivo treatment of mice with mebendazole and thiabendazole. Int J Parasitol 10:143–150

Cornish RA, Bryant C (1976) Changes in energy metabolism due to anthelmintics in *Fasciola hepatica* maintained in vitro. Int J Parasitol 6:393–398

Cornish RA, Behm CA, Butler RW, Bryant C (1977) The in vivo effects of rafoxanide on the energy metabolism of *Fasciola hepatica*. Int J Parasitol 7:217–220

Cornwell RL (1966) Controlled laboratory trials in sheep with the anthelmintic pyrantel tartrate. Vet Rec 79:590–595

Cross BG, David A, Vallance DK (1954) Piperazine adipate: a new anthelmintic agent. J Pharm Pharmacol 6:711–717

Davidse LC (1976) The antimitotic properties of the benzimidazole fungicide carbendazim and a mechanism of resistance to this compound in *Aspergillus nidulans*. Thesis, Landbouwhogeschool, Binnenhaven 9, Wageningen

Davidse LC, Flach W (1978) Interaction of thiabendazole with fungal tubulin. Biochim Biophys Acta 543:82–90

Davis A (1973) Drug treatment in intestinal helminthiases. World Health Organization, Geneva

Davis A (1975) Clinical available antischistosomal drugs. J Toxicol Environ Health 1:191–201

Davis A, Biles JE, Ulrich AM, Dixon H (1981) Tolerance and efficacy of praziquantel in phase II A and II B therapeutic trials in Zambian patients. Arzneimittelforsch 31:568–574

Degremont A, Stahel E (1978) Klinische Bewertung von Ciclobendazol (C-C 2481) bei der Behandlung von Wurmkrankungen des Darmes. Schweiz Med Wochenschr 108:1430–1433

Delatour P, Burgat-Sacaze V (1981) Vers une procedure alternative d'évaluation toxicologique des résidus? Application aux anthelminthiques dérivés du benzimidazole. Recl Med Vet 157:213–218

Delatour P, Lorgue G, Lapras M, Deschanel J-P (1974) Propriétés embryotoxiques (rat) et résidus (ovins, bovins) de trois anthelmintiques dérivés du benzimidazole. Bull Soc Sci Vét Méd Comp 76:147–154

Delatour P, Lorgue G, Lapras M, Richard Y (1976a) Propriétés embryotoxiques et antimitotiques du parbendazole, mebendazole et du cambendazole. CR Séances Acad Sci 282:517–518

Delatour P, Lorgue G, Courtot D, Lapras M (1976b) Tolerance embryonaire de l'oxibendazole chez le rat et le mouton. Recl Med Vet 152:467–470

Delatour P, Debroye J, Lorgue G, Courtot D (1977) Embryotoxicité experimentale de l'oxfendazole chez le rat et le mouton. Recl Med Vet 153:639–645

Del Castillo J (1969) Pharmacology of nematoda. In: Florkin M, Scheer BT (eds) Chemical zoology, vol 3. Academic, New York, pp 521–554

Demoen P, Aelst C van, Loomans J, Verhaegen H, Cree J de, Verbruggen F, Ringoir S (1973) The absorption and urinary excretion of mebendazole after oral administration. In: Clin Res Report, R 17 635/36 Janssen Pharmaceutica, Beerse

De Nollin S, Bossche H vanden (1973) Biochemical effects of mebendazole on *Trichinella spiralis* larvae. J Parasitol 59:970–976

Dicuollo CJ, Miller JA, Colman WF, Kraeer PM, Wong MY (1977) Albendazole metabolic and tissue residue studies in sheep and cattle. In: Proceeding of the 8th international conference of WAAVP, Sydney Juli (Abstract)

Diekmann HW, Bühring KU (1976) The fate of praziquantel in the organism III. Metabolism in rat, beagle dog and rhesus monkey. Eur J Drug Metab Pharmacokinet 2:107–112

Druckrey M, Preussman R, Ivankovic S, Schmähl D (1967) Organotrope carcinogene Wirkungen bei 65 verschiedenen *N*-Nitroso-Verbindungen an BD-Ratten. Z Krebsforsch 69:103–201

Drugs of Today vol 17 (1981) Oxantel pamoate/pyrantel pamoate. In: Leeson PA, Mealy NE (eds) JR Prous, SA, Barcelona, pp 41–42

Düwel D (1977) Fenbendazole. Biological properties and activity. Pest Sci 8:550–555

Düwel D (1979) Summary and evaluation of the worldwide published investigations. Hoechst, Frankfurt

Düwel D, Schleich H (1978) In vivo investigations on the mode of action of fenbendazole. Zentralbl Veterinaermed [B] 25:800–805

Düwel D, Hajdu P, Damm D (1975) Zur Pharmakokinetic von Fenbendazol. Berl Munch Tierärztl Wochenschr 88:131–134

Düwel D, Aguilar FJ, Batte EG, Bürger HJ, Thomas RJ, Zahner H (1981) Therapy in nematode and acanthocephalan infections. In: Slusarski W (ed) Review of advances in parasitology. PWN, Warszawa, pp 507–524

Dunn GL, Gallagher G, Davis LD, Hoover JRE, Stedman RJ (1973) Metabolites of methyl 5(6)-butyl-2-benzimidazole carbamate (parbendazole) structure and synthesis. J Med Chem 16:996–1002

Egerton JR, Campbell WC (1970) The efficacy of 5-isopropoxy-carbonylamino-2-(4-thiazolyl) benzimidazole against helminths of sheep. Res Vet Sci 11:193–195

Egerton JR, Ostlind DA, Blair LS, Eary CH, Suhoyda D, Cifelli S, Riek RF, Campbell WC (1979) Avermectins, new family of potent anthelmintic agents: efficacy of the B^{1a} component. Antimicrob Agents Chemother 15:372–378

Eichler DA (1973) The anthelmintic activity of thiophanate in sheep and cattle. Br Vet J 129:533–543

Eichler DA (1974) The toxicity of thiophanate ("Nemafax") in sheep and cattle. Br Vet J 130:570–576

Eyre P (1970) Some pharmacodynamic effects of the nematodes: methyridine, tetramisole and pyrantel. J Pharm Pharmacol 22:26–36

Fetterer RH, Pax RA, Thompson D, Bricker C, Bennett JL (1980a) Praziquantel: mode of its antischistosomal action. In: Bossche H vanden (ed) The host invader interplay. Elsevier, Amsterdam, pp 695–698

Fetterer RH, Pax RA, Bennett JL (1980b) Praziquantel, potassium and 2,4-dinitrophenol: analysis of their action on the musculature of *Schistosoma mansoni*. Eur J Pharmacol 64:31–38

Friedman PA, Platzer EG (1978) Interaction of anthelmintic benzimidazoles and benzimidazole derivatives with bovine brain tubulin. Biochim Biophys Acta 544:605–614

Friedman PA, Platzer EG (1980a) The molecular mechanism of action of benzimidazoles in embryos of *Ascaris suum*. In: Bossche H vanden (ed) The host invader interplay. Elsevier, Amsterdam, pp 595–604

Friedman PA, Platzer EG (1980b) Interaction of anthelmintic benzimidazoles with *Ascaris suum* embryonic tubulin. Biochim Biophys Acta 630:271–278

Fritz LC, Wang CC, Gorio A (1979) Avermectin B^{1a} irreversibly blocks postsynaptic potentials at the bolster neuromuscular junction by reducing muscle membrane resistance. Proc Natl Acad Sci USA 76:2062–2066

Frohberg H, Schencking MS (1981) Toxicological profile of praziquantel, a new drug against cestode and schistosome infections, as compared to some other schistosomicides. Arzneimittelforsch 31:555–565

Garcia EG (1976) Treatment for trichuriasis with oxantel. Am J Trop Med Hyg 25:914–915

Garcia H, Keefer L, Lyinsky W, Wenyon CEM (1970) Carcinogenicity of nitrosothiomorpholine and 1 nitrosopiperazine in rats. Z Krebsforsch 74:179–184

Garin JP, Kalb JC, Despeignes J, Vincent G (1970) Action des antibiotiques oligo-saccharides sur *Taenia saginata*. J Parasitol 56:112 (No 4, section II, part 1)

Gönnert R, Andrews P (1977) Praziquantel, a new broad-spectrum antischistostomal agent. Z Parasitenkd 52:129–150
Gönnert R, Johannis J, Schraufstätter E, Strufe R (1963) Konstitution und Cestocide Wirkung in der Yomesan-Reiche. In: Medizin und Chemie. Bayer, Leverkusen, pp 540–567
Goodwin LG (1980) New drugs for old diseases. Trans R Soc Trop Med Hyg 74:1–7
Graziani G, Martin GL de (1977 a) Pharmacokinetic studies on levamisole. Drugs Exp Clin Res 2:221–223
Graziani G, Martin GL de (1977 b) Pharmacokinetic studies on levamisole: on the pharmacokinetics and relative bioavailability of levamisole in man. Drugs Exp Clin Res 2:235–240
Hall CA, Kelly JD, Campbell NJ, Whitlock HV, Martin ICA (1978) The dose response of several benzimidazole anthelmintics against resistant strains of *Haemonchus contortus* and *Trichostrongylus colubriformis* selected with thiabendazole. Res Vet Sci 25:364–367
Hamajima F (1973) Studies on metabolism of lung fluke genus *Paragonimus*. VII. Action of bithionol on glycolytic and oxidative metabolism of adult worms. Exp Parasitol 34:1–11
Hashimoto Y, Makita T, Ohnuma N, Noguchi T (1972) Acute toxicity on dimethyl 4,4′-*O* phenylene bis (3-thioallophanate), thiophanate-methyl fungicide. Toxicol Appl Pharmacol 23:606–615
Hecht G, Gloxhuber Chr (1960) Experimentelle Untersuchungen mit *N*-(2′-Chlor-4′-Nitrophenyl)-5-Chlorsalicylamid, einem neuen Bandwurmmittel: toxicologische Untersuchungen. Arzneimittelforsch 10:884–885
Hefferren JJ, Schrotenboer G, Wolman W (1955) Preparation and properties of citric acid and tartaric acid and salts of piperazine. J Am Pharmacol Assoc 44:678–682
Heykants J (1972) The excretion and metabolism of mebendazole (R 17 635) in the dog. In: Biol Res Report, serial no R 17 635/3. Janssen Pharmaceutica, Beerse
Hoebeke J, Neyen G van, Brabander M de (1976) Interaction of oncodazole (R17 934) a new anti-tumoral drug, with rat brain tubulin. Biochem Biophys Res Commun 69:319–324
Hoff DR, Fisher MH, Bochis RJ, Lusi A, Waksmunski F, Egerton JR, Yakstis JJ, Cuckler AC, Campbell WC (1970) A new broad-spectrum anthelmintic: 2-(4-thiazolyl)-5 isopropoxycarbonylamino-benzimidazole. Experientia 26:550–551
Hogg RA (1978) Death after cambendazole dosing. Vet Rec (Nov 18):477–478
Ireland M, Gull K, Gutteridge WE, Pogson CI (1979) The interaction of benzimidazole carbamates with mammalian microtubule protein. Biochem Pharmacol 28:2680–2682
Janssen PAJ (1976) The levamisole story. In: Jucker E (ed) Progress research, vol 20. Birkhäuser, Basel, pp 347–383
Janssen Pharmaceutica (1972) Mebendazole synopsis. Beerse
Johns DJ, Philip JR (1977) Albendazole: safety in sheep. Abstr Pap 8th Int Conf For Adv of Vet Par, Sydney
Junod Ch (1965) Essai de traitement de la trichocéphalose par la diphétarsone. Bull Soc Pathol Exot Filiales 58:653–660
Kaiser JA (1964) Studies on the toxicity of disophenol (2,6-diiodo-4-nitrophenol) to dogs and rodents plus some comparisons with 2,4-dinitrophenol. Toxicol Appl Pharmacol 6:232–244
Kane HJ, Behm CA, Bryant C (1980) Metabolic studies on the new fasciolicidal drug, closantel. Mol Biochem Parasitol 1:347–355
Kass IS, Wang CC, Walrond JP, Stretton AOW (1980) Avermectin B^{1a}, a paralyzing anthelmintic that affects interneurons and inhibitory motoneurons in *Ascaris*. Proc Natl Acad Sci USA 77:6211–6215
Kaushik RK, Katiyar JC, Sen AB (1974) Studies on the mode of action of anthelmintics with *Ascaridia galli* as the test parasite. Indian J Med Res 62:1367–1375
Köhler P, Bachmann R (1980) The possible mode of action of mebendazole in *Ascaris suum*. In: Bossche H vanden (ed) The host invader interplay. Elsevier, Amsterdam, pp 727–730
Köhler P, Bachmann R (1981) Intestinal tubulin as possible target for the chemotherapeutic action of mebendazole in parasitic nematodes. Mol Biochem Parasitol 4:325–336

Lapras M, Deshanel JP, Delatour R, Gastellu J, Lombard M (1973) Accidents tératologiques chez le mouton après administration de parbendazole. Bull Soc Sci Vét Méd Comp 75:53–61
Machemer L (1981) Chronic toxicity of metrifonate. Acta Pharmacol Toxicol [Suppl V] 43:15–28
Malkin MF, Camacho RM (1977) The effect of thiabendazole on fumarate reductase from thiabendazole-sensitive and resistant *Haemonchus conturtus*. J Parasitol 58:845–846
Marriner SE, Bogan JA (1980) Pharmacokinetics of albendazole in sheep. Am J Vet Res 41:1126–1129
Marriner SE, Bogan JA (1981) Pharmacokinetics of oxfendazole in sheep. Am J Vet Res 42:1143–1145
Marsboom R (1973) Toxicological studies on mebendazole. Toxicol Appl Pharmacol 24:371–377
McCracken RO, Stillwell WH, Hudson HM (1982) A possible biochemical mode of action of benzimidazole anthelmintics. Mol Biochem Parasitol [Suppl] 726
Mehlhorn H, Becker B, Andrews P, Thomas H, Frenkel JK (1981) In vivo and in vitro experiments on the effects of praziquantel on *Schistosoma mansoni*. A light and electron microscopic study. Arzneimittelforsch 31:544–554
Mehlhorn H, Kojima S, Rim HJ, Ruenwongsa P, Andrews P, Thomas H, Bunnag B (1983) Ultrastructural investigations on the effects of praziquantel on human trematodes from Asia: *Clonorchis sinensis, Metagonimus Yokogawai, Opisthorchis viverrini, Paragonimus westermani* and *Schistosoma japonicum*. Arzneimittelforsch 33:91–98
Merck (1981) Ivermectin, annotated bibliography, June. Darmstadt
Metcalf RL, Fukuto RB, March RB (1959) Toxic action of Dipterex® and DDVP to the house fly. J Econ Entomol 52:44–49
Metzger H, Düwel D (1974) The development of anthelmintics, based on investigation of metabolism of the liver fluke (*Fasciola hepatica*). Proceedings of the third international congress of parasitology, vol 3, pp 1444–1449. Abstract No. E8(4). Facta publication, Vienna
Meuldermans WEG, Hurkmans RMA, Lauwers WFJ, Heykants JJP (1976) The in vitro metabolism of mebendazole in pig, rat, and dog liver fractions. Eur J Drug Metab Pharmacokinet 1:35–40
Meuldermans W, Hurkmans R, Swijsen E, Heykants J (1977) A comparative study on the excretion and metabolism of flubendazole (R 17 889) and mebendazole (R 17 635) in the rat. In: Preclin Res Report, R 17 889/5. Janssen Pharmaceutica Beerse
Michiels M, Woestenborghs R, Heykants J (1977a) On the absorption and distribution of closantel (R 31 520) in sheep after oral and intramuscular administration. Janssen Research Products Information Service, Beerse
Michiels M, Heykants J, Sneyers R, Wynants J, Marsboom R (1977b) Residual tissue levels of flubendazole in the pig after a single oral administration. In: Preclin Res Report, R 17 889/6. Janssen Pharmaceutica Beerse
Michiels M, Woestenborghs R, Heykants J (1978) Plasma concentrations of closantel in cattle after a single intramuscular or subcutaneous administration. Janssen Research Products Information Service, Beerse
Michiels M, Hendriks R, Heykants J, Bossche H vanden (1982) The pharmacokinetics of mebendazole and flubendazole in animals and man. Arch Int Pharmacodyn Ther 256:180–191
Mirvish SS (1975) Formation of *N*-nitroso compounds: chemistry, kinetics, and in vivo occurrence. Toxicol Appl Pharmacol 31:325–351
Miko M, Chance B (1975) Isothiocyanates, a new class of uncouplers. Biochim Biophys Acta 396:165–174
Moreno MS, Barrett J (1979) Monoamine oxidase in adult *Hymenolepis diminuta* (Cestoda). Parasitology 78:1–5
Mrozik H, Jones H, Friedman J, Schwartzkopf G, Schardt RA, Patchett AA, Hoff DR, Yakstis JJ, Riek RF, Ostlind DA, Plishker GA, Butler RW, Cuckler AC, Campbell WC (1969) A new agent for the treatment of liver fluke infection (fascioliasis). Experientia 25:883

Münst GJ, Kalaganis G, Bircher J (1980) Plasma concentrations of mebendazole during treatment of echinococcosis. Preliminary results. Eur J Clin Pharmacol 17:375–378

Niemegeers CJE (1976) Acute intramuscular and oral toxicity of R 31 520 in mice and rats. Janssen Research Products Information Service

Nordgren I, Bengtsson E, Holmstedt B, Pettersson B-M (1981) Levels of metrifonate and dichlorvos in plasma and erythrocytes during treatment of schistosomiasis with Bilarcil®. Acta Pharmacol Toxicol [Suppl V] 49:79–86

Norton S, Beer EJ de (1957) Investigations on the action of piperazine on *Ascaris lumbricoides*. Am J Trop Med Hyg 6:898–905

O'Brien JJ (1970) Toxicological aspects of some modern anthelmintics. Aust Vet J 46:297–300

Oelkers H-A (1959) Die Chemotherapie der Wurmkrankheiten. In: Jucker E (ed) Progress in drug research, vol 1. Birkhäuser, Basel, pp 159–242

Osteux R, Guerrin F, Lesieur-Demarquilly I (1971) Mode d'action de la pipérazine sur *Ascaris lumbricoides* var. *suum*. II. Etude des contractions musculaires de l'*Ascaris* en présence de pipérazine, de coenzyme A et de l'adénosine-triphosphate. Ann Pharm Fr 29:173–178

Pax RA, Bennett JL, Fetterer RH (1978) A benzodiazepine derivative and praziquantel: effects on musculature of *Schistosoma mansoni* and *Schistosoma japonicum*. Naunyn Schmiedebergs Arch Pharmacol 304:309–315

Phillips JL, Sturman G, West GB (1976) The interaction between anthelmintic drugs and histamine in *Ascaris suum*. Br J Pharmacol 57:417–420

Pong S-S, Wang CC (1979) Specific binding of avermectin B^{1a} to brain synaptosomes. In: Abstract 11th international congress of biochemistry, Toronto, July.

Pong S-S, Wang CC (1980) The specificity of high-affinity binding of avermectin B^{1a} to mammalian brain. Neuropharmacology 19:311–317

Pong S-S, Wang CC, Fritz LC (1980) Studies on the mechanism of action of avermectin B^{1a}: stimulation of release of γ-aminobutyric acid from brain synaptosomes. J Neurochem 34:351–358

Pouplard L (1976) Les anthelmintiques en médicine vétérinaire 9. Les Nématodes. Ann Méd Vét 120:515–529

Prichard RK (1970) Mode of action of the anthelmintic thiabendazole in *Haemonchus contortus*. Nature 228:684–685

Prichard RK (1973) The fumarate reductase reaction of *Haemonchus contortus* and the mode of action of some anthelmintics. Int J Parasitol 3:409–417

Prichard RK (1974) Exploitation of the comparative biochemistry of the host/parasite system with thiabendazole and related anthelmintics. In: Proceedings 3rd international congress of parasitology, vol 3. Facta Publications, Vienna, pp 1446–1447

Prichard RK (1978) The metabolic profile of adult *Fasciola hepatica* obtained from rafoxanide-treated sheep. Parasitology 76:277–288

Prichard RK, Hennessy DR (1981) Effect of oesophogeal groove closure on the pharmacokinetic behaviour and efficacy of oxfendazole in sheep. Res Vet Sci 30:22–27

Prichard RK, Hennessy DR, Steel JW (1978 a) Prolonged administration: a new concept of increasing the spectrum and effectiveness of anthelmintics. Vet Parasitol 4:309–315

Prichard RK, Kelly JD, Thompson HG (1978 b) The effects of benzimidazole resistance and route of administration on the uptake of fenbendazole and thiabendazole by *Haemonchus contortus* and *Trichostrongylus colubriformis* in sheep. Vet Parasitol 4:243–255

Prichard RK, Kelly JD, Bolin TD, Duncombe VM, Fagan MR (1981 a) The effect of iron and protein deficiency on plasma levels and parasite uptake of [^{14}C]fenbendazole in rats infected with *Nippostrongylus brasiliensis*. AJEBAK 59:567–573

Prichard RK, Steel JW, Hennessy DR (1981 b) Fenbendazole and thiabendazole in cattle: partition of gastrointestinal absorption and pharmacokinetic behaviour. J Vet Pharmacol Ther 4:295–304

Prous JR, Mealy NE, Serradell MN, Blancafort P (1982) Annual drug data report, vol 4. Prous JR, SA, Barcelona, p 30

Raeymaekers AHM, Roevens LFC, Janssen PAJ (1967) The absolute configuration of the optical isomers of the broad spectrum anthelmintic tetramisole. Tetrahedron Lett 1467–1470

Rahman MS, Bryant C (1977) Studies of regulatory metabolism in *Moniezia expansa:* effects of cambendazole and mebendazole. Int J Parasitol 7:403–409

Rahman MS, Cornish RA, Chevis RF, Bryant C (1977) Studies of the metabolic changes in parasitic helminths from sheep treated with mebendazole. NZ Vet J 25:79–83

Reiner E (1981) Esterases on schistosomes: reaction with substrates and inhibitors. Acta Pharmacol Toxicol [Suppl V] 49:72–78

Rew RS, Smith C, Conglazier ML (1982) Glucose metabolism of *Haemonchus contortus* adults: effects of thiabendazole on susceptible versus resistant strains. J Parasitol 68:845–850

Robinson HJ, Stoerk HC, Graessle OE (1965) Studies on the toxicologic and pharmacologic properties of thiabendazole. Toxicol Appl Pharmacol 7:53–63

Rogers EW (1958) Excretion of bephenium salts in urine of human volunteers. Br Med J (2):1576–1577

Romanowski RD, Rhoads ML, Colglazier ML, Kates KC (1975) Effect of cambendazole, thiabendazole and levamisole on fumarate reductase in cambendazole-resistant and -sensitive strains of *Haemonchus contortus*. J Parasitol 61:777–778

Roseby FB, Boray JC (1970) The anthelmintic efficiency against *Fasciola hepatica* and the toxicity of BAY 4059 in sheep. Aust Vet J 46:308–310

Rousseau F, Haguenoer J-M, Lesieur D, Gamot AP (1981) Gas-chromatographic determination of levamisole in human plasma. Normalization and reliability of the method. Eur J Drug Metab Pharmacokinet 6:281–288

Sander J, Labar J, Ladenstein M, Schweinsberg F (1975) Quantitative measurement of in vivo nitrosamine formation. IARC Sci Publ 9:123–131

Sano M, Terada M, Ishii AI, Kino H (1981) Effects of avermectin B^{1a} on the motility of various parasitic helminths. Experientia 37:844–846

Sano M, Terada M, Ishii AI, Kino H, Anantaphruti M (1982) Studies on chemotherapy of parasitic helminths (V). Effects of niclosamide on the motility of various parasitic helminths. Experientia 38:547–559

Sasi PK, Raj RK (1975) Effect of piperazine on the level of phospholipid and on the activities of certain enzymes of phospholipid metabolism in human *Ascaris lumbricoides*. Experientia 31:1261–1262

Savin YI, Singin AS, Korolev GK (1977) Synthesis of ^{14}C-piperazine and features of its distribution in animals. Khim Farm Zh 11:26–30

Saz DK, Bonner TP, Karlin M, Saz HJ (1971) Biochemical observations on adult *Nippostrongylus brasiliensis*. J Parasitol 57:1159–1162

Saz HJ (1972a) Comparative biochemistry of carbohydrates in nematodes and cestodes. In: Bossche H vanden (ed) Comparative biochemistry of parasites. Academic, New York, pp 33–47

Saz HJ (1972b) Effects of anthelmintics on ^{32}P-esterification in helminth metabolism. In: Bossche H vanden (ed) Comparative biochemistry of parasites. Academic, New York, pp 445–454

Saz HJ, Lescure OL (1968) Effects of anticestodal agents on mitochondria from the nematode, *Ascaris lumbricoides*. Mol Pharmacol 4:407–410

Schantz PM, Bossche H vanden, Eckert J (1982) Chemotherapy for larval echinococcosis in animals and humans: report of a workshop. Z Parasitenkd 67:5–26

Scheibel LW, Saz HJ, Bueding E (1968) The anaerobic incorporation of ^{32}P into adenosine triphosphate by *Hymenolepis diminuta*. J Biol Chem 243:2229–2235

Selling HA, Vonk JW, Kaars-Sypestyn A (1970) Transformation of the systemic fungicide methyl thiophanate into 2-benzimidazole carbonic acid methyl ester. Chem Ind: 1625–1626

Seubert J, Pohlke R, Loebich F (1977) Synthesis and properties of praziquantel, a novel broad spectrum anthelmintic with excellent activity against schistosomes and cestodes. Experientia 33:1036–1037

Smith TC, Kinkel AW, Gryczko CM, Goulet JR (1976) Absorption of pyrvinium pamoate. Clin Pharmacol Ther 19:802–806

Špaldonová R (1981) Efficacy of febantel on *Trichinella spiralis* larvae in white mice. In: Kim CW, Ruitenberg EJ, Teppema JS (eds) Trichinellosis. Proceedings of the 5th international conference on trichinellosis. Reedbooks, Surrey, pp 323–325

Steiner K, Garbe A, Diekman HW, Nowak H (1976) The fate of praziquantel in the organism. I. Pharmacokinetics in animals. Eur J Drug Metab Pharmacokinet 2:85–95

Striebel HP (1976) 4-Isothiocyanato-4′-nitrodiphenylamine (C 9333 – GO/CGP 4540), an anthelmintic with an unusual spectrum of activity against intestinal nematodes, filariae and schistosomes. Experientia 32:457–458

Strufe R, Gönnert R (1960) Experimentelle Untersuchungen mit *N*-(2′-chlor-4′-nitrophenyl)-5-chlorsalicylamid, einem neuen Bandwurmmittel. Arzneimittelforsch 10:886–890

Strufe R, Gönnert R (1967) Über die Beeinflussung der Bandwurmstoffwechsel durch Arzneimittel. Z Tropenmed Parasitol 18:193–202

Symoens J, Cree J de, Bever WFM van, Janssen PAJ (1979) Levamisole In: Goldberg ME (ed) Pharmacological and biochemical properties of drug substances, vol 2. American Pharmaceutical Association Academy of Pharmaceutical Sciences, Washington DC, pp 407–464

Terada M, Ishii AI, Kino H, Sano M (1982 a) Studies on chemotherapy of parasitic helminths (VII). Effects of various cholinergic agents on the motility of *Angiostrongylus cantonensis*. Jpn J Pharmacol 32:633–642

Terada M, Ishii AI, Kino H, Sano M (1982 b) Studies on chemotherapy of parasitic helminths (VIII). Effects of some possible neurotransmitters on the motility of *Angiostrongylus cantonensis*. Jpn J Pharmacol 32:643–653

Terada M, Ishii AI, Kino H, Sano M (1982 c) Studies on chemotherapy of parasitic helminths VI. Effects of various neuropharmacological agents on the motility of *Dipylidium caninum*. Jpn J Pharmacol 32:479–488

Terada M, Ishii AI, Kino H, Fujiu Y, Sano M (1982 d) Studies on chemotherapy of parasitic helminths (IX). Effects of praziquantel on the motility of various parasitic helminths and isolated host tissues. Experientia 38:549–553

The Merck Index, 9th edn (1976) Rahwag ND (ed) Merck, Darmstadt

The Merck Index (1983) An encyclopedia of chemicals, drugs and biologicals. 10th edition. Merck & Co Inc. Rahways

Theodorides VJ, Chang J, Dicuollo CJ, Grass GM, Parish RC, Scott GC (1973) Oxibendazole, a new broad spectrum anthelmintic effective against gastrointestinal nematodes of domestic animals. Br Vet J 129:97–98

Theodorides VJ, Parish RC, Fuchsman CH, Lee RM (1974) Bromoxanide, a new anthelmintic. Vet Rec (July 27th):84–85

Theodorides VJ, Gyurik RJ, Kingsbury WC, Parish RC (1976) Anthelmintic activity of albendazole against liver flukes, tapeworms, lung- and gastrointestinal roundworms. Experientia 32:702–703

Thienpont D, Vanparijs O, Niemegeers C, Marsboom R (1978) Biological and pharmacological properties of flubendazole. Arzneimittelforsch 28:605–612

Thomas H (1979) The efficacy of amidantel, a new anthelmintic, on hookworms and ascarids in dogs. Tropenmed Parasitol 30:404–408

Tocco DJ, Buhs RP, Brown MD, Matzuk AR, Mertel HE, Harman RE, Trenner NR (1964) The metabolic fate of thiabendazole in sheep. J Med Chem 7:399–405

Tocco DJ, Egerton JR, Bowers W, Christensen VW, Rosenblum C (1965) Absorption, metabolism and elimination of thiabendazole in farm animals and a method for its estimation in biological materials. J Pharmacol Exp Ther 149:263–270

Tollenaere JP, Moereels H, Bossche H vanden (1976) Comparison of the structure-activity relationships of substituted phenols as uncouplers of oxidative phosphorylation in rat liver and *Ascaris* muscle mitochondria. In: Bossche H vanden (ed) Biochemistry of parasites and host-parasite relationships. Elsevier, Amsterdam, pp 629–636

Tollenaere JP, Moereels H, Raymaekers LA (1979) Atlas of the three-dimensional structure of drugs. Elsevier, Amsterdam

Ueno H, Watanabe S, Fujita A (1959) Studies on anthelmintics of common liver fluke. J Jpn Vet Med Assoc 12:301

Ueno H, Watanabe S, Fujita A (1960) Studies on anthelmintics against the common liver-fluke II. Action of bithionol in cattle. J Jpn Vet Med Assoc 13:151–155

Vakil BJ, Dalal NJ, Shah PN, Koti ST, Mankodi NA, Sen HG, Vaidya AB (1977) Clinical evaluation of a new anthelmintic – C 9330 GO/CGP 4540 in human hookworm infection. Trans R Trop Med Hyg 71:247–250

Van Belle H (1972) Kinetics and inhibition of alkaline phosphatases from canine tissues. Biochim Biophys Acta 289:158–168

Van Belle H (1976) Kinetics and inhibition of rat and avian alkaline phosphatases. Gen Pharmacol 7:53–58

Van Belle H, Janssen PAJ (1979) α-Ketoaldehydes, specific catalysts for thiol formation from levamisole. Biochem Pharmacol 28:1313–1318

Vanden Bossche H (1972a) Biochemical effects of the anthelmintic drug, mebendazole. In: Bossche H vanden (ed) Comparative biochemistry of parasites. Academic, New York, pp 139–157

Vanden Bossche H (1972) Studies on the phosphorylation in *Ascaris* mitochondria. In: Bossche H vanden (ed) Comparative biochemistry of parasites. Academic, New York, pp 455–468

Vanden Bossche H (1976a) The molecular basis of anthelmintic action. In: Bossche H vanden (ed) Elsevier, Amsterdam, pp 533–572

Vanden Bossche H (1976b) Effects of levamisole and tetramisole on the acetylcholinesterase activity. Janssen Research Products Information Service. Serial number: R 8299/4, R 12 564/3, Beerse

Vanden Bossche H (1978) Chemotherapy of parasitic infections. Nature 273:626–630

Vanden Bossche H (1980a) Chemotherapy of hymenolepiasis. In: Arai HP (ed) Biology of the tapeworm *Hymenolepis diminuta*. Academic, New York, pp 639–693

Vanden Bossche H (1980b) Peculiar targets in anthelmintic chemotherapy. Biochem Pharmacol 29:1981–1990

Vanden Bossche H, Nollin S de (1973) Effects of mebendazole on the absorption of low molecular weight nutrients by *Ascaris suum*. Int J Parasitol 3:401–407

Vanden Bossche H, Janssen PAJ (1983) Mode of action of known and experimental antifilarial compounds. In: Anand N, Sen AB (eds) Proceedings symposium on "chemotherapy & immunology in the control of malaria, filaria and leishmaniasis", February 17–21, 1981, Lucknow, India. Tata McGraw-Hill, New Dehli, pp 187–201

Vanden Bossche H, Verhoeven H (1982) Biochemical effects of the antiparasitic drug closantel. Proceedings of the British Society for Parasitology. Joint spring meeting 1981. Parasitology 84: (Li) (abstract)

Vanden Bossche H, Claes J, Verhoeven H (1975) The uptake and distribution of mebendazole in *Ascaris suum*. In: Biol Res Report R 17 635, LVD, 2183, Section 11. Janssen Pharmaceutica, Beerse

Vanden Bossche H. Verhoeven H, Vanparijs O, Lauwers H, Thienpont D (1979) Closantel, a new antiparasitic hydrogen ionophore. Arch Int Physiol Biochim 87:851–852

Vanden Bossche H, Verhoeven H, Lauwers H (1980) Uncoupling of liver mitochondria associated with fasciolasis in rats – normalization by closantel. In: Bossche H vanden (ed) The host invader interplay. Elsevier, Amsterdam, pp 699–704

Vanden Bossche H, Senft AW, Steck EA (1981) Antiparasitic agents: mode of action, drug resistance. In: Slusarski W (ed) Review of advances in parasitology. Proceedings of ICOPA IV. Polish Scientific Warszawa, pp 461–480

Vanden Bossche H, Rochette F, Hörig C (1982) Mebendazole and related anthelmintics. In: Garattini S, Goldin A, Hawking F, Kopin IJ (eds) Advances in pharmacology and chemotherapy, vol 19. Academic Press, New York, pp 67–128

Vanhoutte PM, Nueten JM van, Verbeuzen TJ, Laduron PM (1977) Differential effects of the isomers of tetramisole on adrenergic neurotransmission in cutaneous veins of dogs. J Pharmacol Exp Ther 200:127–140

Van Nueten JM (1972) Pharmacological aspects of tetramisole. In: Bossche H vanden (ed) Comparative biochemistry of parasites. Academic, New York, pp 101–115

Verheyen A, Borgers M, Vanparijs O, Thienpont D (1976) The effects of mebendazole on the ultrastructure of cestodes. In: Bossche H vanden (ed) Biochemistry of parasites and host-parasite relationships. Elsevier, Amsterdam, pp 605–618
Verheyen A, Borgers M, Bossche H vanden, Vanparijs O, Lauwers H, Thienpont D (1979) The localization of mitochondrial ATPase in the different tissues of the mature liver fluke *Fasciola hepatica* L. The influence of in vivo administration of closantel, a new antiparasitic hydrogen-ionophore. Biol Cell 35:36 a
Verheyen A, Vanparijs O, Lauwers H, Thienpont D (1980) The influence of closantel administration to sheep on the ultrastructure of the adult liver fluke, *Fasciola hepatica* L. In: Bossche H vanden (ed) The host invader interplay. Elsevier, Amsterdam, pp 705–708
Verhoeven HLE, Willemsens G, Bossche H vanden (1976) Uptake and distribution of levamisole in *Ascaris suum*. In: Bossche H vanden (ed) Biochemistry of parasites and host-parasite relationships. Elsevier, Amsterdam, pp 573–579
WHO (1974) Technical report serial number 542, Geneva
Williamson RL, Metcalf RL (1967) Salicylanilides: a new group of active uncouplers of oxidative phosphorylation. Science 158:1694–1695
Wilson CG, Parke DV, Cawthorne MA (1973) Investigations of the 5-hydroxylation of thiabendazole in rat liver microsomal preparations. Biochem Soc Trans 1:195–196
Wollweber H, Kölling H, Widdig A, Thomas H, Schulz H-P, Mürmann P (1978) Febantel, a new broad-spectrum anthelminthic. Arzneimittelforsch 28:2193–2195
Wollweber H, Niemers E, Flucke W, Andrews P, Schulz H-P, Thomas H (1979) Amidantel, a potent anthelmintic from a new chemical class. Arzneimittelforsch 29:31–32
Yorke RE, Turton JA (1974) The influence of a range of anthelmintic drugs on the respiration of isolated *Hymenolepis diminuta* mitochondria. Z Parasitenkd 45:1–10
Zintz K, Frank W (1982) Ultrastructural modifications in *Heterakis spumosa* after treatment with febantel or mebendazole. Vet Parasitol 10:47–56

CHAPTER 5

Chemotherapy of Gastrointestinal Nematodiasis in Man

P. G. JANSSENS

A. Introduction

Intestinal worms have always been and are still problems for humans. The awareness of practitioners has been generally limited to the helminths occurring within their own field of activity.

This is no longer adequate. Increasing worldwide travel, immigrants, displaced persons, and adopted children from overseas confront doctors everywhere with the higher prevalence and wider diversity of parasites, including intestinal nematodes, found in countries with illiteracy and poor living and sanitation standards (High prevalence and intensity of intestinal parasitism is an index of underdevelopment). The presence of unfamiliar and unknown parasites presents the practitioner with a series of problems.

How can deworming be ensured most favorably? Is the presence of the parasite a serious hazard or simply a nuisance for the carrier? Is the parasite carrier a danger to his relatives and to the community?

Some knowledge of the life cycle, pathogenic potential, and epidemiology of the parasite will enable these and similar questions to be answered and the appropriate decisions to be taken. The presence of a parasite, although an unwanted guest, does not automatically necessitate its elimination. A reasonable decision should be based on the number of worms, their association with others, and their harmful potential.

Hookworms consume the blood of their host and sap its vitality. Roundworms show a tendency for aberrant migration and accumulation; if in large numbers this may end in life-threatening bowel obstruction, or a single worm can abstruct a vital duct. Pinworms are themselves harmless, but the chronic carrier state of anal worms, due to retroinfection, may produce a "pinworm neurosis."

Strongyloides stercoralis is a self-perpetuating infection which can bring about the baffling "larva currens" syndrome or pseudoduodenal ulcer symptoms and, in individuals with a depressed immunity, can lead to hyperinfection and death. *Trichinella spiralis* can cause bouts of fever and a generalized infection ending with the death of persons keen on exotic meat dishes.

By penetrating into unhabited areas or by changing eating habits, man and domestic animals, directly or through vectors, come into contact with novel parasites, which are poorly tolerated by new hosts and produce an unfamiliar pathology: anisakiasis, capillariasis, and oesophagostomiasis, and *Strongyloides fülleborni* and *Ternidens deminutus* infections. A high prevalence of intestinal helminths can produce ill-health. But in undernourished, protein- and calorie-deficient persons helminth infections are potentially the "spark plugs" for serious health deterioration. It has been shown repeatedly that parasites disturb the nitrogen balance and often impair the antibody response after immunization. The combination of protein and calorie deficiencies and the presence of helminths is accompanied by growth and development retardation in the so-called "surviving children," and for a general lowering of working capacity in adults.

The magnitude of the problem of intestinal helminths in human beings is as follows:

	No. of persons infected
Hookworms	1 billion
Pinworms	>500 million
Roundworms	1.3 billion
Strongyloids	90 million
Whipworms	750 million

Reliable information on the relationship of worm load and severity of the symptoms, as assessed for hookworms, is also of interest:

No. of worms	Symptoms
1– 25	No symptoms
25– 100	Light disorders
100– 500	Moderate disorders
500–1,000	Severe disorders
>1,000	Extreme disorders

As a relationship exists between the number of eggs excreted and the number of prolific female worms, it is possible to deduct from the number of eggs per gram of feces (EPG) values a similar kind of relation. Two sets of values are given as examples in Table 2 (Watson 1960; P. G. Janssens, unpublished).

These values are only indicative. They will vary with the prevailing local transmission-bound factors, including the degree of susceptibility, tolerance, or resistance of the population, the way of life, and the environment. However, the disparities are more likely to be as a result of the preconceived opinions of the investigators: parasitologists, epidemiologists, or clinicians.

Table 1. Relationship of egg count and severity of symptoms according to several authors (second set of values in parentheses, unpublished hypotheses by P. G. Janssens)

Severity of symptoms	EPG		
	Hookworms	Roundworms	Whipworms
Very light	< 1,000	< 5,000	< 5,000
Mild	1,000–5,000 (2,000)	5,000–12,000 (10,000)	5,000–12,000 (5,000)
Moderate	5,000–10,000 (5,000)	12,000–50,000 (20,000)	12,000–20,000 (10,000)
Severe	>10,000	>50,000	> 20,000

Agreement on a small number of frames of reference that could be justified would be most welcome, but is still very remote. The main reason is the diversity of technique used for coprological examinations according to understandable individual preferences. It is, however, a pity that no agreement is in sight on the common use of a few standardized practical tests. Such standardization would be invaluable for a correct objective assessment of new anthelmintic drugs.

Anthelmintic drugs were previously identified from empirical observations. Nowadays they result from the screening of numerous chemical compounds in animal models or in vitro. Tomorrow they will be synthesized specifically from the rapidly improving knowledge of the biological and biochemical processes involved in the life cycles of parasites.

In any case, active anthelmintics are increasing rapidly in numbers and in chemical structures. In their final stage of development they need to be submitted to clinical evaluation in man, which should be carried out according to reliable and ethically acceptable protocols. Physicians and public health personnel are consequently confronted with difficult choices between a great variety of available and strongly advertized drugs with contradictory and confusing reports about their efficacy and adverse reactions.

The evidence produced by clinical evaluation can be of doubtful value, as expressed by the well-known dictum: "use the drug as soon as it is released in order to avoid the rapid falloff of its efficacy."

Users of drugs are in need of reliable help in their choices and the balancing of advantages against the potential side effects and hazards. They are also forced to make a decision about the wisdom to withhold or to administer a therapy to persons harboring parasites either isolated or in association.

The assessment of drugs could be much improved. Safeguards such as the use of antibias devices fulfilling the requirements for sound statistical criteria, such as the inclusion of untreated and placebo-treated controls, double-blind trials, multicenter approach, and other acceptable methods in clinical pharmacology.

The poor scientific quality of a number of clinical trials on antiparasitic drugs is related to the quality of the clinical investigation. The investigator should not only be an experienced clinician. A good knowledge of and practical training in medical parasitology, biostatistics, and experimental designs are further basic prerequisites. Collaboration with a statistician is necessary for design, detailed protocol, collection of data and material, tabulation, and interpretation of data. For mass treatment the help of a sociologist can be invaluable in overcoming the problem of participation without excessive dropping-out.

The increasing and unavoidable sophistication of the methodology in trial design and statistical assessment, combined with the sharp increase in legal and ethical obligations, is necessitating more and more a team approach.

Parasitological evaluation is affected by many factors related to the life cycle of the parasite. Many clinical trials will have to be undertaken in endemic areas. Under endemic circumstances attention should be paid to the incubation time of the infective parasite and its prepatent existence in the host.

The three most common, soil-transmitted intestinal helminths lay eggs, to some extent, in amounts proportional to the number of worms. The EPG can be assessed by quantitative methods and egg counts become thus a reasonable base

Table 2. Shortest course between the excretion of a fertile egg in the outside world and its infective stage and between the infection and egg output by a newly infected host

Parasites	Timing	
	From egg to infective stage	From infection to diagnosis
Hookworms	8 days	35–42 days
Pinworms	6 h	15–45 days
Roundworms	9–15 days	60–75 days
Strongyloides	1–3 days	17–28 days
Trichinella	21 days	7 days
Whipworms	21 days	30–90 days

for the evaluation of drug efficacy. Nevertheless the mean EPG data are not absolutely reliable.

The degree of conformity or diversity depends to a large extent on the *methodology* used. A great improvement should follow on appropriate selection of standardized methods. Drug manufacturing companies should strongly recommend that the investigators engaged in clinical trials of their drugs should make use of, in the first instance, the methods selected by experts according to the helminths under investigation, possibly in addition to their own preferred methods. Every investigator sticks to his own methodology and his own scale of assessment. The pharmaceutical companies moreover use different criteria of efficacy, which adds to the confusion.

The daily egg-output can vary substantially [up to 300%: STOLL (1923)] and is moreover subject to seasonal variations in some countries. The count will also differ with the proportion of the stool examined. Collection of 24-h samples is recommended. The egg-laying capacity can on the other hand be only temporarily suppressed by the drug. For these and several other reasons repeated egg counts are essential. Nevertheless data of this type should be regarded as indicative.

The *pretreatment* degree of infection should be established from at least three egg counts on different days. Their average will enable a reliable classification to be made. A correct pretreatment evaluation is of course crucial for a valuable post-treatment assessment of the efficacy of a drug.

The selection of the test cases should avoid the pooling of very light to heavy infections. The mean egg load as a sole parameter involves the risk of masking a poorer reduction in the severe infections. The selection of only moderate infections produces favorable results out of proportion. In evaluating a new drug more attention should be paid to severe infections or at least the results for various grades of infection should be given separately. However, very light infections (< 1,000 EPG) should never be included.

In field trials evaluation is often further complicated by mixed infections. The most typical example is the simultaneous presence in a community or an individual of *Ancylostoma duodenale* and *Necator americanus*. The inconstancy of the activity of several anthelmintics on both hookworms is a well-known fact;

moreover, when several worms are present simultaneously, the presence of the less apparent can be missed at the initial feces examination.

The *post-treatment* assessment needs correct, neither too early nor too late, timing. The EPG after 1–2 weeks can overestimate the efficacy, while after 6–9 weeks it becomes impossible to rule out a reinfection.

EPG values can be determined each time from two counts, at weekly intervals, with the second not later than week 4. The life cycle of the majority of worms lasts no longer than 4–6 weeks. For the majority of the drugs assessment at 14 days is adequate and assessment at 30 days provides a complementary guarantee.

The EPG data, before and after treatment, make it possible to establish the egg output reduction rate (ERR). This rate will be porportionate to the degree of infection and will provide the most accurate results in heavy infections. From the EPG it is impossible to calculate the precise worm population in the host. The EPG indeed cannot provide the number of male or larval worms.

Many factors influence egg production and the average numbers found. Egg output starts with the patent period. Egg production does not occur continuously. Large variations are observed from one day to another and also within one day: therefore reiterated 24-h stool collections are necessary. Egg production is also much lower in winter than in spring, which can be related to the hormonal balance of the host. The consistency of the stools affects the EPG for obvious reasons, the EPG decreasing with dilution. The nutritional condition of the host is another factor. The immune state of the host decreases the egg output inversely with the host's resistance. On the whole older persons have lower EPGs than younger persons. Egg production also decreases when the worm grows older.

Notwithstanding these many disturbing factors, the EPG has an interesting indicative value as a public health tool for helminth control and in drug assessment.

Evaluation is often still too crude and in need of more repeated coprological examinations and more sensitive methods. More stringent and universal criteria would be welcome since the EPG is the key value for the basic assessment parameters: "cure rate" = 100% reduction of EPG or rather a "clearance rate" (CR) and the "egg reduction rate" or ERR.

The CR is based on two formulae:

$$\frac{\text{Number of persons treated} - \text{number not cured}}{\text{Number of persons treated}} \times 100$$

or

$$\frac{\text{Number of persons with an EPG reduction of 70\%}}{\text{Total number of persons}}$$

ERR on:

$$\frac{\text{Original EPG count} - \text{EPG after treatment}}{\text{Original EPG}} \times 100\,.$$

For assessing the efficacy of a new drug the *recovery of worms,* during 4–7 days after drug administration, is insufficiently used. Pouring the feces through sieves under repeated washings and picking the worms out one by one, especially for the smaller worms, such as hook- and whipworms, is indeed an uninviting and rather tedious procedure. Nevertheless recovery of the expulsed worms is of paramount importance for counting, identification, and assessing their degree of vitality or disturbance, the egg or larvae production in the female, the relation of the worm load to the EPG, etc. As opposed to the thousands of sometimes doubtful EPG ratings it does not seem excessive to recommend more often a complementary investigation of the worm expulsion and the degree of maturity of the worms.

Details of the morphology of the eggs are likewise too often drowned in a mass of questionable information about their number. Careful scrutiny of their degree of fertility and vitality would be most useful for epidemiological evaluation.

Coproculture is easy to perform on charcoal or on test tube filter paper (Harada-Mori), but this technique is only casually used, which is a pity. Not only is the correct identity of hookworms indispensable but the identification of the larvae can be a clue to several uninterpretable observations.

The peculiar perianal and perineal localization of the eggs of *Enterobius vermicularis* requires the adhesive tape technique of Graham, provided that the technique is applied soon after getting up in the morning and that the ecological niche is not disturbed by bowel movement or washing.

In the near future, the use of more biologically accountable drugs will enforce the need for closer attention to bioparasitological species differences which might explain some successful or unsuccessful results. At the same time the variations in host tolerance, resistance, or susceptibility will need to be investigated more closely.

The Methodology of Drug Trials

The different stages in the study of anthelmintics have been accurately established. After initial screening for activity, the compound is investigated with regard to its biochemical, pharmacological, toxicological, mutagenic, and carcinogenic characteristics. If the prospects are good, trials in animals are undertaken. In humans the drug is investigated in a small number of healthy male volunteers for absorption, metabolism, distribution, excretion, tolerance, and side effects. A dose-range study is carried out by a clinical parasitologist preferably using a checklist of current clinical and biomedical controls before and after intake of the drug. Recording of the possible side effects must be exhaustive but specific questions should not be asked as it may provoke subjective inputs. Such a checklist should be established from a "protocol" drawn up by a planning group in order to obtain answers to all the questions posed by the objectives. It includes the criteria for selecting convenient candidates, guarding against a high dropout rate. These must also cover the screening tests for admission and the terms of agreement and informed consent.

Clinical observation should consist of a thorough physical examination, including temperature, blood pressure, chest X-rays, ECG, and possibly EEG. It is completed by routine blood, urine, and feces analysis and other tests according to specific needs. This is the baseline for the observations of therapeutic and adverse effects.

The design of the drug administration will be described in detail: presentation, dosage in fixed or variable levels, route, timing and frequency of administration, total duration of treatment, control of quality, stability, storage, dispensing factors affecting absorption (meals and oral administration), supervision of intake of drug and adequate dosage, reactions of patients. Guidelines for the evaluation and management of adverse reactions are useful.

Attention should be paid to the formulation (micronization, etc.) and presentation: too tightly compressed tablets are eliminated as such, chewable presentations are not always appreciated, and oral liquid preparations are too bulky under field conditions, although they are easily administered in children.

Easiness and simplicity of administration are key criteria: single dose regardless of age or weight, drugs needing neither fasting nor purging. It should be kept in mind that overseas the majority of people, including children, enjoy only one meal, which is in the evening: drugs to be taken after breakfast or other meal will be often swallowed on an empty stomach.

Anthelmintic drugs which expel recognizable worms (*Ascaris, Taenia*) are more appreciated than those killing in situ, followed by their digestion and disappearance.

The trial design should include the methodology of standardized data collection, storage, retrieval, analysis, and also definitions of measurements, frequency, timing, statistical approach, randomization, assignment to treatment or control group, and open, single, or double-blind system. The comparison of the deworming effect of a new compound in regard to a drug in current use needs reliable basic data. Provision should also be made for a progress review.

This type of study needs a medical, paramedical, and technical infrastructure with maintenance and supervision facilities capable of supporting this vast array of investigations. This can only be done in hospital even if this imposes a prolonged stay, which will only be accepted by patients with disturbing symptoms (e.g., anemia). However, in readily supervisable groups such as nurses and students, an ambulatory basis can be considered, if dropouts will remain below acceptable numbers.

The problem of assessing the validity and relevance of therapeutic trials with anthelmintics involves some specific matters. They are related to the main purpose of the treatment on a population basis which is, as opposed to the individual therapy, not necessarily a CR of 100%.

In the establishment of the CR, it must be borne in mind that the presence of one fertilized or fertile egg after treatment means failure. A "none or all" result in *S. stercoralis* infections requires reiterated stool examinations, after concentration and/or coproculture, because of the irregularity of the presence of their larvae. For *E. vermicularis* seven to ten examinations on consecutive days 2–3 weeks after the treatment are necessary.

Some investigators make a distinction between a "parasitological cure," i.e., EPG = 0, and a "practical cure" or EPG < 1,000. The health of the worm bearers and the reduction of the worm load to the extent that the spread of infection is reduced below an epidemiological significant transmission level, are, however, the two main objectives.

The ERRs become thus the most important data for assessing the value of a drug, more especially in helminthiases producing symptoms pro rata the number of parasitizing worms. The ERRs also afford a fair idea of the proportion of removal of germs infecting the community.

The removal of the largest possible number of worms from the largest possible number of persons is a responsible approach, especially for children living in a heavily infected environment. Their vitality and in addition that of the whole population will no longer be sapped.

It should never be forgotten that infection with worms is not an unavoidable epiphenomenon of the presence of infective larvae and/or of appropriate vectors in the environment of man. The standard and way of life will increase or decrease the infective contacts: walking barefoot and outdoor domestic, occupational, and even ritual activities may enhance the skin-soil and skin-water contacts. Ill-maintained, neglected toilets will increase the presence and multiplication of soil-transmitted parasites. Environmental sanitation can produce a false sense of security: latrines may become excellent breeding, concentrating, and infective foci. Poor personal hygiene, dirty fingers and fingernails, and soiled anal and bottom region will facilitate direct ano-oral transmission.

In a given country, prevalence and EPG values, being related to diverse environmental conditions, are never uniform. The obvious physical background is furthermore complicated by an ill-understood physiological, nutritional, and immunological background, especially in developing countries. Predictions in a given setup must be checked in typical different endemic conditions. This may even include some understanding about a possible interplay with traditional healers.

The ERR values should be established using an adequate methodology. Standardized direct and/or concentration techniques should not only be selected according to the needs and at the appropriate timing day 15 to day 30, but they should also be supplemented with coproculture and recovery of worms (until day 4), and with 24-h stool samples. One of the most often neglected points is that persons with a low-grade infection such as an EPG $< 5{,}000$ for round- and whipworms and $< 1{,}000$ for hookworms, which has been uniformized by some to an EPG $< 1{,}500$, should be excluded from the pilot trials in order to guarantee a real indicative value for the mean ERR.

These orientating investigations will provide the basic information on which individual or community treatment can be planned. However, their respective objectives and choices will diverge.

Individual therapy aims at relief of symptoms and complaints or a clinical radical cure. The choice of drug will be based on its specific efficacy irrespective of the mode and length of administration.

Community treatment will aim at a lowering or interrupting of the transmission beneath the threshold of the role of the worm as a public health problem. The choice of drug will rest on different criteria: single dose, broad spectrum, cheap, easy to administer by the oral route without side effects, and safe (risk lower than the disease). Eradication is not as yet a practical goal; a significant reduction of the worm burden is a sound objective. Mass treatment is a problem in its own right.

B. Ancylostomiasis

(Hookworm disease, miners's anemia, chlorosis tropicalis, Egyptian chlorosis, uncinariasis, tunnel anemia)

I. Introduction

1. Parasite

Several species of Ancylostominae are parasitic of the intestine in man: *Ancylostoma duodenale* DUBINI 1843, *A. ceylanicum* LOOSS 1911, *Necator americanus* STILES 1902, *A. braziliense* DE FARIA 1910, and *A. malayanum* ALESSANDRINI 1905.

The development of *A. duodenale* and *N. americanus* is identical. The adult worms (1–1.5 cm in length) live in the jejunum, but in heavy infections they may expand into the cecum and the colon. In their usual localization they grasp a plug of mucosa with their chitinized buccal capsule and suck blood from lacerated capillaries.

After mating, the female starts to discharge fertilized, unsegmented transparent eggs into the lumen. Eggs will have reached a four- to eight-cell stage when passed out in the feces.

The L3 infective larvae are attracted by the human skin usually of the foot which they penetrate in 5–10 min (ground itch). Transmission is also possible with foods and drinks or by geophagia. The larvae proceed to the intestine by a roundabout way: they enter the venous or lymphatic system, break through the lung capillaries, and migrate up the bronchi and trachea and down the esophagus and stomach into the jejunum. They differentiate sexually, molt, mature, and copulate and the female lays eggs within 4–6 weeks.

In India and Taiwan, the infective larvae stay in the lungs during the wet season, remain in hypobiosis for between 22 and 40 weeks, and resume their development in the dry premonsoon season: this prepatent period is three to five times in excess of the usual course.

The life span of the adults varies from months to years (15–20 years), but the usual survival is 2–8 years.

The daily egg-output of *A. duodenale*, which exceeds by 2 to 2.5 times the output of *N. americanus*, has been estimated to be between 20,000 and 30,000 eggs per worm. In practice 200–500 eggs/g (EPG) feces corresponds to one-two female hookworms.

2. Host

Hookworms live for years on the host's blood. The main symptom is therefore hypochromic, microcytic anemia and iron deficiency, which appear 2-5 months after the infection. Pallor of the skin and mucous membranes are noticeable (miner's anemia). One *Necator* worm needs from 0.03 to 0.05 ml/day, and one *Ancylostoma* up to 0.15–0.2 ml/day. The blood loss due to *A. duodenale* is five times larger than for the same worm load of *N. americanus*. Consequently the importance of the daily blood loss is directly related to the species and the *number of worms:*

1– 25: little damage: blood loss is compensated for by an increase in hemopoiesis, no symptoms.
25– 100: some damage: light symptoms, a daily loss of some 3 ml blood.
100– 500: considerable damage: moderate symptoms.
500–1,000: serious damage: severe disease up to 100 ml blood loss/day.
>1,000: very extensive damage: very severe disease, erythrocyte count below 1 million/mm^3 and vitamin B_{12} and folic acid deficiencies follow; the anemia can become macrocytic and megaloblastic.

The symptoms vary according to the seriousness of the infection and the nutritional state. In addition to severe pruritus at the site of infection (toes, feet, buttocks) abdominal discomfort, intermittent diarrhea with 10–15 liquid bowel movements, or constipation can be present. Duodenojejunitis is radiologically demonstrable: pseudoduodenal ulcer or cog-wheel pattern of mucosa.

Passage through the lungs can produce a "Loeffler" eosinophilic lung infiltrate, dry cough, dyspnea, but seldomly hemoptysis.

In children retarded physical and mental development and delayed puberty have been reported.

It is generally known that in endemic areas, men may carry hookworms all their lives, but these infections remain relatively mild. There is a continuous incoming stream of parasites; some survive, many die. Obviously man acquires by some sort of mechanism, including a time factor, a certain degree of resistance after repeated infection which prevents an accumulation of worms, but complete immunity is never achieved.

2.1 Clinical Profile of Hookworm Disease

The *baseline symptoms* are:
Chronic anemia, ± severe drop of hemoglobin level
Breathlessness – easy fatigability
Palpitations, tachycardia
Hemic heart murmur
Hypoproteinemia
Hypoalbuminemia
Edema (feet)
Anorexia
Dyspepsia – nausea – epigastric discomfort
Pseudoduodenal ulcer
Diarrhea
Eosinophilia (early stages)
Ground itch at penetration zone of larvae.

3. Diagnosis

The existence of hookworm infections is established by the presence of adult worm, their larvae, or eggs in the feces. This can be demonstrated by a variety of techniques: direct smear (2–3 mg); Kato cellophane thick smear (50–60 mg); concentration methods (sedimentation, brine flotation, formol-ether, SAEX, etc.) with or without egg-counting; or coproculture (Harada-Mori in its Sasa variant-200 mg), which needs an incubator and a waiting time of 8–16 days. The recovery of worms in stools provides the proof.

The choice of the technique must be adapted to the needs. For crude prevalence rates a simple technique will suffice. A drug trial needs, in addition to an appropriate design, with placebo-treated and/or untreated controls, sensitive specific and quantifying parasitological techniques including egg measurements to avoid confusion with *Ternidens deminutus, Trichostrongylus*, or other similar worms such as *Haemonchus contortus*. Culture may be useful. Recovery, identification, and counting of adult worms can provide most useful information.

It must be kept in mind that the time elapsing between skin infection and egg production amounts to 4–6 weeks. In order to avoid interference by reinfection the repeated control examinations must consequently be planned for 14–25–30 days after treatment. The follow-up examinations should be carried out on three consecutive days, as the egg output is not constant. If the risk of reinfection is absent, the follow-up can be extended over longer periods.

The pretreatment egg-load/g (EPG) must be established. The egg output provides an indication of the worm load: the female of *N. americanus* produces some 8,000–10,000 eggs/day and of *A. duodenale* 20,000–30,000 eggs/day. These data can be correlated with the anemia, on condition that the hookworm has been identified and that the iron available in the diet is taken into consideration. Although no consensus has been reached, the EPG provides an idea of the severity of the infection: 1,000, very light; 1,000–2,000, light; 2,000–10,000, moderate; and $>10,000$, heavy infection.

The correct identification of *N. americanus* and *A. duodenale*, which is often neglected, is important as their response to anti-hookworm drugs can vary. Serological tests are not of proven usefulness.

Eosinophilia, hypochromic microcytic anemia, and iron deficiency are useful pointers.

4. Geographical Distribution

Ancylostoma duodenale, the "old-world" hookworm, is resistent to lower temperatures and is present in rural areas of temperate regions as well as in the tropics: in *Europe* – in the Mediterranean coastal areas, and elsewhere mainly in tunnels and mines, in which it has been almost eradicated by control and treatment; in *Asia* – *A. duodenale* is found in the Middle East, northern India, and the Far East: Burma, Indonesia, Malaysia, China, Vietnam, Taiwan, Japan, and Korea; in *Africa* – this species is present in North Africa and some areas of Burundi, Rwanda, and Zaire; and in the *Americas* – its presence has been reported from Mexico, Venezuela, Brazil, Paraguay, and Chile. *A. duodenale* is present also on the northeast coast of Australia and in the South Pacific Islands.

Necator americanus, the "New World" hookworm, dominant in the western hemisphere and in the tropics, is now much more widely spread: in *Asia* – Turkey, Iran, south and east India, Sri Lanka, Malaysia, Thailand, Indonesia, Philippines, Vietnam, China, and Japan; in the *Americas* – southern United States, West Indies, Central America, Mexico, Guatemala, Costa Rica, Panama, Suriname, Colombia, Venezuela, Brazil, Peru, Paraguay, and Argentina; and in *Africa* – Nigeria, Angola, Zaire, Congo, Uganda, Tanzania, Mozambique, Seychelles, Botswana, South Africa, and Madagascar. *N. americanus* is also present in *Europe* – Portugal, Italy, Spain, Romania, and Yugoslavia; in *Australia* (Queensland) and *New Zealand;* and in the *South Pacific Islands* – Papua New Guinea, Fiji, Solomon Islands, Western Samoa, and the Marshall Islands.

Rigid demarcations no longer exist. In almost all of the infected countries both species are present simultaneously, but in variable proportions. As a consequence of this overlapping distribution, the specific helminth has not been completely identified in many surveys, but reported by the generic name "hookworm." They are present from 45° north to 30° south.

5. Prevalence

STOLL (1947) estimated the number of persons infected by hookworm at more than 450 million. If 25% of the world population is still infected, as indeed little if any improvement has been achieved in the tropics, the number of infected persons must have reached at least 1 billion by 1980. Furthermore, ancylostomiasis outranks all other intestinal worm infections in seriousness. Infection rates are a useful danger signal. However, the number of hookworms infecting the host determines the severity of the symptoms: in a single host their number can reach 3,000.

In the tropics hookworm is mainly a rural problem. Nevertheless, many published surveys have been made in urban areas; hence many figures are too low and not representative of the real situation in the countries reported.

Africa:

Angola	53% (5%–100%)
Burundi	10%–12% (Public Health Laboratory, Bujumbura)
Cameroon	39%–53% (Children, Yaounde); 52% (pygmies)
Central Africa	80% (*N. americanus*)
Congo	49.5% (13%–71%). *A. duodenale,* 38%; *N. americanus,* 88%
Egypt	50%, Heleran, 90%; Giza, 42%; Behera (Alexandria), 2.3%
Ethiopia	Children, 89%; adults, 27%–83%; hospitals, 10%
Gabon	45%–59% of suburban schoolchildren, Libreville
Ghana	40% (20%–62%)
Guinea-Bissau	30%–92%
Ivory Coast	58%
Kenya	16%–85%. *N. americanus,* ubiquitous; *A. duodenale,* restricted
Liberia	10%–33%
Mozambique	29% (2%–72%)

Nigeria	Nationwide, urban 12%–21%; rural, up to 70%–80%. 40 million Nigerians are infected with hookworm (predominately *N. americanus*). Benin State, 20%; Northern Province, 5%
Rwanda	1%–10% (*A. duodenale*)
Seychelles	26%
South Africa	20%
Tanzania	Rural Bugojno, Mwanza (Lake Victoria), 82% (*A. duodenale*, 61%; *N. americanus*, 81%). Rural Machui, Tanga, 82% (*A. duodenale*, 39%; *N. americanus*, 94%). Hombolo, Dodoma, 37% (*A. duodenale*, 6%; *N. americanus*, 99%)
Uganda	Teboke, Lango, 51% (*A. duodenale*, 2%; *N. americanus*, 99%)
Zambia	49% (*N. americanus*) (12%–65%)
Zaire	Hospital Mama Yemo, Kinshasa, 38%. Every year 100 children die in Kinshasa from severe anemia resulting from heavy hookworm infection (CERF et al. 1962). Lufira, Katanga, 40%
Asia:	
Arabian peninsula	0.8%
Bangladesh	28%
China	Nationwide, 30% (1949, 100 million) – especially in the north, northeast, and south. Except in the south, where *N. americanus* is predominant, 80% of the hookworms are *A. duodenale*. South China (13 provinces, 1957), average 34%; maximum, 66%; absolute maximum, 98%
India	Bandipur Union, 78%; Bengal, 50%–70% (West Bengal, 80%); Bombay, urban, 69%; Bombay, rural, 80%; Dehli, 86%; Himachel Pradesh, 13.5%; Madras, 90%; Maharashtra State, 94% predominantly *N. americanus*; Punjab, up to 100% *A. duodenale*
Indonesia	Jakarta, 11%; central Java, 22%; west Java, 57%; Sulawesi, 15%
Iraq	Bagdad (rural area), 55%; northern region, 10% (5%–10%); central region, 21% (10%–35%); southern region, 23% (20%–25%)
Iran	Southern provinces, 84%; Khuzestan (southwest Iran), urban <1%–22%; Khuzestan, rural, 5.49%; Strait of Hornuz, 77%; Caspian Sea, 65%
Japan	8%–20%; (1950, 5%; 1977, 0.1%)
Korea	6%
Malaysia	91%
Pakistan	23%; Lahore, 36%

Philippines	31%
Singapore	Urban, 3%–9%; rural, 70%
Sri Lanka	Southwest, 45%; Colombo rural, 60%; urban, 3%–9%
Taiwan	37%–85%
Thailand	Urban, 18%; rural, 28%
Timor	70%
Americas:	
Brazil	28% (40 million infected, 1968); Rio Grande do Norte (littoral), 65%; Paraiba (Favelas), 52%; Amerindians, 74%; Pernambuco, 37%
Colombia (Amazonian)	39%
Costa Rica	Urban, 5% (0%–20%); rural, 14% (6%–24%)
Dominican Republic	9%
French Guyana	16%
Guatemala	2% (1944); 4% (1953); 3% (1980); 2.7% (1981)
Mexico	19% (0%–56%)
Puerto Rico	27%
Suriname	11%; Paramaribo, 36%; Brokopondo, 72%
United States	Texas, 33%; Kentucky, 15%
Venezuela	28%. Sucre, Lo Llanos, Yaracui, up to 70% of which 11% with 100 or more worms
Oceania:	
Papua New Guinea (mostly *N. americanus*)	Star Mountains, 76%; North Fly, 62%; Delta, 43%; Wabo, 78%; Kamea, 78%; West Sepik, 87% (ASFORD et al. 1981)

II. Drugs

Traditional Natural Drugs

Although merely of historical interest, a reference to a few natural drugs will remind the reader that nature has provided some therapeutic principles.

Anacardium occidentale, a member of the Therebinthaceae, better known as the cashew nut, its edible fruit, contains an oil which is effective against Ancylostomidae and also has laxative properties. At a dose of 3–4 g for children and 4–6 g for adults a CR[1] of 60%–65% and an ERR of 78%–99% can be expected.

Diospyros mollis, Griff, a member of the Ebenacea which grows in southeast Asia, produces berries which, when crushed to pulp while still green, show a definite activity against hookworms. This activity is related to a quinone constituent, viz., diospyroquinone (SADUN and VAJRATHIRA 1954). Diospyrol and its derivatives have been tested by SEN et al. (1974) in hamsters infected with *N. americanus* and found active.

1 CR, clearance or cure rate. Clearance would be the most logical choice, but cure is widely used

Chenopodium ambrosioides L., var. *anthelminthicum* Gray (Jerusalem Oak), contains an essence whose principal constituents is "ascaridol," a terpenic peroxide. Oil of chenopodium is highly toxic for nematodes, i.e., hookworms, but is irritant to the gastrointestinal tract. Chenopodium oil can also be administered together with tetrachloroethylene TCE in castor oil (at ratio of 0.6 ml, 3.6 ml, 30 ml).

2. Antibiotics

2.1 Avermectins (Ivermectin)

2.1.1 State of the Art

Dosages below 1 mg/kg ivermectin have been found to have potent activity on at least eight families of nematodes (Filariidae, Oxyuridae, Trichinellidae, Trichiuridae, Heterakidae, Metastrongylidae, Trichostrongylidae, Strongylidae). All stages of development are susceptible to ivermectin: mature and immature worms, hypobiotic and normal L4 larvae, and both benzimidazole-susceptible and -resistant nematode strains.

2.1.2 Assessment

No details are available as yet.

2.1.3 Dosage, Mode of Administration

Dosage is 30–50 µg/kg, in a single oral dose; lower dosages have not been found effective (LARIVIÈRE et al. 1982).

2.1.4 Side Effects

Up to 5 and 10 µg/kg no adverse reactions are encountered. Asthenia, dizziness, and pruritus can follow ingestion of 30–50 µg/kg but disappear spontaneously within 48 h. No hematological, biochemical, ophthalmological, or neurological abnormalities have been observed.

2.1.5 Contraindications, Precautions

Information is lacking.

2.1.6 Comments

The response to a single-dose administration is under analysis, with interesting prospects (LARIVIÈRE et al. 1982). No decision has been taken by the manufacturer at least for use on hookworm.

3. Synthetic Organic Drugs

3.1 Old Timers

3.1.1 Bromo-β-naphthol

This halogenated derivate of β-naphthol (Wormin) is 15 times less toxic than β-naphthol. It is very active against hookworms at the usual dosages: adults, 4–6 g;

Table 3. Treatment of hookworm infection by bromo-β-naphtol

Parasite	Dosage	Number treated	CR	ERR	References
N. americanus	4 g+2 g	241	39	43	HSIEH (1960)
Hookworm	4–6 g	89	68	94	JUTTIJUDATA et al. (1962)
N. americanus	6 g	185	67	–	KOMYA et al. (1960)

12–15 years, 3 g; 7–12 years, 2 g repeated for 2–4 days. The drug is reasonally well tolerated. The CR is about 70% (40%–95%), which is the same as with iodothymol (Thymolan).

3.1.2 Hexylresorcinol

This 1–3-dihydroxy-4-hexylbenzene (Caprokol), a former urinary antiseptic, has anthelmintic properties against hookworms at a dosage of 0.6–0.8 g, for children of 6–12 years, and of 1 g for adolescents and adults. The crystals are hygroscopic. Side effects are common, i.e., irritation of the mucosa of the buccal cavity.

3.1.3 Tetrachloroethylene

3.1.3.1 State of the Art

HALL and SHILLINGER (1925) demonstrated the activity of the halogenated hydrocarbon tetrachloroethylene (TCE) (Didakene, Tetracap) against ancylostomidae. Being more active, less toxic and better tolerated, it became a better choice than carbon tetrachloride, previously recommended by HALL (1921). It is generally accepted that *N. americanus* is more sensitive to TCE than *A. duodenale*.

3.1.3.2 Assessment

This drug, being cheap, is still widely used. Detailed CR and ERR studies with identification of the hookworm species are scarce. Recent available data have been collected in Table 4.

3.1.3.3 Dosage, Mode of Administration

Tetrachloroethylene can be administered as a liquid or in gelatin capsules of 0.2–1.0 ml. A dose of 0.10–0.12 ml/kg, with a maximum of 5–6 ml, is recommended for adolescents and adults. In children 0.2 ml/year of age is recommended. Ideally intake of fats and alcohol should be avoided from 24 h before until 24 h after treatment. On the previous evening a light meal is advisable. The drug should be taken on an empty stomach. The administration was traditionally followed some hours later by a saline purgation until CARR et al. (1954) showed that omission of the purge increased the efficacy of the drug. The treatment has to be repeated, in healthy patients on three consecutive days, or otherwise on alternate days or even with a 4-day interval. Single doses of 4 or 5 ml are more effective than 2- or 3 ml doses at 4-day intervals and can be administered to patients with severe anemia. Other methods of administration have been tried and claimed by their

Table 4. Treatment of hookworm infection by tetrachloroethylene

Efficacy	Dosage	Number treated	CR	ERR	References
≧80%	0.12 ml/kg[a]	80	81	99	JUNG and MACCROAN (1960)
≧70%	3 ml	50	70	–	BAWA et al. (1965)
	0.1 ml/kg	22	77	99	MIGASENA et al. (1978)
≧60%	2–4 ml	43	67	–	SALEM et al. (1965)
	0.1 ml/kg/3 days	16	66	–	KAHN (1966)
≧50%	4 ml	30	53	–	JUTTIJUDATA et al. (1962)
	0.3–3 ml	?	56	–	MISRA et al. (1965)
	4 ml/3 days	?	56	–	ROWLAND (1966)
≧40%	4.5 g (without purge)	17	47	–	YOSHIDA et al. (1960)
≧30%	4.5 g (with purge)	20	30	–	YOSHIDA et al. (1960)
≧20%	4 ml	16	26	–	MACKERRAS (1961)
	1 ml/20 kg	110	29	–	ABDALLAH and SAIF (1963)
≧10%	1.8–2.4 ml	65	18	–	AHMAD and RASOOL (1959)
	0.2 ml/year	190	16	–	HSIEH et al. (1960a, 1961)
	0.6–1.5 ml/2 days	224	14	–	DIGUES LA TONCHE (1962)
<10%	0.6–1.5 ml	334	9	–	DIGUES LA TONCHE (1962)
	3–4 ml	36	3	50–58	YOUNG et al. (1960)

[a] Kilograms body weight

promoters as being superior: emulsified in water by the addition of Tween 80 or similar emulsifiers (MOLINA-PASQUEL et al. 1959), or by an intraduodenal route (SCHREIBER 1959).

3.1.3.4 Side Effects

This drug is unpleasant to take and adverse reactions are frequent. A burning sensation in the epigastric region, nausea, vomiting, abdominal cramps, headache, dizziness, somnolence, and mild inebriation are observed. Patients with severe anemia are prone to collapse.

In order to reduce the adverse reactions, BRUMPT and HO-THI-SANG (1953) recommended administering the drug at midnight: asleep, the patient will remain unaware of the unpleasant effects (?).

3.1.3.5 Contraindications, Precautions

In severely ill patients it is advisable to correct beforehand the anemia (iron administration or blood transfusion), to restore the fluid balance, and to improve the general resistance. Gastrointestinal disturbances, liver disease, alcoholism, nutritional poor status, etc. should be taken into consideration. *Ascaris* worms are stimulated to migrate, which may cause unpleasant or dangerous situations. Their elimination prior to a $Cl_2C{=}CCl_2$ treatment is therefore advisable.

3.1.3.6 Conclusions

For individual therapy TCE is no longer the drug of choice it has been for half a century. It remains, however, a good and cheap treatment against *N. americanus*. For mass treatment its disadvantages are offset by its low cost, ease of administration, and wide experience about possible side effects. An interesting large-scale treatment, involving some 385,000 persons, was carried out in the Dominican Republic by CARR et al. (1954): 0.1–0.12 ml/kg (max. 4–5 ml) was very effective. To achieve a 100% CR two to three doses at 4-day intervals were necessary.

3.1.4 Organophosphorous Compounds

Several organic phosphorous compounds are useful pesticides, some of which also show good anthelmintic activity. At least two have been tested in humans: metrifonate (trichlorfon) and dichlorvos.

3.1.4.1 Metrifonate (*Bayer 2349*) (Trichlorfon)

3.1.4.1.1 State of the Art

Of some 50,000 organic phosphorous compounds synthesized by SCHRADER (1963) a few organophosphorous esters possess anthelmintic activity against Ascaridae of dogs and pigs and have been used in veterinary medicine since 1956. In 1962, CERF et al. tested several compounds on *A. suum* kept in vitro in Ringer solution at 37 °C. For use in man they selected Dipterex (Bayer 2349), a potent inhibitor of nematode cholinesterases.

This compound was introduced as an insecticide by LORENZ in 1952 (LORENZ et al. 1955). It was tried in its crude from (wettable powder worked up in tablets) by CERF (1958) under strict monitoring successively on 15 volunteers, on 40 hospitalized worm-infected patients, and on more than 2,000 people infected with hookworms associated or not with *Ascaris* and/or *Trichuris* infections.

After oral administration, important variations in resorption have been observed. This disparity is related to the physical and galenic presentation: for 50-μm particles the LD_{50} in mice is 125 mg/kg and for 100 μm 200 mg/kg. Consequently the choice fell on a granular polyvinyl chloride formulation in slow-release capsules (CERF et al. 1962).

3.1.4.1.2 Assessment

Table 5. Treatment of hookworm infection with metrifonate (trichlorfon)

Dosage (mg/kg/2 days)	Number treated	CR	References
15	625	91	CERF et al. (1962)
15	24	96 (15 days)	CERF et al. (1962)
15	41	85 (45 days)	CERF et al. (1962)
7.5	40	72	CERF et al. (1962)
20	20	70 (sick children)	CERF et al. (1962)
7.5	90	54	DA CRUZ FERREIRA et al. (1960)
15	20	70	DA CRUZ FERREIRA et al. (1960)

3.1.4.1.3 Dosage, Mode of Administration

A dose of 15 mg/kg administered by the oral route on two consecutive days, without any preparation, produces good results. The drug is available in tablets containing 100 mg active substance; not more than 950 mg should be administered at once. Tablets are to be swallowed whole with some liquid. Opened tins should be used as soon as possible. Discoloration of the tablets indicates that they are no longer suited for use. Exposure of the tablets to high temperatures must be avoided.

3.1.4.1.4 Side effects

Side effects practically absent; light or moderate transient dizziness, abdominal pain, vomiting, and diarrhea are occasionally observed; and symptomatic relief is obtained by atropini sulfas, while oximes (pralidoximine iodide or 2-PAM is an effective antidote in the case of poisoning) are useful for enzyme reactivation. No clinical effects on the CNS are observed, i.e., delayed neuropathy. Since 1967 pure metrifonate has been available, which produces even fewer side effects.

3.1.4.1.5 Contraindications, Precautions

One has to be aware of a rapid complete depression of the plasma cholinesterase, with a recovery to normal levels within days after the last dose, and of a lesser degree of inhibition of the erythrocyte cholinesterase (40%–60% of the pretreatment value), which persists longer, however (5–15 weeks). Treated individuals should be free from recent exposure to organophosphorous insecticides.

3.1.4.1.6 Comments

Metrifonate is a "pro-drug," its therapeutic action being due to its metabolite dichlorvos. Metrifonate can be useful, especially in areas where *S. haematobium* is also present.

3.1.4.2 Dichlorvos

This organophosphorous compound is derived from metrifonate following a rearrangement by deprotonation. It presents good activity against several helminths and is responsible for the insecticidal effect of metrifonate. Administered in slow-releasing pellets of the resin preparation, the safety margin is enhanced, while the efficacy is maintained.

3.1.4.2.1 Assessment

Table 6. Treatment of hookworm infection by dichlorvos

Parasite	Dosage (mg/kg)	Number treated	CR	References
Hookworm (95% *N. americanus*)	6	24	63	PEÑA-CHAVARRIA et al. (1969)
Hookworm	6 V_3[a]	39	77	CERVONI et al. (1969)
Hookworm	6 V_{12}[b]	90	94	CERVONI et al. (1969)
Hookworm	8 V_{12}	7	86	CERVONI et al. (1969)
Hookworm	10 V_{12}	5	100	CERVONI et al. (1969)
Hookworm	12 V_3	26	100	CERVONI et al. (1969)
Hookworm	12 V_3	54	91	CERVONI et al. (1969)
Hookworm	12	63	86	PEÑA CHAVARRIA et al. (1969)

[a] V_3, large pellets [b] V_{12}, small pellets

3.1.4.2.2 Dosage, Mode of Administration

A resin formulation in small pellets at 6 mg/kg is as efficacious as 12 mg/kg in large pellets. Administration is by the oral route.

3.1.4.2.3 Side Effects

Side effects are rather exceptional, although a mild vertigo, abdominal cramp, gastric spasms, and tremor of tongue and lids can occur. The half-life of dichlorvos is only 1–2 min. Statements concerning a possible carcinogenic effect are of a contradictory nature and without proof.

3.1.4.2.4 Contraindications, Precautions

A transient modest depression of the erythrocyte cholinesterase can occur but returns to normal in 1–3 days: this has been the subject of concern to many users, but its practical significance is not clear. It is the likely mechanism by which dichlorvos exerts its toxic effect on the worms.

3.1.4.2.5 Conclusion

Unnecessary alarm and anxiety has discouraged the use of a useful well-tolerated, cheap anthelmintic.

3.1.5 Thymol

This essential oil is present in several plants, such as *Thymus vulgaris* and *Origanum*, but is usually synthesized. Thymol is active against several intestinal parasites, i.e., hookworms. Its administration is cumbersome: three capsules of 0.5–1 g powdered thymol at hourly intervals on an empty stomach for three consecutive days. It is poorly accepted, produces a brown coloration of the urine (thymol-glucuronic acid) and is no longer in use, except as its iodinated derivate (Thymolan). A dosage of 5–6 g (100 mg/kg) produces conflicting CRs: 20%–24% (YOSHIDA et al. 1960), 45% (TAKAMURA 1963), and 86% (MUTALIK et al. 1964).

3.2 More recent Drugs

3.2.1 Albendazole

3.2.1.1 State of the Art

Albendazole has wide-spectrum activity against all major classes of experimental intestinal helminths (*Ascaris suum, Ancylostoma caninum, Toxocara canis, Trichuris vulpis, Syphacia obvelata, Taenia pisiformis, Hymenolepis nana,* and also *Paragonimus kellicotti*). This has provided the incentive to try it out in humans.

3.2.1.2 Assessment

Table 7. Treatment of hookworm infection by albendazole

Efficacy	Parasite	Dosage	Number treated	CR	ERR	References
100%	*Ancylostoma duodenale*	2 mg/kg b.i.d.	3	100	–	GARIN et al. (1980)
	Necator americanus	200 mg repeated after 14 days	7	100	–	PÈNE et al. (1981a)
	N. americanus	200–400 mg	6	100	–	GARIN and MOJON (1980)

Table 7 (continued)

Efficacy	Parasite	Dosage	Number treated	CR	ERR	References
100%	Hookworm	400 mg	5	100	–	CAMILO COURA et al. (1981a)
	N. americanus	200 mg b.i.d.	7	100	–	LUMBRERAS CRUZ et al. (1981)
	N. americanus	100 mg b.i.d./ 3 days	1	100	–	LUMBRERAS CRUZ et al. (1981)
	N. americanus	400 mg	7	100	–	PÈNE et al. (1981a)
	Hookworm	600 mg	18	100	–	RAMALINGHAM et al. (1983)
≧90%	*N. americanus*	10 mg/kg/2 days	–	95	–	AMATO-NETO et al. (1983)
	A. duodenale	2 mg/kg b.i.d. (repeated after 14 days)	39	90	43	EXCLER et al. (1981)
	A. duodenale	400 mg	35	90	–	PÈNE et al. (1981a)
	N. americanus	200 mg b.i.d.	93	96	–	PÈNE et al. (1981a)
	N. americanus	200 mg b.i.d.	21	90	–	MAISONNEUVE et al. (1981)
	Hookworm	400 mg	28	96	97	COULAUD et al. (1982)
	Hookworm	200 mg b.i.d.	10	90	99	BOURDERIOUX and CHEVALIER (1982)
	Hookworm	200 mg b.i.d.	32	97	–	CRUZ LOPEZ (1981)
	A. duodenale	400 mg	28	96	80	ROSSIGNOL (1981)
	Hookworm	400 mg	137	90	98	RANQUE et al. (1982)
	A. duodenale	200–400 mg	39	90	43	MOJON et al. (1982)
≧80%	*A. duodenale*	200–400 mg	38	89	–	GARIN and MOJON (1980)
	N. americanus	2 mg/kg b.i.d. repeated after 14 days	15	80	–	GARIN et al. (1980)
	N. americanus	200 mg b.i.d.	302	89	–	PÈNE et al. (1981b)
		200 mg b.i.d.	93	82	93	PÈNE et al. (1981b)
	N. americanus	2 mg/kg b.i.d.	7	86	–	MAISONNEUVE et al. (1981)
		4 mg/kg	11	82	–	MAISONNEUVE et al. (1981)
	N. americanus	200 mg b.i.d.	18	83	97	BARANSKI et al. (1981)
	A. duodenale	200 mg b.i.d.	8	87	97	BARANSKI et al. (1981)
	N. americanus	4 mg/kg	11	82	–	ROSSIGNOL (1981)
	N. americanus	200 mg b.i.d.	38	89	95	RICHARD-LENOBLE et al. (1982)
	N. americanus	400 mg 200 mg in children	9	89	75	LUMBRERAS CRUZ et al. (1981)
	N. americanus	400 mg	416	87	75	ROSSIGNOL (1981)
	Hookworm	400 mg	102	84	98	COULAUD et al. (1982b)
	N. americanus	400 mg	601	81	97	PÈNE et al. (1982b)
	Hookworm	800 mg	28	84	96	RAMALINGHAM et al. (1983)
≧70%	*N. americanus*	400 mg	144	76	88	KADIO et al. (1982)
	Hookworm	400 mg	88	74	96	SOULA and SIOPATHIS (1982)
	N. americanus	200 mg b.i.d.	29	76	95	RICHARD-LENOBLE et al. (1982)
	N. americanus	10 mg/kg	–	74	–	AMATO NETO et al. (1983)
<70%	*N. americanus*	400 mg	16	63	30	BASTIDAS (1982)
	N. americanus	400 mg	88	56	88	SENTILHES and CARRIE (1982)
	Hookworm	400 mg	33	69	94	RAMALINGHAM et al. (1983)

3.2.1.3 Dosage, Mode of Administration

Doses vary between 4 and 8 mg/kg, as single or repeated doses. The trend is to use 200 or 400 mg respectively for children and adults, but lately a dose of 400 mg, irrespective of age, has been recommended. Administration is by the oral route as 100 mg chewable tablets or a 2% suspension.

3.2.1.4 Side Effects

Slight side effects are observed in about 10% of cases: nausea, epigastric pain, meteorismus, dizziness, pruritus, vomiting, diarrhea, and fever. Biomedical controls remain satisfactory.

3.2.1.5 Contraindications and Precautions

Albendazole has been shown to be embryotoxic and teratogenic in animals; it should not therefore be used during pregnancy.

3.2.1.6 Conclusions

Albendazole, being equally effective against *N. americanus* and *A. duodenale*, appears to be a useful and encouraging acquisition in the treatment of ancylostomiasis, both on a individual and a community basis.[2]

The latest data on the efficacy of a single dose of 400 mg on *N. americanus* provided by ROSSIGNOL and MAISONNEUVE (1984) are interesting. The LR and ERR are resfreelively for light infections (EPG ≦2,000) 91% and 72%, for moderate infections (EPG 2,000–10,000) 70% and 66% and for heavy infections (EPG > 10,000) 67% and 64%.

3.2.1.7 Comments

The spectrum of activity includes gastrointestinal nematodes, lung and other tissue nematodes, several tapeworms, and liver flukes. However, in a single dose its activity on *Trichuris trichiura* is weak-moderate. the chewing of four tablets is not always accepted, nor indeed performed. It is rather arduous to ascertain if the prospects for mass treatment are as bright as the available information. One cannot help thinking that several data have been used over and over again, on different occasions. This impression is not restricted to albendazole; data on other drugs summon identical remarks.

3.2.2 Amidantel (Bay d-8815)

3.2.2.1 State of the Art

Broad anthelmintic activity in animals indicated a possible efficacy against *A. duodenale*, *N. americanus*, *Ascaris lumbricoides*, and *Strongyloides stercoralis* (WOLLWEBER et al. 1979). In dogs a single oral dose of 25 mg/kg reduces the parasite load by 97%–100% in *Ancylostoma caninum*, *Uncinaria stenocephala*, and *Toxocara canis* infections.

---

2 As observed with other drugs results registered are sometimes better in heavy infections (10,000 EPG); the ERR reaches 100%

3.2.2.2 Assessment

RIM et al. (1980) established the efficacy of amidantel on a single blind placebo-controlled study. In 64 patients infected with *A. duodenale* (12–59 years of age), 6 mg/kg produced a CR of 94% and an ERR of 99%. These results were confirmed in a second trial on 76 persons infected with hookworm: the CR was 96% for *A. duodenale* with an ERR of 99%. Yet, amidantel is less, although still substantially, active against *N. americanus:* CR 15% and ERR 65%. No further information has been found. The development of this compound has been discontinued.

3.2.2.3 Dosage, Mode of Administration

The dose is 6 mg/kg by the oral route.

3.2.2.4 Side Effects

Side effects are mild, transient, and dose dependent (over 6 mg/kg body wt): headache, nausea, dizziness, abdominal discomfort, fatigue, and vomiting.

3.2.3 Amoscanate (C. 9333-GO/CGP 4540; Bisconate)

3.2.3.1 State of the Art

Several isothiocyanates display activity against intestinal and systemic nematodes as well as against trematodes. Among these compounds 4-isothiocyanate-4′-nitrodiphenylamine was selected by STRIEBEL (1976) on the basis of its high therapeutic index in experimental filariasis and schistosomiasis. BUEDING et al. (1976) showed that effectiveness was markedly enhanced by reduction of particle size from 30 to 0.5 μm. SEN (1976) established that this compound is highly effective against *N. americanus* adapted to hamsters. DOSHI et al. (1977) obtained CR of 62% and an ERR close to 100% in clinical trials.

3.2.3.2 Assessment

Table 8. Treatment of hookworm infections by amoscanate

Efficacy	Parasite	Dosage	Number treated	CR	ERR	References
100%	*Ancylostoma cluodenale*	1,000 mg × 3 (12 hourly)	7	100	–	VAKIL et al. (1977)
	A. duodenale (Necator americanus) [a]	1,000 mg × 3 (12 hourly)	6	100	–	DOSHI et al. (1977)
	N. americanus (A. duodenale) [a]	1,000 mg × 3 (12 hourly)	5	100	–	VAIDHYA et al. 1977)
	A. duodenale	500 mg × 3 (8 hourly)	11	100	–	VAKIL et al. (1977)
	A. duodenale	250 mg × 3 (8 hourly)	7	100	–	VAKIL et al. (1977)
	N. americanus (N. americanus) [a]	250 mg × 3 (8 hourly)	5	100	–	VAIDHYA et al. (1977)
	N. americanus + A. duodenale	30 mg/kg	20	100	–	GUPTA et al. (1979)

Table 8 (continued)

Efficacy	Parasite	Dosage	Number treated	CR	ERR	References
≧90%	*N. americanus* + *A. duodenale*	250 mg × 3 (12 hourly)	11	91	80–89	GUPTA et al. (197
≧80%	*N. americanus* + *A. duodenale*	1,000 mg × 3 (12 hourly)	8	88	99	GUPTA et al. (197
	N. americanus + *(A. duodenale)* [a]	250 mg × 3 (8 hourly)	15	87	99	DOSHI et al. (197
	N. americanus + *A. duodenale*	250 mg × 3 (4 hourly)	7	86	90–99	GUPTA et al. (197
	N. americanus + *A. duodenale*	125 mg × 3	21	86	90–99	GUPTA et al. (197
	N. americanus + *A. duodenale*	500 mg × 3 (12 hourly)	11	82	90–99	GUPTA et al. (197
	N. americanus + *(A. duodenale)* [a]	125 mg × 3 (4 hourly)	10	80	–	VAIDHYA et al. (1977)
≧70%	*A. duodenale*	125 mg × 3 (4 hourly)	18	78	99	VAKIL et al. (197
	A. duodenale	250 mg × 2 (2 hourly)	11	73	82	VAKIL et al. (197
≧60%	*N. americanus*	30 mg/kg	24	67	78[b] 99[c]	SINGH et al. (198
≧50%	*N. americanus* *(A. duodenale)* [a]	500 mg × 3 (12 hourly)	6	50	88	DOSHI et al. (197
	N. americanus + *A. duodenale*	125 mg × 3 (2 hourly)	25	56	90–99	GUPTA et al. (197
< 50%	*N. americanus*	125 mg × 3 (4 hourly)	6	33	96	DOSHI et al. (197
	A. duodenale	250 mg × 2 (4 hourly)	8	25	–	VAKIL et al. (197
	N. americanus *(A. duodenale)* [a]	125 mg × 3 (2 hourly)	6	–	–	DOSHI et al. (197

[a] *A. duodenale* present in lower percentage. [b] *A. duodenale.* [c] *N. americanus*

3.2.3.3 Dosage, Mode of Administration

Amoscanate is available in tablets of 50, 100, 250, and 500 mg, to be administered orally after overnight fast. Although multiple doses (1,000 mg × 3 at 12-hourly intervals, 500 or 250 mg × 3 at 8- or 4-hourly intervals) cure the majority of persons infected with hookworm, equally *A. duodenale* and *N. americanus*, the single dose of 30 mg/kg is the most useful.

3.2.3.4 Side Effects

On the whole amoscanate produces only mild complaints such as a mild giddiness, sweating, palpitations, vomiting, abdominal pain, diarrhea. However, caution must be advised. On Santa Lucia its use against *S. mansoni* had to be stopped due to jaundice (1%–3%), cholangitis, hypotension, and signs of possible neurotoxicity.

3.2.3.5 Contraindications, Precautions

Mutagenic activation by metabolites of a low order has been detected, but can be prevented by the coadministration of a single oral dose of erythromycin (BATZINGER et al. 1979). It requires the classical precautionary measures.

3.2.3.6 Conclusion

Amoscanate is active in a single dose of 30 mg/kg against hookworm, equally against *A. duodenale* and *N. americanus*. However, the EER is slightly less marked where the pretreatment EPG is higher; the efficacy of the drug is in inverse relation to the worm load. The final decision about its large-scale use will be determined by a more thorough knowledge of its risks.

3.2.4 Bephenium Hydroxynaphthoate

3.2.4.1 State of the Art

Experiments in dogs and cats infected with *A. caninum*, in rats with *Nippostrongylus muris*, and in mice with *Nematospiroides dubius* have shown that bephenium hydroxynaphthoate, a cholinergic agonist, was active against these helminths. GOODWIN et al. (1958) tried it on *Necator americanus* in man in Sri Lanka, by means of a single dose of 2–3 g base, or in multiple doses given on the same or successive days. The compound was found highly effective: very heavy infections were cured and egg counts were reduced to insignificant proportions.

3.2.4.2 Assessment

CAVIER (1973) and DAVIS (1973) made an extensive review of the first trials with bephenium salts in human ancylostomiasis. GOODWIN et al. (1958) showed that the hydroxynaphthoate was the best choice as a standard drug. It was then tried out by a number of clinicians and parasitologists in several parts of the world. These initial attempts were evaluated on different dose schedules with a wide variety of doses, administered once, twice, or three times on single or consecutive days twice a week or at weekly intervals.

The results of nonrandomized studies with a great variety of schedules, such as that on 163 American female mental patients infected with *N. americanus* (YOUNG et al. 1960) and on 95 children with hookworm (JUNG and MACCROAN 1960) are almost impossible to interpret. Their comparative simultaneous trial with TCE serves no other purpose than to arrive at diametrically opposite conclusions with the same drugs; for the former bephenium is superior; for the latter TCE is more efficient. Out of several observations it could, however, be inferred that a single dose of 2.5 g base produced very encouraging results. This interesting lead was explored further and the results of these trials are summarized in Table 9.

The results are very satisfactory on the whole with CRs of about 80% and over. Noteworthy are the excellent results obtained by LAMBOTTE et al. (1960) in Zaire in infants aged 1–3 months and suffering from severe anemia. HULET and KAUFFMANN (1963) obtained, by means of a single dose of 1.25 g base, a CR of 67% in 50 out of 75 infants aged between 6 weeks and 12 months suffering from ancylostomiasis and anemia.

Table 9. Treatment of hookworm infection by bephenium hydroxynaphthoate

Efficacy	Parasite	Number treated	CR	ERR	References
≧90%	*Ancylostoma duodenale*	153	98	–	HAHN et al. (1960)
	A. duodenale	31	93	–	ZAKINE and ZAKINE (1960)
	A. duodenale	25	92	–	SHIGEO-IWATA et al. (1962)
	A. duodenale	30	93	–	AHMAD et al. (1964)
	A. duodenale	239	95	–	NAGATY and RIFAAT (1959)
	A. duodenale	50	92	77	FARAHMANDIAN et al. (1972)
≧80%	*A. duodenale*	74	82	–	AHMAD and RASOOL (1959)
	A. duodenale + *Necator americanus*	500	80	–	LAMBOTTE et al. (1960)
	N. americanus	17	88	–	BECQUET (1963)
	A. duodenale	95	85	–	SALEM et al. (1965)
	A. duodenale + *N. americanus*	74	83	–	AHMAD and GHULAM (1959)
	N. americanus	–	85	–	HULET and KAUFFMANN (1963)
	Hookworm	425	80	–	DEMÉ and SAGNET (1961)
≧70%	*A. duodenale*	34	79	–	MEHROTRA and MALAVIYA (1963)
	A. duodenale	123	79	–	ABDALLAH and SAIF (1963)
≧60%	*N. americanus*	60	62	–	GHYSELS and SARTIAUX (1959)
	N. americanus	–	61	–	HUTTON and SOMERS (1961)
	N. americanus	12	67	–	NAGATY and RIFAAT (1959)
≧50%	*N. americanus*	20	55	–	ROWLAND (1966)
≧40%	*N. americanus*	50	46	–	NINANE and POFFE (1959)
	A. duodenale + *N. americanus*	41	44	–	YOSHIDA et al. (1960)
<40%	*N. americanus*	57	28	–	CHEGE et al. (1974)
	N. americanus	–	16	67	GUNDERS (1960)
	Hookworm	31	16	64	JUNG and MACCROAN (1960)

3.2.4.3 Dosage[3] and Mode of Administration

Bephenium hydroxynaphthoate is available in 5-g sachets, equivalent to 2.5 g base, 1 g bephenium hydroxynaphthoate being equivalent to 500 mg bephenium base. The granules are to be administered in water on an empty stomach. Food should be withheld for at least 2 h. For children it might be advisable to hide the bitter taste with a sweetened or flavored liquid. Half a dose (1.25 g base) appears to be adequate for children under 2 years or weighing less than 20 kg. Neither diet before nor purgation after treatment is necessary.

The total dose is 150 mg/kg for an adult of 50 kg and 300 mg/kg for children of 25 kg. Against *N. americanus* and in heavy infections of *A. duodenale* three doses on consecutive days are advisable and will ensure a 80% worm clearance. Light and moderate *N. americanus* infections are cleared by 2 doses.

3 Doses are expressed as weights of bephenium base

3.2.4.4 Side Effects

Bephenium is fairly well tolerated. Nausea, sometimes vomiting, may occur, especially in young children objecting to the bitter taste. Moreover anorexia, dizziness, abdominal pain, and a mild diarrhea which favors the expulsion of the hookworm are encountered in 7%–10% or more cases, but are mild and transient. The intolerance is more pronounced with the higher doses.

3.2.4.5 Contraindications, Precautions

Bephenium is a safe drug. Pregnancy and very severe anemia in children are not contraindications, but should be taken into consideration for decision.

3.2.4.6 Conclusions

3.2.4.6.1 Individual Treatment

The results of the treatment with bephenium hydroxynaphthoate at a dosage of 2.5 g on three consecutive days are fairly good. However, bephenium is more effective against *A. duodenale* (80%–98% CR) than against *N. americanus* (CR 46%–88%), but with a strong ERR for both.

3.2.4.6.2 Mass Treatment

A single dose, regardless of age or weight in children over 2 years, produces results which make the drug suitable for mass treatment, especially of infants with or without severe anemia. The claims by PAVIOT and NIOGUY (1960) and JUNG and MACCROAN (1960) that TCE is more effective have not been confirmed. However, bephenium hydroxynaphthoate is too expensive for large-scale treatment. There is a good consensus about the good tolerance in spite of a bitter taste and the easy administration as neither fasting nor aperients have to be used. COMMEY and HADDOCK (1970) stated that some hookworms developed resistance against bephenium hydroxynaphthoate: this has not been corroborated.

3.2.5 Bitoscanate

3.2.5.1 State of the Art

Bitoscanate is active against *A. duodenale* and *N. americanus*, and according to HSIEH et al. (1970) more so against *N. americanus*. BHANDARI and SINGHI (1969) obtained a comparable ERR against *A. duodenale* in 90 outpatients, aged between 16 and 63 years with three different protocols: 150 mg × 1, 150 mg × 2 with a 24-h interval, and 150 mg × 3 at 12-h interval, 4 weeks after the treatment. However, a much higher CR (92%) was obtained with the latter regimen, against only 50% and 70% respectively for the two other dosages.

BOTERO and PEREZ (1970) tried bitoscanate against *N. americanus* in 40 ambulatory and 20 hospitalized patients, all of them with an EPG of over 2,000 (maximum, 90,000). The adopted dosage was 100 mg × 3, at 12-h intervals. Only 18 out of the 60 (30%) were cured, but the majority of the remaining 42 showed an ERR of 95%.

3.2.5.2 Assessment

The observations of BHANDARI and SINGHI (1969) and of BOTERO and PEREZ (1970) started a series of therapeutic trials. But MUTALIK and GULATI (1969) and MUTALIK et al. (1970) selected a somewhat different dosage: 200 mg twice at 12-h intervals. Administered to 30 anemic patients, predominantly infected with *N. americanus*, 16 were egg-negative (CR 53%) 4 weeks later and 11 (CR 37%) had an ERR of 95%. Side effects were frequent but mild.

KILALA et al. (1970) in Tanzania tried the selected dosage on 23 persons infected with *N. americanus*, on 2 with *A. duodenale*, and on 7 with mixed infections. On day 30, 13 out of 32 (40%) were negative, 10 out of 32 (30%) had an ERR between 70% and 99%, 6 out of 32 (19%) an ERR between 10% and 69%, and the remaining 3 (10%) showed no reduction at all. Side effects were frequent, but no treatment had to be discontinued. PATEL and OLWENY (1972) treated 40 patients with *N. americanus* and EPGs in excess of 1,000: after 4 weeks, the CR was 78% and in the still infected an ERR of 92% was achieved.

A series of trials are summarized in Table 10.

In children of the 5- to 9-year-old group a dose of 50 mg b.i.d. and for the 10- to 15-year-old group a dose of 100 mg b.i.d. provided CRs of 88% (16 out of 18) and 83% (10 out of 12) (BHANDARI and SHRIMALI 1969). BHANDARI and SHRIMALI also demonstrated that the higher doses used by MUTALIK et al. (1970) do not improve the efficacy.

The lower regimen used by O'HOLOHAN and HUGOE-MATHEWS (1972) in the 4- to 9-year-old group, 50 mg × 1, and 100 mg × 1 in the 10- to 14-year-old group provide less satisfactory results: CR of 34% (17 out of 50), but the ERR is 95%. The observations of these authors on the ERR, which is almost the same irrespective of the pretreatment EPG are noteworthy: at 2,000, 93%; 3,000, 96%; 4,000, 94%; 5,000–10,000, 96%; >10,000, 95%.

Table 10. Treatment of hookworm intection by bitoscanate

Efficacy	Parasite	Dosage	Number treated	CR	ERR	References
100%	*Necator americanus*	100 mg × 3 (12 hourly)	17	100	–	HSIEH et al. (1970)
≧90%	*Ancylostoma duodenale*	100 mg × 3 (12 hourly)	50	92	99	BHANDARI and SINGHI (1969)
	Hookworm	100 mg × 3 (12 hourly)	49	96	–	CHANCO et al. (1972)
≧80%	*A. duodenale* + *N. americanus*	100 mg × 3 (12 hourly)	30	83	98	HSIEH et al. (1979)[a]
	Hookworm	50 mg × 2 (12 hourly)	18	88	72	BHANDARI and SHRIMALI (196[illegible]
	Hookworm	100 mg × 3 (12 hourly)	12	83	92–96	BHANDARI and SHRIMALI (196[illegible]
	A. duodenale + *N. americanus*	100 mg × 3 (12 hourly)	30	83	94	MUTALIK et al. (1970)
	A. duodenale + *N. americanus*	150 mg × 3 (12 hourly)	147	87	93	SHAFEI et al. (1971)

Table 10 (continued)

Efficacy	Parasite	Dosage	Number treated	CR	ERR	References
≧70%	*A. duodenale* + *N. americanus*	100 mg × 3 (12 hourly)	101	74	91	MUTALIK et al. (1970)
	Hookworm	200 mg × 3 (12 hourly)	30	70	70	SHAFEI et al. (1971)
	N. americanus	200 mg × 3 (12 hourly)	40	78	92	PATEL and OLWENY (1972)
	A. duodenale + *N. americanus*	150 mg	1,741	79	–	HOLTZ et al. (1972)
	A. duodenale	150 mg × 2	20	70	96	BHANDARI and SINGHI (1969)
≧60%	Hookworm	100 mg × 3 (12 hourly)	23	65	98	MUTALIK and GULATI (1972)
	Hookworm	300 mg	16	68	–	SHAFEI et al. (1971)
≧50%	Hookworm (*N. americanus*)	100 mg × 3 (12 hourly)	17	52	50–60	GOLDSMID and MACCABE (1972)
	A. duodenale + *N. americanus*	100 mg × 2 (12 hourly)	6	50	77	MUTALIK et al. (1970)
	Hookworm	150 mg × 3 (12 hourly)	30	50	–	SHAFEI et al. (1971)
	N. americanus	200 mg × 2 (12 hourly)	30	53	95	MUTALIK and GULATI (1969)
	A. duodenale	150 mg	20	50	93	BHANDARI and SINGHI (1969)
≧40%	*A. duodenale* + *N. americanus*	100 mg × 3 (12 hourly)	17	47	98	HSIEH et al. (1970)[a]
	N. americanus	100 mg × 3 (12 hourly)	13	46	98	HSIEH et al. (1970)
	A. duodenale + *N. americanus*	100 mg × 3 (12 hourly)	32	40	72	KILALA et al. (1970)
≧30%	Hookworm	100–150 mg	14	36	70–90	BIAGI et al. (1969)
	N. americanus	50–100 mg	50	34	84	O'HOLOHAN and HUGOE MATHEWS (1972)
	N. americanus	150 mg	32	34	70	GAITONDE et al. (1969)
	N. americanus	150 mg	51	35	90	CHITRATHORN et al. (1972)
	N. americanus	100 mg × 3 (12 hourly)	60	30	95	BOTERO and PEREZ (1970)
<20%	*A. duodenale* + *N. americanus*	100 mg × 3 (12 hourly)	16	19	75	POBEE and AMISSAH (1970)
	N. americanus	100 mg × 3 (12 hourly)	24	4	84	JOHNSON (1971)
	N. americanus	3 mg/kg	52	–		CHEGE et al. (1974)

[a] The CR in the same group varies in a nonnegligible manner according to the methodology of the stool examination: with the Stoll method the figure is 90%, but drops to 47% when the Stoll method is combined with the test-tube filter paper cultivation method

3.2.5.3 Dosage, Mode of Administration

The recommended doses are: for adults, 3 × 100 mg at 12-h intervals; for children between 10 and 14 years, 2 × 100 mg at 12-h intervals; and for children between 5 and 9 years: 2 × 50 mg at 12-h intervals. Some authors have obtained good results with single 150 mg doses, which others have been unable to confirm. The drug is available in capsules of 50 mg, to be swallowed after meals. No dietary or other preparation is needed.

3.2.5.4 Side Effects

The drug is taken up in the intestine and circulates. Up to 3–6 h after administration irritation of the gastrointestinal tract and a direct central effect can follow. Complaints are rather frequent – 15%–57%: malaise, abdominal fullness, anorexia, diarrhea (30%), nausea, vomiting, abdominal pain, headache, and dizziness. These side effects are mild or moderate and always transient, but too numerous to make bitoscanate a first choice.

3.2.5.5 Contraindications, Precautions

The still limited experience with regard to a drug with slow elimination and insufficient information on possible harmful effects on the thyroid function indicates that repeated treatments and administration to pregnant or breast-feeding women or to children under five should be avoided. Drivers and persons whose occupation demands mental alertness will also be excluded. It should also be kept in mind that alcohol and coffee increase the risk of adverse reactions.

3.2.5.6 Conclusions

3.2.5.6.1 Individual Therapy

The three-dose regimen of 100 mg at 12-h intervals is generally successful, giving on average a CR of between 70% and 96%.

3.2.5.6.2 Mass Treatment

The administration of a single dose of 150 mg has been used by several authors. GAITONDE et al. (1969) treated 32 persons infected with *N. americanus*. On day 16, a 100% reduction in EPG was obtained in 8 out of 32 (25%) and on day 30 in 11 out of 32 (34%). The remaining had an ERR of 70% or more. In Thailand the efficacy was assessed by CHITRATHORN et al. (1972) in 51 persons infected with *N. americanus*: the CR was only 35% (18 out of 51), the ERR 90%. HOLTZ et al. (1972) used the single dose on 1,724 individuals living on Java and infected with *A. duodenale* and/or *N. americanus*: 1,362 were cured, a CR of 79%. This inconsistency in results precludes indisputable recommendations that only a single-dose regimen is worthwhile.

3.2.5.7 Comments

The available data do not permit a conclusion to be drawn about the respective sensitivity of *A. duodenale* and *N. americanus* to bitoscanate. However, there is a consensus about its excellent ERR for both hookworms, which is an important achievement. This drug is only available in India, where it is produced by Hoechst Pharmaceuticals Ltd., India.

3.2.6 Ciclobendazole

3.2.6.1 State of the Art

This benzimidazole derivative produces its highest activity in the intestinal tract and against intestinal nematodes.

A few attempts to control hookworm have been made with this benzimidazole derivative, but without encouraging results.

3.2.6.2 Assessment

Table 11. Treatment of hookworm infection by ciclobendazole

Efficacy	Parasite	Dosage	Number treated	CR	References
>50%	Hookworm	1,200 mg	25	52	GUGGENMOOS et al. (1978)
<50%	Hookworm	600 mg	26	44	GUGGENMOOS et al. (1978)
		100 mg b.i.d./3 days	13	39	DEGREMONT and STAHEL (1978)
		200 mg b.i.d./3 days	5	20	DEGREMONT and STAHEL (1978)

3.2.6.3 Comments

This substance is closely related to mebendazole; it has the same pharmacological activity, but requires a slightly higher dosage.

3.2.6.4 Side Effects

The only complaints are occasional meteorism, diarrhea, and abdominal spasm.

3.2.7 Fenbendazole

3.2.7.1 State of the Art

This compound is effective against the important gastrointestinal helminths, including *Taenia* spp., in natural and experimental infections of animals. It is well tolerated. It has been used mainly in cattle, sheep, goats, pigs, horses, dogs, cats, etc., but a few trials have carried out in man.

3.2.7.2 Assessment

Table 12. Treatment of hookworm infection by fenbendazole

Parasite	Dosage	Number treated	CR	ERR	References
Necator americanus	100 mg b.i.d./3 days	18	89	80%	SANCHEZ-CARILLO and BELTRAN-HERNANDEZ (1977)
N. americanus	1 g	31	26	–	BRUCH and HAAS (1976)
	1 g 500 mg	20	15	–	BRUCH and HAAS (1976)
Hookworm	30–50 mg/kg	18	83	–	RIM et al. (1975)

3.2.7.3 Comments

The manufacturer limits the use of fenbendazole to veterinary practice. As its efficacy against hookworm is not conclusive and the ERR limited, it is unlikely that this benzimidazole will ever take up a valuable position among the anthelmintics for human use.

3.2.8 Flubendazole

3.2.8.1 State of the Art

Flubendazole is active against hookworms. The results of a large series of trials undertaken in different parts of the world are consistent and justify this assertion, with the exception of the Far East and more specifically Java.

3.2.8.2 Assessment

Tentative treatments started in 1976 and satisfactory CRs were achieved with doses of 200 mg for 3 days by BRUMPT (1976), BECQUET (1976), and GENTILINI (1976). Their results have been confirmed.

Table 13. Treatment of hookworm infection by flubendazole

Efficacy	Parasite	Dosage	Number treated	CR	ERR	References
100%	Hookworm	600 mg/3 days	8	100	–	BOUVIER (1976)
		2 g	3	100	–	BOUVIER (1976)
		2 g	17	100	–	NEYRINCK-VAN KERCKHOV (1976), BALDEZ et al. (1978)
	Hookworm	200 mg t.i.d.	1 (H)	100	–	DA SILVA (1979)
	Hookworm	100 mg t.i.d./2 days	11 (M)	100	–	DA SILVA (1979)
	Hookworm	100 mg t.i.d./2 days	1 (M)	100	–	DA SILVA (1979)
	Hookworm	100 mg b.i.d./3 days	5	100	–	LEÃO (1980)
	Hookworm	100 mg b.i.d./3 days	4	100	–	BLECHMAN et al. (1982)
	Hookworm	100 mg b.i.d./3 days	7 (M)	100	–	KATZ (1980)
	Hookworm	100 mg b.i.d./3 days	5 (H)	100	–	KATZ (1980)
	Hookworm	100 mg b.i.d./3 days	6	100	–	YANGCO and KLEIN (1980)
	Necator americanus	1 g/7 days	6	100	–	COMBESCOT and DUONG (1980)
≧90%	*Ancylostoma duodenale + N. americanus*	100 mg b.i.d./3 days	30	90	–	BRUMPT (1976)
	Hookworm	200 mg/3 days	38	95	–	GENTILINI (1976), DANIS et al. (1980)
	Hookworm	200 mg/4 days	15	93	–	DANIS et al. (1980)
	Hookworm	100 mg b.i.d./3 days	35 (L)	94	99	KATZ (1980)
	Hookworm	100 mg t.i.d./2 days	14	93	99	DA SILVA (1979)
	Hookworm	600 mg/3 days	–	94	–	BOURÉE et al. (1978)
	N. americanus	100 mg b.i.d./3 days	39	97	99	CANESE et al. (1978)

Table 13 (continued)

Efficacy	Parasite	Dosage	Number treated	CR	ERR	References
≧80%	Hookworm	100 mg b.i.d./4 days	54	89	87	BECQUET (1976), BECQUET-LABARRIÈRE (1980)
	Hookworm	400 mg/3 days	5	80	–	BOUVIER (1976)
	N. americanus	900 mg/3 days	8	86	–	PENOT et al. (1978)
	Hookworm	300 mg/2 days	27	82	96	BUNNAG et al. (1980)
	Hookworm	100 mg b.i.d./3 days	8	88	99	DA SILVA (1979)
	Hookworm	100 mg t.i.d./2 days	36 (L)	80	97	DA SILVA (1979)
	Hookworm	100 mg b.i.d./4 days	54	89	87	LABARRIÈRE (1980)
	Hookworm	500 mg b.i.d.	9	89	89	PEÑA-CHAVARRIA (1977)
	Hookworm	500 mg t.i.d.	9	89	95	PEÑA-CHAVARRIA (1977)
≧70%	*N. americanus*	600 mg/3 days	15	75	–	PENOT et al. (1978)
	Hookworm	1 g b.i.d.	9	78	91	PEÑA-CHAVARRIA (1977)
	Hookworm	2 g	10	70	83	PEÑA-CHAVARRIA (1977)
	Hookworm (semirural)	500 mg	51	75	95	ISMAIL and LIONEL (1981)
	Hookworm (urban)	500 mg	19	74	97	ISMAIL and LIONEL (1981)
≧60%	*N. americanus*	200 mg/3 days	66	62	–	NOZAIS (1978)
	Hookworm	1 g	16	62	77	PEÑA-CHAVARRIA (1977)
≧50%	Hookworm	100 mg b.i.d./2 days	2 (M)	50	98	KATZ (1980)
	Hookworm	100 mg b.i.d./2 days	2 (H)	50	99	DA SILVA (1979)
≧40%	Hookworm	100 mg b.i.d./2 days	91	46	88	ARFAA et al. (1979)
	Hookworm	200 mg t.i.d./1 day	63	40	98	DA SILVA (1979)
	Hookworm	200 mg t.i.d./1 day	14 (L)	43	92	DA SILVA (1979)
	Hookworm	100 mg t.i.d./2 days	19	42	83	CABRERA et al. (1980)
<30%	Hookworm	1 g×1	28	21	74	COLAERT (1976)
	Hookworm	2 g×1	26	15	79	COLAERT (1976)

H, heavy; M, moderate; L, light egg load

3.2.8.3 Dosage, Mode of Administration

Flubendazole is available in tablets of 100 mg or in a suspension of 100 mg/5 ml. A total dosage of 600 mg may be necessary. The efficacy appears to be related to the duration of the treatment, with an optimal spread of 3 days. This can be achieved by the administration of 100-mg tablets or 5 ml of a suspension of 20 mg/ml, after morning and evening meals for 3 days. Neither diet nor laxative are necessary. For mass treatment a single standard dose of 200–600 mg has been tried out and found effective in *Ascaris* and *Trichuris* infections and promising against ancylostomiasis. The life of the preparation is limited; the date of expiry must be checked.

3.2.8.4 Side Effects

Flubendazole is practically an inert compound, with a very low resorption. Consequently, tolerance is excellent and complaints are few and transient: headache, nausea, abdominal pain, meteorism, and mild diarrhea. BUNNAG et al. (1980) mention one attack of breathlessness without further explanation. No alterations in the hepatic, renal, and hematopoietic systems were observed and the biological tests remained normal.

3.2.8.5 Contraindications, Precautions

Although neither embryotoxicity nor teratogenecity are on record, it is advisable to restrain from administration during pregnancy. In contrast sickle cell trait or anaemia is not a contraindication.

3.2.8.6 Conclusions

3.2.8.6.1 Individual Therapy

A dose of 100 mg b.i.d. for 3 days procures a CR of some 95% to 100%. The same total dosage administered in 2 days (100 mg t.i.d.) is somewhat less satisfactory. In the Far East the results are generally poor: in Jakarta the CR is only 5.4% (MARGONO et al. 1980). Higher dosages or a more prolonged administration does not ensure better results. The origin of this striking discrepancy is unknown.

3.2.8.6.2 Mass Therapy

The perfect results of a single 2-g dose, claimed by BOUVIER (1976), NEYRINCK and VAN KERCKHOVE (1976) were confirmed neither by PEÑA-CHAVARRIA (1977) nor by COLAERT (1976). Their ERR was only 75%–80% and a significant increase in side effects was observed. In a single dose of 500 mg promising results were obtained recently against hookworm with a much better tolerance (ISMAIL and LIONEL 1981).

3.2.8.7 Comments

Individual treatment aims at a high CR, while mass treatment can be linked to a maximum ERR. Both can be achieved by the use of different goal-adapted dosages.

The EPG load can influence the CR: NOZAÏS (1978) found that, in 66 children living in the outskirts of Abidjan (Ivory Coast), in light infections (< 500 EPG) the CR was 80%, in medium infections (501–3,000 EPG) the CR came down to 58%, and in heavy infections (> 3,000 EPG) the CR was arrested at 46%. It has been established that the CR improves with a treatment spread over more days (ARFAA et al. 1979; BUNNAG et al. 1980). The classic soil-transmitted triad can be controlled by periodic treatment.

3.2.9 Levamisole

3.2.9.1 State of the Art

Levamisole is active against a broad spectrum of human and animal nematodes, including *A. duodenale, N. americanus*, and other Ancylostomidae.

The first results in human hookworm were conflicting. The explanation for the observed variability was given by THIENPONT et al. (1969), when they established that the "levo-isomer" of tetramisole was the active formula. They tried out different treatment schedules in Sulawesi, on 333 adults and children carefully preselected according to the degree of prevalent sanitary conditions. They reached the following conclusions: levamisole is active against *A. duodenale* and *N. americanus* with a CR of 80%; the most advisable dosage is 2.5 mg/kg; levamisole is well tolerated. These conclusions are still valid.

GATTI et al. (1969) confirmed the value of a single dose of 2.5 mg/kg in African schoolchildren. In two groups of children the apparent CRs, controlled after 5 and 15 days, were 86% and 90%, but in a third group, living in a very unsatisfactory environment, the CR was only 32%. A subsequent trial (GATTI et al. 1970) in a similar population, but with a follow-up after 2–3 weeks, brought the CR down to 28%. However, in both trials the mean EPG showed a marked reduction: 68% and 89%, respectively.

3.2.9.2 Assessment

These encouraging results initiated large-scale testing; their results have been summarized in Table 14.

Table 14. Treatment of hookworm infections by levamisole

Efficacy	Parasite	Dosage	Number treated	CR	ERR	References
100%	Hookworm	5 mg/kg	41	100	–	AL SAFFAR et al. (1971)
	Hookworm	5 mg/kg/2 days	9	100	–	AL SAFFAR et al. (1971)
	Ancylostoma duodenale	150 mg	25	100	–	KILPATRICK et al. (1981)
≧90%	*A. duodenale* + *Necator americanus*	2.5 mg/kg	21	90	–	GATTI et al. (1969)
	Hookworm	150 mg b.i.d./4 days	50	92	92	BANNERJEE et al. (1972b)
	A. duodenale	2.5 mg/kg	83	95	98	FARAHMANDIAN et al. (1974)
	A. duodenale	80–120 mg	29	93	–	FARID et al. (1973)
	A. duodenale	150 mg	41	93	–	FARID et al. (1977)
≧80%	Hookworm	2.5 mg/kg	21	86	79	THIENPONT et al. (1969)
	Hookworm	5 mg/kg	22	82	94	THIENPONT et al. (1969)
	A. duodenale + *N. americanus*	2.5 mg/kg	45	87	–	GATTI et al. (1969)
	N. americanus	3.5 mg/kg	21	86	–	VAKIL (1969)
	N. americanus	5 mg/kg	21	86	–	BOUYER (1970)
	N. americanus	6 mg/kg	25	84	–	SAUGRAIN and DELAVAL (1970)
	N. americanus	100 mg/3 days	40	80	92	SINNIAH and SINNIAH (1981)
≧70%	Hookworm	5 mg/kg/2 days	28	75	90	THIENPONT et al. (1969)
	Hookworm	2.5–3.5 mg/kg	2682	70	–	ORBAN (1972)
	N. americanus	160 mg/3 days	35	74	86	SEZI (1974)
	N. americanus	3.5 mg/kg	9	78	–	VAKIL (1969)

Table 14 (continued)

Efficacy	Parasite	Dosage	Number treated	CR	ERR	References
≧60%	Hookworm	5 mg/kg/3 days	43	65	61	THIENPONT et al. (1969)
	Hookworm	3 mg/kg/2 days	60	63	–	BANNERJEE et al. (1972b)
	N. americanus (?)	3 mg/kg	21	67	–	BOUYER (1970)
	N. americanus	5 mg/kg	11	64	–	GENTILINI et al. (1970)
	N. americanus	7 mg/kg	13	62	–	GENTILINI et al. (1970)
	Hookworm	2.5 mg/kg × 2 at 1 week intervals	74	64	–	ASMERA (1974)
		2.5 mg/kg	74	64	–	HUYS et al. (1973)
	Hookworm	2.5 mg/kg × 2 at 4-day interval	45	69	–	HUYS et al. (1976)
	Hookworm	150 mg/4 days	9	67	–	VAKIL et al. (1972)
≧50%	Hookworm	3.5 mg/kg/2 days	45	56	64	THIENPONT et al. (1969)
	N. americanus	7 mg/kg/2 days	23	52	–	GENTILINI et al. (1970)
	N. americanus	100 mg	42	52	90	SINNIAH and SINNIAH (1981)
	A. duodenale	2.5 mg/kg	64	53	–	LÉVAI et al. (1972)
	Hookworm	2.5 mg/kg	78	51	–	COENE (1969)
	Hookworm	2.5 mg/kg/2 days	19	58	–	RADOEV (1974)
≧40%	Hookworm	150 mg	74	43	87	VAN LANDUYT (1973)
	Hookworm	300 mg	73	41	85	VAN LANDUYT (1973)
	Hookworm	150 mg	15	40	18	DE JONCKHEERE (1975)
<40%	*N. americanus*	3 mg/kg	3	33	–	GENTILINI et al. (1970)
	N. americanus	150 mg/2 days	31	32	–	VAKIL et al. (1972)
	N. americanus	8 mg/kg	55	27	–	CHEGE et al. (1974)
	Hookworm	2.5 mg/kg	30	23	68	GATTI et al. (1970)
		2.5 mg/kg/3 days	–	–	89	GATTI et al. (1970)
	N. americanus	4–10 mg/kg	94	18	40	LUCAS and ODUNTAN (1972)
	N. americanus	150 mg/2 days	9	11	86	VAKIL et al. (1972)
	N. americanus	2.5–3.5 mg/kg	19	0%	15%	MILLER (1980)

3.2.9.3 Dosage, Mode of Administration

Due to the remarkably wide safety margin between therapeutic and toxic doses, it is possible to translate the recommended 2.5 mg/kg into the following practical oral doses.

Adults,	>40 kg	1 tablet: 150 mg
Children,	30–40 kg	2 tablets of 50 mg: 100 mg
	20–30 kg	1½ tablets of 50 mg: 75 mg
	10–20 kg	1 tablet of 50 mg: 50 mg

Neither fasting nor purging are necessary.

3.2.9.4 Side Effects

Tolerance is very good. At the recommended dosage less than 10% of persons complain about abdominal pain, headache, dizziness, anorexia, nausea, vomiting, loose stools, floods of tears, or unrest. The first two inconveniences occur most often. The abdominal discomfort, 2–3 h after medication, is probably related to the elimination of the worms.

3.2.9.5 Contraindications, Precautions

Contraindications are unknown. In glucose-6-phosphate dehydrogenase-deficient individuals no modifications of the hemogram have been observed. In pregnancy and serious hepatorenal disease, levamisole should nevertheless be withheld.

3.2.9.6 Conclusions

It is difficult to extract unchallengeable conclusions out of the published results. Dosages vary between 2.5 mg and 7 mg/kg, or 150 mg and 430 mg for adults, and the administration regimens between one single and four oral doses, either on consecutive days or with intervals of up to 4 and even 10 days. The samples may be under 10 or greater than 90. The parasitic diagnosis seldom goes beyond that of "hookworm." Even a specific diagnosis often appears to be only an assumption based on prevalences established on a previous occasion by another author, somewhere in the same country. Egg counts are made using different techniques with variable accuracy. The timing of the follow-up varies between a few day (5–15) and several weeks or months (up to 6) after administration, either on persons remaining in endemic regions or after moving into a noninfectious environment.

The drug sensitivity of *A. duodenale* and *N. americanus* is not identical. It is most unfortunate that too few of the CRs can be related to a species. The efficacy of a single dose of 2.5–3 mg/kg seems better for *A. duodenale* (47%–100%) than for *N. americanus* (0%–80%). ZAMAN and LOH (1974) concluded that a 200-mg dose of levamisole is less effective against *N. americanus*. These data do not enable a general conclusion to be drawn on species sensitivity, nor on a suggestion that the incomprehensible results observed might be due to mixtures of hookworms in varying proportions.

The observations made by LUCAS and ODUNTAN (1972) require careful examination from a different point of view. The selected 199 schoolchildren of villages in the neighborhood of Ibadan (Nigeria) received the drug in a dosage related to their body weight and under strict supervision. The egg counts 2 weeks after treatment made clear that neither larger dose nor repeated administration do improve the moderate CR. Furthermore a follow-up 9 weeks after the administration suggests that results recorded after 1 or 2 weeks are overestimated. It is not unlikely that hookworms may undergo a temporary egg-output suppression, followed by a regain in fertility.

Likewise a scrutiny of the reports on clinical trials focuses attention on the variability of the results according to the environmental, sanitary and living conditions. The percentages of apparent cures after administration of a placebo emphasizes the need for single or double-blind experiments. The observation of negative stools becoming positive after administration of a placebo is a reminder of the possibility of false-negative results.

3.2.9.6.1 Individual Therapy

A single dose of 2.5 mg/kg is likely to provide satisfactory results, especially for *A. duodenale*. It seems, however, advisable to repeat the dose after an interval of 2 weeks in order to overcome a temporary depression of the egg output. It will also increase the CR, particularly for *N. americanus*.

3.2.9.6.2 Mass Therapy

GATTI et al. (1969) underlined the possible value of large-scale administration of levamisole as a new public health measure against soil-transmitted helminthiases.

LECHAT et al. (1974) concluded, from data collected from a control trial in Zairian rural schoolchildren, that 3 months after complete coverage the mean reduction in hookworm prevalence was 57% of its previous level. With only 75% coverage there was a mean reduction to 49% of its previous level. Consequently, an indiscriminate mass treatment of 75% of the target population at 3-month intervals with 2.5 mg/kg is likely to reduce significantly the prevalence and the incidence of hookworm infection.

JANCLOES et al. (1979) tried coverages of 40%, 60%, and 90% in a double-blind single-dose administration of 2.5 mg/kg on 3,267 individuals. The controls after 3, 6, and 9 months showed a decreased prevalence both in the levamisole and control groups, somewhat more pronounced in the levamisole group, but not significantly so. The absence of clear-cut effects against hookworms may be due to the 3-month intervals of the follow-up examinations.

The ERR, which is an acceptable main objective of mass treatment, is quite satisfactory following the recommended dosage of 2.5 mg/kg or 150 mg levamisole. Administration in single oral doses, without fasting or purging, makes this drug suitable for mass administration in all population groups and especially in children. It is the drug of choice for the association of *Ancylostoma duodenale* and *Ascaris*. The administration should be repeated, if possible, every 3 months.

3.2.9.7 Comments

Levamisole is not a first choice for the treatment of ancylostomiasis in an individual patient, although a cure can be successfully achieved. But as a tool in attempts of a mass reduction of soil-transmitted helminthiases in a community, this broad anthelmintic can be considered. The final decision will depend on its availability and its costs.

3.2.10 Mebendazole

3.2.10.1 State of the Art

Mebendazole is active against a large spectrum of worms, including the Ancylostomidae (Strongylidae): *A. duodenale, N. americanus*, and also *A. tubaeforme* ZEDER 1800, *A. caninum* ERCOLANI 1859, *Bunostomum phlebotomum* RAILLET 1900, and *Gaigeria pachyscilis* RAILET and HENRY 1910.

The first published report on the activity of mebendazole on hookworms is from CHAIA and DA CUNHA (1971 a, b). They submitted Brazilian schoolchildren to eight different protocols, out of which a dose of 200 mg b.i.d. for 4 days or 100 mg daily for 6 days provided a cure rate of almost 100%.

GATTI et al. (1972b) and GATTI and VANDEPITTE (1973) tried different schedules in infected African schoolchildren. The better results were obtained with 100 mg of a micronized preparation b.i.d. for 3 days. Out of 52 children 49 (95%) were cured and the egg output was reduced by 99% during a control period of 8 weeks. In a second trial, with a broader protocol, the same doses again provided the best results, 100% cure of 35 children.

The same total amount of 600 mg, administered as 100 mg t.i.d. on two consecutive days, was less successful: CR of 86% 19 out of 22 and ERR of 94%. The drug must be administered in divided doses and over several days. But extension beyond 3 days gives only negligible improvement. Higher dosages and more repeated and prolonged administration do not increase efficacy. BANNERJEE et al. (1972a) and CHAIA and DA CUNHA (1971a, b) obtained CR between 84% and 100% with 200 mg b.i.d. on four consecutive days.

This has been confirmed throughout the tropics in over 50 therapeutic experiments.

3.2.10.2 Assessment

The results enregistered are summarized in Table 15.

Table 15. Treatment of hookworm infection by mebendazole

Efficacy	Parasite	Dosage	Number treated	CR	ERR	References
100%	*Necator americanus + Ancylostoma duodenale*	200 mg b.i.d./4 days	13	100	–	CHOWDURY (1972–1974)
	N. americanus	100 mg b.i.d./3 days	26	100	–	CHAIA et al. (1972)
	Hookworm	100 mg b.i.d./3 days	5	100	–	BEKTHI (1974)
	A. duodenale + N. americanus	100 mg b.i.d./3 days	35	100	–	GATTI et al. (1972b)
	Hookworm	100 mg b.i.d./3 days	11	100	–	DE OLIVIERA/GOMEZ (1974)
	N. americanus	100 mg b.i.d./3 days	36	100	–	LIONEL et al. (1975)
	A. duodenale + N. americanus	100 mg b.i.d./3 days	5	100	–	NGOY and KALOMBE (1975)
≧90%	*A. duodenale + N. americanus*	100 mg b.i.d./3 days	52	94	99	GATTI et al. (1972b)
	Hookworm	200 mg b.i.d./4 days	53	94	–	BANERJEE et al. (1972)
	N. americanus	100 mg b.i.d./3 days	21	95	99	PEÑA-CHAVARRIA et al. (1973)
	N. americanus	100 mg b.i.d./4 days	21	95	99	PEÑA-CHAVARRIA et al. (1973)
	N. americanus	100 mg b.i.d./3 days	14	93	97	CHAIA et al. (1972)
	Hookworm	100 mg b.i.d./4 days	109	94	98	VANDEPITTE et al. (1973)
	Hookworm	100 mg b.i.d./3 days	52	94	99	VANDEPITTE et al. (1973)
	Hookworm	200 mg/3 days	59	93	98	KOSIN (1973)
	Hookworm	100 mg b.i.d./3 days	40	94	–	DE SOUZA et al. (1973a, b)
	Hookworm	100 mg b.i.d./4 days	98	97	–	LORIA-CORTEZ et al. (1973)
	A. duodenale + N. americanus	100 mg b.i.d./3 days	30	97	–	GOLDSMID (1974)
	Hookworm	100 mg b.i.d./3 days	72	94	95	DE SOUZA et al. (1973a, b)
	Hookworm	200 mg b.i.d./2 days + 100 mg b.i.d./ 2 days	30	93	98	SHAFEI (1974)
	N. americanus	100 mg b.i.d./3 days	36	92	–	VERWILGHEN (1974)
	N. americanus	200 mg b.i.d./3 days	30	93	80	CHOWDURY (1974)
	N. americanus	100 mg b.i.d./3 days	42	90	99	ABADI (1974)
	Hookworm	100 mg b.i.d./3 days	17	94	–	HUTCHINSON et al. (1975)
	Hookworm	200 mg b.i.d./4 days	31	94	–	BANZON et al. (1976)
	A. duodenale	100 mg b.i.d./3 days	117	95	99	SOH et al. (1975)
	Hookworm	100 mg b.i.d./3 days	50	92	–	FERNANDEZ (1974)

Table 15 (continued)

Efficacy	Parasite	Dosage	Number treated	CR	ERR	References
	Hookworm	100 mg b.i.d./3 days	12	92	–	DEGREMONT and BAUMGARTNER (1975)
	N. americanus	100 mg b.i.d./3 days	25	92	98	BUNNAG et al. (1978)
	Hookworm	100 mg b.i.d./3 days	41	95	98	JAROONVESAMA et al. (1978
	Hookworm	100 mg b.i.d./3 days	14	93	–	BINA et al. (1977)
	Hookworm	100 mg b.i.d./3 days	20	90	–	KATZ (1977)
	Hookworm	100 mg b.i.d./3 days	30	93	92	SHAFEI (1974)
	N. americanus	100 mg b.i.d./3 days	40	90	–	OTERO et al. (1977)
≧80%	*A. duodenale* + *N. americanus*	100 mg b.i.d./3 days	53	87	98	GATTI and VANDEPITTE (19
	A. duodenale + *N. americanus*	100 mg b.i.d./2 days	22	86	94	GATTI and VANDEPITTE (19
	Hookworm	100 mg b.i.d./3 days	20	85	91	PARTONO et al. (1974)
	Hookworm	100 mg b.i.d./3 days	57	86	86	SHINGAL et al. (1975)
	N. americanus	100 mg b.i.d./4 days	38	87	–	GENTILINI (1974)
	N. americanus	100 mg b.i.d./3 days	23	87	98	BOTERO and PEREZ (1976)
	Hookworm	100 mg b.i.d./3 days	45	73	52	ISLAM and CHOWDURY (19'
	N. americanus	100 mg b.i.d./6 days	34	82	92	SINNIAH and SINNIAH (198
	Hookworm	100 mg b.i.d./3 days	28	86	99	SEAH (1976)
	Hookworm	100 mg b.i.d./3 days	55	85	99	BORDA et al. (1978)
	Hookworm	100 mg b.i.d./4 days	15	87	93	MUSGRAVE et al. (1979)
	Hookworm	200 mg/3 days	27	81	97	STUERCHLER et al. (1980)
	Hookworm	100 mg b.i.d./3 days (semirural)	47	81	95	ISMAIL and LIONEL (1981)
	Hookworm	100 mg b.i.d./3 days (urban)	9	89	99	ISMAIL and LIONEL (1981)

The 12 reports in Table 16 are, however, at variance.

Table 16. Uncommon results of treatment of hookworm infections by mebendazole 100 mg b.i.d./3 days

Number treated	Cure rate	ERR	References
91	70	91	LOUZADA et al. (1973)
25	64	–	KILPATRICK et al. (1981)
24	62	–	AMATO NETO et al. (1973)
12	50	–	BRUMPT (1973)
66	37	75	GORODNER et al. (1977)
50	46	–	GENTILINI (1974)
20	55	86	CONTE et al. (1974)
10	60	–	MONTERO and SANCHEZ (1975)
25	60	95	BORDA et al. (1976)
–	35	–	HUGGINS (1976)
16	37.5	90	DISSANAIKE (1978)
18	61	98	CIMMERMAN et al. (1980)
25	60	–	RICHARD-LENOBLE and GENTILINI (1980)
39	49	88	SINNIAH and SINNIAH (1981)

From the available information it is not possible to find an acceptable interpretation for these diverging results. Again no specific identification beyond the generic "hookworm" is available. Moreover, there is no consensus about the respective sensitivity of *A. duodenale* and *N. americanus*: the first is less sensitive for BRUMPT (1973); the latter for JUWONO and TANTULAR (1973).

Geographical classification gave no clue: the 12 exceptions are evenly distributed over the world map.

3.2.10.3 Dosage, Mode of Administration

Mebendazole is available in tablets of 100 mg or as an oral suspension of 100 mg/5 ml. 100 mg b.i.d. for 3 days of a micronized formulation of mebendazole (of which 90% is in 2- to 3-μm sized particles) is the most recommendable dose. Oral administration includes neither fasting nor purging and chewing up of the tablets is not necesary. However, in diarrheic patients the time of contact may be shortened and thus the efficacy reduced.

3.2.10.4 Side Effects

The safety margin is extremely broad since mebendazole by oral administration is pharmacologically nearly inert. Doses ranging from 100 and 1,200 mg in a single intake or administered on 14 consecutive days produced no significant changes with regard to the placebo controls, over follow-up periods of up to 90 days (BRUGMANS et al. 1971). No adverse drug reactions have been reported, except some complaints of transient abdominal discomfort, giddiness, nausea, gastralgia, vomiting, and diarrhea. In no instance did the treatment have to be discontinued. The complaints appear after the first dose, but diminish and even disappear altogether after subsequent doses. Abdominal pain appears at the time of expulsion of the worms, with which it is related. In massive infections diarrhea disappears with the worms and the consistency of the stools will normalize.

3.2.10.5 Precautions

The potential risk to the fetus should be made known to women taking mebendazole during pregnancy, especially during the first trimester.

3.2.10.6 Conclusions

3.2.10.6.1 Individual Treatment

The crude summary of results enregistered in ancylostomiasis supports the opinion that 100 mg b.i.d. for 3 days is an appropriate dosage. On the whole a CR of between 90% and 99% and an ERR of between 95% and 99% or even a 100% clearance have been ensured.

However, on the whole the infections treated were light and the results are less favorable in heavy infections. SEAH (1976) obtained a 71% CR in heavy infections, against 90% in light and moderate infections, while BORDA et al. achieved 60% and 86%–90%, respectively. HUTCHINSON et al. (1975) focussed attention on a reduced efficacy in mixed infections: 82% against 94% in single infections. This kind of information which might provide indications for a better understanding is not generally available. The standard of living and the level of sanitation do play a role in the risk of reexposure and reinfection and as a consequence in a correct assessment of the efficacy: this type of detail is often missing.

The activity of the drug on immature worms has not yet been proved. Very useful complementary information could be provided by the treatment of a series of heavy infections outside the endemic zones.

3.2.10.6.2 Mass Treatment

The experimental evidence of a prospective broad-spectrum program has since oriented the very first trials toward mass treatment. The careful studies on schoolchildren in Zaire and Rwanda by GATTI et al. (1972b) and VANDEPITTE et al. (1973) were followed by many others. The majority of the published data, even in relatively small groups of children or adults, aimed at drawing up an acceptable and efficient administration protocol suitable for population groups and closed communities (schools, army recruits, etc.).

Interesting preliminary studies have been made by, e.g., CHAIA and DA CUNHA (1971a, b), CHAIA et al. (1972), LOUZADA et al. (1973), LORIA-CORTES et al. (1973), AGUILAR et al. (1973), JUWONO and TANTULAR (1973), KWO and KOSMAN (1973), SOH et al. (1975), BANZON et al. (1976), and BINA et al. (1977). From these the following examples have been selected.

PEÑA CHAVARRIA et al. (1973) assessed the activity of mebendazole against hookworm in Costa Rican hospitalized children and adults. A single dose of 300 mg produced an ERR of 90% 1 month after administration, 100 mg b.i.d. for 2, 3, or 4 days provided identical ERRs of 99.7%–99.9%. The most favorable CR, 95%, was obtained with 100 mg b.i.d. for 3 days.

CHONGSUPHAJAISIDDHI et al. (1978) obtained an overall CR of 76% in Thai children infected with hookworm (95%–97% *N. americanus* and 3%–5% *A. duodenale*). This CR is lower than most other results. In one of the groups (Nakorn-Nayok) even lower unexplained CRs (66%–70%) were determined. The ERR, ranging from 84% to 99%, is in contrast rather high.

The study conducted in Zaire by KRUBWA et al. (1974b) on the effect of mebendazole in schoolchildren as compared with a placebo control resulted in a 90% cure, confirmed by subsequent treatment courses with the recommended dosage at 3-month intervals. KABA et al. (1978) confirmed the benefits of a trimestrial chemotherapy with mebendazole. It is obvious that periodic deworming has a beneficial effect on the nutritional and general health status of preschool and school communities.

RICHARD-LENOBLE et al. (1980) achieved a low CR in a community where reinfestation is permanent, but regular good percentages in normal surroundings.

3.2.10.7 Comments

Ancylostomiasis can be successfully controlled by an extremely well tolerated and accepted administration of 600 mg micronized mebendazole divided into six doses and over 3 days. This interesting possibility is enhanced by the fact that mebendazole is also active against a number of nematodes and cestodes, such as *Ascaris, Trichuris, Enterobius, Trichostrongylus,* and *Strongyloides stercoralis,* and also against *Hymenolepis nana,* although to a lesser extent for the latter.

An ERR of over 90%, a few exceptions proving the rule, makes mebendazole very suitable for a blanket treatment of soil-transmitted and some other helminthiasis. Large-scale trials with single-dose treatment (500–600 mg) ensure highly significant CRs and ERRs in *Ascaris* and *Trichuris* infections along with promising results in ancylostomiasis.

Mebendazole, being efficacious, safe, and inexpensive, meets the basic criteria for polyvalent anthelmintic mass control.

3.2.11 Pyrantel Pamoate

3.2.11.1 State of the Art

CORNWELL and JONES (1968) reported that pyrantel pamoate was very active against *A. caninum* in oral doses of 2.2–8.7 mg/kg pyrantel base (6–25 mg/kg, salt). From 1969 on, the drug has been tried on humans by several authors, in many countries and with impressive results. BUMBALO et al. (1969) showed its efficacy on *E. vermicularis* in the United States. Its efficacy against *Ascaris, T. trichiura,* and hookworm has been shown by HSIEH and CHEN (1970) in Taiwan, by DESOWITZ et al. (1970) in the Cook Islands, by KOBAYASHI (1970) in Japan, by GHADIRIAN et al. (1972) in Iran, by BELL and NASSIF (1971) in Cairo, by CERVONI and OLIVER-GONZALEZ (1971) in Puerto Rico, by VILLAREJOS et al. (1971) in Costa Rica, and by BOTERO and CASTANO (1973) in Colombia. The majority of these trials drew attention to encouraging results in the treatment of hookworm. This potentiality has been widely explored.

3.2.11.2 Assessment

A summary of the trials is given in Table 17.

'able 17. Treatment of hookworm infection by pyrantel pamoate

;fficacy	Parasite	Dosage	Number treated	CR	ERR	References
100%	*Ancylostoma duodenale*	10 mg/kg	2	100	–	GOLDSMID and SAUNDERS (1973)
	Necator americanus	11 mg/kg/2 days	5	100	–	PITTS and MIGLIARDI (1974)
≥90%	*A. duodenale*	10 mg/kg	75	96	92	FARAHMANDIAN et al. (1972)
	N. americanus	20 mg/kg	40	92	–	GHADIRIAN and SANATE (1972)
	A. duodenale	20 mg/kg	40	92	–	GHADIRIAN and SANATE (1972)
	N. americanus	11 mg/kg/3 days	42	93	–	PITTS and MIGLIARDI (1974)
	Hookworm	17.4 mg/kg	41	97	–	SAIF et al. (1971)
	A. duodenale	20 mg/kg		91	–	YOKOGAWA et al. (1970)

Table 17 (continued)

Efficacy	Parasite	Dosage	Number treated	CR	ERR	References
≧80%	*N. americanus* (L)	16 mg/kg (?)	20	80%	–	ZAMAN and LOH (1974)
	N. americanus	22 mg/kg/3 days	143	89%	–	PITTS and MIGLIARDI (1974)
	N. americanus	14 mg/kg	40	82%	–	CERVONI and OLIVER-GONZAI (1971)
≧70%	*N. americanus*	20 mg/kg/2 days	17	70	99	BOTERO and CASTANO (1972, 1973)
	N. americanus	10 mg/kg/3 days	16	75	99	BOTERO and CASTANO (1972, 1973)
	N. americanus	10 mg/kg	40	75	–	GHADIRIAN and SANATI (1972
	N. americanus	10 mg/kg	17	76	–	YOKOGAWA et al. (1970)
	N. americanus	20 mg/kg	14	78	–	YOKOGAWA et al. (1970)
≧60%	*N. americanus* (H)	16 mg/kg (?)	3	66	–	ZAMAN and LOH (1974)
	A. duodenale	20 mg/kg	9	67	–	YOKOGAWA et al. (1970)
	N. americanus (H)	14 mg/kg	8	62	56–70	CERVONI and OLIVER-GONZAI (1971)
≧50%	*N. americanus*	22 mg/kg/3 days	17	57	–	VILLAREJOS et al. (1971)
	N. americanus	22 mg/kg/3 days	33	58	–	GAMBOA et al. (1969)
	A. duodenale	20 mg/kg	12	58	93	GOLDSMID and SAUNDERS (19'
	N. americanus	11 mg/kg	91	54	–	PITTS and MIGLIARDI (1974)
	N. americanus	20 mg/kg/3 days	15	53	97	BOTERO and CASTANO (1972, 1973)
	N. americanus	10 mg/kg/3 days	33	58	85	SINNIAH and SINNIAH (1981)
≦50%	*N. americanus*	10 mg/kg	60	42	–	CHEGE et al. (1974)
	N. americanus	11 mg/kg	26	38	5	VILLAREJOS et al. (1971)
	N. americanus	11 mg/kg/3 days	31	48	–	GAMBOA et al. (1969)
	N. americanus	33 mg/kg/3 days	25	44	–	GAMBOA et al. (1969)
	N. americanus	44 mg/kg/3 days	17	41	–	VILLAREJOS et al. (1971)
	N. americanus	44 mg/kg/3 days	26	48	–	VILLAREJOS et al. (1971)
	Hookworm	20 mg/kg	89	27	73	GOLDSMID and SAUNDERS (19'
	N. americanus	10 mg/kg	41	27	64	SINNIAH and SINNIAH (1981)
	N. americanus	20 mg/kg	38	24	69	SINNIAH and SINNIAH (1981)
	N. americanus	10 mg/kg/2 days	21	14	91	BOTERO and CASTANO (1973)
	Hookworm	10 mg/kg	25	16	67	GOLDSMID and SAUNDERS (19'
	N. americanus	10 mg/kg	12	17	63	GOLDSMID and SAUNDERS (19'
	N. americanus	44 mg/kg	17	5.9	9	VILLAREJOS et al. (1971)
	N. americanus	44 mg/kg	17	5.9	–	PITTS and MIGLIARDI (1974)
	N. americanus	22 mg/kg	17	0	–	VILLAREJOS et al. (1971)

3.2.11.3 Dosage, Mode of Administration

A dose of 20 mg/kg on three consecutive days is effective for heavy infections, while 10 mg/kg on two to three consecutive days suffices for light and medium EPG loads. Pyrantel base is available in chewable tablets of 250 mg pyrantel base or in oral suspension of 50 mg pyrantel base/ml. The drug can be taken after meals without any dietary restriction.

3.2.11.4 Side Effects, Precautions

Pyrantel pamoate is poorly absorbed and consequently free of organ toxicity. The fact that greater amounts are retained in the intestinal tract may, however, induce gastrointestinal side effects.

Complaints are frequent in some individuals (16%–39%), but always mild and transitory; these are mainly low-grade abdominal or epigastric discomfort or cramps at the time of the passing of the worms, i.e., headache, nausea, anorexia, vomiting, dizziness, diarrhea, and gas cramps. Biological monitoring reveals no significant changes.

3.2.11.5 Contraindications

Although no teratogenic effects have been observed, it is advisable to withhold the drug from pregnant women and children below 1 year of age. It should not be used with piperazine, an antagonist.

3.2.11.6 Conclusions

Due to the fact that the initial investigations were made using dosages expressed in mg/lb or on protocols starting from the lowest active dose against experimental *A. caninum* infections and doubling at every step, we now have 11, 17.4, 22, and 33 mg/kg. Low ranges of activity, even after 3-day courses, preclude a logical interpretation. The most surprising observation is the extremely poor results registered for the highest doses, 44 mg/kg.

The comparative efficacy of pyrantel against *A. duodenale* and *N. americanus* permits no indisputable conclusions to be made. HSIEH and CHEN (1970) made use of a single oral dose of 10 mg/kg in 35 patients with *A. duodenale* and in 21 with *N. americanus*. Stools were negative 4 weeks after treatment in 32 of the *A. duodenale* group, CR 91%, and in 15 of the *N. americanus* group, CR 71%, implying that *A. duodenale* might be more sensitive. VILLAREJOS et al. (1971), GAMBOA et al. (1969), and others claim that the efficacy on *N. americanus* is poor to moderate, which fits with their results, but is contradicted by the observations of many other authors.

YOKOGAMA et al. (1970) treated patients with *N. americanus* with 10 mg or 20 mg/kg: 17 on the first and 14 on the second dosage; the CRs were practically identical: 76% and 78%. Patients with *A. duodenale* were administered 20 mg/kg; 11 out of 14 were freed of infection, CR 90%.

BELL and GOULD (1971), in their pilot study in Kenya, treated 55 inpatients infected generally with *A. duodenale* with five different dosages from 2.2 to 34.8 mg/kg, with optimal results at 17.4 mg/kg. The results increased with the higher dosage but the greatest reduction (93.5%) obtained with the highest dosage was only 2.9% higher than that achieved with half that dose: hence the choice of 17.4 mg/kg. With regard to the evacuation of hookworms, pyrantel pamoate acts rapidly, and reaches 85%, leaving thus a residuum of ovipositing females.

SAIF et al. (1971) made use of a single oral dose of 17.4 mg/kg pyrantel base in 41 patients. The CR was established on three negative stools and cultures after 10–12 and 15–17 days. At the last control 40 out of 41 were negative, CR 97%. It was observed that the fecal blood loss fell rapidly after treatment.

CERVONI and OLIVER-GONZALEZ (1971) administered about 14 mg/kg (6.5 mg/lb) to bearers of *N. americanus* in Puerto Rico, which provided an overall CR of 82%. They observed, however, some variations in connection with the EPG load: in light infections (500–2,499) the CR was 87% and the ERR 50%–60%; in medium infections (2,500–4,999) the CR was 87% and ERR 86%; and in heavy infections (>5,000) the CR was 62% and ERR 56%–70%. The results were the most beneficial in the medium EPG range.

3.2.11.6.1 Individual Treatment

A regimen of 10 mg/kg on two to three consecutive days can be recommended for light and moderate infections, but must be increased to 20 mg/kg for 3 days in severe infections.

3.2.11.6.2 Mass Treatment

GHADIRIAN and SANATI (1972) claimed good results at the village level with a single 20 mg/kg dose (CR, 92%). But MIGASENA et al. (1978) observed a much lower CR (37%) after 20 mg/kg for 2 days, although the ERR obtained was 83%. Because mass treatment usually aims at multiple infections, pyrantel pamoate, since it is ineffective against *T. trichiura*, cannot be recommended as a first choice.

3.2.11.7 Comments

The results reported in ancyclostomiasis are quite variable. This uncertainly could be related to a different sensitivity of hookworm strains, but such a guess needs objective confirmation. Some of the poorer results are simply baffling.

3.2.12 Oxantel and Pyrantel

3.2.12.1 State of the Art

Oxantel is very active against whipworms in animals. HOWES (1972) reported a CR of 63% after a single dose of 10 mg/kg and an ERR of 91%. Consequently it seemed indicated to try it out also in humans. LIM (1974) evaluated the efficacy of a single dose of 10 mg/kg oxantel pamoate in *Trichuris trichiura* and obtained a CR of 91% and an ERR of 98%. KALE (1975) tested the drug for hookworm and with 10 mg/kg obtained a CR of 45% and 58% with 20 mg/kg.

Obviously, oxantel has never been used against hookworm as such, but rather to widen the spectrum of pyrantel to whipworms through a combination of pyrantel with oxantel.

3.2.12.2 Assessment

A limited number of investigations provide some specific information about the activity of the oxantel-pyrantel combination on hookworm.

Table 18. Treatment of hookworm infection by oxantel and pyrantel

Efficacy	Parasite	Dosage (of each component)	Number treated	CR	ERR	References
100%	Hookworm	15 mg/kg	4	100	–	LEE and LIM (1978)
	Hookworm	15–20 mg/kg	8	100	–	LIM (1978 a, b)
≧90%	Hookworm	20 mg/kg/2 days	–	95	–	AGUILAR (1976)
			–	96	–	BERTI et al. (1976)
	Hookworm	10 mg/kg	45	96	99	LIM (1978 a, b)
	Hookworm	10 mg/kg	21	95	–	RIM et al. (1981)
≧80%	Hookworm	10 mg/kg	–	89	–	CHO (1976)
	Hookworm	20 mg/kg/2 days	44	84	77	KALE (1977)
	Hookworm	10–20 mg/kg/3 days	32	84	–	GARCIA (1978)
	Necator americanus	10 mg/kg/3 days	47	83	90	SINNIAH and SINNIAH (1981)
≧70%	Hookworm	15 mg/kg	–	73	–	CABRERA and SY (1978)
	Hookworm	10 mg/kg	22	73	–	CABRERA and CRUZ (1980 b)
≧50%	Hookworm	20 mg/kg	–	58	–	KALE (1977)
	N. americanus	10–20 mg/kg/3 days	17	53	94	DISSANAIKE (1978)
<50%	Hookworm	10 mg/kg	–	45	–	KALE (1977)
	N. americanus	10 mg/kg	54	35	70	SINNIAH and SINNIAH (1981)
	Hookworm	20 mg/kg	74	24	89	MARGONO et al. (1980)
	N. americanus	10–20 mg/kg	11	18	79	DISSANAIKE (1977)

3.2.12.3 Dosage, Mode of Administration

Oxantel and pyrantel is available as an oral suspension containing 50 mg pyrantel and 50 mg oxantel per milliliter. A single oral dose of 10–15 mg/kg of each component will suffice in the majority of intestinal worm infections. In heavy infections 20 mg/kg of each, possibly on two consecutive days, may be necessary. For children less than 6 kg in weight, the latter dose should never be exceeded.

3.2.12.4 Side Effects

Absorption and general toxicity is identical to that of pyrantel. In about 25% of patients some mild and transient complaints such as abdominal discomfort or pain, headache, or nausea occur. Vomiting may occur, and also dizziness, loose bowel motions, and diarrhea. None of these warrants withdrawal of the drug. In the post-treatment period no significant differences are observed in hemopoietic, hepatic, and renal functions. However, after much higher doses than that recommended, SGOT and SGPT levels may become elevated.

3.2.12.5 Contraindications, Precautions

Tolerance is good and no teratogenic effects have been observed. Nevertheless administration of the drug to persons with hepatic or renal insufficiency or pregnant women should be discouraged.

3.2.12.6 Conclusion

3.2.12.6.1 Individual Treatment

This combination, produced for the purpose of multiple infections and mass treatment, has no place in the individual treatment of hookworm disease.

3.2.12.6.2 Mass Treatment

Oxantel and pyrantel is an association, made up with the aim of widening the spectrum of activity of pyrantel and in no way of improving activity against hookworm, which it obviously does not. In consequence its use must be reserved for mass campaigns against soil-transmitted helminths.

3.2.12.7 Comments

The final choice of a drug for mass treatment must fulfil several requirements, among others cost. The data collected enable oxantel and pyrantel to be taken into consideration for mass treatment.

3.2.13 Tiabendazole

3.2.13.1 State of the Art

Tiabendazole has a broad spectrum of anthelmintic activity, including moderate activity against *A. duodenale* and *N. americanus* and very interesting activity against cutaneous larva migrans *(A. braziliensis, A. caninum)*.

Since 1962 ancylostomiasis has been treated with doses of 25–50 mg/kg, in single or divided doses, with divergent results: good for BUI-QUOC-HUONG et al. (1962), poor for VILLELA et al. (1962), and complete failure for HUANG and BROWN (1963), ISWARIAH and NARAYANA-RAO (1964), and several others.

CAMPBELL and CUCKLER (1969) gathered over 1,000 hookworm-infected persons treated with different doses of tiabendazole. The overall CR was 52%. In the absence of species diagnosis it is impossible to form an opinion about a relative efficacy, if any, on *A. duodenale* and *N. americanus*.

3.2.13.2 Assessment

The only available data on ERR are from BOTERO (1965) and SABHARWAL et al. (1966). Even with doses of 50 mg/kg for 3 days, the ERR does not always cross the 90% threshold.

Table 19. Treatment of hookworm infection by tiabendazole

Efficacy	Parasite	Dosage	Number treated	CR	ERR	References
100%	Hookworm	25 mg/kg/2 days	9	100	–	ESCOBAR (1964)
	Hookworm	25 mg/kg/b.i.d./3 days	21	100	–	CHANCO and PAGUIO (1964)
	Hookworm	25–30 mg/kg/b.i.d./5 days	53	100	–	FRANZ et al. (1965)
≧90%	Hookworm	50 mg/kg/t.i.d.	10	90	–	CHOWDURY et al. (1964)
	Hookworm	25 mg/kg/5 days	16	94	–	ESCOBAR (1964)
	Hookworm	25 mg/kg	21	95	–	CHANCO and PAGUIO (1964)
	Hookworm	25–30 mg/kg/3 days	43	91	–	FRANZ et al. (1965)
	Hookworm	100 mg/kg	20	95	99	SABHARWAL et al. (1966)
	Hookworm	50 mg/kg/3 days	20	95	99	SABHARWAL et al. (1966)
≧80%	Hookworm	25–50 mg/kg/2 days	40	85	–	BUI-QUOC-HUONG et al. (1962)
	Hookworm	25 mg/kg	79	83	–	ESCOBAR (1964)
	Hookworm	25 mg/kg/2 days	26	88	–	ESCOBAR (1964)
	Hookworm	25 mg/kg/b.i.d./3 days	11	82	82	BOTERO (1965)
	Hookworm	50–60 mg/kg/2 days	7	85	–	ASSHAUER and MOHR (1966)
≧70%	Hookworm	30 mg/kg/2 days	7	71	–	IWATA et al. (1963b)
	Hookworm	50 mg/kg	57	79	–	ESCOBAR (1964)
	Hookworm	50–60 mg/kg/5 days	8	75	–	FRANZ et al. (1965)
	Hookworm	50–60 mg/kg/5 days	24	79	–	ASSHAUER and MOHR (1966)
	Hookworm	25 mg/kg/3 days	20	75	92	SABHARWAL et al. (1966)
≧60%	Hookworm	50 mg/kg/1–3 days	22	68	–	SHAH and ZAMAN (1964)
	Hookworm	50 mg/kg	47	66	–	ESCOBAR (1964)
	Hookworm	25–36 mg/kg/t.i.d./2 days	13	66	–	FRANZ et al. (1965)
	Hookworm	25–30 mg/kg/b.i.d./3 days	30	67	–	FRANZ et al. (1965)
	Hookworm	50–60 mg/kg/3 days	10	60	–	FRANZ et al. (1965)
	Hookworm	25 mg/b.i.d./2 days	13	62	–	VAKIL et al. (1965)
≧50%	Hookworm	150 mg/kg	4	50	–	CHOWDURY et al. (1964)
	Hookworm	50 mg/kg	25	56	–	CHANCO and PAGUIO (1964)
	Hookworm	50 mg/kg	20	30	76	SABHARWAL et al. (1966)
	Hookworm	25 mg/kg/b.i.d./3 days	20	30	73	SABHARWAL et al. (1966)

3.2.13.3 Dosage

The usual 25 mg/kg, either in a single dose or twice daily, by oral administration for 2–3 days, produces interesting CRs. Whenever doses of 50 mg/kg are used in mass treatment, the total amount should never exceed 3 g.

3.2.13.4 Side Effects

Mild and transient complaints are not uncommon: headache, anorexia, nausea, epigastric discomfort, vomiting, vertigo, drowsiness, and more occasionally pruritus, skin rashes, xanthopsia, diarrhea, hypoglycemia, hypotension, and slowing of the pulse rate. It is rather difficult to decide how far tiabendazole as such, rather than as an indirect reaction against drug-killed parasites, is responsible for the adverse reactions. Their importance and frequency increase with dosage, and also with a single compared with a split administration, but decrease when doses are taken after meals.

3.2.13.5 Contraindications, Precautions

Tiabendazole should not be given to anemic, dehydrated, and malnourished patients. Liver or kidney disorders are a contraindication. It should be remembered that mental alertness may become depressed. Although no teratogenic, mutagenic, or carcinogenic activity has been observed, tiabendazole should not be given during pregnancy or breast feeding.

3.2.13.6 Conclusion

Tiabendazole is not and will never become a drug of choice for the treatment of hookworm infections. It is, however, useful to know that such activity exists whenever tiabendazole is used in mixed infections.

III. Drug Combinations

1. Bephenium Hydroxynaphthoate and Tetrachloroethylene

Bephenium is more effective against *A. duodenale* and TCE against *N. americanus*; it was therefore rational to try out a combination of the two drugs in the treatment of the frequently mixed hookworm infections. Hsieh et al. (1961) recommend the administration during the same morning of 2.5 g bephenium base, followed by 5 ml TCE, each followed by a gulp of water. This technique is suitable for mass treatment since the side effects are transitory, slight, and rare.

Dutta (1970), practicing in India, achieved excellent parasitological results in a series of 20 patients (ERR, 100%), but was disturbed by the frequency of adverse reactions: giddiness (75%), vomiting (40%), and diarrhea (20%). It might be attributed to an additive effect of the side effects of both or related to an unusual proportion of very sensitive individuals in poor health.

Adam and Janssens (1965) has been using this combined treatment routinely in Antwerp without disturbing reactions. However, bephenium is too expensive for mass treatment and newer drugs are more efficient.

2. Tiabendazole and Levamisole

2.1 State of the Art

This combination has been tried out, taking into account that tiabendazole is highly active on *Strongyloides stercoralis* and levamisole on *A. lumbricoides* and *A. duodenale* in single doses.

2.2 Assessment

Table 20. Treatment of hookworm infection by a combination of tiabendazole and levamisole

Parasite	Number		Cured	CR	Reference
Necator americanus	168	200	175	87%	Gentilini et al. (1971)
Ancylostoma duodenale	2				
Hookworm	30				

2.3 Dosage, Mode of Administration

Tiabendazole, 50 mg/kg, and levamisole, 5 mg/kg, were given to 114 patients simultaneously and to the remaining 86 separately, viz, levamisole after breakfast and tiabendazole after lunch. The CR in both groups was identical.

2.4 Side Effects

The untoward reactions observed are those produced by tiabendazole. They have been slightly more frequent after simultaneous administrations: 22% against 12%. They appear 2–3 h after intake, but do not persist longer than 8–12 h.

2.5 Comments

This drug combination, which can be administered at once, is effective in hookworm infections and also ensures the control of *Ascaris* and *S. stercoralis*.

3. Tiabendazole and Pyrvinium Pamoate

3.1 State of the Art

The rationale of this drug association can be inferred from an attempt to reduce the dose and side effects of tiabendazole by compensating the loss of activity through the addition of a compound with a complementary spectrum of efficacy.

3.2 Assessment

Table 21. Treatment of hookworm infection by a combination of tiabendazole and pyrvinium pamoate

Parasite	Dosage	CR	Reference
Hookworm	2 tablets b.i.d./6 d	90%	Atra et al. (1965)

3.3 Dosage, Mode of Administration

Each tablet contains 375 mg tiabendazole and 150 mg pyrvinium pamoate.

3.4 Side Effects

Tolerance is poor, but the 21% side effects can be reduced to 4% by daily administration of two tablets spread over 12 days.

3.5 Comments

Although some kind of synergism has been claimed, the final results obtained, also in associated helminthiases, are too poor or too irregular to warrant recommendation of this protracted schedule for further use.

4. Tinidazole and Flubendazole

4.1 State of the Art

HUGGINS (1979a) studied this combination in an attempt to broaden the spectrum of activity against the common intestinal parasitoses and giardiasis.

4.2 Assessment

Table 22. Treatment of hookworm infection by a combination of tinidazole and flubendazole

Parasite	Dose	Number treated	CR	Reference
Hookworm	Tinidazole 175 mg, Flubendazole 100 mg } 2–3 days	16	81	HUGGINS (1979)

4.3 Side Effects

Complaints are limited to distended stomach (15%) and headache (10%).

4.4 Comments

This association gives a CR of 90% in ascariasis, 80% in amoebiasis and enterobiasis, 70% in trichiuriasis, and 95% in giardiasis, which is interesting progress in the treatment of a broad-spectrum of intestinal parasitoses. Investigations on similar combinations might disclose useful new approaches.

5. Flubendazole and Levamisole

In the search for a reliable single-dose schedule for mass treatment of polyparasitism an association of 500 mg flubendazole and 50 mg levamisole has been investigated by ISMAIL and LIONEL (1981). Table 23 shows the results obtained in a semirural (a) and an urban community (b).

Table 23. Treatment of hookworm infections by a combination of flubendazole and levamisole

Number treated	CR	ERR
52 (a)	77	99
23 (b)	70	93

Side Effects

Side effects are minimal and mild: 2.4% complained of vomiting. The quarterly follow-ups after three quarterly treatments showed side effects as follows:

After first treatment	After second	After third treatment
34% (a)	29%	27%
19% (b)	7%	7%

In this short-term clinical trial no benefit was observed by the addition of levamisole to flubendazole.

6. Mebendazole and Pyrantel

6.1 State of the Art

This composite make-up aims at combining the more specific pharmacological activities of both compounds: the slow-acting but effective anti-whipworm properties of mebendazole and the paralysing effect of pyrantel. Mebendazole can induce erratic ascariasis, which is reduced by pyrantel, thus eliminating a psychological adverse effect of erratic migrations.

6.2 Assessment

Table 24. Treatment of hookworm infection by a combination of mebendazole and pyrantel

Drug combination	Number treated	CR	Reference
Mebendazole 200 mg/3 days + Pyrantel 600 mg/3 days	26	100	PURNOMO et al. (1980)

6.3 Dosage, Mode of Administration

The combination is supplied as tablets with 150 mg mebendazole and 100 mg pyrantel pamoate, or 200 mg and 60 mg respectively. Dosage: either one tablet for three consecutive days, or as a single dose to be repeated after 2 and 4 weeks.

6.4 Contraindications

The combination is contraindicated in the first trimester of pregnancy.

7. Piperazine and Tiabendazole

Table 25. Treatment of hookworm infection by a combination of piperazine and tiabendazole

Drug combination	Number treated	CR	Reference
Piperazine hexahydrate 750 mg + Tiabendazole 375 mg	32	91	FERNANDES and CARCIA (1976)

IV. General Comments

Ancylostomiasis is an insiduous, troublesome infection sapping the vitality even if it can become a self-limiting infection. As no multiplication occurs within the host, only a continuous entry of infective larvae will maintain or enlarge the infection. Hosts can show a biological capacity to resist a nonmassive infection and even to limit the blood loss in the presence of an adequate amount of physiologically available iron in the diet.

These defense mechanisms as well as the circumstances favoring the soil transmission justify mass control campaigns. However, up to now no drop in incidence has been achieved, the only exception being in the southern United States. The number of people with hookworm infection lies somewhere between 630 million (STOLL 1962) and 1 billion (1982).

It is always possible that better drugs will become available. In the meantime individual treatment is no great problem. There is a choice of active drugs. The different responses of *A. duodenale* and *N. americanus* can be overcome by repeated or mixed treatments, possibly combined with a change to a different compound.

In mass treatment, the objective is not absolute cure, but "the removal of the largest possible number of worms from the largest possible number of persons." The decreasing egg output will reduce drastically the number of available infective larvae and the prevalence to below the critical transmission level. This can be achieved by some of the existing drugs, suitable for use in single doses: albendazole (400 mg), amidantel (6 mg/kg), bephenium hydroxynaphthoate (2.5 g), levamisole (150 mg), and mebendazole (600 mg). The final choice will be made on acceptability, tolerance, easy and indiscriminate administration, broad spectrum in intestinal helminthiases, and last but not least cost.

C. Anisakiasis

Introduction

The herring worm was first recognized by VAN THIEL et al. (1960). He discovered a parasitic structure in an eosinophilic phlegmon in the wall of the small intestine of a man; the worm was later identified as *Anisakis marina* [= *Filocapsularia marina* (VAN THIEL 1966)]. Similar infections were encountered later on among consumers of raw or inadequately preserved or cooked fish in Japan, Alaska, western Europe, and along the Pacific coast of the Americas.

Anisakiasis is an infection of man by larvae of the family Anisakidae. Up to now three "types" of anisakine larvae have been recognized in contaminated humans: *Anisakis, Phocanema,* and *Contracaecum.*[4] But the taxonomy of the third-stage larvae (L3) of these "aquatic ascarids," with some 24–30 genera, is still open to controversy.

1. Parasite

The adult *Anisakis* and *Phocanema* worms occur in the stomach and intestinal tract of marine mammals, seals, sea lions (Pinnipedia), dolphins, and mainly toothed whales (Cetacea).[5]

4 The identification of *Contracaecum osculatum* in a case of anisakiasis from Kiel is, according to VAN THIEL (1976), doubtful. Moreover *Contracaecum* is unlikely to be able to penetrate the human digestive tract and is not at all pathogenic (OISHI et al. 1974)

5 Anisakidae also live in the stomach or intestine of fish, amphibians, reptiles, and even birds. These are unrelated to any known human disease

The *morphology* of these large aquatic-transmitted ascarids is characterized by the presence of a mouth surrounded by three lips, a typical pharynx consisting of an anterior club-shaped muscular pharynx, and a posterior cylindrical predominantly glandular ventriculus with a valve apparatus. The ventriculus bears also one or more blind pouches or ceca. *Anisakis* has no anteriorly projecting cecum, which is present in *Phoconaema*.

The eggs are excreted with the feces into the water, sink to the sea floor where they molt twice, and hatch at 5°–7 °C in 20–27 days. The L2 are ingested by planktonic crustacea, especially euphausids (krill). In the North Sea these first intermediate hosts are *Meganyctiphanes norvegica, Thysanoëssa inermis*, and *T. raschii*. In Japanese waters the first intermediate hosts are *Euphausia pacifica, T. raschii*, and *T. longipes*. The percentage of the infected euphausids ranges from 0.2% to 4.0%. The euphausids remain on or near the sea bottom during the day, but rise during the night toward the upper layers, where they may become the prey of pelagic night feeders.

Sea fishes, such as herrings, and squids which may ingest infected euphausids, can become second intermediary hosts. In their hemocoelom the larvae have molted into infective L3 which are liberated in the stomach. They make their way into the body cavity, encapsulate there, and grow. They can penetrate into the somatic muscles of living fishes, invasion which occurs mainly after their death. In newly caught fish VIK (1964) found 0.5% larvae in the muscular tissue, but this ratio rose to 10%–13.5% after 3–4 days. Gutting and curing of the fish at sea thus limits the muscular invasion, while postponement until after disembarking increases the number of clinical anisakiases.

These secondary intermediate hosts belong to the food chain (fish-fish; squid-squid; fish-marine mammals; fish-man). The marine mammals become infected by ingesting fish or squid containing L3 larvae. Fish and squids are "transport hosts" in which the Anisakidae remain unaltered. Man also becomes infected by eating raw or partly raw fish containing L3 larvae: green herring swallowed as such (the Netherlands and Belgium); *gravlaks* of salmon or herring (Norway); *suchi, sunomono, shinesiba,* and *sashimi* fillets from mackerel, cod, and squid and *izushi*, raw or slightly salted cod roes (Japan).

The L3 larvae in man measure 20 × 0.4 mm. They have teeth at their anterior end and a general ascarid structure with an excretory pore near the head, lateral chords in a Y-shape, a ventriculus between the pharynx (esophagus) and intestine, and three anal glands near the rectum.

2. Host

The L3 larvae are liberated in the stomach of man. They can be expelled by vomiting or migrate actively up the esophagus toward the posterior oropharynx or the tonsillar bed without invading the tissues, causing only some local discomfort. They can also move into the intestine and start off a pathological reaction on their invasion of the tissues.

It must be mentioned that the seat of the tissular inflammatory reaction is the small intestine in the Netherlands and the stomach in Japan.

In the majority of human infections a single larva is recovered. If the larvae survive long enough they may molt from L3 to L4, but they will never mature.

Humoral antibodies develop only after penetration of the tissues. It has been demonstrated that sensitization increases the severity of the reaction, which can be mild, but also anaphylactic and fulminant.

In man, infection by anisakine larvae produces heterogeneous reactions according to their localization and the host's own reactivity. Within 12 h after the infecting meal reaction can start and be limited to a slight irritation followed by expulsion in a vomit. The infecting larvae produce an eosinophilic phlegmon at an early stage, which will later turn into a granulomatous reaction. The edematous lesion containing the larva can become interspersed by petechial hemorrhages, possibly ulcerate, and even necrotize.

This reaction to the larva was at first interpreted as a hypersensitivity reaction to the penetration of another larva near the site of a former larval invasion. In experimental infections, a primary reaction has been observed around the site of penetration of a single *Anisakis* larva, in the absence of local hypersensitivity. It is well known that some individuals react against the fortuitous invasion of living organisms or the presence of their secretions. The larvae may also elicit cellular reactions, simulating tumors.

3. Clinical Manifestations

Complaints can be limited to a slight local irritation, followed by coughing up or expulsion in the stool of the causative larva. Pharyngeal discomfort appearing shortly after the consumption of raw fish is due to the attachment of larvae in the rhinopharyngeal area, provoking mild edema and inflammation, disappearing after the removal of the larva. Invasion of the stomach or intestinal wall will produce severe, acute gastric, or intestinal complaints.

Gastric lesions, acute or more chronic, are the most common pathological condition. Within 12 h after swallowing the larvae, complaints of nausea, vomiting, epigastric pain, and hematemesis start. On X-ray examination, one or more ulcers is visualized. With the aid of a "mucosal relief method" the worm can be directly demonstrated. On gastroscopy it is possible to establish the presence of the motile larva in the gastric mucosa and, together with some adroitness and luck, to remove it under direct visual control.

If the acute condition is overlooked, chronic gastric anisakiasis follows. The patient complains about vague epigastric pain, nausea, vomiting, and blood-streaked vomitus. Clinically and radiologically the symptoms mimic chronic gastritis, peptic ulcer, and pseudotumor. The early eosinophilic phlegmonous stage is transformed in a granulomatous reaction.

In the small bowel, the acute diffuse interstitial edema accompanied by a phlegmonous infiltrate rich in neutrophils, lymphocytes, plasmocytes, and mainly eosinophils can evolve into an eosinophilic abscess in which the parasite will be present. This simulates an acute abdomen, with violent abdominal colics, nausea, vomiting, resembling appendicitis, regional enteritis, etc. The edema of the intestinal wall may produce incomplete obstruction. As a result of only nonspecific R_x changes, the patient runs the risk of undergoing laparotomy as an emergency. For that matter the very first anisakiasis diagnosis has been made on such surgically resected tissues.

A small amount of tinted ascitic fluid is present. Under a fibrinous exudate a diffusely thickened and edematous intestinal wall, corresponding to the eosinophilic phlegmon, will be found. The mesenteric lymph nodes are hyperplastic.

Except for lesions of the cecum, the colon is not involved. If perforation occurs, the parasite may be found in an extraintestinal localization.

4. Diagnosis

Morphological identification of larvae, either recovered free after expulsion (vomitus or stool) or histopathologically in resected tissues provides an answer. The latter approach is not easy, but trained parasitologists are able to identify genera and species from sections.

Anamnestic evidence of consumption of raw or undercooked fish is a good starter for a presumptive diagnosis: eosinophilia in up to 30%–35% of cases is also helpful.

Immunological techniques [complement fixation test (CFT) and immunofluorescence technique (IFT) the latter the more sensitive] on two serum samples (the first taken 1 week after the onset and the second in the 3rd or 4th week) and electrophoretic and enzymological reactions may also be helpful (CAIN and RAJ 1980). An intradermal (ID) test using somatic and excretory-secretory antigen has been used in Japan for epidemiological studies.

5. Geographical Distribution, Prevalence

The Netherlands are the cradle of this parasitosis. This infection is rather exceptional and limited to the short period of the traditional consumption of lightly salted raw young (green) herring.

From 1955 through 1968, 160 proven or highly suspected cases have been reported in the Netherlands (POLAK and KAMPELMACHER 1967; BIJKERK 1969; RUITENBERG 1970) with a peak of 51 cases in 1967. The enforcement of governmental regulations, making provision for freezing all raw herring at −20 °C and keeping it at least 24 h at this temperature before release for consumption, resulted in a decrease to three and seven cases in 1969 and 1970. Since then anisakiasis has not been observed again (BIJKERK 1969, 1970, 1971).

In the western European and North Sea foci single proven cases have been diagnosed in West Germany, Denmark, England, Norway, and Belgium.

The prevalence is much higher in the northern Pacific, among the Alaskan Eskimos, and especially in Japan. Japanese connoisseurs and people in general enjoy *sashimi, sushi*, and other carriers of anisakine larvae.

Since ASAMI et al. (1965) established the existence of anisakiasis in Japan, it has become obvious that it constitutes a serious health problem there. The number of recorded cases in 1972 was 487 (OSHIMA 1972), with 363 localized in the stomach, or 74.5% against 2.4% in the Netherlands. More species of fish (122) have been found infected. The parasite carriers also include sea mammals, Cetacea (toothed and baleened whales), Pinnipedia (seals), and dolphins. Anisakiasis occurs throughout Japan, but is more prevalent in coastal areas and affects male adults more, who are fond of raw marine food washed down with alcohol. Cases have been detected in Malaysia (CHO 1977) and Korea (CHO 1980). Along the Pacific coast of South America, *ceviche* is a favorite delicacy which causes anisakiasis in Chile and Peru. Cases were also reported from Western United States (KLIKS 1983).

The distribution of the causative worms is cosmopolitan, but the disease is limited to those eating raw fish or squid.

6. Treatment

Whenever feasible, treatment is instrumental removal of the anisakine larvae, especially when the infection has a gastric location. No anthelmintic drugs have been tried, as their efficacy is dubious. Attempts to reduce the anaphyllactoid reaction by antihistamines could avert the number of surgical resections.

7. Prevention

The immediate removal of the guts of fish substantially decreases the number of infective larvae migrating into the muscular tissues. The freezing of fish at −20 °C immediately after netting, for at least 24 h and preferably for 60 h, has been very successful in the Netherlands.

D. Ascariasis

I. Introduction

Ascaris lumbricoides, the commonest helminth parasite of man, is a fairly large roundworm. The adult worm lies free in the lumen of the small intestine but can find its way into all the possible apertures and ducts and can even break through tissues due to wanderlust and strength. *Ascaris* is a community-loving worm: up to a 1,000 have been found in one host.

Ascaris has parasitized man for well over 3,000 years. Its abundance and its great size points at the likelihood that ascaris might have been the first intestinal parasite known by man. Aristoteles mentions roundworms in his observations, but its presence in man dates much futher back. Human excrements, some 2,000–2,200 years old and discovered in prehistoric salt mines in the Austrian Alps, have contained eggs of *A. lumbricoides* and *Trichuris trichiura* in amounts up to 1,000/g.

Ascaris represents nearly one half of man's helminthiases. About one in every four people in the world (±1.3 billion) is infected. Every infected person hosts on average six worms: thus some 8 billion Ascaris worms must live in human beings. It should be noted that the worm burden is higher in children. In the Philippines, CABRERA (1975) observed an average worm load of 18.9 in children and 8.2 in adults.

1. Parasite

The *adult worms* are large: the male measures 150–310 mm in length and 2–4 mm in diameter; the female 200–490 mm and 3–6 mm respectively. Their weight varies between 4.5 and 9 g. Their mouth has three large prominent lips with dentiferous ridges along the inner rim: the tiny denticles makes it possible to differentiate *A. lumbricoides* and *A. suum*. The esophagus is simple and muscular. The posterior end of the male is curved, the tail is bluntly pointed, and the gubernacula are absent. The vulva in the female is located at the anterior one-third of the body length. The ovaries are extensive and the uteri may contain up to 27 million eggs.

The worms lie free in the lumen of the jejunum and ileum. They feed on the semidigested food of the host. The unusual fecundity of the female facilitates diagnosis and assessment of the worm load. The life span of *Ascaris* is between 9–24 months.

The *eggs* are passed with the feces. They measure 50–70 μm × 40–60 μm, are spheriodical with a thick transparent outer shell surrounded by a proteinaceous coat with an irregularly mammilated surface contributed by the uterine wall, and are yellowish-brown tinted by bile pigments while moving in the intestine. When deposited on the soil, they are unsegmented and may remain dormant for months or years. Among the numerous eggs, some 15% are infertile, particularly those laid in the early stages of oviposition or those from still unfertilized females. These eggs are longer and narrower (90 × 40 μm–88–94 × 40–44 μm), their shell is thinner, their outer coat is less regular, and their contents look unhealthy.

When conditions are favorable after a minimum 9–15 days[6] the fertilized ova develop the active first-stage rhabditoid larvae (L1) inside their shell. Still inside the egg they molt into second-stage larvae (L2), which are infective, a quite exceptional situation for nematodes.

After ingestion the infective eggs hatch in the stomach or duodenum (they need high CO_2 concentration; low redox potential; pH, ±7.0, temperature, 37 °C): the L2 larvae liberate themselves through an indistinct operculum. They penetrate the intestinal wall with the aid of a lytic enzyme and the majority enter venulae of the portal system. Some penetrate directly into the mesenterium or the peritoneal cavity, from where they reach, after a journey lasting 3–4 days, the liver, the liver circulation, and thus the heart. Others enter the lymphatic vessels, move into the mesenteric lymph nodes, and reach the same right heart cavities along the lymph duct. Finally some become lost and end up in unusual locations (spleen, brain, eye, etc.).

The standard infective larvae are pumped through the pulmonary artery and its capillary ramifications into the lung, which on average is reached in 1 week. The L2 break through the capillary walls and penetrate into the air spaces, where they molt twice (on the 5th and 10th days). The fourth-stage larvae (L4) migrate up the bronchi to the trachea and the epiglottis. At the aerodigestive junction they

6 The "Bodenheimer formula" offers a way of forecasting the number of days needed at a given temperature (WHO 1967): $S = \frac{C}{T-t}$, where S is the speed or number of days needed for attaining the larval stage, C is the sum of degree-days or "sum of heat" necessary for the completion of development (varies between 140 and 200), T is effect on mean temperature over 24 h, and t is the lowest temperature compatible with development (10 °C) e.g., Bujumbura 22 days, Ngozi 25 days

can be coughed up and swallowed or will pass directly into the esophagus. From the esophagus they descend into the stomach and reach the intestine. During this journey back to the intestine, their basic biotope, the surviving larvae have increased tenfold in size. A final molt brings the larvae to adulthood, which is attained 25–29 days after infection. They live mainly in the jejunum (87%) or in the ileum (12%) and a few (1%) in ectopic localizations, such as the appendix and bile duct.

Eggs appear in the feces some 60–75 days after exposure. The female *Ascaris* is a tremendous egg-layer. Careful estimates put the egg production of one worm at between 200,000 and 240,000 eggs/24 h (BROWN and CORT 1927). During its lifetime one female worm may produce some 146 million eggs. Egg production fluctuates with the age of the worms, the intensity of infection, and even from day to day. The daily egg production per female worm may vary. On six consecutive days it may vary between 73,000 and 227,000. Moreover, it has been ascertained that the intestine is a good mixer: stirring stools before examination does not improve *Ascaris* egg-counts.

Egg counts (EPG) over several days, followed by recovery of worms after administration of a vermifuge, put the worm: EPG ratio between 2,500 and 3,600, with a likely mean of 2,900. FARID et al. (1966) found a mean EPG of 1,500 (283–3,200)/worm.

In assessing the worm burden the following EPG criteria are generally agreed upon: light, $<10{,}000$; moderate, 10,000–50,000; and heavy, $>50{,}000$.

The sex ratio is near unity, according to the World Health Organization. But male worms are lost more easily, so that as a result the number of female worms will be higher. After 2 years the number of worms decreases as a result of the appearance of a limiting mechanism. In a given community 50% of the eggs are excreted by 5% of its members (CORT and STOLL 1931). Finally, the 2.64 billion female *A. lumbricoides* worms in man excrete an astronomical number of eggs daily.

There is no evidence that *A. suum* is significantly involved in the epidemiology of human ascariasis. TAKATA (1951) reported transitory experimental infections with *A. suum*. Four students infected with *A. suum* on the occasion of the annual carnival 10–14 days later developed anorexia, nausea, and vomiting followed by breathlessness, dyspnea, lung infiltrates, asthmatiform attacks, and eosinophilia; the symptoms were halted by piperazine.

2. Host

Transmission usually follows the ingestion of dirt, beverages, and/or food contaminated with embryonated eggs in kitchen gardens or by soiled hands. Vegetables and fruit (lettuce, radish, cabbage, strawberries, etc.) grown on contaminated soil and eaten unwashed or uncooked are the classical way of contagion. Night-soil diluted in water used as manure for vegetable crops leads to heavily contaminated products on the market. ANUAR and RAMACHANDRAN (1977) found all samples of lettuce from 12 markets in Penang (Malaysia) positive for eggs. Children run a high risk of infection by playing in egg-laden earth, which can contaminate their fingers and toys and they run an even higher risk, when engaging in dirt eating. In endemic regions children often defecate indiscriminately in or around the houses, are wiped with dirty rags, are scrubbed with leaves or corncobs, or clean themselves by dragging their buttocks on the grass. They fulfil all the conditions for transmission.

Infection may also follow inhalation of wind-borne embryonated eggs suspended in dust. BOGOJAWLENSKI and DEMIDOVA (1928) found eggs in the nasal mucosa in 3.2% of egg-positive children. Transplacental migration is possible, but extremely rare (CHU et al. 1972).

Contamination follows two patterns: (1) 5–9 years of age, yard exposure, and (2) all ages, vegetables contaminated by nightsoil. In some countries (Iran, China, Korea, Philippines, Tunisia) the prevalence may consequently be higher in adults.

Soil in which eggs have been laid remains a real danger for months and even years; *Ascaris* eggs are extremely resistant. Drying only delays the development. MUELLER (1953) infected a strawberry plot with *Ascaris* eggs and succeeded in producing an autoinfection in six consecutive years. BRUDOSTOV et al. (1971) demonstrated by self-infection that in Samarkand after 10 years 30.7%–52.7% of eggs were still infectious. Such observations are numerous: e.g., eggs kept between $-4°$ and 10 °C surviving for 4 years in a moist environment.

The resistance of *Ascaris* eggs is, owing to the lipid layer on the egg shell, amazing. They embryonate successfully in 2.4% formaldehyde (only 7%–10% are killed), in potassium bichromate, and in a 50% solution of HCl, of HNO_3 or of H_2SO_4.

Ascaris eggs thrive better in moist than in dry ground: sand is favorable; silt is acceptable; clay is unfavorable. The optimal temperature ranges between 20° and 25 °C with an upper limit of $\leqq 18$ °C ($\geqq 40$ °C kills the fertilized eggs) and a lower inhibiting limit of $\leqq 18$ °C. Moisture should be around 80% (70%–100%), the being minimum 8%. A shady environment is advantageous.

The survival of eggs has been studied in different environmental conditions. Eggs settle on a layer of particles at a depth of 40 cm by passive penetration. Survival on the surface is 23–29 days and on vegetable leaves 24–35 days; at a depth of 10–20 cm it reaches 1 ½ years, but at 40–60 cm up to 2 ½ years, and under snow (-23 °C) a 40-day survival has been observed.

Direct sunlight is detrimental. The highest mortality occurs during the hot dry season (soil temperature $\geqq 40$ °C). Consequently a distinct seasonality has been observed. During the dry season, eggs disappear rapidly in sandy ground, new infections are rare, and the loss of worms is continuous: the prevalence remains unchanged but the worm load decreases. Whenever the rainy season is short, so will be the transmission period. The infections start with the rains, are accompanied by an increasing occurrence of pneumonitis and eosinophilia, and produce the false impression of a seasonal pathology.

3. Pathology

In order to infect an host the parasite must cross several barriers: site of entry, liver sinusoids, pulmonary tissues, etc. During this larval migration the host will react. The response will vary, not only with the tissues or organs involved, but also with the number of migrating larvae and the grade of tolerance, sensitivity, or immunity of the host.

The mechanical crossing of tissue barriers is facilitated by the appropriate lytic enzyme armament of the larvae. These mixed stimuli are followed by an aspecific reaction to the injury, possibly combined with a somewhat more specific reaction. As a rule the penetration of the intestinal mucosa by the L2 stage induces little damage and the passage through the liver arouses no harm to the hepatocytes. Occasionally a transient focalized pseudotuberculoid granulomatous reaction and some inflammatory foci may appear. Heavy infections, or zoonotic infections trapped in the liver *(A. suum)*, may produce hepatomegaly.

The breaking through the lung capillaries may produce petechial hemorrhages at the larval emerging places in the alveoli. The molting from L2 into L3 larvae occurs in the lung and can produce hypersensitivity reactions. A localized passage of numerous L3 larvae will produce small bleeding pools, followed by congestion, edema, and pneumonitis. If a bacterial superinfection occurs this can end in a severe pneumonia or bronchopneumonia. Granulomas arise around trapped larvae. A serous severe alveolar exudation appears in heavy infections.

The metabolites freed by the molting of larvae, as well as adult metabolites, may produce allergic and general reactions in hypersensitive individuals: fever, urticarial rashes, eye pain, restlessness, asthma, eosinophilia, and more specifically Loeffler syndrome. This syndrome is characterized by low-grade fever, pruritis, retrosternal discomfort, irritative cough, dyspnea, bronchial spasms, and blood-stained sputum. On X-rays a subclavicular homogeneous infiltrate with a clear-cut border, usually in the right lung, appears but fades away after 6–12 days. A leukocytosis of 20,000–25,000, of which 30%–70% is due to eosinophils, points toward a parasitic etiology.

KOINO (1923), after self-infection by ingestion of 2,000 infective eggs, developed a severe pneumonia between day 6 and day 17. A specific treatment on day 50 was followed by the expulsion of 667 worms, but only 38 mm in length.

It needs to be mentioned that, due to the seasonality of *A. lumbricoides* transmission in dry countries, a seasonal pneumonitis caused by larval ascariasis may occur. It has been observed in Saudi Arabia (GELPI and MUSTAFA 1967, 1968).

Larvae ending up in abnormal migration routes will become blocked in unusual organs such as the brain, spinal cord, eyeball, and kidney. They will produce tissue reactions which may be followed by dramatic symptoms according to the intensity and the localization of the reaction. The adult worms do not, in their regular intestinal localization, produce untoward effects. They feed on the liquid contents of the ileum and, apart from this derivation of nutrients, they occasionally suck blood.[7]

In the intestinal mucosa several receptors react to the presence of foreign metabolic substances secreted by living adults. They interfere with normal peristalsis, produce spasms, and generate flattening of the intestinal villae, hypertrophy of the muscle layers, shortening of the depth of the crypts, and secretory changes through which the mucosa acquires a corrugated appearance. *A. lumbricoides*

7 The presence of a number of *Ascaris* worms in a poorly nourished community will precipitate the appearance of "protein-calorie malnutrition" (PCM) in the children: five female worms produce 1 million eggs daily, which means a loss of 4.2 mg N_2

also produces antienzymes for trypsin and chemotrypsin. As a result volatile fatty acids are excreted in the urine.

4. Immunity Reactions

The Ascaridae stimulate a nonsterilizing immune response. Its kinetics correlates with the life cycle. Each developmental stage induces its own reaction. The host response depends on the host's own physiological inborn or acquired characteristics.

The inducing factor is undoubtedly chemical, viz., foreign metabolic substances released by the molting process of the larvae, secreted by the living parasites or liberated by dead parasites. These *Ascaris* antigenic substances are not only immunogenic but also allergenic. Antigen-antibody complexes have been demonstrated in the lung parenchyma of animals experimentally infected with *A. suum*.

An interesting item is the regulating mechanism limiting the intensity of reinfection. This partial resistance to invasion depends on a nonsterilizing immunity. Several mechanisms may be involved in this hindrance such as interference with the hatching of L2 and its penetration into the intestinal mucosa, further immobilization and destruction of L2 in the lung tissue, or maturation arrest of L4 in the intestine. However logical, those are mere hypotheses which do not as such explain the increasing resistance to reinfection with age.

Ascaris lumbricoides produces humoral and cell-mediated antibodies. From day 5 after contamination the immunoglobulin content rises, reaches a maximum on day 15 to day 25, and decreases after day 90. IgM, type III, is the most specific (PHILLS et al. 1972). They are more an indicator of immune reorganization than protective antibodies. Higher levels of IgG will follow. The strongest antigenic stimuli are roused by the larval stage. This could be put to use for the diagnosis of recently acquired infections (NAKASATO 1974).

The IgE level rises but these reagins, produced by plasma cells in the Peyer plates of the small intestine, only measure a global parasitism.

Heterophilic anti-A and anti-B isoagglutinins may appear: in tissues and excretions of ascarids group-like A-B antigens are indeed present.

On the cellular level, the number of T cells will increase during the first days of infection. The production of mediators is intensified and induces a delay in the migration of lymphocytes and macrophages. During the migration of the larvae lymphocytes are transformed into lymphoblasts, and incubation with sheep erythrocytes produces rosettes on day 5 and day 6 (LEIKINA and POLETAEVA 1980).

5. Symptoms

Ascaris lumbricoides is well adapted to man. Single or light infections seldom produce symptoms. Moreover, the correlation between the presence of eggs in stools and vague complaints is difficult to ascertain.

The baseline symptoms, when the worm load is important ($\geqq 100$ worms) and the host hypersensitive, are during the migration phase: fever, chills, dyspnea, paroxysmal cough, asthmatic attacks, pneumonitis (on X-ray – mottling to larger infiltrates), and eosinophilia.

The intestinal localization can be accompanied by irritability, restlessness, insomnia, convulsions in children, anorexia, nausea, vomiting, abdominal discomfort, and live worms discharged in the stools and through the mouth, nose, urethra, and umbilicus (the naval), which causes consternation in the victim and the victim's next to kin and neighbours.

The mechanical and traumatic disturbances produced by these wandering worms are even more important. Their tendency to fasten onto the victim and pass through minute openings, to invade ectopic places such as the ampula Vateri, biliary and pancreatic ducts, appendix, lacrymal duct, nasal cavity, Eustachius tube, and larynx produces ill-defined, disturbing symptoms. This erratic migration can follow on from the administration of certain anthelmintics.[8] Their perforation of the umbilical string, Fallopian tubes, placenta, and urethra leads to even more alarming situations.

The intestinal subobstruction in the terminal ileum or at the ileocecal valve due to overcrowding of the worms or their knotting up due to a bolus after the intake of anthelmintics such as tetrachloroethylene (TCE), or following fever or a peppery diet, is more dramatic. These masses of intertwined worms produce colicky pains in the epigastrium, with anorexia and nausea, abdominal discomfort, intestinal spasms, intussusception, volvulus, and obstruction, which can lead to an untimely end. The clew of worms can be visualized by X-rays. Perforation and peritonitis are rare occurrences. In some countries *Ascaris* obstruction is a important item in acute abdominal surgery [India, 5% (CHOWDURY 1971); South Africa, up to 15% (LOUWE 1974)].

In the absence of a heavy worm load, *Ascaris* worms seldom cause illness, but can lower resistance and elicit and aggravate PCM in undernourished children. *Ascaris* infections are detrimental on the growth of undernourished preschool children. They provoke malabsorption of macronutrients and vitamin A. In addition, *Ascaris* deprives its host of a substantial amount of nutrients, particularly the most essential and richest, which are diverted toward the mass egg production of *Ascaris*.

Gut parasites can bind enzymes of the host to their surface membranes and consequently either enhance or inhibit the enzyme activity. They can also release intrinsic digestive enzymes at their surface. Antienzymes have been isolated from intestinal helminths such as *A. suum*, viz., antitrypsin and antichemotrypsin, located in its cuticle (CHAPPEL 1980). These findings are certainly important in relation to some digestive disturbances; they need further investigation.

The striking improvement of the nutritional status of *Ascaris*-infected children after deworming (GUPTA et al. 1974) is justification for periodic mass treatment of children. VENKATACHALAM and PATWARDHAN (1953) calculated that the presence of some 25 worms deprives the host every day of about 4 g protein from a diet that is often already low in proteins and thus reduces the proteinemia to critical levels.

In conclusion, a typical clinical profile does not exist in ascariasis. Ascariasis often remains unrecognized. In hypersensitive individuals allergic local and gen-

8 Wanderlust and ectopic migrations of adult worms may be induced by changes in body temperature and by the introduction in the bowel of irritating drugs

eral reactions may appear during the larval migration stage. Some systemic disorders appear with a greater frequency:

Digestive:	colics, nausea, vomiting
Respiratory:	nocturnal spastic cough
Neurological:	convulsion, meningism
Surgical complications:	obstruction of bile or pancreatic duct and of intestine

6. Diagnosis

1. *Parasitological* evidence is fairly easy to obtain, due to the dimension and the mobility of the adult worm and the unusual fecundity of *A. lumbricoides* (200,000 eggs/day).

a) Adult worms of this size are easily found and counted in stools or they turn up from various orifices. The evacuation of *Ascaris* never goes unnoticed. But the prepatent period is 2 months.
b) Since the number of eggs is seldom less than 100 to 50 mg feces, a 1-min examination is sufficient. Fresh stools, especially small samples, must be protected against drying. The characteristic mamillated normal fertilized eggs[9] will be detected easily by direct smear or Kato cellophane thick smear. Concentration methods are only useful for assessment of intensity by counting the eggs (EPG) by flotation, the Master or Stoll method.
c) Larvae can be found in sputum or gastric aspirate.
d) On histological slides differential diagnosis can be difficult. *A. suum, Toxocara canis, T. cati, Toxoascaris leonina* look alike.

2. *Biomedical signs* are useful in systemic infections, e.g., lung syndrome. Leukocytosis (up to 80,000) with >3,000 eosinophils (91%) can be present. SGOT, alkaline phosphatases and lactic dehydrogenase are increasing. The presence of "volatile fatty acids, with a branched carbon chain" in fresh urine is 98% specific, but needs gas chromatography and double benzol extraction (SOPRUNOVA et al. 1973).

3. *Immunological techniques*. The available antigens lack specificity. They can nevertheless be used in agar-cell diffusion, immunoelectrophoresis, the hemagglutination test, indirect immunofluorescence test, etc.

4. *Radiological examination*. On a roentgenograph, after a barium meal, the adult worms can be visualized in the bowel. In the lungs mottling (2–3 mm in diameter) can be present.

7. Geographical Distribution

Ascaris lumbricoides is not only the commonest but also the most cosmopolitan worm of man. STOLL (1947) estimated the number of parasitized persons at about 650 million, or roughly one in every fourth individual of a total population of 2,166 million. In 1980, this latter figure amounted to 4,415 million and, since no

9 Unfertilized eggs, longer along one axis, are decorticated, smooth, and transparent, which results from the absence of the outer mamillated coat

real drop in prevalence has been observed, the present number of *Ascaris* bearers can be roughly guessed at about 1 billion (1.1–1.3 billion).

Ascariasis is more abundant in a primitive sanitary environment and in persons little concerned with personal hygiene. As a result this parasitosis occurs mainly in the poorer socioeconomic classes and more specifically in children.

All the continents are infected to varying degrees. The main foci are localized in specific environments. In Africa, the numbers of infected amount to some 200 million; in South and Central America 100 million; in Asia 640 million, 335 million of which are in China; in Australia-Oceania 6 million; in Europe 32 million; in the United States over 3 million; and in the USSR 20 million, 13 million of which are in European and 7 million are in Asian countries. The grand total exceeds 1 billion.

Taking into account a mean worm load of six per infected person and an average weight of 6.75 g (4.5–9.0 g) per worm, astonishing and even frightening figures of the number and weight of *A. lumbricoides* worms in man are attained: 6,000 million worms, with a weight of 40,500 tonnes, corresponding to 675,000 human adults. By extending this parasitological arithmetic to the high egg production the figures are even more impressive: each female *Ascaris* worm produces 5 g eggs annually, which, for an initial sex ratio of nearly 1 : 1, adds up to an egg mass of 15,000 tonnes (for some 3,000 million female worms) of biological materials of the highest quality withdrawn from destitutes in need of good nutrients.

8. Prevalence

Africa:

Varies widely from country to country and also within a given country. The patchy distribution is in accordance with the environment and way of life.
Benin State: 20%; north region, 6%
Burundi: 87% (0–4 years of age); schoolchildren, 45%; adults, 32%
Cape Verde: 7%–71%
Cameroun: Yaounde, 80%–90% (children); forest area, 72%–75%; pygmies 57%
Central Africa an Republic: 53%
Egypt: 3%–43%; Cairo, 12%; Nuta region, 2%
Ethiopia: 58%
Gabon: 30%–77% (rural)
Ivory Coast: 24%
Kenya: 25%
Mozambique: 0.3%–86%
Rwanda: 30%–60% (Butare)
San Tomé-Principe: 65%–93%
Tanzania: 40%–45% (Mwanza)
Togo: 23% (Lomé)
Tunesia: 71% (Cape Bon)
Zaire: Ndjili, 83% (6–15 years of age); population in general, 67%; Kimuenza, 58%; Lower Zaire, 57%
Zambia: 3.7%
Zimbabwe: 2.7%; Burma Valley, 2.2%; Harari, 6.6%; Inyanga, 0.2%

America:

South and Central

- Brazil: 58%–68%, viz., 46 million Brazilians living in backward areas; e.g., Rio Grande do Norte, 57%
- Chile: 0.3%–21% (1970–1980)
- Colombia: 9%–59%
- Costa Rica: urban, 16% (6%–31%); rural, 27% (7%–46%)
- Dominican Republic: rural, 13%
- French Guyana: 18%
- Guatemala: 42% (1953), 73% (1980)
- Mexico: 26% (11%–84%) (1976); 18% (Hospital Infantil)
- Peru: 68% (Madre de Dios)
- Puerto Rico: 30%–50%
- Suriname: 9%–79%
- Venezuela: 44%; Costa and Cordillera, 60% (5%–22% >10,000 EPG or ten worms); Amerindians, 95%

North

- United States: out of 3 million stool specimens, more than 2% (centers for Disease Control, 1978)
- Rhode Island, 3.5%; Pennsylvania, 6.7%; Ohio, 2.2%; Nebraska, 2.6%; West Virginia, 3.0%; South Carolina, 3.1%; in coastal South Carolina school children (5–12 years of age), 21%–39%; Georgia, 2.3%; Kentucky, 3.5%; Tennessee, 3.0; Wyoming, 4.8%; Washington State, 2.1%; Oregon, 2.4%; California, 2.6%; Hawai, 2.7%; Guam, 8.9%

Asia:

- China, 54% (16%–18%) in 15 provinces and municipalities; Beijing, 43% (2,461 persons); Shangai, 36% (1,421 specimens)
- India: Dehli, 20%; Bandipur Union, 1.9%; Himachal Pradesh, 33%
- Indonesia: Java, 75%; Jakarta, 64% (orphans); Sulawezi, 13%; Surabaja, 26%
- Iran: Central Iran, 98% (children); Ispahan, 81% (65%–89%); Khorasan, 26%; rural Khuzestan, 2%–36%; urban Khuzestan, 3%–22%
- Japan: 6.5% (63% in 1949; 0.7% in 1971; 0.4% in 1980)
- Malaysia: 90%
- Philippines: Leyte, 83%–94%; Victoria (laguna), 83%; average, 80%
- South Korea: 68% (56% in 1970; 15% in 1979); 3% higher in spring
- Taiwan: 40%–75%; average 50%
- Thailand: 20%
- USSR: 7 million
- Vietnam: 35% (Saigon)

Australia-Oceania:

- Cook Islands: 40%–60%
- Kar-Kar Islands: 57%
- Marshall Islands: 38% (Micronesia)

Papua New Guinea: 59%. Star Mountains, 6%; North Fly, 2%; Delta, 56%; Nato, 25%; Kamea, 51%; West Sepih, 1%
Polynesia: 5%–13%; Noumea, 4%–12%

Europe:
France: 46% (postwar)
Germany: 52% (postwar)
Hungary: 5%–9% (focalized)
Italy: 75% (children at Ropano); 40% (toddlers, Napoli)
Netherlands: 45% (postwar)
Poland: 3.4%–8% (Poznan, schoolchildren)
Portugal: 20%–96%; Coimbra, 41% (22%–67%)
USSR: Georgia, 58%

A *prevalence* of up to 70% or more is not uncommon, but varies widely in any one country according to the population sample and to the existence of an *Ascaris* friendly environment. Furthermore, transmission being seasonal, the period of the inquiry is not irrelevant. In addition, the distribution is patchy. It has been generally agreed to set the level of high endemicity at >60% and of low endemicity <20%.

The available information is only indicative, as the role of the population group and of the selected landscapes or ecosystems is determinant.

II. Drugs

Ascaris infections are so widespread and the adult worms so easily detected by the naked eye that a number of anthelmintics of natural origin have been tried out and found efficient over the past centuries.

1. Traditional Drugs

Until quite recently some traditional drugs were indeed widely in use. *Semen contra*, which stands for "semen contra vermes," is composed of the dried unexpanded flower heads of *Artemisia cina* Berg, common in southern USSR, Afghanistan, Turkistan, and the Arabo-Caspian region, or *Artemisia herba alba* Asso, the African variety abundant among others in Marocco and southern Algeria. From these Compositae essential oils can be extracted, among which *Santonine*, a sesquiterpene lactone, is a poison for the nervous system. The recommended dosage was 10 mg/year of age on three consecutive days.

Other drugs of natural origin are *ascaridol*, extract of *Chenopodium ambrosioides* var. anthelminthicum, *pyrethrines*, extract of *Chrysanthenum cinerariaefolium* Visani, and *kainic acid*, extract of *Digenea simplex*. The latter has a synergistic effect on santonine [(10 mg kainic acid + 50 mg) santonine provides a cure rate of 85%–100% (IWATA et al. 1963 a) or only 37.3% (19/51) (KOBAYASHI 1970)]. The side effects, headache and xanthopsia, are almost the same as with santonine.

These traditional drugs cannot match the modern synthetic drugs in efficiency. Nevertheless they should neither be forgotten nor discarded totally: in less affluent communities, especially those living in remote rural zones, they may be the only drugs available. Moreover, their active principles as well as their mode of action can still be an inspiration for modern pharmacologists.

2. Antibiotics

Hygromycin B is active against *Ascarididea*. Neither this antibiotic, nor others known to show an activity against nematodes (Antibiotic G 418, Destomycin, Netropsin, Aspiculamycin, Anthelmycin), have been tested out or put into use against human ascariasis.

3. Synthetic Organic Drugs

3.1 Old Timers

Some synthetic products such as tetrachloroethylene have been used especially in combination with halogenated hydrocarbon, ascaridol (1:6), and the alkylated phenol derivatives, especially hexylresorcinol [a single oral dose of 100 mg/year up to 10 years (1 g for adults), followed 2 h later with a saline purgative] or thymol. Their period of popularity belongs to the past.

3.1.1 Phenothiazine and Derivatives

The antihelmintic properties of thiodiphenylamine against ascarids in swine were recognized by HARWOOD et al. 1938. This olive to grayish-green powder, insoluble in water and oxidized in air, has been recommended for the treatment of human enterobiasis (oxyuriasis) by MANSON-BAHR (1940) and later on also against roundworm.

Phenothiazine varies in toxicity with the animal species (DESCHIENS 1946), but in man the therapeutic index of 1:4 is very unsatisfactory. A drug too toxic for use in serious diseases should not been considered against worms such as *A. lumbricoides* and *E. vermicularis*. Liver damage, hemolytic anemia, photosensitivity, etc. can occur even after a cautious administration.

With a view to reducing the toxicity several derivatives of phenothiazine (methyl-, ethyl-, tetrachloro variants) have been investigated by DESCHIENS (1946) and several others, including the 1-hydroxyphenothiazine (CAVIER 1963). None has been found satisfactory.

Based on some structural analogy, synthetic antihistamines such as promethazine have been tried, but found practically inactive and poorly tolerated.

3.1.2 Stilbazium Iodide

This pyridine derivative has been found active in ascariasis by SWARTZWELDER et al. (1962): after 50–70 mg/kg per 1–3 days the ERR was 97%. The poor results are combined, according to HSIEH et al. (1963) and HUANG and BROWN (1964), with frequent intolerance phenomena (vomiting, abdominal colics).

3.1.3 Organophosphorous Compounds

3.1.3.1 State of the Art

SCHRADER et al. synthesized some 50,000 organic phosphorous compounds between 1938 and 1944 (SCHRADER 1963). Several appeared to be excellent pesticides. Some also possess anthelmintic activity against nematodes in animals (Ascaridae of pigs and dogs) and also against trematodes.

Following studies in vitro on *A. suum* in Ringer at 37 °C, CERF et al. (1962) selected trichlorfon (metrifonate) for human use. Later on dichlorvos was tried by PEÑA-CHAVARRIA et al. (1969) and CERVONI et al. (1969).

3.1.3.2 Assessment

Table 26. Treatment of *Ascaris* infection by organophosphorous compounds

Dosage (mg/kg)	Number treated	CR	ERR	References
Metrifonate (Trichlorfon)				
15–17/2 days	1,209	66%–86%	–	CERF et al. (1962)
Dichlorvos				
6	24	56	47	PEÑA-CHAVARRIA et al. (1969)
12	36	78	84	PEÑA-CHAVARRIA et al. (1969)
6 V_3[a]	14	100	–	CERVONI et al. (1969)
6 V_{12}[a]	49	76	–	CERVONI et al. (1969)
10 V_{12}	5	80	–	CERVONI et al. (1969)
12 V_3	7	71	–	CERVONI et al. (1969)
12 V_3	78	79	–	CERVONI et al. (1969)

[a] V_3 is a formulation with large and V_{12} with a smaller size of pellets. The active substance released by 6 mg V_{12} is nearly the same as that released by 12 mg V_3

3.1.3.3 Dosage, Mode of Administration

See Sect. B.II.3.1.4.1.3.

3.1.3.4 Side Effects

See Sect. B.II.3.1.4.1.4.

3.1.3.5 Contraindication – Precautions

See Sect. B.II.3.1.4.1.5.

3.1.3.6 Conclusions

The organophosphorous compounds are active against ascariasis with, according to CERVONI et al. (1969), a decreasing efficacy from single to triple infections. Dead worms are recovered in washed post-treatment stools.

Notwithstanding several interesting characteristics suitable for mass deparasitization, these compounds present risks for a fraction of the population. Furthermore they are less satisfactory against ascaridiasis than piperazine.

3.1.4 Piperazine Derivatives

3.1.4.1 State of the Art

In the thesis of MEHREZ (1947) and in the publications of DESCHIENS et al. (1954) a basic observation of P. Giroud is mentioned. In 1942 he noted that a patient undergoing piperazine treatment was cleared of his long-standing enterobiasis. It was followed up by MEHREZ (1947), and more specifically for ascariasis by FAYARD (1949). The latter used a 3% syrup of which he recommended five teaspoonfuls after supper and another five the following morning. The drug was well tolerated and worms were expelled alive. This was confirmed by CAVIER and GAULIN (1951) and MOURIQUAND et al. (1953). DESCHIENS et al. (1954) focused attention on the spectrum of activities of the compound.

Piperazine salts are indeed very active against both mature and immature roundworms and pinworms, but are almost without activity against the other intestinal helminths. The first therapeutic attempts were made with the hexahydrate derivate, which is, however, potentially unstable and due to its unpleasant taste rather inacceptable. Several salts, such as phosphate, citrate, and adipate, are easily produced. A number of pharmaceutical firms boosted different salts, which were used by different clinicians. This resulted in a succession of conflicting claims and counterclaims according to the more or less stringent criteria applied and strong personal feelings. The investigations of GOODWIN and STANDEN (1958) are based on solid ground, and as such are accepted as conclusive.

GOODWIN and STANDEN (1958) produced strong evidence, from the comparative activity of the current piperazine salts, administered as a single 3- or 4-g dose, that the efficiency of piperazine preparations is directly related to their base content and that no outstanding differences can be obtained by virtue of a different acidic radical. This is clearly demonstrated in Table 27.

Table 27. Comparative efficacy of different piperazine salts against *Ascaris* worms

Dosage	Salts	Number treated	CR
3 g	Citrate (tablets)	77	76
	Phosphate (tablets)	103	76
	Adipate (tablets)	92	76
	Sebacate (tablets)	58	86
	Stearate (tablets)	56	86
4 g	Citrate (tablets)	91	84
	Citrate (syrup)	237	87
	Phosphate (tablets)	28	89
	Adipate (tablets)	28	82

3.1.4.2 Assessment

Nevertheless a number of assays have been carried with different salts, on varying dosages according to weight or age and on a variety of administration regimens.

Table 28. Short review of the efficacy of piperazine derivatives in varying administration regimens against *Ascaris* infection

Efficacy	Dosage	Number treated	CR	ERR	References
100%	2–4 g/5 days	35	100	–	ALBOS-MARTINEZ and ARCE (19
≧90%	0.5–2 g/3 days	15	93	–	BROWN (1954)
	2 g/3 days	16	94	–	HOEKENGA (1955)
	3.6 g/2 days	11	91	–	HANNA and SHEHATA (1955)
	3 g/3 days [a]	479	94	–	BUDZHE et al. (1959)
	4 g/1 day	36	94	–	RICCI and CORBO (1957)
	75 mg/kg/2 days	80	97	–	BRUMPT and HO-THI-SANG (195
	120 mg/kg	10	90	–	HALEEM et al. (1971)
	140 mg/kg (max.3 g)	17	94	–	SWARZWELDER et al. (1955)
	200 mg/kg	34	94	–	NINANE et al. (1957)
≧80%	0.5–2 g/2 days	13	85	–	BROWN (1954)
	0.5–2 g/4 days	15	87	–	BROWN (1954)
	2 g/5 days	18	89	–	HOEKENGA (1955)
	3.6 g	21	81	–	HANNA and SHEHATA (1955)
	4 g	50	88	–	CAMPOS et al. (1968)
	6 g [a]	322	85	–	BUDZHE et al. (1959)
	4.5 g/2 days [b]	251	82	–	BUDZHE et al. (1959)
	900–1,500 mg/6 days	196	86	–	ROELS-BROADHURST and DE MA (1957)
	40 mg/kg/2 days [c]	?	86	–	YANAGISAWA et al. (1957)
	50–156 mg/kg/3–7 days	25	88	–	SWARZWELDER et al. (1955)
	120 mg/kg	28	89	–	HATCHUËL et al. (1973)
	65–70 mg/kg/3 days	–	89	–	CABRERA et al. (1960)
≧70%	1–4 g	44	75	–	ATCHLEY et al. (1956)
	2–3 g	66	73	–	GOODWIN and STANDEN (1954)
	3–6 g	33	79	–	FARID et al. (1966)
	2–4 g	94	78	–	RODRIGUES et al. (1967b)
	4 g	41	70	72	BELL and NASSIF (1971)
	4 g	13	70	96	VAKIL and DALAT (1975)
	150 mg/kg	48	75	96	SARGENT et al. (1976)
	4 g	206	75	97	MILLER and ARFAA (1975)
	100 mg/kg	50	76	–	HUGGINS et al. (1958)
	3–4 g		75–90		HUYS et al. (1973)
<70%	150 mg/kg	461	66	90	MILLER et al. (1978)
	150 mg/kg	214	57	73	MILLER and KATZ (1975)
	150 mg/kg	51	57	–	KOBAYASKI (1980)
	60 mg/kg/5 days	22	64	–	AMATO-NETO and CORREA (195
	100 mg/kg/7 days	105	59	–	COUTELEN et al. (1956)
	350 mg/years of age/10 days	30	67	–	BASNUEVO et al. (1953)
	75 mg/kg	26	54	83	WINSOR and TOTTEN (1976)
	100 mg/kg/2 days	21	43	96	WERSHING et al. (1975)
	100 mg/kg	108	33	–	LEVI et al. (1972)

[a] Children: 300 mg/year [b] Children: 100–150 mg/year [c] Maximum 4 g

They have been reported in detail by CAVIER and HAWKING (1973). Some have been extracted in Table 28, in order to provide a brief overview.

3.1.4.3 Dosage, Mode of Administration

The WHO Expert Committee (1967) recommended recording the dose of piperazine as its hexahydrate equivalent. Hexahydrate contains 44% base. The single-dose treatment is 75 mg/kg, with a maximum of 2 g under 20 kg body weight, of 3 g over 20 kg, and of 4 g in adults. A similar regimen of 50–75 mg/kg on two successive days increases the CR to over 90%. Only oral administration has to be considered, but poses problems of stability and palatability.

Piperazine hexahydrate is potentially unstable, sebacate, and adipate are distasteful, stearate is tasteless but soapy, and citrate and phosphate are slightly acid, but not unpleasant. For the solid chewable preparations (wafers of 500 mg) the choice of the salt is important in view of the rather large oral dosages needed. For mass treatment liquid formulations, which are as effective as tablets, make the drug more acceptable and palatable.

Solutions should be chosen in preference to suspensions, which tend to form a sediment on storage. Tablets are not always swallowed; 4 g piperazine means eight tablets of 500 mg, and the control of correct in-take is almost impossible when confronted with a continuous flow of persons. Neither prior fasting nor cathartics or enemas are necessary.

3.1.4.4 Side Effects

Piperazine is a safe anthelmintic; the wide range between therapeutic and toxic doses gives a reassuring therapeutic index. Adverse reactions are uncommon, trivial, and transient. They may include abdominal discomfort, nausea, vomiting, loose stools, and diarrhea. Some individuals react to piperazine treatment with urticarial reaction and fever, which are to be attributed at least partially to liberation of sensitizing material by the intoxicated worms. But some individuals are or can become hypersensitive to piperazine as such, namely nurses, manufactory workers, etc. This individual sensitivity can be detected by patch-testing and relieved by antihistaminic drugs.

Besides transient neurological effects toxic central nervous system disturbances may occur by overdosage. Such a situation can be brought about by replacing a teaspoon with a spoon by mistake; the supposed 4 g or 75 mg/kg goes up to 12 g or 225 mg/kg. The alarm signals of neurotoxicity are somnolence, nystagmus, vertigo, respiratory depression, incoordination, weakening of tendons and reflexes, muscular weakness or myoclonic contractions, convulsions, epileptic seizures, and corresponding EEG changes (BETTECKEN 1957; ELIACHAR et al. 1960; CHAPTAL et al. 1963; VANNESTE et al. 1975; and several more).

3.1.4.5 Contraindications, Precautions

Long-standing liver and renal disease, jaundice, a history of neurological abnormalities (epileptic seizures, myoclonic contractions, etc.), and pregnancy in the first trimester are some of the many conditions in which piperazine is contraindicated.

3.1.4.6 Conclusions

3.1.4.6.1 Clinical Use

The recommended dose of 75 mg/kg (maximum 3.5–4 g), for 1 or 2 days, gives satisfactory results. If a cure is not achieved, the treatment can be repeated until successful. Piperazine is obviously a good standard drug, easy to administer, and cheap.

3.1.4.6.2 Mass Treatment

This inexpensive drug is active on a single dose, ensures expulsion of the worms, and is well tolerated: all are important factors from a psychological point of view. It is a good choice for blanket treatment. The efficiency of the different salts offers the possibility of selection on acceptability and cost. Moreover, the administration of a saline or mild purgative, while complicating the mass treatment, does not improve the results.

Many attempts at mass piperazine administration have been made. BIAGI and RODRIGUES (1960) treated the village Astape in Southeast Mexico monthly with 100 mg/kg. Participation was 98.9% and after the first treatment the CR was 97%. The number of worms collected dropped to zero in the 8th month.

Feasibility does not depend on efficacy, but on the recurrent expenses. FARID et al. (1966) achieved a CR of 79% in farmers of the Nile Delta with a single dose of 6 g, reduced to 3 g for those under 40 kg. POND et al. (1970) recorded a CR of 88% in Indian schoolchildren after five quarterly drug administrations of 3 g piperazine citrate. SARGENT et al. (1972) compared in schoolchildren in coastal South Carolina the activity of a regular dose of piperazine citrate repeated after 45 days and one and half times such a dose repeated after 60 days. Both groups finished with a CR of 100%, the first group after four treatments, the second after three. However, the reinfection rates observed at 60-day intervals indicate a need for retreatment after 45 days and an increase of the recommended dose by 50%. In a follow-up report in the same community, DUDLEY and LEASE (1973) brought the prevalence down to 6% after two mass treatments at a 60-day interval. After continuation of the scheme for another school year the prevalence dropped to 0.6% and the ERR attained 97%. In a control group with pyrantel pamoate treatment an ERR of 97.5% was achieved.

In a population of children ROELS-BROADHURST and DE MAYER (1957) tried a monthly administration regimen. They made use of the inexpensive piperazine citrate syrup, easily acceptable as soon as the children become used to the aniseed flavor. In a community close at hand, the 3-g dose can be divided over 3 days. The ERR reached 98% after 9 months.

Piperazine and its derivates remain suitable for mass and periodic blanket treatments against *A. lumbricoides*.

3.1.4.7 Comments

Piperazine salts are good standard drugs against ascariasis. They present a series of advantages: easy administration, excellent tolerance, very low toxicity, and inexpensive. They are still a good choice for mass treatment in certain specific situations, e.g., when produced locally.

3.2 Newer Drugs

3.2.1 Albendazole

3.2.1.1 State of the Art

This benzimidazole derivate, in a single oral dose of 2.5–10 mg/kg, has been found a safe and broad-spectrum anthelmintic in sheep and cattle (THEODORIDES et al. 1976). Consequently it has been rational to try it out for human use. GARIN (1980) found that albendazole was extremely well tolerated in a single dose, as high as 8 mg/kg, or as repeated doses at the same level for seven consecutive days.

3.2.1.2 Assessment

The available results in humans with ascariasis are summarized in Table 29.

Table 29. Treatment of *Ascaris* infection by albendazole

Efficacy	Dosage	Number treated	CR	ERR	References
100%	400 mg	41	100	–	PENE et al. (1981b)
	400 mg	5	100	–	LUMBRERAS CRUZ et al. (1981)
	400 mg	11	100	–	AYAD EL-MASRY et al. (1983)
	400 mg	6	100	–	RAMALINGHAM et al. (1983)
	600 mg	14	100	–	RAMALINGHAM et al. (1983)
	800 mg	12	100	–	RAMALINGHAM et al. (1983)
	4 mg/kg	9	100	–	MAISONNEUVE et al. (1981)
≧90%	400 mg	49	96	99	PENE et al. (1982a)
	400 mg	50	92	99	BARANSKI et al. (1981)
	400 mg	10	90	–	CAMILO-COURA et al. (1981a)
	400 mg	42	95	99	BOURDERIOUX and CHEVALIER (1982)
	400 mg	32	91	98	SOULA and SIOPATHIS (1982)
	200 mg b.i.d.	13	92	99	BARANSKI et al. (1981)
	200 mg b.i.d.	42	95	97	CRUZ-LOPEZ (1981)
	400 mg	99	97	99	ROSSIGNOL (1981)
	200 mg (children)	72	90	98	PENE et al. (1981a)
	400 mg	49	94	93	BASTIDAS (1982)
≧80%	400 mg	18	88	–	CAMILO-COURA et al. (1981b)
	400 mg	136	88	96	SENTILHES and CARRIE (1982)
	400 mg	35	83	95	COULAUD et al. (1982b)
	400 mg	17	82	94	COULAUD et al. (1982b)
	400 mg	8	87	99	COULAUD et al. (1982b)
	200 mg b.i.d.	55	82	96	RICHARD-LENOBLE et al. (1982)
≧70%	200 mg b.i.d.	27	78	–	RICHARD-LENOBLE et al. (1982)
	200 mg b.i.d.	7	71	–	SALAZAR SCHETTINO and HARO ORTEGA (1981)
≧50%	100 mg b.i.d.	12	58	–	SALAZAR SCHETTINO and HARO ORTEGA (1981)

3.2.1.3 Dosage, Mode of Administration

For human use the drug is available as 100-mg chewable tablets or a 2% suspension. A single dose of 4 mg/kg (200–300 mg in adults) is suitable for individual treatment of ascariasis; however, a 400-mg single dose in adults and 200 mg in children has been recommended.

3.2.1.4 Side Effects

See Sect. B.II.3.2.1.4.

3.2.1.5 Contraindications, Precautions

See Sect. B.II.3.2.1.5.

3.2.1.6 Conclusions

3.2.1.6.1 Clinical

The drug is still under observation on the basis of a uniform protocol in a multicenter study, which includes 18 units spread over France, West Africa, Latin America, and the Far East and numbering 1,000 single and mixed infections.

In a recent overview, ROSSIGNOL and MAISONNEUVE (1984) noted on day 15–16 after a single dose of 400 mg the following CR and ERR: light infections (EPG <2,000) 96% and 38%; moderate infections (EPG 2,000–10,000) 85% and 80%; severe infections (EPG >10,000) 100%.

3.2.1.6.2 Mass Treatment

Its spectrum of activity covering soil-transmitted and a number of other worm species places albendazole among the suitable candidates for mass therapy. Mass therapy, which has to make allowance for multiple infections, requires 8 mg/kg and in the presence of strongyloidiasis and hymenolepiasis an administration extended over three consecutive days.

3.2.2 Amidantel

This compound is active against *Ascaris*, but is no longer on the market for human ascariasis.

3.2.3 Bephenium Hydroxynaphthoate

3.2.3.1 State of the Art

Although bephenium is known to be effective in ascariasis (GOODWIN et al. 1958), it is not as active as against hookworms. Its activity will be useful in lowering the *Ascaris* worm burden, whenever it coexists with hookworm.

3.2.3.2 Assessment

Following the demonstration by GOODWIN et al. (1958) of activity of bephenium against *Ascaris* and the careful assessment of a minimum dose by JAYEWARDANE et al. (1960) numerous attempts have been made to ascertain its practical value in ascariasis. The CR varies for the same dose of 2.5 g base from 18% to 95%.

Table 30. Treatment of *Ascaris* infection by bephenium hydroxynaphthoate

Efficacy	Dosage	Number treated	CR	ERR	References
100%	2.5 g/2 days	7	100	–	JUTTIJUDATA et al. (1962)
≧90%	2.5 g (pellets)	15	93	–	AHMAD et al. (1964)
	1.75 g	12	92	–	AHMAD et al. (1964)
	2.5 g	20	95	–	LYNGDOH et al. (1962)
	1.66 g/2 days	49	94	–	JAYEWARDANE et al. (1960)
≧80%	2.5 g	78	82	–	HAHN et al. (1960)
	2.5 g	56	80	–	JAYEWARDANE et al. (1960)
	2.5 g	8	87	–	JUTTIJUDATA et al. (1962)
	2.5 g	60	83	–	AL-ISSA and WAHAB (1971)
	2.5 g	50	83	16	FARAHMANDIAN et al. (1972)
	1.25 g/2 days	55	89	–	JAYEWARDANE et al. (1960)
≧70%	2.5 g	16	75	–	MARX and TONTHANIEN (1961)
	2.5 g (granules)	11	73	–	AHMAD et al. (1964)
	2.5 g/2 days	–	77	–	COSTA et al. (1966)
	1.25 g	56	71	–	JAYEWARDANE et al. (1960)
≧60%	2.5 g b.i.d.	–	65	91	HSIEH et al. (1960b)
≧50%	2.5 g	–	50–80	95–97	HSIEH et al. (1960b)
	2.5 g	12	50	–	YOSHIDA et al. (1960)
	2.5 g	–	56	–	UCHIDA et al. (1964)
	2.5 g	–	50	–	COSTA et al. (1966)
	2.5 g	50	53	62	FARAHMANDIAN et al. (1972)
<50%	1.25 g	9	33	–	AHMAD et al. (1964)
	0.625 g	4	25	–	AHMAD et al. (1964)
	–	17	18	–	FARID and MIALE (1962)
	2.5 g	45	29	–	SALEM et al. (1968)
	2.5 g	12	43	98	VAKIL et al. (1965)
	1.25–2.5 g/1–7 days	44	48	–	HSIEH et al. (1960)

3.2.3.3 Dosage, Mode of Administration

JAYEWARDENE et al. (1960) tried eight different modalities of administration on 396 schoolchildren with varying degrees of *Ascaris* infestation. The clear-cut conclusion was that 1.25 g bephenium base was the minimum dose providing optimum results, i.e., an ERR of 80% or more, when the initial EPG count was 20,000 or more. The passing of worms starting ½ h after treatment and continuing for up to 3 days raised some problems for the school heads. The bitter unpleasant taste of the drug gives rise to vomiting and a refusal by many.

In practice, the dosage recommended for hookworm will be the only one put into use, viz., 2.5 g bephenium base.

3.2.3.4 Side Effects

See Sect. III.3.2.4.4.

3.2.3.5 Contraindications, Precautions

See Sect. III.3.2.4.5.

3.2.3.6 Conclusion

3.2.3.6.1 Clinical

Bephenium is not suitable for use in the individual treatment of ascariasis.

3.2.3.6.2 Mass Treatment

Whenever bephenium hydroxynaphthoate is selected for treatment of ancylostomiasis in a community, its efficacy against *Ascaris* will be an extra benefit.

3.2.3.7 Comments

Activity against *A. lumbricoides* is moderate and the CRs are very uncertain, ranging between 18% and 100% for similar dosages. Furthermore the side effects are frequent: vomiting occurs in 11%–39% of the patients.

Bephenium can be helpful when hookworms and *Ascaris* coexist.

3.2.4 Cambendazole

3.2.4.1 State of the Art

3.2.4.2 Assessment

Table 31. Treatment of *Ascaris* infections by cambendazole

Efficacy	Dosage	Number treated	CR	References
100%	25 mg/kg	5	100	MARTIRANI and RODRIGUES (1976)
≧80%	25 mg/kg/2 days	10	80	MARTIRANI and RODRIGUES (1976)
	25 mg/kg/3 days	6	83	MARTIRANI and RODRIGUES (1976)
<80%	5 mg/kg	8	63	MARTIRANI and RODRIGUES (1976)

3.2.4.3 Comments

This compound is active against ascariasis. However, its use has been probably discontinued for unknown reasons. It is not improbable what the rapid development of resistance against cambendazole by several nematodes is an underlying reason.

3.2.5 Ciclobendazole

3.2.5.1 State of the Art

In a clinical pilot-study DEGRÉMONT and STAHEL (1978) observed that the highest activity of ciclobendazole was in the intestinal tract, followed by 75% excretion with the feces, and established that it was active against *Ascaris*.

3.2.5.2 Assessment

Table 32. Treatment of *Ascaris* infection by ciclobendazole

Efficacy	Dosage	Number treated	CR	ERR	References
100%	200 mg b.i.d./3 days	9	100	–	DEGRÉMONT and STAHEL (1978)
≧90%	100 mg b.i.d./3 days	30	93	–	DEGRÉMONT and STAHEL (1978)
	600 mg	51	98	–	GUGGENMOOS et al. (1978)
	1,200 mg	44	98	–	GUGGENMOOS et al. (1978)
	200 mg b.i.d./3 days	69	88	98	STÜRCHLER et al. (1980)
	1,000 mg	109	88	98	STÜRCHLER et al. (1980)

3.2.5.3 Dosage, Mode of Administration

100 mg b. i. d. for 3 days guarantees excellent results against ascariasis. Doubling the dosage to 200 mg b. i. d. for 3 days does not improve the results. A single dose of 600 mg produces an interesting CR.

3.2.5.4 Side Effects

See Sect. B.II.3.2.6.4.

3.2.5.5 Contraindications, Precautions

See Sect. B.II.3.2.6.5.

3.2.5.6 Conclusions

3.2.5.6.1 Clinical Use

Ciclobendazole is an efficient anthelmintic in ascariasis at a well-tolerated dose.

3.2.5.6.2 Mass Treatment

The available data show that ciclobendazole is a suitable drug for use in communities, since it produces a satisfactory CR after a single dose of 600 mg or 1,000 mg.

3.2.6 Fenbendazole

3.2.6.1 State of the Art

Fenbendazole is an efficient anthelmintic against gastrointestinal nematodes in cattle, calves, and sheep. An orientating clinical study in man indicated that a single dose of 200 mg was active against *Ascaris* and well tolerated (HAAS and BRUCH, unpublished).

3.2.6.2 Assessment

Table 33. Treatment of *Ascaris* infection by fenbendazole

Efficacy	Dosage	Number treated	CR	References
100%	1 g	7	100	BRUCH and HAAS (1976)
	600 mg b.i.d./3 days	2	100	SANCHEZ CARILLO and BELTRAN HERNANDES (1977)
≧80%	30–50 mg/kg	31	84	RIM et al. (1981)
	1 g 500 mg	5	80	BRUCH and HAAS (1976)

3.2.6.3 Dosage, Mode of Administration

The dosage has not been established: a single dose of 1.5 g is not better than 1 g; moreover tablets and suspension provide the same results. But, whenever the dosage is split into two administrations, many do not take the second dose.

3.2.6.4 Side Effects

Ascaris worms start moving and can be vomited.

3.2.6.5 Conclusions

It is unlikely that this benzimidazole will have a place among the anthelmintics for human use.

3.2.7 Flubendazole

3.2.7.1 State of the Art

During the past decade, the search for broad-spectrum drugs, efficient against soil-transmitted helminths, easy to administer, safe, and ensuring a high ERR has focussed interest on the benzimidazoles. Among them flubendazole, a parafluoro derivative of mebendazole, has been found to be particularly worthwhile. Owing to its limited solubility in the gastrointestinal tract, after oral administration, flubendazole does not produce acute or chronic neither toxic nor behavioral effects in laboratory animals. In all species investigated the LD_{50} was higher than 2,560 mg/kg (THIENPONT et al. 1978). No teratogenic and embryotoxic effects have been observed. In human volunteers the absorption was equally limited and the tolerance good.

The orientation studies of BECQUET (1976), BRUMPT (1976), BOUVIER (1976), GENTILINI (1976), and COLAERT (1976) among others were extremely encouraging concerning the CR and ERR in ascariasis.

3.2.7.2 Assessment

During the period 1978–1980 a great number of clinical and field trials were carried out, which largely confirm the first optimistic conclusions. They are summarized in Table 34.

Table 34. Treatment of *Ascaris* infection by flubendazole

Efficacy	Dosage	Number treated	CR	ERR	References
100%	100 mg b.i.d./3 days	45	100	–	BECQUET (1976)
	100 mg b.i.d./3 days	17	100	–	GENTILINI (1976)
	100 mg b.i.d./3 days	23	100	–	BLECHMAN et al. (1982)
	100 mg b.i.d./3 days	25	100	–	WERSHING et al. (1979)
	100 mg t.i.d./3 days	3	100	–	DA SILVA (1979)
	100 mg t.i.d./3 days	23	100	–	KATZ (1980)
	100 mg t.i.d./2 days	2	100	–	DA SILVA (1979)
	100 mg t.i.d./2 days	20	100	–	KATZ (1979)
	200 mg b.i.d./1 day	17	100	–	ARFAA et al. (1979)
	200 mg t.i.d./1 day	6	100	–	DA SILVA (1979)
	200 mg t.i.d./1 day	2	100	–	LEAO (1980)
	200 mg/3 days	14	100	–	NOZAIS (1978)
	200 mg/3 days	17	100	–	DANIS et al. (1980)
	250 mg b.i.d./2 days	23	100	–	WERSHING et al. (1979)
	300 mg/2 days	34	100	–	KAN (1983)
	300 mg b.i.d.	5	100	–	BUNNAG et al. (1980)
	300 mg/2 days	3	100	–	BUNNAG et al. (1980)
	400 mg	2	100	–	BOUVIER (1976)
	500 mg b.i.d.	22	100	–	WERSHING (1972)
	500 mg b.i.d.	7	100	–	PEÑA-CHAVARRIA (1977)
	500 mg t.i.d.	24	100	–	WERSHING et al. (1979)
	500 mg t.i.d.	8	100	–	PEÑA-CHAVARRIA (1977)
	500 mg t.i.d.	24	100	–	WERSHING et al. (1979)
	1,000 mg	22	100	–	PEÑA-CHAVARRIA (1977)
	1,000 mg b.i.d.	8	100	–	PEÑA-CHAVARRIA (1977)
	2,000 mg	9	100	–	PEÑA-CHAVARRIA (1977)
≧90%	100 mg	42	90	97	WERSHING et al. (1979)
	100 mg b.i.d.	31	97	99	ARFAA et al. (1979)
	100 mg b.i.d./2 days	45	96	99	ARFAA et al. (1979)
	100 mg b.i.d./2 days	11	91	–	LEÃO (1980)
	200 mg	21	91	–	BRUMPT (1976)
	200 mg	40	90	99	KAN (1983 a)
	200 mg	31	97	99	ARFAA et al. (1979)
	200 mg t.i.d.	29	93	–	KATZ (1979)
	300 mg/2 days	48	90	–	CABRERA et al. (1980)
	300 mg/2 days	34	94	99	KAN (1983 a)
	300 mg b.i.d.	27	93	98	BOTERO (1980 b)
	500 mg	47	94	99	KAN (1983 a)
	500 mg	22	98	98	LIONEL et al. (1980)
	500 mg	43	97	99	KAN (1983 a)
	600 mg	33	97	99	KAN (1983 a)
	2,000 mg	48	97	99	COLAERT et al. (1976)
≧80%	100 mg b.i.d./3 days	9	89	–	LEÃO (1980)
	200 mg	47	89	97	LIONEL et al. (1980)
	200 mg/3 days	30	87	–	SCHENONE et al. (1977)
	300 mg/2 days	76	82	96	MARGONO et al. (1980)
	300 mg/2 days	48	89	–	CABRERA et al. (1980)
	1,000 mg	50	84	96	COLAERT (1976)
	2,000 mg	25	88	95	NEYRINCK and VAN DE KEIRKHOVE (1976)
≧70%	200 mg/3 days	31	77	–	NOZAIS (1978)
	300 mg/3 days	18	78	–	PENOT et al. (1978)
≧60%	600 mg	5	60	–	BOUVIER (1976)

3.2.7.3 Dosage, Mode of Administration

Flubendazole is available in tablets of 100 mg or a suspension of 20 mg/ml for oral administration. Neither diet nor purging are required. The dose is identical for children and adults: one tablet or 5 ml suspension morning and evening for 3 days. The efficacy period does not exceed the time limit indicated on the bottle.

3.2.7.4 Side Effects

See Sect. B.II.3.2.8.4.

3.2.7.5 Contraindications, Precautions

See Sect. B.II.3.2.8.5.

3.2.7.6 Conclusions

3.2.7.6.1 Individual Treatment

The oral administration of 200 mg, twice in 1 day with an interval of 12 h, provides CRs of between 97% and 100%. Since the studies of SCHENONE et al. (1977), CANESE et al. (1978), NOZAÏS (1978), BECQUET and LABARRIÈRE (1980), and DANIS et al. (1980), the efficacy of this dosage has become indisputable. Higher doses, applied by PENOT et al. (1978) and BOUVIER (1976), have not improved the outcome. Expulsion of worms starts from the 1st day on, but does not provoke erratic migration of the *Ascaris*. It is one of the better anti-*Ascaris* drugs.

3.2.7.6.2 Mass Treatment

The administration will be limited to a single dose of 200 mg, which can be repeated after weeks or months. The CR will be around 90%, but the important ERR will reach 97%–99%, which is quite satisfactory.

3.2.7.7 Comments

The majority of *Ascaris* infections are eradicated by a dosage of 200 mg b. i. d. at a 12-h interval. A single dose of 200 mg produces a CR of 89%–97% and an ERR of between 97% and 99%, which are very satisfactory for mass treatment. Effective, safe, and easy to administer are qualities which place flubendazole among the valuable assets in the control of intestinal nematodes.

3.2.8 Levamisole

3.2.8.1 State of the Art

The remarkable anthelmintic properties of tetramisole, an aminothiazole derivative, were discovered by THIENPONT et al. (1966) and confirmed in humans by DO NASCIMENTO et al. (1966), RODRIQUEZ et al. (1966), AMATO NETO et al. (1967), and several others: on the whole the CR in ascaridiasis varied between 52% and 88%. However, the real breakthrough came when THIENPONT et al. (1969) demonstrated that the helminthic activity was mainly due to the laevorotatory isomer, which in a dose of 2.5 mg/kg sharply increased the CR from about 50% to 90%. This fact was confirmed by GATTI et al. (1969), LIONEL et al. (1969), and DÜRR (1969).

3.2.8.2 Assessment

An impressive number of *Ascaris* infections have been treated throughout the world between 1969 and 1978. Their results are summarized in Table 35.

Table 35. Treatment of *Ascaris* infections by levamisole

Efficacy	Dosage	Number treated	CR	ERR	References
100%	2.5 mg/kg	22	100	–	GATTI et al. (1970)
	2.5 mg/kg	104	100	–	LEVAI et al. (1972)
	2.5 mg/kg	26	100	–	MILLER (1976)
	2.5 mg/kg	54	100	–	AL-ISSA and WAHAB (1971)
	3 mg/kg	58	100	–	DAN et al. (1973)
	3.5 mg/kg/2 ×	106	100	–	THIENPONT et al. (1969)
	5 mg/kg	74	100	–	THIENPONT et al. (1969)
	5 mg/kg	41	100	–	AL SHAFFAR et al. (1971)
	5 mg/kg	13	100	–	BOUYER (1970)
	3–7 mg/kg	21	100	–	BOUYER (1970)
	3–7 mg/kg	16	100	–	GENTILINI et al. (1970)
	40–80–120 mg [a]	14	100	–	FARID et al. (1973)
	50–100–150 mg [b]	20	100	–	FARID et al. (1973)
	150 mg	38	100	–	VAKIL and DALAL (1975)
	40–60–80 mg/2 × (week)	111	100	–	LIONEL et al. (1969)
≧90%	2.5 mg/kg	250	92	99	GATTI et al. (1969)
	2.5 mg/kg	54	96	83	FARAHMANDIAN et al. (1977)
	2.5 mg/kg	113	97	97	CRUZ-LOPEZ and ALCANTARA (1980)
	2.5 mg/kg	65	92	–	HUGGINS (1970)
	2.5 mg/kg	1,000	94	98	HUYS et al. (1973)
	2.5 mg/kg	25	96	–	LENGYEL et al. (1973)
	2.5 mg/kg	208	95	98	MILLER and KATZ (1975)
	2.5 mg/kg	30	93	–	ORA et al. (1976)
	2.5 mg/kg	196	90	99	MILLER and ARFAA (1975)
	3.5 mg/kg	29	93	–	VAKIL (1969)
	2.5–3.5 mg/kg	60	90	–	KUZMICKI et al. (1972)
	2.5–3.5 mg/kg	1,098	94	–	ORBAN (1972)
	4–10 mg/kg	199	95	55	LUCAS and ODUNTAN (1972)
	2.5 mg/kg	85	98	–	ASMERA (1974)
	2.5 mg/kg	64	98	–	NAGATY et al. (1978)
	40–80–120 mg	161	92	–	LIONEL et al. (1969)
	40–80–120 mg	83	99	–	FARAHMANDIAN et al. (1974)
	40–80–120 mg	50	96	–	DE OLIVERA et al. (1971)
	40–80–120 mg	126	93	–	DE PAULO CASTRO et al. (1970)
	40–80–120 mg	65	93	–	HUGGINS (1970)
	40–80–120 mg	246	97	–	NAGATY et al. (1978)
	50–100–150 mg	17	94	99	VAKIL et al. (1972)
	50–100–150 mg	36	97	–	FREIRE et al. (1969)
	50–100–150 mg	362	94	–	CABRERA et al. (1971)

[a] 50 mg (10–20 kg), 100 mg (21–40 kg), 150 mg (>40 kg)
[b] 40 mg (10–20 kg), 80 mg (21–40 kg), 120 mg (>40 kg)

Table 35 (continued)

Efficacy	Dosage	Number treated	CR	ERR	References
	50–100–150 mg	453	92	98	MILLER et al. (1978)
	50–100–150 mg	117	97	99	PEÑA-CHAVARRIA and VILLAREJOS (1975)
	50–100–150 mg	51	94	99	DE JONCKHEERE (1973)
	50–100–150 mg	450	95	–	EVDOKIMOV and NTIBARUTAYE (1970)
	150 mg	30	97	–	DE SOUZA et al. (1972)
≧80%	2.5 mg/kg	23	87	92	THIENPONT et al. (1969)
	2.5 mg/kg	3,000	87	92	THIENPONT et al. (1969)
	2.5 mg/kg	140	89	–	NITZULESCU (1971)
	2.5 mg/kg	46	82	97	SARGENT and CHAMBERS (1976)
	3 mg/kg	68	89	–	LAIGRET et al. (1969)
	40–80–120 mg	93	86	–	AMATO-NETO et al. (1969)
	40–80–120 mg	45	88	–	SCHMITZ and KNACKFUSS (1971)
	50–100–150 mg	943	88	–	CABRERA et al. (1971)
	150 mg	27	85	97	VAN LANDUYT (1973)
	2.5 mg–25 mg	60	88	–	BIAGI (1980)
	300 mg	37	84	95	VAN LANDUYT (1973)
<80%	2.5 mg/kg	108	70	–	DUFEK and KALIVODA (1973a, b)
	2.5 mg/kg	28	71	96	WIMOR-TOTTER (1976)
	2.5 mg/kg	24	67	90	WERSHING et al. (1975)
	2.5 mg/kg	308	70	–	COENE (1969)
	3.6 mg/kg	30	66	–	GUIMARAES et al. (1971)
	40–80–120 mg	–	68–95	–	HALL et al. (1970)
	80–150 mg	100	78	–	LEVI et al. (1972)
	150 mg	41	78	98	CERVONI and OLIVER-GONZALES (1975)

3.2.8.3 Dosage, Mode of Administration

The suitable dose is 2.5 mg/kg in a single peroral administration, without dietetic preparation or purgatives.

3.2.8.4 Side Effects

See Sect. B.II.3.2.9.4.

3.2.8.5 Contraindications, Precautions

See Sect. B.II.3.2.9.5.

3.2.8.6 Conclusions

3.2.8.6.1 Individual Treatment

Levamisole is the drug of choice in ascariasis: a single dose of 2.5 mg/kg without food restriction or laxatives provides a CR of 90%–100%, while the side effects are rare, transient, and never alarming.

3.2.8.6.2 Mass Treatment

Levamisole possesses a wide anthelmintic spectrum of activities, but is ineffective against *Trichuris trichiura* and *Enterobius vermicularis:* therefore its usefulness in mass campaigns against helminths remains limited.

3.2.8.7 Comments

Levamisole has been an important advance in the drug treatment of ascariasis and other intestinal helminthiasis. Up to a certain point it has been a pioneer in the field of modern anthelmintic drugs. The analysis by MOENS et al. (1978) of ten clinical studies, using a common protocol, performed in the Bahamas, Brazil, Costa Rica, Iran, Israel, Puerto Rico, the United States, and Zaire, in a total of 830 people, mainly children infected with ASCARIS, confirms this conclusion. With dosages of 50 mg (10–20 kg), 100 mg (21–40 kg), and 150 mg (>40 kg) a CR of 91% and an ERR of 98% was produced.

3.2.9 Mebendazole

3.2.9.1 State of the Art

A drug taken up by *Ascaris*, active against a great number of nematodes and cestodes and known to be a highly efficient individual and industrial dewormer in pig farms, was of itself a candidate for use in humans (BRUGMANS et al. 1971). It was the more so that this drug, poorly absorbed from the intestinal tract, was almost pharmacologically inert. After the administration of 200 mg for 3 days the plasma levels never exceeded 30 ng/ml (DEMOEN et al. 1973).

From 1971, the value of mebendazole in ascariasis has been confirmed by CHAIA and DA CUNHA (1971 a, b), BANNERJEE et al. (1972a), GATTI et al. (1972b), CHAIA et al. (1972), and VAN DE PITTE et al. (1973). These studies also showed that a micronized formulation improved the CR.

3.2.9.2 Assessment

The first interesting results were confirmed by an impressive series of different dose regimens, summarized in Table 36.

Table 36. Treatment of *Ascaris* infection

Efficacy	Dosage	Number treated	CR	ERR	References
100%	100 mg	4	100	–	BEKHTI (1974)
	200 mg	11	100	–	PEÑA-CHAVARRIA et al. (1973)
	200 mg	16	100	–	VAKIL et al. (1975)
	200 mg	52	100	–	MUTTALIB et al. (1981)
	200 mg	44	100	–	CABRERA (1980)
	400 mg	10	100	–	VAKIL et al. (1975)
	100 mg b.i.d./2 days	40	100	–	SHAFEI (1974)
	100 mg b.i.d./3 days	52	100	–	GATTI et al. (1972b)
	100 mg b.i.d./3 days	31	100	–	CHAIA et al. (1972)
	100 mg b.i.d./3 days	116	100	–	VAN DE PITTE et al. (1973)

Table 36 (continued)

Efficacy	Dosage	Number treated	CR	ERR	References
	100 mg b.i.d./3 days	48	100	–	DE SOUZA et al. (1972)
	100 mg b.i.d./3 days	3	100	–	BRUMPT et al. (1973)
	100 mg b.i.d./3 days	35	100	–	GATTI and VAN DE PITTE (1973)
	100 mg b.i.d./3 days	10	100	–	GOLDSMID (1973)
	100 mg b.i.d./3 days	42	100	–	KRUBWA et al. (1974b)
	100 mg b.i.d./3 days	5	100	–	RUAS (1973)
	100 mg b.i.d./3 days	18	100	–	DE OLIVEIRA GOMES (1974)
	100 mg b.i.d./3 days	35	100	–	SHAFEI (1974)
	100 mg b.i.d./3 days	8	100	–	BIAGI et al. (1974)
	100 mg b.i.d./3 days	143	100	–	ABADI (1974)
	100 mg b.i.d./3 days	19	100	–	HUTCHINSON et al. (1975)
	100 mg b.i.d./3 days	50	100	–	FERNANDEZ (1974)
	100 mg b.i.d./3 days	40	100	–	NGOY and KALOMBO (1975)
	100 mg b.i.d./3 days	35	100	–	MONTERO and SANCHEZ (1975)
	100 mg b.i.d./3 days	74	100	–	CHONGSUPHAGAISIDDHI et al. (1978)
	100 mg b.i.d./3 days	3	100	–	BUNNAG (1976)
	100 mg b.i.d./3 days	41	100	–	JAROONVESAMA et al. (1978)
	100 mg b.i.d./3 days	11	100	–	DISSANAIKE (1978)
	100 mg b.i.d./3 days	25	100	–	MARTINS and GABURI (1974)
	100 mg b.i.d./3 days	18	100	–	DE OLIVEIRA GOMES (1974)
	100 mg b.i.d./3 days	13	100	–	PALACIOS Y SAUCEDO (1973a, b)
	100 mg b.i.d./3 days	84	100	–	CASTRO et al. (1973)
	100 mg b.i.d./3 days	20	100	–	LEE and LIM (1978)
	100 mg b.i.d./4 days	109	100	–	GATTI et al. (1972b)
	100 mg b.i.d./4 days	16	100	–	PEÑA-CHAVARRIA (1973)
	100 mg b.i.d./4 days	109	100	–	VAN DE PITTE et al. (1973)
	100 mg b.i.d./4 days	8	100	–	BRUMPT (1973)
	100 mg b.i.d./4 days	87	100	–	LORIA-CORTES et al. (1974)
	100 mg b.i.d./4 days	30	100	–	KUZMICKI et al. (1979)
	100 mg t.i.d./2 days	6	100	–	BRUMPT (1973)
	200 mg/2 days	25	100	–	SEO et al. (1978)
	200 mg/3 days	128	100	–	KOSIN (1973)
	200 mg/3 days	30	100	–	SEO et al. (1978)
	200 mg b.i.d./2 days	2	100	–	GENTILINI (1974)
	200 mg b.i.d./2 days	40	100	–	SHAFEI (1974)
	200 mg b.i.d./2 days	51	100	–	CHAIA and DA CUNHA (1971a, b)
	200 mg b.i.d./3 days	9	100	–	BRUMPT (1973)
	200 mg b.i.d./3 days	22	100	–	CHAIA and DA CUNHA (1971a, b)
	200 mg b.i.d./4 days	18	100	–	CHAIA and DA CUNHA (1971a, b)
	200 mg b.i.d./4 days	9	100	–	VAKIL et al. (1975)
	400 mg/3 days	1	100	–	GENTILINI (1974)
	600 mg	45	100	–	GUGGENMOOS et al. (1978)
≧90%	100 mg	18	94	–	CHAIA and DA CUNHA (1972)
	100 mg	43	93	93	JUWONO and TANTULAR (1973)
	100 mg	28	97	–	VAKIL et al. (1975)
	100 mg	70	94	98	PARTONO et al. (1974)
	100 mg	18	94	–	CHAIA and DA CUNHA (1971a, b)
	100 mg	39	90	–	SEO et al. (1978)
	200 mg	32	94	–	SEO et al. (1978)
	300 mg	15	99	–	PEÑA-CHAVARRIA et al. (1973)
	300 mg	30	97	–	SEO et al. (1978)

Table 36 (continued)

Efficacy	Dosage	Number treated	CR	ERR	References
	400 mg	17	94	–	CABRERA et al. (1980)
	600 mg	24	92	–	CABRERA et al. (1980)
	600 mg	51	94	–	CABRERA et al. (1980)
	75 mg/2 days	32	91	99	GATTI and VAN DE PITTE (1973)
	100 mg/×2 (48 h)	82	99	–	CHAIA and DA CUNHA (1971 a, b)
	100 mg/×2 (week)	26	96	–	CHAIA and DA CUNHA (1971 a, b)
	100 mg/×3	50	98	–	KUZMICKI et al. (1979)
	100 mg b.i.d./2 days	10	99	–	PEÑA-CHAVARRIA et al. (1973)
	100 mg b.i.d./3 days	22	99	–	PEÑA-CHAVARRIA et al. (1973)
	100 mg b.i.d./3 days	91	91	98	LOUZADA et al. (1973)
	100 mg b.i.d./3 days	40	97	–	LATONIO (1973)
	100 mg b.i.d./3 days	89	97	99	PARTONO et al. (1974)
	100 mg b.i.d./3 days	100	98	–	DE SOUZA et al. (1973 a, b)
	100 mg b.i.d./3 days	62	95	98	LIONEL et al. (1975)
	100 mg b.i.d./3 days	284	94	99	SOH et al. (1975)
	100 mg b.i.d./3 days	74	91	99	BOTERO-PEREZ (1976)
	100 mg b.i.d./3 days	42	95	–	DEGRÉMONT and BAUMGARTNER (1975)
	100 mg b.i.d./3 days	208	99	–	CARRIÉ (1978)
	100 mg b.i.d./3 days	77	94	–	FOBA-PAGOU et al. (1978)
	100 mg b.i.d./3 days	34	99	–	BINA et al. (1977)
	100 mg b.i.d./3 days	60	99	–	STÜRCHLER et al. (1980)
	100 mg b.i.d./3 days	34	94	99	CIMERMAN et al. (1980)
	100 mg b.i.d./3 days	121	90	–	RICHARD-LENOBLE and GENTILINI (1980)
	100 mg b.i.d./3 days	21	95	–	ASPÖCK et al. (1977)
	100 mg b.i.d./3 days	54	94	91	FAHRAMANDIAN et al. (1977)
	100 mg b.i.d./4 days	85	98	99	GATTI and VAN DE PITTE (1973)
	200 mg b.i.d.	46	97	–	CHAIA and DE CUNHA (1971 a, b)
	200 b.i.d./2 days	28	97	–	VAKIL et al. (1975)
	200 mg/4 days	93	97	–	PAVLOVSKI and CHODERA (1975)
	200 mg b.i.d./4 days	53	94	–	BANNERJEE et al. (1972 a)
≧80%	100 mg/3 days	53	87	98	GATTI and VAN DE PITTE (1973)
	100 mg/3 days	22	86	94	GATTI and VAN DE PITTE (1973)
	100 mg b.i.d./3 days	42	83	–	AMATO-NETO et al. (1973)
	100 mg b.i.d./3 days	86	87	–	SINGHAL et al. (1975)
	100 mg b.i.d./3 days	68	87	99	SEAH (1976)
	100 mg b.i.d./3 days	22	86	–	SCHENONE et al. (1974)
	100 mg b.i.d./3 days	31	87	–	WERSHING et al. (1975)
	100 mg b.i.d./4 days	580	82	–	BANZON et al. (1976)
	100 mg b.i.d./4 days	27	85	99	CIMERMAN et al. (1980)
	200 mg/4 days	5	80	–	GENTILINI (1974)
<80%	100 mg	20	45	80	GATTI and VAN DE PITTE (1973)
	200 mg/2 days	34	59	89	GATTI and VAN DE PITTE (1973)
	100 mg b.i.d.	66	72	–	CHAIA and DA CUNHA (1971)
	100 mg b.i.d./2 days	22	76	67	WERSHING et al. (1975)
	100 mg b.i.d./3 days	100	78	–	HUGGINS (1976)
	100 mg b.i.d./3 days	13	69	99	AGUILAR et al. (1973)
	100 mg b.i.d./3 days	44	41	–	KABA et al. (1978)
	100 mg	21	48	97	WERSHING et al. (1973)
	300 mg	24	58	99	WERSHING et al. (1973)

3.2.9.3 Dosage, Mode of Administration

The optimal and most-used regimen is the oral administration of 100 mg b.i.d. for 3 days. It should be noted, however, that this dosage is selected because it is equally efficient against hookworm and whipworm. But lower dosages and even single doses of 100 mg or 200 mg gives CRs of between 94% and 100% for ascariasis.

A single dose of 600 mg is convenient, acceptable, efficient, and not too costly for mass treatment aiming at multiple infections (Cabrera et al. 1980).

3.2.9.4 Side Effects

See Sect. B.II.3.2.10.4.

3.2.9.5 Contraindications, Precautions

See Sect. B.II.3.2.10.5.

3.2.9.6 Conclusions

3.2.9.6.1 Clinical Treatment

Mebendazole is as efficient as levamisole in the treatment of ascariasis, but does possess a wider spectrum of activity and is consequently more suitable for multiple infections.

3.2.9.6.2 Mass Treatment

The undoubted value of a single dose against other, especially the main soil-transmitted, nematodes (ancylostomiasis and trichiuriasis), and the absence of adverse reactions, makes mebendazole, a first-choice drug for mass treatment.

3.2.10 Pyrantel Pamoate

This cyclic amidine with broad-spectrum activity in animals, both on mature and immature nematodes, has justified its use in veterinary practice. Its pamoic salt was tried out by Bumbalo et al. (1969) against *Enterobius vermicularis* in mentally retarded children and produced a CR of 96%. This success was an incentive to investigate its activity against *A. lumbricoides*.

Desowitz et al. (1970) administered 5 mg/lb (11 mg/kg) of an oral suspension (5 mg/ml) to schoolchildren in the Cook Islands. After a single dose the CR was 86% after 1 week and 92% after 6 weeks. On a 2-day regimen the CR was 97% after 1 week. Hsieh and Chen (1970) treated 55 persons with ascariasis, living in a village in south Taiwan, with a single dose of 10 mg/kg, given as tablets, and achieved a CR of 98% at a follow-up 4 weeks later.

Villarejos et al. (1971) tried pyrantel pamoate in Costa Rica. With a single dose of 5 mg/lb in oral suspension, the CR was 99% after 30 days and with doses of 10 mg/lb and 20 mg/lb it was 100%. Similar doses repeated on three consecutive days uniformly guaranteed a CR of 100%.

3.2.10.1 Assessment

The demonstration of the efficacy of pyrantel pamoate against *A. lumbricoides* has been confirmed by several authors throughout the world. Some of the studies are summarized in Table 37.

Table 37. Treatment of *Ascaris* infections by pyrantel pamoate

Efficacy	Dosage	Number treated	CR	ERR	References
100%	10 mg/kg	30	100	–	DE SOUZA et al. (1972)
	10 mg/kg	62	100	–	AL-ISSA and WAHAT (1971)
	10 mg/kg (suspension)	47	100	–	PITTS and MIGLIARDI (1974)
	10 mg/kg (tablets)	21	100	–	PITTS and MIGLIARDI (1974)
	10 mg/kg (tablets)	154	100	–	PITTS and MIGLIARDI (1974)
	10 mg/kg	39	100	–	BELL and NASSIF (1971)
	8.5–10 mg/kg	79	100	–	RIM and LIM (1972)
	10 mg/kg	205	100	–	GHADIRIAN et al. (1972)
	10–15 mg/kg	7	100	–	GENTILINI et al. (1976)
≧90%	2.5 mg/kg	40	90	88	BELL and NASSIF (1971)
	5 mg/kg	40	90	98	BELL and NASSIF (1971)
	5 mg/kg	85	97	–	KOBAYASHI (1970)
	10 mg/kg	48	98	90	FARAHMANDIAN et al. (1971)
	10 mg/kg	291	94	–	PITTS and MIGLIARDI (1974)
	10 mg/kg	72	90	78	FARAHMANDIAN et al. (1972)
	11 mg/kg	42	93	98	CERVONI and OLIVER-GONZALES (1971)
	11 mg/kg	47	95	99	PEÑA-CHAVARRIA and VILLAREJOS (1975)
	11 mg/kg	34	97	99	SARGENT and CHAMBERS (1976)
	11 mg/kg	17	94	–	MILLER et al. (1978)
	10 mg/kg/2 days	38	97	–	DESOWITZ et al. (1970)
	10 mg/kg	55	98	99	HSIEH and CHEN (1970)
	10 mg/kg	1,324	91	–	ARFAA and GHADIRIAN (1977)
	10 mg/kg	34	95	99	STÜRCHLER et al. (1980)
≧80%	10 mg/kg	103	80	–	LEVI et al. (1972)
	10 mg/kg	63	89	–	KOBAYASHI (1970)
	11 mg/kg	11	87	91	Miller et al. (1976)
	11 mg/kg	42	81	96	CERVONI and OLIVER-GONZALEZ (1975)
≧60%	11 mg/kg	23	65	88	WERSHING et al. (1975)

3.2.10.2 Dosage, Mode of Action

A single dose of 10 mg/kg is standard against *A. lumbricoides*. Pyrantel pamoate is available in an oral suspension of 250 mg base/5 ml or as chewable tablets of 250 mg. Efficacy remains undiminished within the given time limit.

3.2.10.3 Side Effects

See Sect. B.II.3.2.11.4.

3.2.10.4 Contraindications, Precautions

See Sect. B.II.3.2.11.5.

3.2.10.5 Conclusions

3.2.10.5.1 Individual Therapy

At the recommended single dose efficacy is extremely good and its use is fully justified.

3.2.10.5.2 Mass Treatment

BOTERO RAMOS (1974) tried pyrantel pamoate in the suburban and rural population of the Heliconia township (Colombia), among which 76% were bearers of *A. lumbricoides*, 56% with an EPG >20,000 and 98% with more than one intestinal worm species. Ten milligrams per kilogram were administered for 3 days to 2,745 individuals, over 1 year of age, belonging to 420 families. This treatment was followed by the expulsion of a huge number of *Ascaris* worms. After 1 month the prevalence was down from 76% to 14%. The follow-up of 416 persons 5 months later showed a rise to 62%, indicating a very important reinfection.

The reinfection risk has also been underlined by CERVONI and OLIVER-GONZALEZ (1975). Reexamination of 31 cured individuals on day 20, day 175, and day 210 gave a reinfection rate of 10%, 50%, and 77%, respectively.

In addition to the risk of rapid reinfection, pyrantel pamoate, being inactive against trichiuriasis, is not a good choice for mass treatment. This deficiency has been made up by combination with oxantel (see below).

3.2.10.6 Comments

Pyrantel is a reliable choice for individual deworming of ascariasis, but not for mass treatment.

3.2.11 Pyrantel and Oxantel

3.2.11.1 State of the Art

The major shortcoming of pyrantel as a broad-spectrum anthelmintic is its lack of activity against *Trichuris trichiura*. Oxantel, closely related to pyrantel, is active against *T. trichiura* (LIM 1974; GARCIA 1978; RIM et al. 1976; LEE et al. 1976; PAUL and ZAMAN 1976; BERTI et al. 1976; CHO 1976; DISSANAIKE 1978), but without a significant effect on hookworm and threadworm. Oxantel as such produces a CR of 97% at a 10 mg/kg dosage in ascariasis (LIM 1978b). In order to broaden the activity spectrum the manufacturers have sought a solution in a combination of oxantel pamoate and pyrantel pamoate.

3.2.11.2 Assessment

The value of this combination has been tested in multiple nematode infections, in several areas with a high prevalence of trichiuriasis and with the roundworm as the most common fellow worm. The specific activity of pyrantel and oxantel on *A. lumbricoides* is summarized in Table 38.

Table 38. Treatment of *Ascaris* infection by pyrantel and oxantel

Efficacy	Dosage	Number treated	CR	ERR	References
100%	15 mg/kg	10	100	–	Lee and Lim (1978)
	15 mg/kg/b.i.d.	12	100	–	Cabrera and Sy (1978)
	15 mg/kg/2 days	10	100	–	Lee and Lim (1978)
	15–20 mg/kg	67	100	–	Lim (1978a, b)
	15–20 mg/kg/3 days	21	100	–	Dissanaike (1978)
	20 mg/kg	10	100	–	Lee and Lim (1978)
	20 mg/kg/2 days	10	100	–	Lee and Lim (1978)
	20 mg/kg/2 days	15	100	–	Cabrera and Sy (1978)
≧90%	10 mg/kg	43	97	–	Lim (1978a, b)
	10 mg/kg	75	97	99	Lim (1978a, b)
	10 mg/kg	60	95	73	Cabrera et al. (1980)
	10 mg/kg	30	97	–	Rim et al. (1981)
	15 mg/kg	150 (rural)	97	–	Cabrera and Sy (1978)
	15–20 mg/kg	31	97	–	Chanco and Vidad (1981)
	15–20 mg/kg/3 days	31	97	–	Garcia (1978)
	20 mg/kg/2 days	55	91	95	Kale (1977)
	30 mg/kg	50	96	99	Zahedi (1980)
≧80%	50 mg of each	47	89	–	Canzonieri et al. (1977)

3.2.11.3 Dosage, Mode of Administration

The combination of pyrantel and oxantel is available in an oral suspension, containing 50 mg base of each compound per milliliter.

The recommended single dosage of 15 mg/kg of each will suffice for ascariasis. In children of less than 6 kg a dose of 20 mg of each substance will not be exceeded. For heavy infestations and especially in the presence of *N. americanus* it is advisable to repeat the administration on two or three consecutive days.

3.2.11.4 Side Effects

See Sect. B.II.3.2.12.4.

3.2.11.5 Contraindications, Precautions

See Sect. B.II.3.2.12.5.

3.2.11.6 Conclusion

Pyrantel and oxantel is efficient against *A. lumbricoides*, but its use should be reserved for mass campaigns.

3.2.12 Tiabendazole

3.2.12.1 State of the Art

The broad-spectrum anthelmintic activity of this benzimidazole derivative includes *A. lumbricoides*. However, its application is of a much greater interest against *Strongyloides stercoralis*, larva migrans, trichostrongylosis, and trichinosis. Its ovicidal and larvicidal properties, including activity against immature worms, should be kept in mind whenever one is faced with problems related to migration in unusual organs.

3.2.12.2 Assessment

The results of the many trials are uncommonly variable and difficult to interpret due to the differences in their setup. Since the index experiments carried out by BUI-QUOC-HUONG et al. (1962), using daily dosages of 25 or 50 mg/kg, the efficacy of tiabendazole on ascariasis has been demonstrated.

In the Table 39 some usuable results are summarized.

Table 39. Treatment of *Ascaris* infections by tiabendazole

Efficacy	Dosage	Number treated	CR	ERR	References
100%	120–150 mg/kg	11	100	–	CHANCO and PAGUIO (1964)
	50 mg/kg	7	100	–	PAPASARATHORN et al. (1964)
	1 g/3 days	10	100	–	ISHIZAKI et al. (1963)
	50 mg/kg/t.i.d.	6	100	–	CHOWDURY et al. (1964)
≧90%	25 mg/kg	30	97	–	CHANCO and PAGUIO (1964)
	25 mg/kg/b.i.d.	22	95	–	CHANCO and PAGUIO (1964)
	50 mg/kg/2 days	14	99	99	BOTERO (1964)
	25–50 mg/kg/3–5 days	42	98	–	FRANZ (1965)
	25 mg/kg/5 days	32	94	99	ESCOBAR (1964)
≧80%	25–30 mg/kg/b.i.d./ 3 days	24	86	–	FRANZ (1965)
	25 mg/kg	145	80	91	ESCOBAR (1964)
≧70%	25 mg/kg/b.i.d.	7	71	–	SALEM et al. (1968)
	25 mg/kg/b.i.d./ 3 days	14	78	99	BOTERO (1964)
	50 mg/kg/3 days	12	75	–	CHOWDURY et al. (1964)
	50 mg/kg	9	77	–	CHANCO and PAGUIO (1964)

Table 39 (continued)

Efficacy	Dosage	Number treated	CR	ERR	References
	50 mg/kg	47	79	13	FARAHMANDIAN et al. (1977)
	50 mg/kg	199	72	94	ESCOBAR (1964)
≧60%	50 mg/kg	6	69	69	BOTERO (1964)
	25 mg/kg/2 days	77	68	88	ESCOBAR (1964)
	1 g 250 mg	14	64	–	SALUNKHE et al. (1964)
	1 g 250 mg	14	64	–	VAKIL et al. (1965)
	1 g 250 mg b.i.d.	28	67	–	SALEM et al. (1968)
	1 g 500 mg	8	62	–	IWATA et al. (1963b)
	2 g	24	66	–	SALEM et al. (1966)
≧50%	50 mg/kg (chewable tablets)	14	50	95	BOTERO (1964)
	50 mg/kg (chewable tablets)	10	50	–	CHOWDURY et al. (1964)
	1 g	9	55	–	IWATA et al. (1963b)
	2 g	6	50	–	ISHIZAKI et al. (1963)
	1 g 250 b.i.d./2 days	22	59	99	VAKIL and DALAH (1975)
	2 g 500 mg	20	55	–	SALUNKE et al. (1964)
	2 g 500 mg	24	54	–	VAKIL et al. (1965)
<50%	25 mg/kg/2 days	20	35	76	HUANG and BROWN (1963)
	25 mg/kg/2 days	4	25	–	CHOWDURY et al. (1964)
	25 mg/kg/b.i.d./2 days	21	33	85	WERSHING et al. (1975)
	25 mg/kg	8	25	–	CHOWDURY et al. (1964)
	750 mg	9	44	–	IWATA et al. (1963b)
	1 g	3	–	–	ISHIZAKI et al. (1963)
	1 g 250 mg/b.i.d.	22	36	–	VAKIL et al. (1965)

3.2.12.3 Dosage, Mode of Administration

The recommended dosage is 25 mg/kg b. i. d. for one or on two consecutive days, with a maximal daily dose of 3 g. The 2-day treatment guarantees slightly better results. Tiabendazol is presented as tablets or a suspension containing 100 mg/ml. Neither dietary precautions nor laxatives are needed.

3.2.12.4 Side Effects

See Sect. B.II.3.2.13.4.

3.2.12.5 Contraindications, Precautions

See Sect. B.II.3.2.13.5.

3.2.12.6 Conclusions

3.2.12.6.1 Clinical

CRs of between 33% and 95% point to an inconstancy, which rules out tiabendazole for the individual therapy of ascariasis.

3.2.12.6.2 Mass Treatment

Whenever the multiple infections include a substantial percentage of *Strongyloides stercoralis*, tiabendazole will also be able to reduce significantly the roundworm load.

3.2.12.7 Comments

Tiabendazole is not to be used in ascariasis as such.

III. Drug Combinations

Although ascariasis does not actually pose a therapeutic problem, several authors with various intentions have tested different combinations of drugs. For the sake of completeness a few are mentioned here.

1. Flubendazole and Tinidazole

The dose ratio is: flubendazole 100 mg, tinidazole 175 mg. HUGGINS (1979) obtained a CR of 90% (36:40).

2. Flubendazole and Levamisole

The makeup is: flubendazole, 500 mg; levamisole, 50 mg. ISMAIL and LIONEL (1981) achieved a CR of 93% in a rural area (number treated, 75) and of 92% in urban surroundings (number treated: 60) and in both an EER of 99%.

3. Levamisole and Mebendazole

A combination of levamisole, 50 mg, and mebendazole, 100 mg, administered on three consecutive days gave ISEBAERT (1970) a CR of 95% and an ERR of 99%.

4. Mebendazole and Pyrantel

The association of mebendazole, 200 mg, and pyrantel, 60 mg, on three consecutive days brings about a CR of 100% (PURNOMO et al. 1980).

In both mebendazole associations the purpose is to guard against erratic wandering about of *Ascaris* worms.

5. Piperazine and Pyrvinium

The combination of 75 mg/kg piperazine hydrate and 2.5 mg/kg pyrvinium pamoate 2.5 mg/kg (as a suspension of 750 mg and 25 mg/5 ml respectively or tablets containing 750 mg and 25 mg) provided interesting results: CR of 86% (BECK 1966). A suspension of 750 mg piperazine and 25 mg pyrvinium/5 ml, at a dose of 0.5 ml/kg for 2 days, ended the *Ascaris* infection in 15 out of 30 persons: CR 50% and ERR 85% (BOTERO et al. 1966). There are obviously by now more powerful anthelmintics available.

6. Piperazine and Tiabendazole

The administration of a combination of 750 mg piperazine hydrate and 375 mg tiabendazole per 10 ml, pro rata 5 ml b. i. d. on a 3-day schedule, produced a CR of 92% (number treated, 242) in *Ascaris* infections (FERNANDEZ and GARCIA 1976). The total dose amounted to 3,750 g piperazine hydrate and 1,875 g tiabendazole. On a schedule of 5 ml b. i. d. on three consecutive days the CR was 90% (FILHO et al. 1971) for a total dose of 2.25 g piperazine hydrate and 1.125 g tiabendazole.

E. Enterobiasis

(Synonyms: oxyuriasis, pinworm disease, seatworm infection).

I. Introduction

Enterobius vermicularis (LINNAEUS 1758; LEACK 1853[10]) is most probably the most common nematode of man which only infects man.[11] It has been a human parasite for the major part of human history and its ova have been identified in coprolites, about 10,000 years old, discovered in the Danger Caves, Utah. HOEPPLI (1959) traced it back to the beginnings of recorded history in writings from Indian, Graeco-Roman, and Arabic origin. He found highly descriptive names for it in the Far-Eastern cultures, next to bizarre accounts of its presumed life cycle and transmogrification. In the majority of countries the popular names for this worm are plentiful.

Enterobiasis is more common in the affluent and centrally planned than in the developing countries. The worm lives better in temperate than in tropical zones. Underwear, bedclothes, and bedding play a role in the maintenance of the infection.

Although commonplace, *E. vermicularis* is not unimportant. It causes discomfort, infection, and mental stress in millions of persons anxious to obtain treatment.

1. Parasite

Enterobius vermicularis worms are small whitish cylindrical worms, pointed at both ends, and with a smooth cuticle. The mouth is bordered by three lips without a buccal capsule. The esophagus contains a conspicuous muscular bulb at its posterior end. The cephalic cuticular inflations continue as lateral projecting alae, which are useful landmarks for the recognition of the threadworm in tissue sections.

The adult male measures 2–5 mm in length and 0.1–0.2 mm in diameter. Its posterior end is strongly curved ventrally. Its appearance is completed by a single

10 *Oxyurus vermicularis* L. 1758

11 The *Guinness Book of Records* puts the threadworm as the second most common affection for man, following the common cold (GUINNESS SUPERLATIVES LTD. 1977)

spicule of about 70 μm without a gubernaculum, and by conspicuous caudal alae supported by papillae.

The female measures 8–13 mm in length and 0.3–0.5 mm in diameter. The vulva opens midventrally at one-third to two-thirds of the body length. The posterior end has paired lateral alae almost to the anus, but its long slender sharply pointed tail extends to one-third of the total length. This typical feature gave rise to the profusion of vernacular names. A gravid uterus contains thousands of eggs.

The eggs measure 50–60 × 20–32 μm, are ovoid and flattened on one side and have a smooth semitransparent thin shell, composed of an outer very sticky albuminous layer, two chitinous layers, and an inner lipoidal membrane. It contains a late-stage morula or L1 larva.

Life Cycle

The eggs, containing the L1 rhabditiform larvae (145 × 10 μm) are swallowed by the host, pass through the stomach, and hatch in the duodenum. These larvae lodge in the crypts of the ileum, molt two to three times, and the immature young worms migrate towards the cecum, where they feed on epithelial cells, bacteria, and other intestinal contents, reach sexual maturity, and copulate. The male dies after copulation, disintegrates, and passes out with the feces. The fertilized female attaches itself loosely to the mucosa of the cecum and appendix and remains there until gravidity is reached. The gravid female migrates within the colon and rectum, especially when the host is at rest in a comfortably warm environment, during the evening and night, for instance, in bed. It can then emerge on the perianal and perineal skin. While crawling around, the worm contracts violently in the cooler surroundings and leaves behind a trail of numerous sticky eggs. The number of deposited eggs is estimated to be from 4,600 to 16,000, with an average of 11,000 per female. She can burst and release all the eggs at once. After oviposition the female dies. The interval between ingestion and sexual maturity is 15–49 days. The life span of the female does not exceed 8 weeks (35–53 days). CRAM (1943) stated that after ingestion of pinworm eggs, female worms migrate out of the anus 15–28 days later. But AKAGI (1973) observed, after autoinfection, their appearance after 45–45 days. A follow-up limited to 21 days is therefore insufficient for assessment. Eggs are killed within a few days in a dry environment, but remain viable up to 2 months under suitable moisture and temperature (not lower than 23 °C) conditions. The life cycle is essentially an indoor occurrence.

2. Host

2.1 Epidemiology

Contamination takes place by ingestion of eggs. These may be carried under the fingernails as a result of perianal scratching and transmitted with the soiled fingers into the mouth. This direct ano-oral autoinfection is common. Indirect infection may result from oral contact with soiled food, eating utensils, glasses, cigarettes, towels, beddings, nightclothes, underwear, carpets, toys, bedpans, lavatory seats, etc.

Up to 50,000 eggs/m^2 have been counted on household surfaces (especially lavatories and dormitories). They arise from dust-borne infections through the mouth or nose (occasionally a pinworm may be present in the nose). This transmission mode has been often been underestimated.

Reinfection is not only a common occurrence, but "retroinfection" by larvae hatching on the perianal skin and migrating directly back into the anus has been assumed. This premises that the perianal folds remain unclean for periods to allow the hatching, which is most unlikely. If it did really occur, infection would be more common in adults. In any case when autoinfection is brought to an end the infection dies out.

It will be remembered that *E. vermicularis* is an almost exclusively human worm. Dogs and cats are free from pinworms.

As a result of domestic contamination enterobiasis is a major problem in orphanages, kindergartens, boarding schools, mental hospitals, asylums, and similar overcrowded closed communities. It is also a family infection, both in the lower and higher socioeconomic groups. The latter are more prone to "pinworm neurosis." Group infections also occur among homosexuals and such-like inconstant free communities.

2.2 Pathology

The adult worms congregate mainly in the ileocecal and appendicular lumen, although they may be present from the stomach to anus in very heavy infections. The damage resulting from the loose attachment of the adults to the mucosa does not exceed mild inflammation or minute ulceration, which may become secondarily infected. The majority of the claims about an enterobiasis etiology of appendicular disturbances disregard the fact that the lumen of the appendix is a usual localization for *E. vermicularis*.

As a matter of fact one-third of the threadworm bearers remain completely symptomless. In the remaining two-thirds the symptoms are as a rule negligible.

The inconveniences result from the movement of the wandering females, the very irritant nature of their secretions, and the desposition of the sticky eggs on the perianal skin or on neighbouring organs, such as the vulva.

The discomfort in the perianal region is the most common and major symptom. The pruritus ani may lead to secondary pyogenic infection and often to disturbed sleep. In turn this will be followed by general irritability, loss of appetite, and tiredness. In the majority of cases, even in infected children, not more than 5% will show symptoms attributable to the pinworm.

About 20% of infected girls and women will develop pruritus vulvae, vulvovaginits, but rarely endometritis, and will complain about discharge. The female worm can indeed wander into the vulva, provoke a mild irritation there, or exceptionally penetrate into the vagina, uterus, oviduct, and even the peritoneal cavity. In these localizations the worm encysts and ends up in a granuloma.

2.3 Clinical Profile

Symptoms can be absent or negligible. In 10%–20% of cases they are mild and indefinite: perineal discomfort, pruritus ani or vulvae, and mild catarrhal colitis are the cardinal features. Other symptoms are enuresis, tenesmus, disturbed sleep, irritability, poor appetite, and other added complaints. It should, however, be remembered that in a given closed community 64% of infected, but also 52% of noninfected control persons complain about anal pruritus. The wide variety of secondary symptoms ascribed to enterobiasis: (enuresis, tooth-grinding, nose-picking, poor appetite, etc.) underlines the risk of a faulty diagnosis. *E. vermicularis* is, however, so widespread that to relate anything unusual with the presence of the pinworm is unwarranted.

In heavy infections mild catarrhal inflammation of the bowel may indeed appear and become accompanied by nausea and diarrhea. Many publications mention the presence of *E. vermicularis* in mesenteric abscesses, in liver and other ectopic granulomata, and in urinary tract disturbances, but disregard the fact that, with the exception of transit via the female genital tract, they can be explained by merely coincidental occurrences. Lastly the symptoms are not dependent on the number of worms but rather on the personality of the subject. Nervous children and neurotic adults are more prone to develop symptoms than quiet ones.

2.4 Immunology

Not much is known about the defense mechanisms of the host except that some individuals become tolerant, while others become sensitized to the secretions of the worm and to the sticky eggs. It should be remembered that gravid females dying after oviposition can burst and liberate all their eggs and their milieu interieur at once. The host may develop some response to threadworm infestation. Heavy infections are accompanied by slight eosinophilia. A local reaction follows the intradermal administration of *Enterobius* antigen in infected individuals. The prevalence of infection decreases in older children and adults, which suggests some sort of acquired resistance.

3. Diagnosis

The presence of *E. vermicularis* can be suspected whenever small threads are seen in the stools. Detection of eggs and threadworm is best carried out by the Scotch adhesive tape method (GRAHAM 1941). The sampling of the anal and perianal area should be carried out on at least two occasions. The swabbing should be done in the morning before defecation and bathing. Eggs can also be found under fingernails. The tapes are placed adhesive face down on a slide and examined Stool examination as such detects only 2% of the infections. *Eosinophilia* is at most moderate and worthless for diagnosis.

4. Geographical Distribution

Enterobius vermicularis is a cosmopolitan nematode, which may infect up to 100% of the individuals in some foci. STOLL (1947) estimated the number of threadworm infections roughly at 209 millions or some 7% of the world population. If this level of infection has remained constant their number in 1983 cannot be less than 309 million and more probably over 500 million. The ratio of infected persons in western Europe has been estimated at 16% or 60 millions. On the basis of the prescriptions for threadworm and over-the-counter sales the percentages for the United Kingdom have been assessed at 30%–40% (in 1973, 370,000, and in 1975, 354,000 prescriptions).

5. Prevalence

It is impossible to produce an accountable overview of the prevalence of enterobiasis. It has been observed that this infection is more prevalent in some regions than in others, e.g., in Germany the prevalence was higher in Hamburg and Rostock than in Leipzig, Nürnberg, and St. Gallen. In the United States it is more common in Caucasians than in darker-skinned persons (CRAM 1943).

It is common knowledge that enterobiasis is a group infestation, very common in children, especially schoolchildren, but minimal under 2 years of age. Its prevalence is high under crowded conditions such as closed communities, orphanages, asylums, hospitals, boarding schools, and family circles. Statistics are often only backed up by such groups and communities. Institutions for children are preferential study groups, but yield abnormally high figures: Italy, 80%; Iran, 95%; Netherlands, 100%; New York, 56%–78%; and United States, 88% (MATHIES 1961). The same remark also applies for confined adults: Belgium, 64%; Brazil, 45%; Sao Paulo, 77%.

The following figures underline the importance of reliable information about the sample selection: Belgium 31%–97% (boarding school children, 75%–97%; long-term hospital patients, 78%; army recruits, 31%); Brazil (Minas Gerais) children, 24%; adults, 7%; rural, 16%; urban, 29%; Chile, 88% (boarding school children and personnel, 44%); Ecuador, Guayaquil in pediatric hospital, 9.5%; Italy (Abruzzo rural) children, 80%; Korea (Kwangwha island), 65%; Labrador, 24%; Mexico, 9%–12%; Papua New Guinea, 5%–17%; Philippines 80% (rural, 10%; urban, 62%–75%); Singapore, 21% (children); Taiwan, Taipei City, orphans, 42%; preschool children, 44.5%; schoolchildren, 53.4%; Zambia, 0.9%; Zimbambwe, Burma Valley, 0.6%; Gabon, 10.6%; Harare, 0.14%; Inyanga, 1.1%. These data confirm the point at issue: figures relative to prevalence are at their best a rough estimate.

As a rule, under identical conditions of exposure, enterobiasis is more frequent in rural areas and in temperate climates. Tropical and more specifically arid climates are less suitable surroundings.

II. Drugs

1. Drugs of Natural Origin

Such an ancient widespread, often disturbing, and easily identifiable worm infection could not remain without attempts at treatment. The majority of the folkore modes of treatment may be relegated, along with the introduction of salted pork fat into the rectum, to the pages of history.

Oil of chenopodium, or rather its active principle ascaridol, is weakly active against *E. vermicularis*. However, combination with tetrachloroethylene (1:6) enhances their mutual vermicidal properties and provides the possibility of relief in the absence of better drugs.

Digenea simplex, a popular vermifuge in Japan, with kainic acid as an active principle, is not as such very effective. In association with santonin and piperazine hydrate its efficacy is enhanced. Under the name "TED3," a syrup containing 5 mg kainic acid, 50 mg santonin, and 2 g piperazine hydrate for every 15 ml has been produced. It was administered by IWATA et al. (1963 a) in a daily 10-ml dose for 3 days in 135 schoolchildren infected with *E. vermicularis*. The CR was 63%. This promising combination has been displaced from the market by the newer drugs.

2. Antibiotics

Oxytetracycline has been tried since 1951 against enterobiasis and rather successfully. Doses of 10 mg/kg or 1–2 g in children for 7 days provide a CR of 90%–96% (LOUGHLIN et al. 1951; LOUGHLIN and MULLIN 1955; GOETERS 1955 a; OWINGS 1955). This treatment is much too expensive and lengthy.

Other *tetracyclines* ensure similar results.

Macrolides: *erythromycine and carbomycin* (Magnamycin) are less efficient than oxytetracyline (MACCOWEN et al. 1953; BUMBALO und GUSTINIA 1955).

Paromomycin (YOUNG and FREED 1956) is active against *E. vermicularis*.

Spiramycin (Rovamycin), although inactive in enterobiasis, enhances the activity of diphetarsone (SCHNEIDER et al. 1960).

On the whole, whatever the CR achieved, the available antibiotics are too expensive and produce too many untoward effects to be of practical use.

3. Synthetic Organic Products

3.1 Old Timers

3.1.1 Benzoylmetacresol (Cresentyl)

At a daily dose of 3–5 g for adults and 2 g for children, administered on an empty stomach and for 4–5 days the outcome is in no way overwhelming.

3.1.2 Diphetarsone (Bemarsal)

SCHNEIDER et al. (1960) observed the disappearance of *E. vermicularis* in a women and a child who were treated for amoobiasis with the spiramycin-diphetarsone salt. After a systematic and successful trial in 32 persons (CR 94%), he investigated the role of both components. Only diphetarsone was active. A group of five children was administered 500 mg t. i. d. for 3 days, which was repeated after 1 week, and the results were excellent up to the 5th–6th week. A second group of 23 children received 1.5 g in one dose for 14 days with the same good result. It was extremely well tolerated.

As a conclusion the author proposed 1 g daily for 7 days, which has been tried out successfully.

3.1.3 Gentian Violet and Crystal Violet

These dyes derived from triphenylmethane are a mixture of derivatives of rosaniline. Since WRIGHT and BRADY (1940) and DESCHIENS (1943) demonstrated their anthelmintic potential in enterobiasis, they have been the current drug for many years. A daily dosage of 10 mg/year of age for five consecutive days provides a CR of 71% (BROCK et al. 1952). After a second course the CR can reach 94%.

3.1.4 Phenothiazine

This compound has been recommended in human enterobiasis by MANSON-BAHR (1940). The usual dosage is 8 g daily for 5 days in adults; 2 g/day for 7 days in children between 4 and 8 years of age; and 1 g/day for 1 week in children under 4 years of age. Side effects nearly always arise. Phenothiazine is toxic for the blood and liver. It has no place in modern chemotherapy.

3.1.5 Promethazine (Phenergan)

From 1956 onwards, several investigators, impressed by structural analogies between phenothiazine and some antihistaminic drugs, investigated the activity of promethazine against enterobiasis. The CR of 97% obtained by AVERY (1956) after 125 mg administered on going to bed was not confirmed by COUTELEN et al. (1956). SADUN et al. (1956) obtained a CR of 44%, BROWN et al. (1956a) 33%, MILLER et al. (1957) 20%, and BUMBALO et al. (1957) only 5%, although these authors were using similar doses. The overall results point toward poor and irregular activity.

3.1.6 Urethane Group

Miscellaneous compounds of a rather toxic group of weedkillers, insecticides, and nitrogen-mustard-like substances, have been tried against *E. vermicularis*, with limited success. Lubisan, Egressin, etc. belong to the past.

3.1.7 Organophosphorous Compounds

The successful use of organophosphorous compounds in veterinary medicine has led some investigators to extend their use to human parasitic infections. Metrifonate has been used by FERREIRA et al. (1960), BEHEYT et al. (1961), and CERF et al. (1962). TALAAT (1964) obtained a CR of 92% (22 out of 24) in enterobiasis. These compounds never came into use in enterobiasis. See also Sects. B.II.3.1.4.1.4 and B.II.3.1.4.1.5.

3.1.8 Stilbazium Iodide (Monopar)

This derivative of pyridine, a broad-spectrum anthelmintic with low toxicity, was found active in enterobiasis. JEFFERY et al. (1963) and SWARZWELDER et al. (1963), using a single dose of 10 mg/kg,obtained a CR of 100%. With doses of 5 or 3 mg/kg, the CRs are respectively 83% (SWARZWELDER et al. 1963) and 76% (BUMBALO and GEIST 1964). As better drugs have since been discovered, stilbazium iodide has only had a temporary and restricted circulation.

3.2 Newer Drugs

3.2.1 Albendazole

Albendazole has been tried out successfully by GARIN (1980). He obtained 100% CR with a single dose of 50 mg or 100 mg. This has been confirmed by ROSSIGNOL (1981) with a single dose of 200 mg (children) or 400 mg (adults); all of the 26 persons infected with whipworms were cured. The 400-mg dose produced a CR of 100% for BASTIDAS (1982).

3.2.1.1 Side Effects, Contraindications, Precautions

See Sects. B.II.3.2.1.4 and B.II.3.2.1.5.

3.2.1.2 Conclusion

Albendazole is an effective drug for enterobiasis. However, the dosage should be more explicit: 400 mg is obviously excessive.

3.2.2 Ciclobendazole

The efficacy of this benzimidazole in enterobiasis is very satisfactory at a dose of 100 mg, to be repeated after 1 week. BÄCHLIN and DEGRÉMONT (1979) obtained a cure rate of 100% in 50 children in a day nursery. Three out of the 50 toddlers were found reinfected 4–6 weeks later, which is a usual occurrence. No side effects were observed. See also Sects. B.II.3.2.6.4 and B.II.3.2.6.5.

3.2.3 Fenbendazole

Fenbendazole, which displays a high degree of safety in animals and of effectiveness against all developmental stages of nematodes, was used in man at a dosage of 100 mg b.i.d. after meals by BHANDARI and SINGHI (1980). Out of 25 patients, 22 showed negative results at a follow-up at day 11, a CR of 88%. Relief from pruritus ani was observed at the same percentage.

3.2.3.1 Side Effects

A burning sensation on micturition was recorded in 16% (4 out of 25).

3.2.3.2 Contraindications, Precautions

See Sects. B.II.3.2.7.4 and B.II.3.2.7.5.

3.2.3.3 Conclusion

Fenbendazole is a potentially useful drug, but not yet available for use in humans.

3.2.4 Flubendazole (Fluvermal)

3.2.4.1 State of the Art

Enterobiasis needs a safe, efficacious, cheap anthelmintic, and, if possible, combined with broad-spectrum activity. The potency and good tolerance of flubendazole led to its being tried out.

3.2.4.2 Assessment

Table 40. Treatment of *E. vermicularis* infections by flubendazole

Efficacy	Dosage	Number treated	CR	References
100%	100 mg	22	100	TORHOUDT (1974)
	100 mg	10	100	BRUMPT (1976)
	200 mg	74	100	SCHENONE et al. (1977)
	100 mg b.i.d./3 days	38	100	BECQUET (1976)
≧90%	100 mg	27	96	TORHOUDT (1974)
	100 mg	21	90	DE WULF (1975)
	200 mg	73	95	ROMBAUT et al. (1975)
	100 mg	25	92	ARADA et al. (1978)
≧80%	100 mg	62	87	ROMBAUT et al. (1975)
	100 mg	55	85	VANDERDONCKT et al. (1975)
	200 mg	16	87	GENTILINI (1976)

3.2.4.3 Dosage, Mode of Administration

A single dose of 100 mg provides excellent results. Bearing in mind that larvae lodge in the crypts of the ileum, it is logical to repeat the treatment after 7–10 days.

3.2.4.4 Side Effects

See Sect. B.II.3.2.8.4.

3.2.4.5 Contraindications, Precautions

See Sect. B.II.3.2.8.5.

3.2.4.6 Conclusions

Flubendazole is a reliable anthelmintic in enterobiasis.

3.2.5 Mebendazole

3.2.5.1 State of the Art

The fact that a single 100-mg dose of mebendazole is efficacious against *E. vermicularis* and can be administered as well to toddlers as to adults with very slight side effects has aroused the interest of the medical profession.

3.2.5.2 Assessment

An impressive number of clinical studies have been carried out. However, with the possibility in view of simultaneously attaining maximum benefit against the other intestinal helminths, a wider range of dosages has been investigated.

Table 41. Treatment of *E. vermicularis* infection by mebendazole

Efficacy	Dosage	Number treated	CR	References
100%	100 mg	100	100	FIERLAFIJN (1971)
	100 mg	13	100	GOLDSMID (1974)
	100 mg	3	100	DEGRÉMONT and BAUMGARTEN (1975)
	100 mg	94	100	LORMANS et al. (1975)
	100 mg	62	100	JAROONVESAMA et al. (1978)
	100 mg	24	100	KRASA and KAUPENY (1977)
	100 mg	21	100	CHO et al. (1977)
	100 mg	7	100	GORODNER et al. (1977)
	100 mg b.i.d./3 days	28	100	CHAIA et al. (1972)
	100 mg b.i.d./3 days	18	100	DE SOUZA et al. (1973a, b)
	100 mg b.i.d./3 days	38	100	AMATO-NETO et al. (1973)
	100 mg b.i.d./3 days	25	100	DE SOUZA et al. (1973)
	100 mg b.i.d./3 days	21	100	DE OLIVEIRA GOMEZ (1974)
	100 mg b.i.d./3 days	–	100	HUGGINS (1976)
	100 mg b.i.d./3 days	29	100	BIAGI et al. (1974)
	100 mg b.i.d./3 days	30	100	FERNANDES (1974)
	100 mg b.i.d./3 days	45	100	OTERO DOMINGUEZ et al. (1977)
	100 mg b.i.d./4 days	2	100	BRUMPT (1973)
	200 mg (C)[a]	56	100	BRUGMANS et al. (1971)
	200 mg b.i.d.	41	100	CHAIA and DA CUNHA (1971a, b)
	200 mg b.i.d./2 days	31	100	CHAIA and DA CUNHA (1971a, b)
	200 mg b.i.d./4 days	17	100	CHAIA and DA CUNHA (1971a, b)
≧90%	75 mg (C)	63	92	BRUGMANS et al. (1971)
	100 mg (C)	148	91	BRUGMANS et al. (1971)
	100 mg	20	95	BEKHTI (1974)
	100 mg	45	98	PARTONO et al. (1974)
	100 mg	50	92	LEPERCQ (1974)
	100 mg	74	96	MILLER et al. (1974)
	100 mg	25	96	YALCINKAYA (1977)
	100 mg	110	98	COSTANZO (1975)
	100 mg	151	98	LENGYEL et al. (1978)
	100 mg	73	98	SZORADY et al. (1976)
	100 mg	455	99	ALEKSEEVA and PUCENKO (1980)
	100 mg	43	96	MATHIES (1973)
	100 mg	111	97	LECOMTE-RAMIOUL (1975)
	100 mg	70	94	VAN OLPHEN and NABBEN (1974)
	100 mg	43	91	FIERLAFIJN and VAN PARIJS (1973)
	100 mg	750	98	BALAGOPAL (1974)
	100 mg/2 days (C)	27	93	BRUGMANS et al. (1971)
	100 mg b.i.d./3 days	12	92	LOUZADA et al. (1973)
	100 mg b.i.d./3 days	107	91	SOH (1975)
	5 mg/kg/3 days	122	93	LIAN and ZI (1972)
	5 mg/kg/3 days	20	90	LOPEZ MONTERO and CALZADA SANCHEZ (1975)
	5 mg/kg/3 days	53	96	CASTRO et al. (1973)
	5 mg/kg/3 days	144	93	SCHENONE et al. (1974)
	200 mg	36	92	RUAS (1973)

Table 41 (continued)

Efficacy	Dosage	Number treated	CR	References
≧80%	100 mg (A)[b]	51	88	Brugmans et al. (1971)
	100 mg (A)	25	84	Arada et al. (1978)
	100 mg/1–2 days	100	81	Narmada et al. (1974)
	100 mg/3 days (C)	24	88	Brugmans et al. (1971)
	200 mg (A)	45	89	Brugmans et al. (1971)
	100 mg b.i.d.	20	85	Bhandari and Singhi (1980)
≧70%	25 mg (C)	73	77	Brugmans et al. (1971)
≧60%	50 mg (C)	215	62	Brugmans et al. (1971)

[a] C, children
[b] A, adults

Some of these studies were open trials, but the majority had the support of a double-blind study. Closed communities and families expectedly received most attention.

3.2.5.3 Dosage, Mode of Administration

Oral administration of 100 mg without preparation or post-treatment measures is the only requirement.

3.2.5.4 Side Effects

See Sect. B.II.3.2.10.4.

3.2.5.5 Contraindications, Precautions

See Sect. B.II.3.2.10.5.

3.2.5.6 Conclusions

3.2.5.6.1 Clinical

A single dose of 100 mg is nearly always efficacious, especially so when repeated 1 week later, and is practically devoid of side effects.

3.2.5.6.2 Mass Treatment

For eradication of enterobiasis in closed communities, this single, non-weight-depending standard dose of mebendazole is a first choice. Its efficacy is not substantially increased by higher or repeated doses. Lecomte-Ramioul (1975) tried a monthly administration of 100 mg. The CR reached 93% in the 3rd and 85% in the 9th month.

3.2.6 Piperazine

3.2.6.1 State of the Art

In 1942 Giroud observed the disappearance of enterobiasis in a patient under piperazine treatment for hyperuricemia. Mehrez (1947) and Deschiens et al. (1954) demonstrated the efficacy of piperazine in enterobiasis. It has become standard treatment for *E. vermicularis*, especially under the influence of Brown et al. (1956b). The activity of piperazine derivatives against ascariasis enhances the value of this inexpensive drug.

3.2.6.2 Assessment

The multiplicity of the proposed derivatives of this diethylene-amine compound and the variation in dosages expressed in milligrams per year of age, per pound or kilogram body weight, or in grams according to weight cause confusion. The compounds in use are hydrate, citrate, phosphate, and adipate, all of which transform into piperazine hexahydrate. The dosage can thus be based on the latter, and Brown (1969) provided a useful table on the basis of body weight groups (see Sect. 3.2.6.3).

It has been shown by Ricci and Corbo (1956), Swartzwelder et al. (1957a), Goeters (1955b), and Mathies (1961) that prolonged treatment is more effective. However, no agreement has been reached about the relative efficacy of a continuous or a renewed administration after 1 week.

Table 42. Treatment of *E. vermicularis* infection by piperazine and its derivatives

Efficacy	Dosage	Number treated	CR	References
Administration of fixed dose per body weight group				
100%	2 –2.5 g/14 days	24	100	Sadun et al. (1956)
≧90%	0.5–2 g/14 days	39	97	Brown and Chan (1955)
	0.5–2 g/ 7 days[a]	24	92	Brown and Chan (1955)
≧80%	0.5–2 g/10 days	57	89	Brown and Chan (1955)
≧70%	2 –3 g	50	74	Chandra et al. (1951)
Administration of a dose individualized for body weight				
100%	60–70 mg/kg/14 days (max. 2 g)	26	100	Bumbalo and Plummer (195
≧90%	50 mg/kg/ 7 days	150	97	Rachelson and Ferguson (1
	60 mg/kg/ 7 days	22	95	Mathies (1961)
≧80%	60–80 mg/kg/ 7 days	38	89	Biguet et al. (1953)
	60–70 mg/kg/ 7 days (max. 2 g)	47	85	Bumbalo and Plummer (195
	±83 mg/kg/10 days	58	84	Howie (1955)
Administration of an individualized dose per year of age				
≧80%	250 mg/year of age/7 days[b]	42	83	White and Standen (1953)
≧50%	100 mg/year of age/7 days[b]	35	54	White and Standen (1953)

[a] Dose renewed after 1 week
[b] Administered ×3; but variations of weight/year of age are considerable: an analysis based on dose/weight shows that over 50 mg/kg the CR is 97%

3.2.6.3 Dosage, Mode of Administration

A dose of 50–75 mg/kg given orally, with a maximum of 4 g, is obviously correct. The hexahydrate contains 44% base. In order to simplify the administration, BROWN's table (1969) can be used (Table 43).

Table 43. Doses per body weight of solid and liquid formulations of usual piperazine derivatives

Weight of patient (kg)	Piperazine hexahydrate (g)	Piperazine (citrate) syrup (ml)
7	0.250	2.5
8–14	0.500	5.0
15–30	1.000	10.0
30	2.000	20.0

3.2.6.4 Side Effects

See Sect. B.II.3.2.9.4 and be aware of the risk of CNS involvement.

3.2.6.5 Contraindications, Precautions

See Sect. B.II.3.2.9.5.

3.2.6.6 Conclusions

This standard treatment of enterobiasis has become obsolete, except in situations characterized by lack of modern drugs.

3.2.7 Pyrantel Pamoate

3.2.7.1 State of the Art

BURIEL et al. (1969) showed that pyrantel pamoate in a single dose of 10 mg/kg procures a CR of 98%, a fact confirmed by BUMALO et al. (1969). These observations initiated a series of studies on its efficacy compared with that of the current anthelmintics.

3.2.7.2 Assessment

Table 44. Treatment of *E. vermicularis* infection by pyrantel pamoate

Efficacy	Dosage	Number treated	CR	References
100%	10 mg/kg	21	100[a]	CHO et al. (1977)
≧90%	10 mg/kg	86	98	BURRIEL et al. (1969)
	10 mg/kg (suspension)	28	96	BUMBALO et al. (1969)
	10 mg/kg	43	96	GUARNIERA et al. (1969)
	10 mg/kg	50	96	CHANDRA (1977)
	10 mg/kg	20	90	ALEXANDER et al. (1970)

Table 44 (continued)

Efficacy	Dosage	Number treated	CR	References
≧90%	10 mg/kg	120	95	SANATI and GHANDIRIAN (1971)
	10 mg/kg	50	94	CARNEY et al. (1971)
	10 mg/kg	450	98	ALEKSEEVA and PUCENKO (1980)[b]
	10 mg/kg (suspension)	245	99	PITTS and MIGLIARDI (1974)
	10 mg/kg (tablets)	217	95	PITTS and MIGLIARDI (1974)
	10 mg/kg	50	94	CHANDRA (1977)
	10 mg/kg	390	91	HARFOUCHE et al. (1974)
	10 mg/kg	249	93	LUMBRERAS et al. (1974)
	5 mg/kg/4 days	118	99	LIAN and ZI (1981)
≧80%	10 mg/kg	43	84	RIM and LIM (1972)
≧70%	250–500 mg	100	79	MASSIF et al. (1974)
	180–250 mg (tablets)	89	63	CHRICE et al. (1975)

[a] But success on day 14 was followed by progressive return to the original level from day 19 on

[b] Twice, at an interval of 2 weeks

3.2.7.3 Dosage, Mode of Administration

A single dose of 10 mg/kg is effective. The drug is available as an oral suspension containing 250 mg/spoon or chewable tablets of 250 mg. A useful schedule is as follows:

6 months – 2 years	½ spoon	½ tablet
2 months – 6 years	1 spoon	1 tablet
6 months – 12 years	2 spoons	2 tablets
12 years	3 spoons	3 tablets

3.2.7.4 Side Effects

See Sect. B.II.3.2.11.4.

3.2.7.5 Contraindications, Precautions

See Sect. B.II.3.2.11.5.

3.2.7.6 Conclusions

3.2.7.6.1 Clinical

Pyrantel pamoate is obviously an interesting and efficacious drug against *E. vermicularis*.

3.2.7.6.2 Mass Treatment

The wide spectrum and easy administration of pyrantel pamoate make it a suitable drug for the treatment of families and communities. The choice of the drug will depend on its price and possible side effects. It should be kept in mind that the relapse rate is very high and occurs quite early.

3.2.8 Pyrvinium Pamoate (Vanquin, Povan)

3.2.8.1 State of the Art

This anthelmintic of the cyanine group has been in use for about 20 years. Since it is virtually nonabsorbed its activity is confined to intralumen elements. ROYER (1956) and SAWITZ and KARPINSKI (1956) drew attention to the potential value of this compound. BECK et al. (1959) established its efficacy against *E. vermicularis* at a dose of 2 mg/kg for 7 days and observed that a simple dose of 5 mg/kg was just as efficacious. This was confirmed by BIGUET et al. (1952), BUMBALO et al. (1958) and many other authors. KOMIYA et al. (1962), BECK (1964), and NISHIMURA et al. (1965) obtained similar good results after the administration of a single 1- to 2-mg/kg dose. 7.5 mg pyrvinium pamoate corresponds to 5 mg pyrvinium base.

3.2.8.2 Assessment

Table 45. Treatment of *E. vermicularis* infections with pyrvinium pamoate

Efficacy	Dosage	Number treated	CR	References
100%	2 mg/kg	125	100	NISHIMURA et al. (1965)
	5 mg/kg	18	100	BIGUET et al. (1952)
	5 mg/kg	61	100	ROYER and BARONIKOFF (1962)
	5 mg/kg (tablets)	77	100	ROYER and BARONIKOFF (1962)
	5 mg/kg	17	100	BUMBALO et al. (1958)
	5 mg/kg	43	100	MATHIES (1969)
	5 mg/kg	35	100	MATHIES (1973)
	5 mg/kg	18	100	CHO et al. (1977)
	7 mg/kg	28	100	SANDERS and HALL (1960)
	7.5 mg/kg	40	100	ADIAO et al. (1961)
≧90%	1 mg/kg	294	98	KOMIYA et al. (1962)
	2 mg/kg	188	99	KOMIYA et al. (1962)
	2 mg/kg	100	98	BECK (1964)
	5 mg/kg	505	97	ALEKSEEVA and PUCENKO (1980)[a]
	5 mg/kg	100	96	BECK et al. (1959)
	5 mg/kg (capsules)	49	94	KOMIYA et al. (1960)
	5 mg/kg	123	90	DONOSO and ATHIAS (1961)
	5 mg/kg (capsules)	128	99	SUZUKI et al. (1961)
	5 mg/kg (syrup)	45	91	SUZUKI et al. (1961)
	5 mg/kg	150	98	DESAI (1962)
	5 mg/kg	55	93	GARIN (1962)
	5 mg/kg	42	93	FARID (1963)
	5 mg/kg	73	97	MAKA (1963)
	5 mg/kg	94	97	FRITZ (1965)
	5 mg/kg	76	97	HAYASHI et al. (1976)
	5 mg/kg/x 2, 7-day interval	52	94	DAVIS (1966)
	10 mg/kg	28	93	RODRIGUES et al. (1960)
≧80%	2 mg/kg	14	86	NISHIMURA et al. (1965)
	5 mg/kg (syrup)	35	88	KOMIYA et al. (1960)
≧80%	5 mg/kg	133	83	SALEM et al. (1961)
	5 mg/kg	44	86	ERICKSEN (1964)
	5 mg/kg	48	89	MOST (1963)

Table 45 (continued)

Efficacy	Dosage	Number treated	CR	References
	5 mg/kg	51	80	DAVIS (1965)
	5 mg/kg	–	81	GUARNIERA et al. (1969)
	5 mg/kg	20	85	ALEXANDER et al. (1970)
≧60%	5 mg/kg	100	60	NASSIF et al. (1974)
	5 mg/kg	50	70	CARNEY et al. (1971)

[a] Twice, at an interval of 2 weeks

3.2.8.3 Dosage, Mode of Administration

The efficacy against enterobiasis of 5 mg/kg, the dose applied most often, approaches 100%, but 2 mg/kg is also sufficient (KOMIYA et al. 1962). The possibility of a residual infection justifies a second administration after 2–3 weeks. The drug is available in coated tablets, capsules with 50 mg base, or a suspension of 10 mg base/ml for oral administration.

3.2.8.4 Side Effects

The patient should be warned that feces and underwear will possibly be stained red post-treatment and that photosensitization is possible. Gastrointestinal irritation, nausea, vomiting, cramps, and diarrhea are observed after the larger doses. The possibility of the Stevens-Johnson syndrome has been mentioned by COURSIN (1966).

3.2.8.5 Contraindications, Precautions

Although not absorbed from the intestinal tract, pyrvinium pamoate should be used with caution in persons with renal or hepatic dysfunction.

3.2.8.6 Conclusions

3.2.8.6.1 Clinical

The consensus about a dosage of 5 mg/kg is manifest. However, the value of 1 or 2 mg/kg dosages may have been overlooked. Several newer drugs commercially available have reduced its use.

3.2.8.6.2 Mass Treatment

Pyrvinium pamoate is efficient and useful for treatment in closed communities and families with children. It is one of the drugs of choice in enterobiasis.

3.2.9 Tiabendazole (Mintezol)

3.2.9.1 State of the Art

The broad-spectrum activity of this substituted benzimidazole against nematodes includes *E. vermicularis*. It has been confirmed continuously since 1963. The efficacy of tiabendazole compares well with that of other enterobicides, but is not ovicidal (MULLIN and IMPERATO 1969).

3.2.9.2 Assessment

Table 46. Treatment of *E. vermicularis* infection by tiabendazole

Efficacy	Dosage	Number treated	CR	References
100%	25 mg/kg	33	100	CHANCO and PAGUIO (1964)
	50 mg/kg/2 days	29	100	MOST et al. (1965)
≧90%	25 mg/kg b.i.d./2 days	51	98	MOST et al. (1965)
	25 mg/kg b.i.d./2 days	49	98	DAVIS (1965)
	25 mg/kg b.i.d./2–3 days	256	94	CAMPBELL and CUCKLER (1969)
	25 mg/kg b.i.d., repeated on day 7	47	93	MATHIES (1969)
	50 mg/kg	31	90	ESCOBAR (1964)
	25 mg/kg b.i.d., repeated on day 7	51	94	DAVIS (1966)
	25 mg/kg b.i.d., repeated on day 7	75	96	DAVIS (1969)
≧80%	50 mg/kg	108	81	MOST et al. (1965)
	25 mg/kg b.i.d., repeated on day 7	26	85	MULLIN and IMPERATO (1969)
	25 mg/kg b.i.d., repeated on day 14	75	84	MULLIN and IMPERATO (1969)
≧70%	25 mg/kg b.i.d	21	72	MULLIN and IMPERATO (1969)
≧50%	25 mg/kg b.i.d	141	55	MOST et al. (1965)

3.2.9.3 Dosage, Mode of Administration

Quite satisfactory results are given by 25 mg/kg b. i. d., after meals and repeated after 1–2 weeks.

3.2.9.4 Side Effects

See Sect. B.II.3.2.13.4.

3.2.9.5 Contraindications, Precautions

See Sect. B.II.3.2.13.5.

3.2.9.6 Conclusions

Tiabendazole is active against threadworm even on a 1-day schedule. However, the side effects are so frequent (up to 30%) and so troublesome that its use should be at least restricted to multiple infections. Even for this purpose alternative better-tolerated drugs are readily available.

III. Drug Combinations

Irregularities in the outcome of many therapeutic attempts, although obviously due in part to poor delivery and control, lead to the use of two or more enterobicidal drugs in combination. *Oil of chenopodium* and *TCE* was followed by *"TED 3"*, and *diphetarsone-spiramycin.*

This latter association is in fact the chemical salt generated by the reaction of diphetarsone (acid) and spiramycin (base). It is used against amebiasis, but also cures persons chronically infected by pinworms. *Flubendazole* (100 mg) in combination with *tinidazole* (175 mg) b.i.d. gave HUGGINS (1979a) a CR of 80% (8:10). A syrup containing 750 mg *piperazine* and 25 mg *pyrvinium*/5 ml provided, at a dose of 0.5 ml/kg for 2 days, a cure of 30 out of 30 (BOTERO et al. 1966). A suspension of 750 mg *piperazine* and 375 *tiabendazole*/10 ml, after administration of 5 ml for 5 days, cleared 35 out of 35, a 100% CR (FERNANDES and GARCIA 1976). The combination of *mebendazole* and *pyrantel pamoate*, 5 mg/kg of each, was successful in 116 of 119 infections, a CR of 98% (LIAN and ZI 1981).

The excellent efficacy ensured by several of the newer drugs makes it obvious that the drug combinations are superfluous efforts against enterobiasis.

IV. Comments

Speaking from experience, the main point is the absolute necessity to treat all the members of the family or the community in order to avoid reinfection. It can be difficult to convince those without complaints: they are nonetheless dangerous parasite reservoirs.

As the larvae lodging in the crypts of the ileum are not destroyed by current drugs, while autoinfection provides a new generation, it is advisable to repeat the treatment after 1–2 weeks. There is no proof that administration on seven consecutive days guarantees better results.

Chemoprophylactic sanitation is possible provided there is generalization of the chemotherapy and an allowance is made for possible reinfection by fingers, etc. and also by dust-bearing eggs.

F. Gnathostomiasis

[Yangtse Edema, Tua Chid (Thailand)]

I. Introduction

Gnathostoma worms infect animals in different parts of the world (Africa, America, Asia). Their life cycle requires passage through a *Cyclops*, followed by passage through a freshwater fish. Man is an accidental host, becoming infected by eating raw, poorly cooked, or marinated parasitized fish. Being an abnormal host the parasite will not reach maturity, but the L3 larvae migrate subcutaneously, producing a creeping eruption, and through all kinds of tissue, causing a visceral larva migrans syndrome. As these larvae may survive as long as 12 years, symptoms may reappear periodically.

1. Parasite

The sexually mature worms live in the stomach of feline or canine carnivores (dog, cat, tiger, etc.). They are embedded in small nodules of hyperplastic gastric mucosa. In these tumor-like growths, the gnathostoma have a pink and stout body with a swollen head bulb covered with four circles of stout spines. The anterior half is covered with rows of flat-toothed spines followed by a bare portion. Numerous tiny spines cover the posterior half.

The males measure 11–31 mm; the females measure 11–54 mm; both have a blunt posterior end.

The eggs escape through an apical opening in the nodules and pass with the feces. They are yellowish-brown, measuring 69 µm (62–79 µm) by 39 µm (36–42 µm). The outer shell is finely granulated and shows a typical polar cap at one end.

If the unembryonated eggs are deposited in fresh water, they will hatch in 7 days at 27°–31 °C. The L1 larvae swim actively and must be ingested by a *Cyclops*. In the copepod the L1 larvae pass into the hemocele, where they molt into L2 within 7–10 days. For further development they must be ingested by a secondary intermediate host, such as fish (Ophicephalus, etc.), frogs, and aquatic rodents.

The L2 larvae pierce the gastric wall and migrate to the muscles or connective tissues, where they molt into L3 larvae. The larvae, infective to a definitive host, are encysted in muscle. This part of the life cycle is completed within 1 month.

The infection of the definitive hosts follows eating infected fish. It can also occur in paratenic hosts (amphibians, snakes, rodents, birds). The digestion of muscle and cyst wall sets the parasite free. The L3 larvae passes through the stomach wall into the peritoneal cavity, migrates through the liver to the skeletal muscles and connective tissue, and penetrates the stomach again 3 months later from the serosal side, becoming embedded in the gastric mucosa. Six months later full maturity is achieved in a normal host, but of course not in man, in whom these larvae may survive and migrate for as long as 10–12 years.

The whole cycle lasts approximately 1 year.

2. Host

The infection of man follows the eating of raw or poorly cooked freshwater fish, chicken, and pork, which are carriers of L3 in their muscle. Within 24–48 h after ingestion a dramatic abdominal condition, mimicking an acute abdomen not unlike that seen in anisakiasis, may occur and is accompanied by leukocytosis due to eosinophilia that can affect up to 90% of the leukocytes.

The epigastric discomfort is accompanied by nausea, salivation, vomiting, flushing, pruritus, and urticaria, all of which disappear spontaneously.

The migrating immature larvae produce the pathology. Subcutaneous swelling can appear 3–4 weeks later and start "wandering". This creeping eruption moves about 1 cm/h and lasts 10–14 days, but can reappear intermittently at intervals of 2–6 weeks.

The migrating larvae may invade and disturb the liver, respiratory tract, eyes, cervix, remaining internal organs, and even the CNS. In the latter, eosinophilic meningoencephalites can produce paraplegia and cerebral hemorrhages: the CSF will be bloody or xanthochromatic. Death can follow. It is, however, an exceptional evolution. The same is true about the production of intestinal nodules [only five cases have been published (CHITANONDH and ROSEN 1960)].

In the respiratory organs, edema of the larynx, spontaneous pneumothorax, and hemoptysis are possible complications.

3. Diagnosis

Obviously some effort should be made to diagnose the still masked parasitosis, by means of specific immunodiagnostic tests or serological techniques, as larvae in a blind alley can survive for years. Larvae can be extracted from the skin lesions and identified.

4. Geographical Distribution

Gnathostoma infect various animals in Africa, the Americas, the Middle East, and Asia. They belong to a variety of species, e.g., *G. spinigerum* in domestic pigs.

Human gnathostomiasis occurs, with the possible exception of Mexico, only in Asia. Cases have been observed occasionally in Burma, China, India, Indonesia, Malaysia, and Papua New Guinea. The main foci are Japan (Kyushu, Shikoku, South Honsu) and Thailand.

II. Drugs

To date the activities of several newer anthelmintics have been established: tiabendazole, 45 mg/kg, for at least 7 days; mebendazole, 200 mg t. i. d., for 28 days levamisole, 2.5 mg/kg or 150 mg b. i. d. for several days; but no systematic assessment has been made. Inasmuch as the immature larvae survive for years, during which they can cause damage to many organs, it seems imperative that more attention should be paid of the problem of chemotherapy.

G. Intestinal Angiostrongyliasis

I. Introduction

Infection in man by *Angiostrongylus costaricensis* (MORERA and CESPEDES 1971),[12] a nematode parasitic of Central American rodents which lives in small branches of the mesenteric arteries in the ileocecal regions, was reported in 1967 (CESPEDES et al.). The clinical syndrome had, however, been observed in Costa Rican children since 1952.

1. Parasite

The filiform adults are tapered toward both ends. The caudal extremity is curved ventrally. The round cephalic extremity is devoid of a buccal capsule. The cuticle is smooth and transparent, except at both ends, where it is finely striated and thicker. The excretory pore is slightly posterior to the esophagointestinal junction.

The male measures 20 mm (17–22 mm) by 0.28–0.31 mm. The copulatory caudal bursa has two slender striated, equal spicules and one gubernaculum. The

12 Reclassified in 1972 by CHABAUD as a new genus *Morerastrongylus, M. costaricensis*

female measures 33 mm (28–42 mm) by 0.32–0.35 mm. The anus and vulva are located near the conical posterior end.

The adults inhabit the mesenteric arteries and lay their eggs in the tissue or the capillaries of the wall of the ileocecum. The thin-shelled ovoid eggs embryonate in the tissue and L1 larvae (0.27 mm/14–15 μm) migrate into the intestinal lumen and pass with the feces into the outside world. They are very active. The intermediate host *Vaginulus plebeius* feeds on rat feces. The L1 larva molts on day 4 into a L2 nonmotile larva, which grows from day 4 until day 10 (0.37 mm/ 36 μm), and molts again on day 11–14 into the L3 larva, which matures on day 16–19 and becomes free and active again.

The infective L3 larva is taken up by the definitive host, usually rats and occasionally man, which eat the slug or vegetables contaminated with mucous secretion of the slug. The L3 larva passes from the stomach into the intestine, penetrates the lymphatics and lymph nodes, molts, and undergoes sexual differentiation. The young adults migrate to the arterioles of the ileocecal region, their definitive habitat where they reach maturity and oviposition occurs. A few may get lost into the liver, kidney, or lungs.

The common reservoir hosts are the ommivorous *Rattus rattus* and *Sigmodon hispidus* (cotton rat): 24% of the older and bigger ones may be infected. Other less important final hosts are the herbivorous *Oryzomys fulvescens, Liomys adspersus*, and *Zygodontomys microtinus*, with an infection rate up to 3%.

2. Host

The adult worms cause thrombosis in the arteries in which they are living, while the eggs and larvae, unable to hatch in man, degenerate and produce a granulomatous reaction in the wall of the appendix, cecum, ascending colon, and terminal ileum and also in the regional lymph nodes. The thickened wall may partially or completely obstruct the lumen or become necrotic with the possibility of perforation.

This reaction produces a painful indurated tumor-like mass in the fossa iliaca dextra, in the area of the appendix, and arousing right-sided tenderness on rectal examination. The local symptoms are accompanied by a prolonged fever of 38°–38.5 °C lasting for 2–4 weeks, anorexia, vomiting, diarrhea, and occasionally bowel subobstruction.

On roentgenography examination the filling defects in the ileocecal region are perceptible and the walls are rigid or spastic. Sterling's sign, a brusque contraction of the cecum, is observed by fluoroscopy.

In man, the majority of infections occur in rural children of the school age group (6–13 years), followed by the preschool age group. The male:female ratio is 2:1.

3. Diagnosis

In endemic areas the symptoms are pointers, but the signal is the leukocytosis, in the 20,000–30,000 range, due to an eosinophilia of up to 70% or more. Since the parasites, including the eggs and larvae, remain in the tissue, a stool examination will provide no useful information. Serological evidence can be obtained by gel diffusion or latex-precipitation tests against specific antigens.

4. Geographical Distribution

This abdominal angiostrongyliasis has been reported in Venezuela, Panama, Costa Rica, Honduras, El Salvador, and Southern Mexico.

5. Prevalence

After the syndrome had been recognized in man, an abnormal host, 10–30 patients have been diagnosed every year. During the 10-year period 1966–1975, 116 cases were observed in Costa Rica's National Children's Hospital (LOREA-CORTES and LOBO-SANAHUJA 1980). Since 1967 the number has increased, which may be related to a steady expansion of the intermediate host population. Slugs are becoming a major pest in agriculture. The monthly distribution shows a consistent increase during the wettest months (September–November), corresponding with the activity of the slugs.

II. Drugs

1. State of the Art

This parasitosis has only recently come to the attention of the medical profession. Due to the pseudotumoral symptomatology in the ileocecal region surgical resection has understandably been the therapeutic approach. However, drug therapy could be useful, especially in the early stages. Nonetheless the destruction of the parasites might induce a strong unwanted local reaction. Up to now only tiabendazole has been tested.

2. Tiabendazole

The standard procedure has been 75 mg/kg/3 per days, repeated four times. The concurrent administration of diethylcarbamazine (DEC), 6 mg/kg, during 3 weeks does not improve the results.

III. Angiostrongyliasis

State of the Art

Angiostrongylus cantonensis CHEN 1935 is a nematode of rats, occasionally infecting man, but unable to develop to maturity in the human host. The L3 larvae show a tendency to migrate to the brain and rarely to the eyes or lungs.

The involvement of the CNS is the most striking clinical manifestation, with the eosinophilic meningitis due to the localization of the L3 larvae under the arachnoid where they die some time later (marked pleiocytosis for 92% eosinophils in the CSF). This eosinophilic meningoencephalitis, and also the eye and lung localization, is most certainly the exception after infection.

Premonitory gastrointestinal symptoms, with eosinophilia, are rare. The *geographical distribution* of angiostrongyliasis is much wider than the western Pacific, Tahiti, and Southeast Asia. Cases occur also in Madagascar, Japan, and Cuba. Infection follows eating parasitized raw terrestrial and aquatic snails (e.g., *Achatine*), slugs, or freshwater prawns.

Several drugs have been tested experimentally on infected rats or on larvae in vitro. Levamisole has been found very active against the larvae (MOREAU and LAGRAULET 1972). In rats, tiabendazole produced good results. Avermectin B_{1a} might be useful. On *A. malaysiensis* infection in rats, mebendazole and flubendazole (10 mg/kg per 5 days) were effective (AMBRE and MAK 1981).

H. Intestinal Capillariasis

I. Introduction

In 1963 a case of severe gastroenteritis was reported from northwest Luzon. This "Pudoc Mystery disease" or "non-vibrio cholera" reached epidemic proportions: 1300 sick and 90 deaths in Tagudin, Ilocos Sur, during 1967–1968 (SINGSON 1969). Since 1969 the situation has become endemic with some ten cases a year or small epidemics. It is likely that the present situation is a return to the state of affairs prevailing before 1963, when this protein-losing enteropathy occurred unrecognized in the Philippines and elsewhere. *Capillaria philippinensis* (CHITWOOD et al. 1964) was identified as the cause of this syndrome.

1. Parasite

Capillaria philippinensis is one of the smallest intestinal nematodes of man.[13] Its anterior and posterior ends are of the same length. The males measure 2.3–3.9 mm by 23–28 µm. The single spicule is 200–300 µm in length and its spine-free sheathy may reach 440 µm. The male has small caudal alae. The females are 2.3–5.3 mm long with a diameter of 29–47 µm. The vulva opens behind the esophagus. The uterus may contain unembryonated thick-shelled eggs (containing a mucoid coat), embryonated thin-shelled eggs, and embryos without a shell.

Both varieties pass in the feces. They are peanut shaped with flattened bipolar plugs and measure 36–45 µm by 21 µm. Differentiation from *Trichuris trichiura* is based on its smaller size, more ovoid shape, and absence of protuberant plugs.

Life Cycle

It has been shown experimentally that some species of brackish or fresh-water fish are possible intermediate hosts. Both in the Philippines and Thailand a number of species can be infected. The life cycle has been established in laboratory animals. A similar cycle is assumed to occur in man.

Eggs passed out with feces embryonate in water within 5–10 days dependent on the ambient temperature. Fed to fish, they hatch in the intestine. The emerged larvae (130–150 µm) grow up to 250–300 µm in 2–3 weeks. Administered by stomach tube to Mongolian gerbils *(Meriones unguiculatus)* the infective larvae develop into adults in 10–11 days. The fertile females can generate larvae 2 weeks

13 Of some 250 known *Capillaria* species, four have been identified in man: *C. hepatica, C. cutanea, C. aerophila,* and *C. philippinensis*

later. These larvae are the origin of a second generation of adults which will produce eggs, passing out in the feces of the infected gerbils from day 25 postinfection.

As long as the infection persists a few larviparous females are always present; they maintain and increase the population level. This internal autoinfection mechanism is obvious, since adults, larviparous adults, and larvae at all development stages are simultaneously present (CROSS et al. (1972). It is part of the life cycle. From gerbils infected with only two to three larvae, up to 7,000 worms were recovered postmortem.

An important observation is the variability of the course of infection in animals. In gerbils, the infection ends with death after progressive emaciation. In monkeys the infection persists for many months without producing ill effects. In rats, the infection is transient and symptom free.

Freshwater fish which could be infected in the Philippines, among others, are *Hypselotris bipartita* and *Elotris melanosoma* (CROSS et al. 1972) and in Thailand, *Cyprinus capio, Gambusia holbrookii*, and *Puntius gonionotus* (BHAIBULAYA et al. 1979). Fish-eating birds which were successfully infected in Thailand are *Amaurornis phoenicurus* and *Ardeola bacchus* (BHAILBULAYA and INDRANGARM 1979) and in Taiwan, *Bulbulcus ibis, Nyticorax nyticorax*, and *Ixobrychus sinensis*. These herons and egrets could be reservoir hosts.

2. Host

Contamination follows ingestion of raw, preserved, and undercooked fish. The defense mechanisms of man must be low, since the parasite load builds up by internal autoinfection even from a light initial infection. Relapses are common and in some persons extremely frequent (812 out of 1219 or 67%) and 11 recurrences were seen in 6 patients (SINGSON 1974).

Clinical Manifestations

At the onset the signals are: recurrent dull epigastric or generalized abdominal pain and distension, intermittent diarrhea, and borborygmus. The evolution engenders an intractable diarrhea, with five to ten voluminous watery and fatty stools a day. The protracted diarrhea leads to a severe dehydration. Electrolytic and protein depletion follow, which in turn produce malaise, anorexia, nausea, and vomiting.

The protein-losing enteropathy and malabsorption are followed by loss of weight, somewhat compensated by edema, anasarca, ascites, or followed by emaciation. Muscle-wasting, hypotension, and heart failure may follow. The disease ends in death for some 12% (120 out of 1,500 cases) or in frequent relapses for others.

The plasma levels of Ca (3.7–5 mEq), K (2.6–3.6 mEq), carotene, and proteins (4.6 g%) become dangerously low. Severe hypokalemia can lead to death from cardiac arrest, which can be corrected by coconut water, oral potassium solution, or KCl, 40 mEq/g per liter intravenously. IgM and IgG levels are lowered, while IgE increases.

3. Diagnosis

Intestinal capillariasis can be identified by the presence of eggs, larvae, or adult *C. phillipinensis* in direct smears, formalin-ether concentration, etc. At autopsy 200,000 worms have been recovered from 1 liter of intestinal contents. The ovoid eggs with their obviously more flattened plug at both ends, their more square, coarser pitted shell and smaller size can be easily differentiated from those of *Trichuris trichiura*. A direct smear after a formalin-ether concentration suffices.

4. Geographical Distribution

Endemic foci of intestinal capillariasis have been detected in villages bordering the China sea on the northern and western coast of Luzon, and in northeastern Mindanao, and have been identified since 1973 in scattered areas of Thailand.

Taking into consideration the diversity of species of fish that can be experimentally infected, and the possible role of fish-eating birds, migratory birds included in the dissemination, the geographical distribution of capillariasis must be much more widespread.

5. Prevalence

Over 1,500 people have been found infected (aged 2–84 years), but mostly middle aged (20–40 years), with two males for one female. In one village north of Manila the prevalence reached 32%: 227 out of 700 inhabitants (DETELS et al. 1969). Since the first observed epidemic, several hundred new cases have been reported. The mortality can be checked by early diagnosis and chemotherapy.

II. Drugs

This serious intestinal parasitosis was only discovered recently. Only a few drugs have been tentatively administered, simultaneously with an appropriate supportive therapy for the replacement of fluids, depleted electrolytes, and lost proteins. Dithiazanine iodide was the first drug, but is no longer in use. Tiabendazole, levamisole, and the benzimidazoles have successfully taken over.

1. Flubendazole

1.1 Assessment

Although 100 mg/10 days has been found effective, patients have experienced relapses (CROSS et al. 1980).

1.2 Conclusion

Flubendazole is efficacious, but not a better drug than mebendazole (see below).

2. Levamisole

2.1 State of the Art

Levamisole shows activity against capillariasis.

2.2 Assessment

Table 47. Treatment of intestinal capillariasis by levamisole

Dosage	Number treated	CR	References
2.5 mg/kg/22 days	4	100	SINGSON and BANZON (1969)
2.5 mg/kg/30 days	11	91	SINGSON and BANZON (1969)
150 mg/30 days	10	100	SINGSON and BANZON (1969)
150 mg/30 days	21	53	SINGSON et al. (1974)
Old infections	14	64	
New infections	7	72	

2.3 Dosage

Dosage is either 2.5 mg/kg or 150 mg/30 days.

2.4 Side Effects

See Sect. B.II.3.2.8.4.

2.5 Contraindications, Precautions

See Sect. B.II.3.2.8.5.

2.6 Conclusions

Although levamisole is efficacious it is not a first choice.

3. Mebendazole

3.1 State of the Art

Human intestinal capillariasis was an unknown disease before the 1967 epidemic. The attempts at treatment were based on its position among the Trichuridae. Mebendazole was tried on 32 patients and found effective.

3.2 Assessment

Table 48. Treatment of intestinal capillariasis by mebendazole

Efficacy	Dosage	Number treated	CR	References
100%	200 mg b.i.d./30 days	24[a]	100	SINGSON et al. (1974)
	200 mg b.i.d./20–30 days	33[a]	100	SINGSON et al. (1975)
	200 mg b.i.d./10 days followed by 250 mg/10 days	19	100	SINGSON et al. (1977)
	200 mg b.i.d./15 days	21	100	SINGSON et al. (1977)
	500 mg/16 days	11	100	CROSS (1983, personal communication)
≧90%	200 mg b.i.d./30 days	65	95	SINGSON et al. (1975)
	200 mg b.i.d./30 days	32[b]	91	SINGSON et al. (1975)
≧70%	100–200 mg/20–30 days	83	70	SINGSON et al. (1975)
≧60%	200 mg b.i.d./30 days	8	63	SINGSON et al. (1974)
<50%	200–300 mg/10–14 days	26	42	SINGSON et al. (1975)

[a] New infections [b] Old infections

3.3 Dosage

In new infections, 400 mg d.d., either as a single or divided dose (200 mg b.i.d.) is administered during 20 days, but for relapses this time is prolonged to 30 days.

3.4 Side Effects

See Sect. B.II.3.2.10.4. Tolerance of the higher dosages and over a longer period is good.

3.5 Contraindications, Precautions

See Sect. B.II.3.2.10.5.

3.6 Conclusions

Mebendazole stops diarrhea within 2–4 days. Borborygmi and edema can persist for 10–14 days. Appetite improves and body weight increases. Clinical improvement is dramatic. Mebendazole is the drug of choice for intestinal capillariasis. Moreover, mebendazole simultaneously ensures the disappearance of *Ascaris*, *Trichuris*, and hookworm.

4. Pyrantel Pamoate

The only available information for pyrantel pamoate is the appearance of atypical ova in the feces following the administration of pyrantel (Kan 1979).

5. Tiabendazole

5.1 State of the Art

This compound induces early disappearance of complaints but does not achieve a radical cure.

5.2 Assessment

Table 49. Treatment of intestinal capillariasis by tiabendazole

Efficacy	Dosage	Number treated	CR	References
100%	25–50 mg/kg or 1 g/70 days[a]	1	100	Singson et al. (1974)
≧80%	25 mg/kg/3–4 weeks; control, 4 months	24	88	Whalen et al. (1971)
≧70%	25 mg/kg/3–4 weeks; control	14	79	Whalen et al. (1971)
<50%	25–50 mg/kg or 1 g/70 days or 1 g/30 days	36[b] 37	46 46	Singson et al. (1974) Singson et al. (1974)

[a] At the start the dose is administered on ten consecutive days followed by a dose every other day for 4 months

[b] Old infections

5.3 Dosage

Dosage is 25–50 mg/kg, with a maximum of 1 g, over long periods (Sect. B.II.3.2.13.4).

5.4 Side Effects

See Sect. B.II.3.2.13.4. Side effects are mild and transient and disappear in a few days without treatment.

5.5 Contraindications, Precautions

See Sect. B.II.3.2.13.5.

5.6 Conclusions

Tiabendazole is less effective against the adults entrapped in the crypts of Lieberkühn; this entails a very prolonged treatment. Many patients do not complete such a lengthy therapy.

III. General Comments

Mebendazole is very effective at a dosage of 400 mg/day for 20 days. It cuts the relapses down to a minimum and produces no side effects. The clinical improvement is dramatic. From the 1st day of treatment a striking feeling of wellbeing is experienced and diarrhea stops within 2–4 days. Eggs disappear from the 5th day on, but larvae and adults persist up to the 20th day. Nevertheless, a drug of similar efficiency on a shorter schedule would be welcome.

J. Oesophagostomiasis

I. Introduction

Oesophagostomiasis (also known as helminthoma, nodule worm infection, pimply gut, helminthic pseudotumors, or abscesses of the bowel) is a rare infection of the intestine or abdominal cavity of man by *Oesophagostomum.* This strongyloid nematode normally inhabits the large intestine of primates, pigs, and ruminants.

Oesophagostomum apiostomum WILLACH 1891; RAILLET and HENRY 1905 is the most common species found in man. *O. stephanostomum* STOSSICH 1904, a parasite of the gorilla, has been reported in man in Uganda, and also in Brazil (THOMAS 1910). *O. bifurcum* CREPLIN 1849 has been identified in nodules of the colon in northern Ghana.

1. Parasite

The adult *Oesophagostomum* worm lives in the lumen of the bowel of its definitive hosts (monkeys, swine, cattle, sheep, goats). These nematodes resemble hookworms. The cuticle presents characteristic prominent transverse striations and a transverse groove on the ventral surface of the cervical region. At its anterior extremity the cuticle is thickened and dilated to an ovoidal cephalic swelling. The buccal capsule opens forward, is cylindrical rather than globose, and carries ten sharply pointed cuticular "leaf crown" elements surrounding the mouth opening.

At the base of each chord a lateral body is present. Every quarter of the worm contains a few large muscle cells. In the intestine only a few multinucleated cells, lined with microvilli, are present. The reproductive organs are confined to the posterior two-thirds of the worm.

The male measures 8–10 mm by 300–350 μm and has a well-developed symmetrical bell-shaped copulatory bursa, adorned with long typically curved spicules, characteristic for the species. The female measures 8.5 mm by 295–325 μm. The vulva is in a slightly anterior position to the anus. These features ensure differentiation from hookworms. The medium-sized eggs measure 60–63 μm by 27–40 μm. They are thin shelled, colorless, and broadly ovoid in shape with wide round poles, and contain 16–32 blastomeres.

Life Cycle[14]

The eggs are passed with the stools. They hatch in the soil and molt twice to become L3 infective larvea. These remains exsheathed and enter the host by the oral route and will exsheath on the 1st day that they reach the small intestine. They lay on day 3 either in the lumen or coiled up in the depth of the mucosa. The majority remain in the small intestine; others move into the cecum and colon. They bore a passage into the submucosa or muscularis muscosae. They enclose themselves in cysts, visible to the naked eye as fine granulations on the mucosa. The fourth molt is achieved around the time of the encystation. Between day 6 and day 8 the L4 larvae migrate back from the cysts of the lumen. At about day 15 L5 larvae appear and may be passed in the feces. On day 21 females are not yet gravid. On day 30, 98% of the worms are mature and the females are laying eggs.

The prepotent period is 28–30 days. The period of potency 77–157 days.

The immunity status of the host can suppress or cause large fluctuations in the egg production. The egg count is higher in spring and summer than in winter.

More exhaustive knowledge about the existence and/or the arising of hypobiosis is badly needed.

2. Host

The *Oesophagostomum* worm may be hampered in its emergence by a strong reaction of the host. This produces multiple nodules in the wall of the lower ileum and colon, tumor-like solitary masses in the ileocecal region, and even abscesses of the overlying abdominal wall. Death of the worm is followed by calcification. This will bring about a fortuitous finding on a roentgenogram of the abdomen.

14 The life cycle of *O. apiostomum* has not been worked out completely in its normal simian host. But the evolution of *O. columbianum* in sheep and goats and *O. venulosum* in lambs has been studied experimentally

ANTHONY and MCADAM (1972) in a postmortem observation in Uganda, report the presence of such nodules spread along the length of the colon which could have easily been mistaken for carcinomatosis.

Abdominal pain, localized in the right lower quadrant, will increase gradually but without provoking nausea, vomiting, or diarrhea. It corresponds to a mass on the palpation of the fossa iliaca dextra. Multiple helminthomata, up to 100 or even more, may extend along the length of the colon and initiate intussusception or incarceration of a hernia. Since man is an accidental host, the *Oesophagostomum* worms are unable to complete their life cycle. Thus larvae may become locked in the cyst. The rupturing of the nodule into the lumen of the bowel can give rise to bleeding, dysenteric disorders, and bacterial superinfection. If the nodule ruptures into the abdominal cavity peritonitis may ensue.

3. Diagnosis

Diagnosis is arduous. Eggs appear in the feces 30–40 days after infection. If eggs are present in the stool, daily sampling fluctuates greatly. They can easily be mistaken for hookworm. Eosinophilia is the rule for the common intestinal worms. No specific immunodiagnostic tests are available. The roentgen examination will show defects quite indistinguishable from many other specific and aspecific lesions, i.e., carcinoma, Crohn's disease, tuberculoma, and ameboma.

4. Geographical Distribution

About 50 cases of human esophagostomiasis have been reported in indigenous and expatriate residents of tropical Africa, both East (KAMINSKY and NDINYA-ACHOLA 1977) and West Africa (HAAF and VAN SOEST 1964), and a few isolated infections in Indonesia, Philippines, China, and Brazil have been recorded.

5. Prevalence

Infection in man can reach 4% in some foci of northern Nigeria. *Oesophagostomum* is not uncommon in northern Ghana and in the lake Omo region (Kenya). All of the foci are in dry savanna. Transmission from man to man is possible: household infections have been recorded.

II. Drugs

1. Specific Anthelmintic Treatment

In man no active drug has been identified. But on the basis of experience in animals it can be expected that besides CCl_4 and TCE, levamisole and tiabendazole can be recommended.

2. Surgical Treatment

The nodules, usually 4–6 cm in diameter, and accompanying inflammatory masses remain a problem for the surgeon. Puncture and aspiration may offer a theoretical possibility for an etiological diagnosis (worm bathing in thick sterile pus) and also for a rapid resolution of the nodules. But exeresis of the suspected masses will be the rule.

K. Strongyloidiasis

I. Introduction

Strongyloides stercoralis (BAVAY 1876); STILES and HASSEL 1902 is a member of the family Strongyloididae (order Rhabdiasoidea). It is also known as *Anguillula stercoralis* BAVAY 1876. This worm was discovered by NORMAND in 1876 in diarrheic stools of French soldiers in Cochin China (South Vietnam). In addition to its clinical manifestations in man, this small nematode bridges the gap between free-living and parasitic modes of life. Both life cycles may alternate depending on the environmental conditions. *S. stercoralis* worms can maintain a parasitic life cycle or repeat free-living generations in decaying fruit and other vegetal debris. They can find a way into animals and man and their adaptation is facilitated by their former feeding conditions, which can open new evolutionary avenues. Up to a certain point this justifies their classification as "pioneering parasites." Other primates, cats, dogs, and various mammals can become infected. Reciprocally man becomes contaminated in Africa by *S. fülleborni*, a parasite of primates.

1. Parasite

1. *The parthenogenetic females* constitute practically the parasitic generation as parasitic males are either absent or extremely rare. They are among the smallest nematodes parasites of man, but are strongly embedded in its tissues. They anchor themselves with their buccal capsule to the mucosa of the duodenum, jejunum, or ileum or burrow their anterior ends into the submucosa. Localization in the respiratory, biliary, or pancreatic system is exceptional. They measure 2.0–2.5 mm in length with a diameter of 40 µm (30–75 µm) and are transparent and filiform. Their cuticle is finely striated and their tail pointed. The buccal capsule is small (smaller than the buccal capsule of the hookworm), and the mouth is surrounded by three small lips. The esophagus is long and cylindrical, lacks a posterior pharyngeal bulb, and joins the midgut in its anterior third, which ends in a ventral anus. The vulva opens in the posterior third. The paired oviducts and uteri are divergent and contain only a few eggs (10–20) at a time. Several dozen eggs are released daily in the submucosa or in the lumen of the gut.

The parasitic male is met only exceptionally and measures only 0.7 mm × 40 µm. The eggs are ovoid, grayish-green, and with a thin transparent shell. They measure 50–60 × 30–35 µm and are partially embryonated. The short, thick L1 larvae hatch within the submucosa or during their passage through the gut. These L1 rhabditoid larvae, 300–380 µm long and 20 µm in diameter, characterized by a club-shaped anterior portion of the esophagus, are very active, escape into the lumen, and pass out with the feces. The L3 larvae, free-living filariform larvae measure 490–630 µm × 20 µm. They develop no further unless they find access to a new host, by skin penetration or ingestion, or are able to become free-living adults.

2. *The free-living females* are shorter and stouter (1 mm × 0.06 mm) and have a double-bulbed short rhabditiform esophagus. The position of the vulva is about equatorial and the uteri contain more eggs. *The free-living male* is ventrally curved, measures 0.7–0.9 mm by 40–50 µm, and has a rhabditiform esophagus, two spicules, and a gubernaculum (chitinous sheath in which the spicules can slide up and down). The tail is pointed. Transmission is almost exclusively interhuman. Chimpanzees and dogs have been found infected, but their role as reservoir is negligible for the time being. *S. fülleborni* is common in primates and children in parts of tropical Africa (PAMPIGLIONE and RICCIARDI 1971).

1.1 Life Cycle

Several dozen partially embryonated eggs are produced daily and deposited in the mucosa or submucosa of the jejunum and upper ileum. The L1 rhabditiform larvae hatch in situ and pass out in the feces and thus into the soil. They can either develop there directly into infective L3 filariform larvae (490–630 µm), which await penetration of the skin, or molt in the soil into free-living sexual mature male and female worms. This indirect cycle starts in the presence of as yet unknown favorable conditions. Lastly the rhabditoid larvae may molt in infective larvae in the intestine, which enables the penetration of the perianal skin and autoinfection to take place.

1.2 The Homogenic, Direct Parasitic Cycle

The L1 larvae feed in the soil, molt twice, and become infective filariform larvae (the development is similar to that of hookworms, but the pharynx is longer, while the sheath and notched forked tail are lacking). They can survive in the soil for several weeks, but their resistance to desiccation is slight. Inversely they are also destroyed by too much moisture.

When they come into contact with human skin or oral mucosa, they penetrate the neighboring small dermal blood vessels and are carried by the venous blood through the right heart into the lungs. They break through the wall of the capillaries into the alveolar spaces and molt twice and the adolescent worms travel up the respiratory tree to the pharynx.

Once swallowed, they descend through the esophagus and stomach and mature in the small intestine. Some authors are of the opinion that fertilization occurs in the lung and/or respiratory and intestinal tract. Nevertheless, the female is able to produce eggs by parthenogenesis, which are present 17 days after penetration. However, silent egg-laying periods of up to 5 days make daily examination compulsory for several days. If eggs or larvae are ingested directly, the lung migration does not take place. The larvae burrow directly into the mucosa of the intestine and become mature in situ.

1.3 The Autoinfective Cycle

Some rhabditiform larvae develop into filariform infective larvae while still in the intestinal tract. These invade the mucosa of the ileum or colon, pass into the portal system, and start a complete internal migration, returning via the lungs, upper respiratory tract, and esophagus to the duodenum, and complete their life cycle without an outside passage. This "endo-autoinfection" leads to hyperinfection.

By a variant mechanism the filariform infective larvae developed in the intestine may penetrate immediately through the skin of the perianal region. This "exo-autoinfection," is more common than genuine autoinfection. In this way a *S. stercoralis* infection can persist for decades in persons living outside endemic regions.

If the resistance of the host is very poor or lowered by steroid therapy, immunosuppressive drugs, or immunodepressing diseases, hyperinfection will take place via either a normal or an autoinfective cycle, and end in extreme hyperinfections: both filariform larvae and gravid females are found throughout the body of the host, viz., in portal areas, hepatic lobules, lymphatics, pulmonary arteries, alveoli, etc. Death may follow.

1.4 The Indirect, Heterogenic, Free-Living Cycle

Whenever the external environmental conditions are favorable, one or more successive free-living generations may take place between parasitic generations. But the basic mechanism which determines the return to a free-living cycle is unknown. Some evidence suggests that parasitic females are haploid: if this is taken for granted these haploid larvae will produce parasitic females, while diploid larvae should generate free-living adults.

Rhabditiform larvae will only be able to fulfil, within 24–48 h, the speedy sequence of four molts, into male and female worms if they are deposited in a moist, warm, well-aerated topsoil rich in organic nutrients. These conditions are present only in the tropics and subtropics. After fertilization, partly embryonated eggs are laid. The L1 rhabditiform larvae will hatch, feed on bacteria and organic matter, and molt repeatedly to become nonfeeding infective larvae or to pass through the stages leading to a free-living adult. If the environmental conditions are favorable, whatever that means, several free-living generations may succeed each other.

2. Host

2.1 Epidemiology

Infection follows cutaneous penetration after contact with contaminated soil. This implies favorable environmental conditions for the larvae: lack of sanitary facilities, use of human nightsoil as fertilizer, promiscuous defecation, walking barefoot, etc.

Another mode of infection is the ingestion of infective larvae, present on fingers, drinking vessels, cigarettes, etc., and penetration through the buccal mucosa, followed by the classical migration or direct passage into the intestinal canal. Autoinfection is a not unusual mechanism for maintaining strongyloidiasis over the years.

On the whole, the ecology of the free-living stages is insufficiently known, including their resistance to excessive humidity or desiccation, and to changes in temperature and other environmental conditions. It has been observed that low or high temperature are not well tolerated: rhabditiform larvae do not resist longer than 10 h at 8 °C or at 40 °C, and filariform larvae not more than 1 week.

The survival of *S. strongyloides* is most probably short. The long-lasting infections [15–20–35 years and even more (GROVE 1982)] are not the expression of long-living worms, but of persistent autoinfection, which can maintain the parasitism almost indefinitely.

2.2 Pathology

The *invasion* of infective larvae through the skin produces a so-called "ground-itch" at the site of entry, expressed by itching, swelling, slight hemorrhages, or remaining asymptomatic. This cutaneous phase lasts only 2 days. However, in sensitized individuals the penetration will be accompanied by more severe pruritus, erythema, edema, and petechial hemorrhages. Long-standing autoinfection will be accompanied by a creeping eruption of the "larva currens" type.

The *migration* of the infective larvae induces mainly lung symptoms. The pulmonary phase, starting 1 week after infection, follows the breaking out of the larvae into the air sacs, which produces hemorrhages and leukocytic infiltration, resulting in bronchitis and pneumonitis. This phase is accompanied by a burning sensation in the chest, a nonproductive cough, and rales. The reaction may delay the migration and can even block some larvae in the lungs. The arrested larvae mature on the spot and produce pneumonitis. The clinical picture is similar but not identical to that of the Loeffler syndrome in ascariasis. Other larvae may invade the pleural and pericardial cavities and produce pleuritis and pericarditis.

Concurrent viral and bacterial infections of the lungs may result in more extensive lesions, or in reactivation of quiescent lesions. Confusion with lung tuberculosis or viral pneumonitis does occur.

The burrowing of the adults and the laying of their eggs in the depths of the crypts of duodenal and jejunal epithelium, without crossing the muscularis mucosae, characterizes the intestinal phase appearing after 3 weeks. It produces edema and irritative inflammation leading to fibrosis, atrophy, and flattening of the wall. Sometimes ulceration, necrosis, sloughing of patches of the mucosa, and hemorrhagic enteritis will follow. It brings about abdominal complaints such as a burning sensation, which grows worse 20–30 min after a meal, accompanied or not by nausea, vomiting, and anorexia. Combined with loss of elasticity of the duodenum and jejunum, on X-rays producing a honeycomb appearance of this part of the gut (in about 10%), a presumptive erroneous diagnosis of duodenal ulcer is almost unavoidable, if a parasitic etiology has been overlooked.

Heavy infections cause intractable mucous diarrhea and dehydration. More moderate infections produce mostly alternating diarrhea and constipation. Slight infections may remain practically symptom free, except for occasional discomfort, mild diarrhea, and transitory creeping eruptions.

Erratic migration of infective larvae produce local granulomatous reactions in the lymphatic tissues, liver, gallbladder, myocardium, pleura, brain, urogenital tissues, etc. This haphazard dissemination of larvae is especially frequent in individuals deficient in cell-mediated immune response or under immunosuppressive treatment (including cytostatica, corticosteroids). This emphasizes the serious risk involving a disregard for the presence of even a few larvae in the stools, which may persist for many years. Clinicians should look out carefully for this helminthiasis whenever confronted with immunodepression or planning immunosuppression in individuals who have been exposed to the risk of a *S. stercoralis* infection.

2.3 Clinical Profile

Nearly half of infected persons have neither complaints nor symptoms.

Cutaneous symptoms at the site of penetration – ground itch pruritus, erythema, urticaria, and petechiae – are dependent on the number of larvae and sensitivity of the patient.

Pulmonary symptoms are related to the passage of larvae through the respiratory system: dyspnea, rales, pneumonitis, hemoptysis, irritation of the upper respiratory way, cough, eosinophilic lung infiltrates (up to 5%).

Intestinal symptoms occur when a worm is anchored in the mucosa of the duodenum and jejunum: hunger pain, cramps, diarrhea.

A late creeping skin eruption of the larva currens type may appear after some 10 years or more. It is due to a persistent previously unrecognized but self-perpetuating autoinfection.

One should beware of disregarding the significance of the presence of larvae especially in immunodepressed or -suppressed persons: they may develop a lethal hyperinfection, with intractable diarrhea, dehydration, and emaciation.

The *seriousness* of the infection can be rated as follows:

Very light	< 100 larvae/g
Light	101– 500/g
Moderate	501–1,000/g
Heavy	> 1,000/g
Severe	>10,000/g

2.4 Immunology – Defense Mechanisms

Man is possessed of several defense mechanisms. He has a natural resistance to foreign species, such as *S. ratti*, which are checked at the skin level. But man can become parasitized by *S. fülleborni* von Linstov 1905, normally a parasite of monkeys in Africa and the southwest Pacific.

Age resistance is a biological rule. The skin of children is a weaker barrier for *S. stercoralis*. The immunity residual to a previous infection must be rather weak, since autoinfection can go on for years. Hypersensitivity can arise and produce general and local reactions such as the "larva currens."

The immunity produced in man has not yet been thoroughly investigated. In animals (rats, cats, dogs), active immunity can also be induced by repeated infections of heat-killed filariform larvae or of antigens extracted from infective larvae and adults.

3. Diagnosis

The clinical symptoms are not conclusive, but suggestive: early cutaneous, pulmonary and/or intestinal irritation, and eosinophilia. Later on, larva currens occurs.

The parasitological evidence is usually easily obtainable. Findings in freshly passed stools or after concentration methods may include, in addition to the larvae, which are usually rhabditoid and occasionally filariform, eggs to be differentiated from those of hookworms and *Trichostrongylus*. In stools kept for a period of over 36 h even adult worms can be present. Larvae can also be found in sputum, duodenal fluid, and urine. Stool examination is based on direct smear, thick cellophane smear (the Kato technique), and concentration methods, such as zinc sulfate centrifugal flotation or the Saex method. Culturing larvae to their infective stage is carried out on charcoal (larvae are recovered with a soft brush from the condensation drops on the lid) or on filter paper strips (Harada-Mori technique, with Sasa's modification), which is the most dependable method for correct identification. The differential diagnosis of *S. fülleborni* can be performed on eggs: 53 × 35 µm (48–61 × 30–40 µm) or on free-living adults. Serological tests and complement fixation or indirect fluorescent antibody test methods, making use of the cross-reacting filaria-antigens, are sometimes helpful, especially in pulmonary pathology and late-stage symptoms.

4. Geographical Distribution

Strongyloidiasis is a cosmopolitan parasitosis and a member of the soil-transmitted helminthiasis group. The infective larvae penetrate through the skin in a way similar to hookworm. Therefore their endemic zones coincide, without being superposable. The free-living stages are favored by warmth and by moisture of the soil; consequently their prevalence will be higher in tropical and subtropical regions than in a temperate climate. Their preference for a humid environment results in a patchy distribution: abundant in favorable surroundings, scarce in semiarid and arid regions. On the other hand the temperature and humidity prevailing in deep mines fosters the existence and persistence of underground foci in temperate regions. The presence of strongyloidiasis is also to a large extent dependent on low sanitary standards, but the holidays of the affluent and the educated in "folkloristic hideways" equally present identical risks.

Strongyloidiasis is found in all age groups, but real misery is the fate of the immune-deficient.

With a focal distribution and a great variability within the foci, strongyloidiasis is present in all the continents:

Africa:

The infection is present over the whole area of Africa's tropical zones: Benin, Cameroun, Congo, Ethiopia, Gabon, Madagascar, Malawi, Republique Centro-Africain, Togo, Zambia, Zaire, the Maghreb and the Nile valley; it is limited in Egypt to some foci.

America:

South America, mainly Brazil, Colombia, Suriname; Central America and the Caribbean; southern states of the United States.

Asia:

Middle East, Iran; central and south China; Southeast Asia, Vietnam; Japan and all of the tropical areas of this continent.

Europe:

Mainly southern and eastern regions: Bulgaria, Italy, Greece, Iberian peninsula, Romania, southern Poland, southern regions of the USSR; Yugoslavia and microfoci in underground mines.

Oceania:

Larger islands of the Pacific Ocean.

5. Prevalence

The wide distribution of strongyloidiasis is compensated by a rather low prevalence. Moreover its presence is very irregular, due to a strong dependency on environmental conditions and on contact modalities with contaminated soil or water. Its distribution is parallel to that of hookworm, but notwithstanding its free-living multiplication, *S. stercoralis* is, with some exceptions (China), rarer than hookworm. Their coexistence is not usual.

In temperate climates only sporadic infections occur and prevalence is below 1% except in institutionalized groups (mental homes, institutions for retarded children, prisons, camps), where prevalences may reach 25% or more. DANESCU and TOMA (1978) have investigated a strain adapted to temperate zones.

In the tropics the figures vary between 3% and 30%. The available data are dependent on the sampling methods and on the choice of the clusters.

STOLL (1947) estimated the number of infections at 35 million. Taking into account the increase in world population, mainly in countries with poor sanitation, nowadays the number of infections will not be less than 88–90 million and will still be increasing.

Africa:

Cameroun: 7.8%–16.6% (labor) and 7.5%–16% (schoolchildren, Douala)
Congo (Brazzaville): 76.6% (children)
Ethiopia: 6%
Nigeria: Kwara State, 1.1%; Benin State, 2%; Northern Province, 4%
Rwanda: 1.9%. For the period 1950–1960 estimated at >150,000
Zaire: Lower Zaire, 25% (17%–30%), but a Kibambi focus with 61%; Djili, according to age groups: <1 year, 2.2%; 1–5 years, 17.4%; 6–15 years, 20%; >15 years, 15.2% (KRUBWA et al. 1974a); Kinshasa, 4.8% [men, 3.7%; women, 8.2% (ORBAN 1972)]. In the whole of Zaire the number was assessed at between 500,000 and 600,000 (1950–1960) (JANSSENS 1965)
Zambia: 13.3%
Zimbabwe: ±1% (Burma Valley, 0.3%; Gaboona, 1%; Harare, 0.8%; Inyanga, absent)
S. fülleborni is sometimes the commoner species

America:

Brazil, 38%–85% in some foci; Colombia, 15%–20%; Costa Rica, urban, 0.7% (0%–3%); rural 1.6% (0%–45%); Mexico, 4% (0%–16%); Suriname, 1.4% to 25%–40%; United States, East Kentucky (children), 4%; New York (mentally retarded), 17%

Asia:

Iran, Caspian Sea area, 10%; Philippines, up to 85%, Papua New Guinea (*Strongyloides* sp.): Star Mountains, 1%; North Fly, 13%; Delta, 1%; Wabo, 42%; Kamea, 78%

II. Drugs

Strongyloidiasis has been a headache for the therapeutist for many years. No natural or traditional compounds have been of value. The first synthetic product with some activity was Gentian violet; dithiazanine followed, but had to be withdrawn due to severe side effects and even fatal poisoning. Bephenium hydroxynaphthoate was found ineffective.

1. Synthetic Drugs

1.1 Old Timers

1.1.1 Gentian Violet (Crystal Violet)

1.1.1.1 State of the Art

Gentian violet is a mixture in variable proportions of the tetra-, penta-, and hexamethyl derivates of rosaniline, with the pentamethyl derivative predominating. Readily soluble in water it gives a violet solution. Gentian violet possesses anthelmintic activity (WRIGHT and BRADY 1938).

1.1.1.2 Assessment

The use of gentian violet against *S. stercoralis* has been underlined by RIZZOTTI (1952). After one treatment 34% were freed of the infection (13 out of 38), 26% (10 out of 38) needed two series, 16% (6 out of 38) needed three, and 24% (9 out of 38) even needed four series. He used the following schedule: 60 mg t. i. d. for 16 days, or rather up to a total of 3 g or 50 capsules of 60 mg: hence the 16 days.

This was confirmed by TANAKA et al. (1960) on Okinawa, but without giving any figures, and by SAN JUAN (1962) in Rio de Janeiro.

It became generally agreed that administration of a 0.5% or 1% solution by duodenal intubation provides a higher CR. SCHREIBER (1959) using 15 ml of a 1% solution achieved a CR of 82% (14 out of 17) and even 90% (28 out of 31). Intravenous administration has been also tried, but the use of a 0.5% solution has given conflicting results: a CR of 91% (41 out of 45) by PALMER (1950) and complete failure (0 out of 15) by BROWN et al. (1957).

1.1.1.3 Dosage, Mode of Administration

Capsules or enteric-coated tablets of 30 or 60 mg are available for oral administration. The solutions have to be prepared extemporaneously. The schedule is 60 mg t. i. d., after meals, for 8–10 days and repeated over three to four courses, separated by rest periods of 1 week; or, daily intraduodenal intubation of similar dosages. Intravenous administration has never been justified.

1.1.1.4 Side Effects

Untoward reactions include nausea, vomiting, abdominal pain, diarrhea, headache, and vertigo. Gentian violet is no longer in use.

1.1.2 Bephenium Hydroxynaphthoate

1.1.2.1 State of the Art

The localization of *S. stercoralis* in the gut at the same level as hookworm has justified some expectations concerning possible bephenium activity against strongyloidiasis. Its lesser efficacy against *N. americanus* somewhat reduced the prospects.

1.1.2.2 Assessment

Salem et al. (1965) demonstrated in four cases that 2.5 g bephenium base has no effect on *S. stercoralis*.

1.1.2.3 Dosage, Mode of Administration

See Sect. B.II.3.2.4.3.

1.1.2.4 Side Effects

See Sect. B.II.3.2.4.4.

1.1.2.5 Contraindications, Precautions

See Sect. B.II.3.2.4.5.

1.1.2.6 Conclusion

Bephenium hydroxynaphthoate is without anthelmintic activity against *S. stercoralis*.

1.1.3 Basic Bismuth Carbonate

Deschiens and Benex (1957) found basic bismuth carbonate capable of inhibiting the development of *S. stercoralis* and *S. fülleborni* in coproculture and suggested a possible use for it in strongyloidiasis. No results in man have been published.

1.1.4 Dithiazanine Iodide (Telmid, Delvex)

This dicarbocyanine derivate is an intense blue-violet powder with very poor solubility and therefore without significant absorption. In the intestinal lumen the drug level is high and the stools are stained blue and eliminate the drug.

1.1.4.1 State of the Art

The antihelmintic properties of diathiazanine iodide were demonstrated by MacCowen et al. (1957) and its value in the treatment of strongyloidiasis was ascertained by Correa (1958), Miller et al. (1958), and Brumpt and Ho-Thi-Sang (1959).

1.1.4.2 Assessment

Table 50. Treatment of *Strongyloides stercorolis* infection by dithiazine iodide

Efficacy	Doses	Number treated	CR	ERR larval RR	References
100%	200 mg t.i.d./5 days	23	100	–	VINKE and VAN DER SAR (19:
	600 mg/7 days	–	100	–	CORREA (1958)
	600 mg/5 days	–	100	–	AGUILAR (1959)
≧90%	20 mg/kg/10 days (max. 600 mg)	16	94	–	BASNEUVO et al. (1959a, b)
	200–600 mg/8 days	45	93	78	GUERERO et al. (1960)
	200 mg t.i.d/21 days	20	90	–	SWARTZWELDER et al. (1957b
	100 mg t.i.d/7 days	–	94	–	CORREA (1958)
	600 mg/21 days	100	90	–	FIGUERIDO MENDES et al. (1S
	25 mg b.i.d/2–3 days	–	96	–	CAMPBELL and CUCKLER (196
≧70%	400–600 mg/5 days	–	77	–	VILLAREJOS and SALDANA (19
	15–20 mg/kg/14 days	–	71	–	NAVARRO-HILDAGO and URIE (1962)
	30 mg/kg/3 days	14	71	–	CERF (1958)
≧60%	6–20 mg/kg/7 days	12	67	–	WANG and GALLI (1965)
	200 mg/ t.i.d./14 days	148	60	–	JANSSENS (1971)
≧50%	200 mg t.i.d/7 days	7	57	–	BRUMPT and HO-THI-SANG (1S
	600 mg/5 days	–	52	–	FARID (1964)
	20 mg/kg/2 days	44	50	–	CERF (1958)
<50%	10 mg/kg/5 days (max. 100 mg)	–	33	–	MEJIA and BIAGI (1959)
	20 mg/kg (max. 600 mg)	57	14	–	MILLER et al. (1958)

1.1.4.3 Dosage, Mode of Administration

The drug is supplied as enteric-coated, 100-mg tablets. Three doses of 200 mg repeated daily for 5–14 days have been agreed upon. Overdosages have obviously been due to confusion about the dosage fixed at 40 mg/kg and even 20 mg/kg corresponding with 2.4 g or 1.2 g, instead of 0.6 g for an adult.

1.1.4.4 Side Effects

When administered in enteric-coated tablets side reactions have been generally mild, infrequent, evanescent, and limited to headache, nausea, vomiting, and diarrhea. But, administered as such, dithiazanine easily leads to intolerance: striking nausea, vomiting, abdominal disturbances, diarrhea, dizziness, headache, fever, allergic reactions, urticaria, edema, albuminuria. Higher absorption occurring in some individuals can be assessed by the appearance of a bluish-green urine and a bluish discoloration of the conjunctiva, some of the many signals which indicate that the treatment should be stopped.

Dithiazanine has been used widely and successfully for several years, due to the fact that practitioners have learned ways of limiting complaints and of reducing side effects.

Two lessons can be learned from this experience: dyes to be taken orally irritate the mucosa of the digestive tract and the unpleasant secondary reactions can be avoided by its administration in enteric-coated tablets.

Resorption and metabolism of dyes vary from individual to individual. They are also undoubtedly dependent on the state of the mucosa. An abnormal degree of absorption can be assessed by the appearance of a bluish-green urine and a bluish discoloration of the white of the eyes, nail beds, etc. These signals which indicate that the treatment should be stopped have not always received the needed attention.

Severe lesions of the mucosa markedly enhance the crossing of the intestinal barrier. This systemic invasion will produce severe dysfunction and greenish-gray staining of several organs (kidney, heart, liver), and can lead to death. Between 1960 and 1968, eight deaths were associated with dithiazanine (ABADIE and SAMUELS 1965). These fatalities were the reason for the withdrawal of dithiazanine from the list of accepted drugs.

1.1.4.5 Contraindications, Precautions

Contraindications are at present irrelevant.

1.1.4.6 Conclusion

Dithiazanine is undoubtedly a good polyvermicide and was the first really active drug against strongyloidiasis. However, its ratio of harm: efficacy is unacceptable since the anthelminthiasis is only disturbing on the whole. Its withdrawal from the market was a sound decision. It is astonishing that such a potentially dangerous drug has been used by some in combination with TCE without accident.

1.1.5 Pyrvinium Pamoate (Povan, Vanquin)

1.1.5.1 State of the Art

BROWN and STERMAN (1958), MEIRA et al. (1961), and WAGNER (1963) have shown that pyrvinium is effective against *S. stercoralis*. Pamoate emerged as the preferable form. The treatment schedule must be more prolonged than for enterobiasis, since the drug must enter the crypts where the worms live.

1.1.5.2 Assessment

Table 51. Treatment of *Strongyloides stercoralis* by pyrvinum pamoate

Efficacy	Dosage	Number treated	CR	References
≧90%	2.6 mg/kg/7 days	12	92	WANG and GALLI (1965)
≧80%	5 mg/kg t.i.d/5 days	18	83	WAGNER (1963)
	5 mg/kg t.i.d/7 days[a]	–	80	BROWN and STERMAN (1958)
	5 mg/kg t.i.d/5 days	10	80	TANAKA et al. (1965)
≧70%	3–10 mg/kg t.i.d/3–5 days	34	76	WAGNER (1963)
<50%	5–10 mg/kg/3 days	20	15	MEIRA et al. (1961)

[a] Pyrvinium chloride was used

1.1.5.3 Dosage, Mode of Administration

Pyrvinium pamoate is available in tablets containing the equivalent of 50 mg base and a suspension containing 50 mg base in each 5 ml. The dosage of 5 mg/kg t.i.d. for 5 days appropriate for adults should also be adopted for children. The published details do not generally make it clear whether the doses are expressed in pyrvinium base or in its pamoate, although the ratio is 5:7.5.

1.1.5.4 Side Effects

See Sect. B.II.3.2.8.4.

1.1.5.5 Contraindications, Precautions

See Sect. B.II.3.2.8.5.

1.1.5.6 Conclusion

Although efficient, the use of pyrvinium pamoate will be only occasional: it has been displaced by tiabendazole.

1.2 Newer drugs

1.2.1 Albendazole

1.2.1.1 State of the Art

Albendazole has shown a broad spectrum of activity against some nematodes, trematodes, and platyhelminths parasitizing various animals. Moreover, the LD_{50}, after oral administration, is greater than 5 g/kg in mice and 1.5 g/kg in rats. These data have led to this drug being tried in humans, and indeed its tolerance is good and the results on several intestinal helminths encouraging.

1.2.1.2 Assessment

Table 52. Treatment of *Strongyloides stercoralis* infection by albendazole

Efficacy	Dosage	Number treated	CR	References
100%	200 mg b.i.d/3 days	7	100	CAMILO-COURA et al. (198
	20 mg/kg/3 days, repeat after 2 weeks	2	100	MOJON and PIENS (1982)
90%	16 mg/kg/3 days, repeat after 2 weeks	10	90	MOJON and PIENS (1982)
≧80%	2–8 mg/kg/b.i.d./3 days, repeated after 2 weeks	8	87	ROSSIGNOL (1981)
	8 mg/kg/b.i.d/3days, repeated after 2 weeks	8	87	MOJON et al. (1981)
	1,200 mg (3 × 400 mg?)		88	FERNANDEZ ORTEGA (19
	16 mg/kg/3 days, repeated	7	86	MAISONNEUVE et al. (198
≧70%	800 mg/3 days	66	77	COULAUD et al. (1982a)
≧60%	400 mg/3 days, repeated after 2 weeks	5	60	MOJON et al. (1981)
	400 mg/3 days, repeated after 2 weeks	5	60	MAISONNEUVE et al. (198
	20 mg/kg/5 days	5	60	MOJON and PIENS (1982)

Table 52 (continued)

Efficacy	Dosage	Number treated	CR	References
≧50%	400 mg	6	50	PENE et al. (1981)
	200 mg b.i.d/3 days	12	50	BARANSKI et al. (1981)
≧40%	4 mg/kg b.i.d	9	44	MOJON et al. (1981)
	8 mg/kg/3 days	9	44	MAISEONNEUVE et al. (1981)
	400 mg/3 days	25	48	PENE et al. (1981b)
	400 mg	25	44	ROSSIGNOL (1981)
≧20%	100 mg/b.i.d/3 days	4	25	LUMBRERAS CRUZ et al. (1981)
	2–8 mg/kg/b.i.d/3 days	21	24	ROSSIGNOL (1981)
<20%	2 mg/kg b.i.d	8	12.5	MOJON et al. (1981)
	4 mg/kg/5 days	8	12.5	MAISONNEUVE et al. (1981)
	4 mg/kg, repeated after 2 weeks	3	–	GARIN (1981)
	8 mg/kg/b.i.d	4	–	MOJON et al. (1981)
	16 mg/kg/3 days	6	17	MOJON and PIENS (1982)

1.2.1.3 Dosage, Administration

Albendazole is available in chewable tablets containing 100 mg or 200 mg of active substance and a suspension containing 100 mg/ml. The dosage should be 16 mg/kg or 800–1,000 mg daily for adults, repeated on three consecutive days.

1.2.1.4 Side Effects

See Sect. B.II.3.2.1.4.

1.2.1.5 Contraindications, Precautions

See Sect. B.II.3.2.1.5.

1.2.1.6 Conclusion

Albendazole has, in the most favorable situations, only a very limited effect on *S. stercoralis*, provided the treatment is repeated after 2 weeks.

The negative outcome of some 37% of the placebo controls reduces the value of the available data and argues against the claim that this drug does represent a worthwhile acquisition for the control of strongyloidiasis.

The most recent data show that 800 mg in a single dose for three consecutive days gives a CR of 77% (COULAUD et al. 1982a), against 45% following 400 mg once a day for three consecutive days (PÈNE et al. 1982a). However, control for 6–9 months is no guarantee of a full cure, as larvae of endogenous origin may reappear after 18–21 months.

1.2.2 Cambendazole[15]

1.2.2.1 State of the Art

The structure of cambendazole is similar to that of tiabendazole but is, due to its slower metabolization, ten times more active. Consequently, it has been tried out

15 ICN – USA FARMA, Saõ Paulo

as a new broad-spectrum anthelmintic in cattle (HOFF et al. 1970 and BAKER and WALTERS 1971) and in sheep (EGERTON and CAMPBELL 1970).

An assay in human strongyloidiasis was undertaken by MARTIRANI and RODRIGUES (1976) and RODRIGUEZ et al. (1977).

1.2.2.2 Assessment

Table 53. Treatment of *Strongyloides stercoralis* infection by cambendazole

Efficacy	Dosage	Number treated	CR	Reference
100%	5 mg/kg	40	100	BICALHO et al. (1983)
	5 mg/kg	29	100	RODRIGUES et al. (1977)
	8 mg/kg/3 days	3	100	RODRIGUES et al. (1977)
	12.5 mg/kg/2 days	4	100	RODRIGUES et al. (1977)
≧90%	5 mg/kg	40	95	BARANSKI et al. (1978)
	5 mg/kg	40	95	DE OLIVEIRA GOMES (1977)
	5 mg/kg	39	97	CIMERMAN et al. (1980)
	5 mg/kg	33	91	AMATO NETO et al. (1978)
	5 mg/kg	100	90	HUGGINS (1979b)
≧80%	2.5 mg/kg	24	83	RODRIGUES et al. (1977)
≧70%	25 mg/kg	4	75	RODRIGUES et al. (1977)

1.2.2.3 Dosage, Mode of Administration

An efficient dosage is 5 mg/kg by the oral route, preferably 2 h after light supper. Cambendazole is available in 180-mg tablets.

1.2.2.4 Side Effects

Tolerance is good. Complaints are occasional (< 10%): anorexia, nausea, vomiting, vertigo, colics, and diarrhea.

1.2.2.5 Contraindications, Precautions

No information on contraindications is available (cf. tiabendazole?).

1.2.2.6 Conclusion

Cambendazole seems a useful anthelmintic in the management of *S. stercoralis* infections. However, so far it has only been tried out in Brazil.

1.2.3 Fenbendazole

1.2.3.1 State of the Art

This benzimidazole derivative is known to possess anthelmintic activity against both immature and adult stages of gastrointestinal nematodes in bovine, ovine, and domestic animals. It has only been tried against strongyloidiasis by one team.

1.2.3.2 Assessment

Table 54. Treatment of *Strongyloides stercoralis* infection by fenbendazole

Dosage	Number treated	CR	Reference
100 mg b.i.d./3 days	14	29	SANCHEZ-CARRILLO and BELTRAN-HERNANDEZ (1977)

1.2.3.3 Comments

Fenbendazole is too slightly active against *S. stercoralis* to be of prospective value.

1.2.4 Flubendazole

1.2.4.1 State of the Art

Its broad-spectrum activity has led to it being testing against *S. stercoralis.*

1.2.4.2 Assessment

Table 55. Treatment of *Strongyloides stercoralis* infection by flubendazole

Efficacy	Dosage	Number treated	CR	Reference
≧60%	2 g	5	60	BOUVIER (1976)
	200 mg/3 days	5	60	DANIS et al. (1980)
	600 mg/3 days, repeated	–	67	BOURÉE et al. (1978)
≧50%	200 mg/3–4 days	11	55	GENTILINI (1976)
	600 mg/3 days	–	54	BOURÉE et al. (1978)
	200 mg/4 days	6	50	DANIS et al. (1980)
≧40%	200 mg/3 days (>12 years)	33	42	PENOT et al. (1978)
	300 mg/3 days (>12 years)	15	46	PENOT et al. (1978)
	600 mg/3 days	10	40	BOUVIER (1976)
	100 mg/b.i.d./3 days	28	39	BOURÉE et al. (1982)

1.2.4.3 Dosage, Mode of Administration

See Sect. B.II.3.2.8.3.

1.2.4.4 Side Effects

See Sect. B.II.3.2.8.4.

1.2.4.5 Contraindications, Precautions

See Sect. B.II.3.2.8.5.

1.2.4.6 Conclusion

Flubendazole is neither a useful short-course anthelmintic in strongyloidiasis nor a good substitute for tiabendazole in the hyperinfection syndrome.

1.2.5 Levamisole

1.2.5.1 State of the Art

Levamisole has acquired a valuable reputation among the broad-spectrum anthelmintics. It was therefore logical to try it out also against *S. stercoralis*.

1.2.5.2 Assessment

Table 56. Treatment of *Strongyloides stercoralis* infection by levamisole

Efficacy	Doses	Number treated	CR	Larval RR[a]	References
100%	3.5–7 mg/kg	3	100	–	BOUYER (1970)
	150 mg	6	100	–	DE JONCKHEERE (1975)
	80–150 mg	5	100	–	SCHMITZ and KNACKFUSS (1971)
≧90%	2.5 mg/kg	28	90	–	LUCAS and ODUNTAN (1972)
≧80%	2.5 mg/kg	5	80	–	GENTILINI et al. (1970)
	2.5 mg/kg	8	87	–	LEVAI et al. (1972)
	3 mg/kg	16	81	–	SEZI (1974)
≧70%	2.5 mg/kg	40	75	–	GATTI et al. (1972b)
	2.5 mg/kg	122	75	–	ORBAN (1972)
	150 mg	11	73	80	VAN LANDUYT (1973)
	300 mg	9	78	96	VAN LANDUYT (1973)
≧60%	2.5 mg/kg repeated after 2 weeks	8	62	–	ASMERA (1974)
≧50%	2.5 mg/kg[b]	16	56	–	GATTI et al. (1972)
	2.5/kg[c]	62	55	63	GATTI et al. (1972)
	2.5 mg/kg	6	50	–	DUFEK and KALIDOVA (1973b)
≧40%	2.5 mg/kg	91	41	–	COENE (1969)
<40%	2.5 mg/kg	147	32	41	KRUBWA et al. (1974a)
	100 mg t.i.d.	18	22	–	ANDRADE FREIRE et al. (1969)

[a] RR, reduction rate
[b] D- and L-tretamisol
[c] Mass treatment on a quaterly schedule; CR after the first: 50–56%, after the second, 38%; and after the third, 50%

1.2.5.3 Dosage, Mode of Administration

For obvious reasons only the usual dose of 2.5 mg/kg or 150 mg has been retained. See Sect. B.II.3.2.9.3.

1.2.5.4 Side effects

See Sect. B.II.3.2.9.4.

1.2.5.5 Contraindications, Cautions

See Sect. B.II.3.2.9.5.

1.2.5.6 Conclusions

Levamisole deserves some credit as an anthelmintic in strongyloidiasis. In mass-treatment trials, on a quarterly administration schedule, the results have, however, not produced substantial consistent differences after 9 months (JANCLOES et al. 1979). This lack of demonstrative benefit in mass control should nevertheless not overshadow the successes achieved in the individual treatment with a single dose of roughly 2.5 mg/kg. Besides the reduction of larvae passing with the stools (MANDOUR and OMRAN 1976), the rapid and complete immobilization in vitro of filariform larvae after 1 h contact with 10 mg levamisole/100 larvae is an important element in the estimation of its value in the control of hyperinfections.

Furthermore, ISEBAERT (1970) drew attention to the fact that the addition of 50 mg levamisole to 100 mg mebendazole improved the efficacy of the latter.

1.2.6 Mebendazole

1.2.6.1 State of the Art

GATTI et al. (1972b) and VANDEPITTE et al. (1973) assessed the potentiality of mebendazole against strongyloidiasis. Its vermicidal activity was boostered significantly when a micronized preparation was used.

1.2.6.2 Assessment

Table 57. Treatment of *Strongyloides stercoralis* by mebendazole

Efficacy	Doses	Number treated	CR	Larval RR[a]	References
100%	100 mg b.i.d./3 days	5	100	–	GATTI et al. (1972)
	100 mg b.i.d./3 days	2	100	–	ASPÖCK et al. (1977)
≧90%	200 mg/2 days or 100 mg/4 days	11	91	–	PEÑA-CHAVARRIA et al.(1973)
≧80%	100 mg b.i.d./3 days	6	83	–	VANDEPITTE et al. (1973)
	100 mg b.i.d./3 days	8	88	–	GOLDSMID (1974)
	100 mg b.i.d./3 days (C)[b]	40	82	–	SHAFEI (1976)
	100–200 mg b.i.d./2 days	30	80	–	SHAFEI (1974)
	200 mg b.i.d./3 days (A)[b]	60	82	–	SHAFEI (1976)
	300 mg b.i.d./3 days (A)	50	84	–	SHAFEI (1976)
≧70%	100 mg b.i.d./3 days	3	75	–	DEGREMONT and BAUMGARTNER (1975)
	100 mg b.i.d./3 days	4	75	–	JAROONVESAMA et al. (1978)
≧60%	100 mg b.i.d./4 days	20	65	–	LORIA CORTES et al. (1974)
	100 mg b.i.d./4 days	21	67	–	MUSGRAVE et al. (1979)

Table 57 (continued)

Efficacy	Doses	Number treated	CR	Larval RR[a]	References
≧50%	100 mg b.i.d./3 days	4	50	71	VANDEPITTE et al. (1973)
	100 mg b.i.d./3 days	13	54	–	RICHARD-LENOBLE and GENTILINI (1980)
	100 mg b.i.d./3 days	6	50	–	CHAIA and DA CUNHA (1971a,
	100 mg b.i.d./3 days	32	50	82	CHONGSUPHAJAISIDDHI et al. (1978)
<50%	75 mg/2 days[c]	12	40	–	GATTI et al. (1972)
	100 mg b.i.d./3 days	24	42	–	KRUBWA et al. (1974b)
	100 mg b.i.d./3 days	30	47	–	SHAFEI (1974)
	100 mg b.i.d./4 days	17	29	71	GATTI et al. (1972)
	200 mg b.i.d./4 days	18	27	–	GENTILINI (1974)
	100 mg/2 days	23	22	–	CHAIA and DA CUNHA (1971a,
	200 mg b.i.d./3 days	17	18	–	GENTILINI (1974)
	100 mg × 2 (1 week)	17	12	–	CHAIA and DA CUNHA (1971a,
	200 mg b.i.d.	22	14	–	CHAIA and DA CUNHA (1971a,
	200 mg/2 days	7	0	–	CHAIA and DA CUNHA (1971a,
	200 mg/4 days	13	8	–	CHAIA and DA CUNHA (1971a,

[a] RR, reduction rate. [b] C, children; A, adults. [c] Nonmicronized

1.2.6.3 Dosage, Mode of Administration

See Sect. B.II.3.2.10.3.

1.2.6.4 Side Effects

See Sect. B.II.3.2.10.4.

1.2.6.5 Contraindications, Precautions

See Sect. B.II.3.2.10.5.

1.2.6.6 Conclusions

The usual dosage, 100 mg b. i. d. for 3 days, provides inconstant CRs, varying between 40% and 100%. Any attempt at interpretation, taking into account the possible great variability of factors and a number of individualized assumptions, would be probably misleading. The micronized presentation should, however, be further carefully investigated.

Mebendazole is certainly not the drug of choice for strongyloidiasis. But in mixed infections the high level and broad-spectrum activity of mebendazole justifies it as first choice. Its relative efficacy against *S. stercoralis* requires careful stool control in mixed infection before proceeding to a complementary administration of a specific drug.

1.2.7 Pyrantel Pamoate

1.2.7.1 State of the Art

The interesting prospects presented by pyrantel pamoate as a broad-spectrum anthelmintic do not yet include strongyloidiasis.

1.2.7.2 Assessment

A single dose of 11 mg/kg did not produce worthwhile results in 13 children infected with *S. stercoralis* in the southern Cook Islands (DESOWITZ et al. 1970). This has been confirmed by GHADIRIAN and SANATI (1972) in 38 Iranian patients after a single dose of 10 mg/kg and in 6 after 20 mg/kg: none of them was cured. In mass treatment of a rural population in Colombia BOTERO-RAMOS (1974) observed an apparent reduction from 19% to 10%–11%. None of them was cured. No therapeutic action was observed by KATZ et al. (1972) after the administration of 10 mg/kg for 3 days.

1.2.7.3 Dosage, Mode of Administration

The dose, 10 or 20 mg/kg, has to be repeated on three consecutive days.

1.2.7.4 Side Effects

See Sect. B.II.3.2.11.4.

1.2.7.5 Contraindications, Precautions

See Sect. B.II.3.2.11.5.

1.2.7.6 Conclusions

Owing to the fact that the activity of pyrantel pamoate on *S. stercoralis* is not really significant, this drug has no place in individual treatment. On the contrary some benefit may be expected in mass treatment.

1.2.8 Oxantel and Pyrantel

No information is available.

1.2.9 Tiabendazole (Mintezol)

1.2.9.1 State of the Art

Tiabendazole emerged as a breakthrough in the treatment of strongyloidiasis and so far remains unchallenged. FRANZ (1963) demonstrated the activity of tiabendazole on *S. stercoralis*, but the main contribution has been made by Brazilian authors: VILLELA et al. (1962), RODRIGUEZ DA SILVA et al. (1968), CROCE et al. (1963), GOMEZ FERRAZ et al. (1963), and CHAIA and DA CUNHA (1966).

1.2.9.2 Assessment

Table 58. Treatment of *Strongyloides stercoralis* infection by tiabendazole

Efficacy	Dosage	Number treated	CR	References
100%	50 mg/kg (A)[a] and 30 mg/kg (C)[a]	38	100	VILELA et al. (1962)
	50 mg/kg/2 days	3	100	BOTERO (1965)
	25 mg/kg/2 days	1	100	PAPASARATHORN et al. (1964)
	25 mg/kg/5 days (C)	13	100	ESCOBAR (1964)
	50 mg/kg	20	100	JORGE and BARBOSA (1964)
	25–37 mg/kg/2 days	28	100	FRANZ (1965)
	25–37 mg t.i.d./2 days	7	100	FRANZ (1965)
	25–30 mg b.i.d./3 days	15	100	FRANZ (1965)
	25 mg b.i.d./2 days	17	100	MOST et al. (1965)
	25 mg b.i.d./2 days	30	100	BEZJAK (1968)
	12.5 mg b.i.d./3 days	3	100	BOTERO (1965)
	40–60 mg/kg/2 days	3	100	ASSHAUER and MOHR (1966)
	40–60 mg/kg/5 days	10	100	ASSHAUER and MOHR (1966)
≧90%	25 mg/kg/5 days	11	91	CROCE et al. (1963)
	25 mg b.i.d.	50	90	GOMEZ-FERRAR et al. (1963)
	25 mg/kg b.i.d.	38	97	CARRIE (1968)
	50 mg/kg (A)	39	93	CHAIA and DA CUNHA (1966)
	50 mg/kg	51	96	FRANZ et al. (1965)
	25–30 mg/kg b.i.d./5 days	25	92	FRANZ et al. (1965)
	50–60 mg/kg/3–5 days	10	90	FRANZ et al. (1965)
	25–30 mg/kg b.i.d./3 days	20	95	FRANZ et al. (1965)
	25–40 mg/kg/2 days	25	96	NAUENBERG et al. (1970)
	50 mg/kg/2 days	41	93	JANSSENS et al. (1966)
	25 mg b.i.d./3 days	42	93	GROVE (1982)
≧80%	25 mg/kg/2 days	15	87	CROCE et al. (1963)
	25 mg/kg/2 days	10	80	BOTERO (1965)
	25–50 mg/kg/1–3 days	19	89	COWDHURY et al. (1964)
	25 mg/kg (C)	28	86	ESCOBAR (1964)
	25 mg/kg/2 days	21	86	ESCOBAR (1964)
	50 mg/kg (C)	36	89	ESCOBAR (1964)
	50 mg/kg	78	86	DOMART et al. (1967)
	30–50 mg/kg/1–2 days	6	83	GARIN et al. (1965)
	25 mg/kg/2 days	10	80	BOTERO (1965)
≧70%	30 mg/kg	8	75	CHAIA and CUNHA (1966)
	25 mg/kg/2 days	4	75	ESCOBAR (1964)
	50 mg/kg	13	77	ESCOBAR (1964)
	25 mg/kg/2 days	56	70	MOST et al. (1965)
≧60%	50 mg/kg	11	64	RODRIGUEZ DA SILVA et al. (1968)
	50 mg/kg/3 days	29	69	RODRIGUEZ DA SILVA et al. (1968)
	50 mg/kg	10	60	FRANZ et al. (1965)
<60%	50 mg/kg	22	54	CROCE et al. (1963)
	25 mg/kg b.i.d.	21	48	CROCE et al. (1963)
	50 mg/kg	36	58	RODRIGUEZ DA SILVA et al. (1968)

[a] A, adults; C, children

1.2.9.3 Dosage, Mode of Administration

The recommended dosage of 25 mg/kg twice daily on two consecutive days ensures the best CR, but a single dose of 50 mg/kg also guarantees good results. The maximum daily dosage is 3 g. Tiabendazole suspension should be administered after meals.

1.2.9.4 Side Effects

Tolerance is inconstant. Dizziness, anorexia, nausea, and vomiting are the most frequent complaints. Headache, epigastric distress, pruritus, giddiness, drowsiness, and diarrhea are less frequently encountered. Some patients excrete a metabolite which imparts an asparagus odor to their urine, disappearing within 24 h after completion of the therapy. Many other troubles have been related to tiabendazole, including transient leukopenia, crystalluria, rashes, and liver dysfunction, such as severe intrahepatic cholestasis. One should be aware of possible intolerance, but it occurs only occasionally and the side effects are generally light.

1.2.9.5 Contraindications, Precautions

No teratogenic effects have been observed. Nevertheless the drug should be withheld from pregnant and lactating women. Patients should be cautioned against engaging in occupations requiring complete mental alertness, including driving a motor vehicle. On rare occasions *Ascaris* worms are set in motion and may leave by natural exits, such as the mouth and nose.

1.2.9.6 Conclusions

Tiabendazole is still the drug of choice for strongyloidiasis. In the presence of mixed infections, one should remember that next to a specific CR of 95%, tiabendazole gives a CR of 55%–85% for ascariasis and hookworm, but only 15%–35% for trichiuriasis. As a rule early failures remain as such in the following stool controls, but early cures may be misleading: larvae of endogenous origin may reappear after several months (6–18 months).

III. Drug Combinations

1. Cambendazole and Mebendazole

HUGGINS (1977–1978) tried the simultaneous administration of cambendazole, 3 mg/kg, and mebendazole, 5 mg/kg, and compared the CR after a single dose and following a 3-day course.

Table 59. Treatment of *Strongyloides stercoralis* infection by a combination of cambendazole and mebendazole

	Number treated	CR	References
Cambendazole 3 mg/kg + mebendazole 5 mg/kg	25	95%	HUGGINS (1977/1978)
Cambendazole 3 mg/kg + mebendazole 5 mg/kg for 3 consecutive days	20	90%	HUGGINS (1977/1978)

2. Cambendazole, Mebendazole, and Tinidazole

The combination was provided in either a suspension containing per 5 ml: 112 mg cambendazole, 120 mg mebendazole, and 1.2 g tinidazole or in tablets, containing: 50 mg cambendazole, 134 mg mebendazole, and 500 mg tinidazole (HUGGINS 1979, 1980). Both 20 children and 20 adults had a CR of 90%.

2.1 Side Effects

Side effects are nausea, cephalalgy, and vertigo.

2.2 Conclusion

Although the CRs with this combination are surprisingly good, further information is not available. The reason for this lack of interest in these mixed compounds may the rather low prevalence of strongyloidiasis.

L. Ternidens or False Hookworm Infection

I. Introduction

1. Parasite

Ternidens deminutus[16] RAILLET and HENRY 1909 lodges in the colon of man. The adults are very similar to human hookworms in size and appearance. Their eggs, almost identical to those of the human hookworm, are larger and have usually reached the eight-cell stage when they pass out in the feces.

2. Host

The infection route is probably oral, by means of unclean hands, contaminated food, water, eating utensils, and drinking vessels. Up to now all attempts of experimental infection with this worm, obviously a parasite of primates other than man, have failed.

Man is merely a symptomless parasite-carrier of only a few worms. However, *T. deminutus* may cause ulceration of the intestinal wall, from the duodenum to the colon, and produce blood loss. If the worm load is high, anemia may follow.

In the normal simian hosts adults become encapsulated in nodules. This has not been observed as yet in man. However, the epidemiology and pathology, established only in eastern Africa and the Comoro Islands, is badly in-need of elucidation.

3. Diagnosis

Eggs can be found in the feces by direct or concentration methods. For obvious reasons they will often be mistaken for hookworm or *Trichostrongylus* spp. They measure 84(70–94) × 51(47–55) μm and usually contain eight cells.

16 *Tridontophorous deminutus* RAILLET and HENRY 1905

Culture to the infective stage (Harada-Mori or similar test tube filter paper methods) makes possible correct identification by differentiation of the infective filariform larvae. The recovery of the worm after treatment is equally reliable.

4. Geographical Distribution

Ternidens deminutus is a parasite of primates and monkeys (inter alia, baboons). The first infection in man was discovered on the island of Mayotte in the Comoro Islands. The main focus in humans has been identified in Zimbabwe, but infections have been found over large areas of southern and eastern Africa mainly as local occurrences: Malawi, Mozambique, Uganda, Tanzania, Transkei, Zambia, and Zaire.

5. Prevalence

In Zimbabwe, prevalences are: Burma Valley, 5.2%; Gatoone, 0.7%; Harare, 3.7%; and Inyanga, 8.2%. But in some regions the percentages of infections are said to reach 40%, 60%, and even over 80%. These high rates of infection are observed in the neighborhood of high-rate infections among baboons. More information about the situation in other countries would be welcome.

II. Drugs

All available information has been gathered by GOLDSMID (1972). The usual older drugs are inactive: oil of chenopodium (SANDGROUND 1931), carbon tetrachloride (SANDGROUND 1931 and WEBB 1937), and TCE (SANDGROUND 1931).

Among the newer ones the results in Table 60 have been observed.

Table 60. Treatment of ternides infections by current anthelmintics

Drug	Dosage	Number treated	CR	ERR	References
Bephenium hydroxynaphthoate	2.5 g		88	–	GOLDSMID (1972a, b)
Bitoscanate	100 mg × 3 (12-h interval)	9	22	58	GOLDSMID and MACCABE (1972)
Pyrantel pamoate	20 mg/kg	10	90	50	GOLDSMID and SAUNDERS (1972)
Pyrantel pamoate	10 mg/kg	2	100	–	GOLDSMID and SAUNDERS (1972)
Tiabendazole	10 mg/kg	–	91	–	GOLDSMID (1972a, b)

III. Comments

Pyrantel pamoate is to be recommended although the ERR is low. It is, however, likely that other compounds active against hookworms may achieve similar results. Tiabendazole has been used at an unusually low dosage but with good results.

M. Trichinosis

(Trichiniasis, trichinellosis)

"...and the swine, though he divides the hoof and the cloven footed, yet he cheweth not the end; he is unclean to you" (Lev. 11:4–7).

I. Introduction

Infection by *Trichinella spiralis* (OWEN 1835) RAILLET, 1896 may produce an acute disease characterized by a classical triad of myalgia, palpebral edema, and eosinophilia. This infection is often asymptomatic or expresses itself only by transient, nonspecific symptoms related to the encysted larvae in muscle.

1. Parasite

The short-lived adults are attached to or embedded in the mucosa of the intestine of pigs, rats, bears, and other carnivorous animals, including man. They are minute, threadlike worms (male measures 1.4–1.6 mm, female 3–4 mm) and of uniform diameter (40–60 μm), except a slightly thicker posterior portion.

The ovoviviparous female deposits 200–2,000 larvae in the intestine during its lifetime. The larvae penetrate the lymphatic of blood vessels and travel toward the skeletal muscles, where they encyst. The encysted larvae are capable of transmission to a new host 17–21 days after infection.

The ingested cysts are digested by the gastric juices, and the larvae emerge and invade the mucosa of the duodenum and jejunum. They undergo a number of molts and develop into adult worms.

2. Host

2.1 Epidemiology

Man becomes contaminated by consuming raw or undercooked infected meat. In 75% of the cases the source is the enzootic infection of domestic swine (raw pork meat, dried pork sausages,[17] ground beef adulterated with infected pork), but the meat of dogs, cats, and even horses[18] can also be the origin of the contamination. It is the synanthropic or domestic cycle in close connection with the backyard butcher. In the sylvatic or feral cycle the main source is meat of brown bears, polar bears, wild boars, bush pigs, warthogs, foxes, eskimo dogs, seals, walrus, and whales. The mode of infection of whales, of horses, and of dromedaries is still a matter for conjecture.

2.2 Pathology

During the *"enteral phase,"* both larvae and adult worms produce petechial hemorrhages, edema, traumatic damage, and chronic inflammation of the intestine:

17 The biggest trichinosis epidemic (705 cases) was reported among German prisoners of war in internment in Ireland, after having eaten uncooked pork sausages

18 Since Horses are herbivorous, the only possible source of infection could be infected rats grinded with the grains during processing to compact food for transportation (BOURÉE et al. 1979)

the villi are swollen and hyperemic. The secretion of mucin is excessive, Peyer's patches become prominent, and loops of the bowel are dilated.

These symptoms appear between 12 h and 2–12 days after eating infected meat. Their severity varies with the number of ingested viable parasites.

Gastroenteritis characterizes the early enteric phase. Light infections induce a transient diarrhea. In more severe infections the diarrhea will be accompanied by anorexia, tiredness, weakness, and abdominal discomfort. However, in some cases constipation replaces diarrhea. This initial abdominal syndrome is usually benign in character and occurs during the 1st week. During the abdominal syndrome the antibody level against adults in maximal and may induce a "self-cure phenomenon" (STEWART 1955). A delayed abdominal syndrome has been observed in 35% of cases (OZERETKOVSKAYA 1968).

During the *"migration or dispersal phase"* leading to the muscular invasion, a protean symptomatology can develop. The intestinal symptoms may persist in some 30% of cases for a while, but will be associated with urticarial rashes, facial edema on day 5–7, swelling of the eyelids, myalgia, and flame-shaped hemorrhages under the nails. The myocardium may be involved and produce transient weakness of the pulse, palpitations, and systolic murmurs. The nervous system may be affected, producing not only muscular paralysis but also encephalitis, meningitis, encephalomeningitis, hemiplegia, and coma. Pulmonary manifestations are not uncommon, with dyspnea, chest pain, pulmonary edema, bronchopneumonia, and lung infiltrates of the Löffler type seen on X-rays of the chest. Nephritis can be present in severe infections.

The majority of the infections are light with less than ten larvae/g of muscle. In severe infections the number of cysts per gram of muscle may reach several hundreds. However, the severity of the disease is linked to a large extent with the reactivity of the patient; death may follow infection with only 100 larvae/g, which occurs between the 4th and 6th week. Recovery is the rule, convalescence sets in at about the 5th week but myalgia may persist for months. The vast majority of trichinous infections in man are "subclinical."

2.3 Clinical Profile

1. Trichinosis occurs within 24 h after ingestion of contaminated food and produces gastro intestinal symptoms of a similar nature to food poisoning.

2. Migration of the larvae causes soreness of the muscles; edema of the upper eyelids (day 10); remittent fever, lysing after 1 week; profuse sweating, loss of weight; subconjunctival, retinal, and subungeal hemorrhages; respiratory disturbances; neurological disorders; and myocardial failure.

3. Diagnosis

Eosinophilia, starting at about day 10 and with its acme in the 3rd–4th week, is a useful pointer. The number of leukocytes reaches, in percentage terms, 25%–50% and even 80%; and in absolute figures 4,000 eosinophils/mm^3 is not unusual. The presence of larvae and adult worms in the stools is exceptional. Larvae may be detected in striated muscle and picked up by biopsy or at autopsy from the 4th week on. Serodiagnosis is extremely helpful. In addition, use can be made of complement fixation (CF), latex agglutination (LA), and bentonite floccula-tion tests (BFT); countercurrent electrophoresis (CEP); indirect immuno-fluorescence (IFA); and enzyme-linked immunosorbent assay (ELISA).

4. Geographical Distribution

The distribution of trichinosis is cosmopolitan, but infection is rare in popula-tions abstaining from pork (Jews, Moslims) and is furthermore always focal-ized.

Europe:
- Eastern and central: Bulgaria, Czechoslovakia, Germany, Hungary, Poland (northeast), Romana, USSR, and Yugoslavia
- Western: Denmark, Finland, Spain, Sweden, and Switzerland

Mediterranean area:
- Algeria, Egypt, Greece, Italy, Lebanon, Portugal, and Turkey

America:
- North: Arctic regions (Eskimos), Canada and the United States (New York, Louisiana, Rhode Island)
- Central and South: Argentina, Chile, Mexico, Venezuela (?), and West Indies (Bahamas)

Asia:
- Afghanistan, China, India, Iran, Indonesia, Japan, Kampuchea, Laos, Philippines, Thailand, and Vietnam

Africa:
- Kenya, Senegal, and Tanzania

Pacific area:
- Aleutian, Hawai, Japan, and New Zealand

5. Prevalence

It is almost impossible to obtain reliable data on the prevalence of trichinosis in man. Piecemeal information about the presence of *Trichinella spiralis* cysts at postmortem examination is available. Early in the twentieth century European figures were: Posen, 6.9%; Berlin, 5.6%; and Denmark, 3%, but decreased to about zero in 1913–1915. Persistent urban trichinosis is related to backyard butchers. Recently 3.9% of the necropsies in elderly Polish people were found positive but in the Netherlands 1100 corpses were negative (1967). For the United States, the figures amounted to 14% in 1894 and 5.3% in 1901; out of 12,000 diaphragms collected in 1931–1943, 16% were positive, but of 8,000 diaphragms collected in 1966–1970 in 50 states only 4% (2.2% after age adjustment) showed cysts (ZIMMERMANN et al. 1973). Between 1947 and 1975, 6, 749 cases were re-ported, viz., 232/year, with a mortality of 1.9%. The actual trend is of approxi-mately 100 cases of trichinosis each year.

Another source of information is a surveillance system aiming at detecting outbreaks and monitoring epidemiological trends. In Poland, between 1946 and 1970 13,288 cases were registered, viz., a mean of 532/year, of which 78% or 15% were in the Bialystok region.

A common means of follow-up of the trends in urban trichinosis has been trichinoscopy of pig carcasses in slaughterhouses. In the Federal Republic of Germany, in 1976, trichinoscopy yielded 1:90 million examinations. It only detects infection of or above one to two larvae/g muscle (VIRCHOW 1866) and is now replaced by the more reliable ELISA technique. Nowadays small epidemic outbreaks are more related to backyard butchers and sylvatic sources, so that the available data are without much practical value.

A new source of epidemics is connected with package tourism and exotic meals such as "giant-*mechoui*" of pork (BOURÉE et al. 1976). Imported trichinosis should be suspected in refugees, tourists, and diplomats.

II. Drugs

Since Cobbold (1879) stated that it was absurd to try to kill muscle-dwelling *T. spiralis* by chemotherapy and GOULD (1945) came to the conclusion that there was as yet no specific treatment of trichinosis, much headway has been made. The exhaustive overview and critical examination by CAMPBELL and BLAIR (1974) of all the compounds tried out on *T. spiralis* infections provide an excellent background for available and useful drugs.

An important point in the assessment of therapeutic agents is to remember that the same species can be a definitive and intermediate host and that infective larvae, adults, and migrating and encysted larvae are located in different organs. Consequently it is necessary to distinguish between their activity against the enteral, migrating, and muscular stages. After ingestion of contaminated meat the larvae are liberated in the stomach and pass into the small intestine. During the first 24 h the larvae do not yet attain the mature worm status.

The migratory phase takes places between day 9 and day 21 and, after which the encystment starts. The present discussion is limited to the enteral phase, where the worms and their larvae are within easy reach of a peroral administered compound. An active drug administered during an appropriate space of time will suffice.[19] However, the fact that adult female worms, still alive 2 weeks after infection, are expulsed spontaneously must also be kept in mind.

1. Synthetic Organic Drugs

1.1 Old Timers

Among the compounds presumed active, but without proof of activity within tolerated dosages, betanaphthol, hexylresorcinol, metronidazole, phenothiazine, TCE, and thymol are worth mentioning. As the number of drugs with unequivocal efficacy is steadily increasing, their importance is now at most minor.

1.2 Newer Drugs

The discovery by CAMPBELL (1961) that tiabendazole is active on infected mice and rats was a breakthrough. This has been an incentive to widen the therapeutic

19 Killing the encysted larvae (muscular phase) requires effective plasma levels of poorly absorbed drugs, in higher dosages, or a selection of drugs with a stronger penetrating capacity, and on a more prolonged administration schedule

field with a number of other anthelmintics such as diethylcarbamazine (DEC) dithiazanine (no longer in use), metyridine, piperazine, and tetramisole; further organophosphorous compounds (bromofos, fenthion, haloxon, metrifonate), ethanol (table wine, Irish whiskey), and more specially benzimidazoles (cambendazole, flubendazole, mebendazole, parbendazole).

Yet, out of this selected list only a small number are available for use in man during the enteral phase: piperazine salts, cambendazole, flubendazole, levamisole, mebendazole, pyrantel pamoate, and tiabendazole. Some differences of opinion exist about the usefulness of drug administration after the migratory phase is well on its way. The number of worms is reduced by an efficient treatment during the enteral phase. But the discharge of larvae by gravid females takes place mainly within 15 days after infection. Some gravid worms may, however, persist for months (CARTER 1949). Suppression of the larviposition, also during a possible prolonged phase, is acceptable in presumptive cases which are part of a trichinosis outbreak. This protection by a specific treatment against muscle invasion during the enteral phase stands for "prophylaxis" in trichinosis.

1.2.1 Cambendazole

Table 61. Treatment of trichinosis by cambendazole

Assessment Dosage	Number treated	CR	Reference
200 mg b.i.d./5 days	45	100	CAMPBELL and HARTMAN (1968)

1.2.2 Clofazole

This *o*-chlorophenyl-benzimidazole, a Soviet drug, has been used with interesting results.

1.2.3 Assessment

Table 62. Treatment of trichinosis by clofazole

Dosage	Number treated	CR	Reference
25 mg/kg/5–7 day	11	100	OZERETSKOVSKAYA et al. (1976)

1.2.4 Fenbendazole

State of the Art

Fenbendazole is known to be active in pigs against both immature worms and the migratory phase, at a dosage of 20–50 mg/kg/5–7 days.

1.2.5 Flubendazole

1.2.5.1 State of the Art

This drug, closely related to mebendazole, is active against the three stages. Eradication of *T. spiralis* is achieved as long as larvae and adults remain in the gastrointestinal tract.

1.2.5.2 Assessment

Table 63. Treatment of trichinosis by flubendazole

Dosage	CR	Reference
300 mg/5 days	100	Bourée et al. (1979)

1.2.5.3 Conclusions

Experience in man has been to limited for useful conclusions.

1.2.6 Levamisole

A dose of 2.5 mg/kg kills adults in the intestine (Ozeretskovskaya 1968).

1.2.7 Mebendazole

1.2.7.1 State of the Art

Ozeretskovskaya et al. (1976) found mebendazole quite effective in the prepatent period of the infection. This observation has since been corroborated by several other authors.

Mittermayer et al. (1978, 1979) obtained satifactory results. Vujosevic et al. (1979) observed a prompt defervescence of fever and a general relief of symptoms. Klein et al. (1981) claim a successful outcome in the early invasion stage. The number of cases reported in the literature is still rather small.

1.2.7.2 Assessment

Table 64. Treatment of trichinosis mebendazole

Dosage	Number treated	CR	References
2.5 mg/kg or 300 mg daily/7 days	79	100	Ozeretskovskaya et al. (1976)
100 mg t.i.d./4 days followed by 200 mg b.i.d./6 days	12	100	Vusojevic et al. (1979)
100 mg t.i.d./6–8 days (total dose, 1.8–2.4 g)	18	100	Klein et al. (1980)
100 mg b.i.d./5 days etiotopic prophylaxis (late stage)	45	100	Klein et al. (1981)
200 mg b.i.d./5 days	30	84	Klein et al. (1980)
200 mg t.i.d./4 days followed by 400–500 mg t.i.d./10 days	–	–	Sonnet and Thienpont (1977)
100 mg t.i.d./4 days followed by 200 mg b.i.d./6 days	4	–	Mittermayer et al. (1978, 1979)

LEVIN (1983) reported a successful treatment of subacute trichinosis by a prolonged administration of 400 mg mebendazole every 6 h (total dose of 77 g with side effects limited to a Herxheimer reaction).

1.2.7.3 Dosage, Mode of Administration

During the enteral phase a dosage of 200 mg b.i.d. on five consecutive days will provide satisfactory results. The addition of steroids is recommended particularly in severe infections. Attempts to control the muscle stage should be made according to the schedule recommended by THIENPONT (1976) and SONNET and THIENPONT (1977). It guarantees effective plasma levels of the drug. An initial dosage of 200 mg t.i.d. for 4 days will be followed by a stepwise increase to 400–500 mg t.i.d. for 10 days (total amount of 15 g). The simultaneous administration of prednisolone to alleviate the muscular pain is advisable. Etiotropic prophylaxis is effective. Only 5 out of 37 cases started in late stages developed a light infection. In the control group 22 out of 38 fell ill (57.8%).

1.2.8 Pyrantel Pamoate

Pyrantel pamoate is efficacious at 10 mg/kg against adults in the intestine (OZERETSKOVKAYA et al. 1981). No further information is available.

1.2.9 Tiabendazole

1.2.9.1 State of the Art

CAMPBELL (1961) and CAMPBELL and CUCKLER (1964) showed that tiabendazole has some degree of efficacy in infected mice and rats. The drug kills immature worms in the intestine, inhibits reproduction, and also kills the early migrating larvae.

The efficacy in man of tiabendazole was confirmed in 1964 by STONE et al. (50 mg/kg on two consecutive days), by SPAETH et al. (30 mg/kg b.i.d. for seven consecutive days), by KEAN and HOSKIN (25 mg/kg b.i.d. for 5–7 days). According to the Russian authors, this drug is highly effective against the sylvatic strains and the malignant forms. It was the first drug used with good results against *T. spiralis* and the steadfastness of the results over the years provides reliable evidence.

1.2.9.2 Assessment

Table 65. Treatment of trichinosis by tiabendazole

Dosage	Number treated	CR	References
25 mg/kg/5–7 days	148	99	OZERETSKOVSKAYA et al. (1976)
25 mg/kg/5–9 days (maximum 3 g)	25	84	UNDEUTSCH et al. (1981)
500 mg t.i.d./5 days (total dose, 7.5 g)	21	–	KLEIN et al. (1981)
35–30 mg/kg/5 days	–	100	BOURÉE et al. (1976)

1.2.9.3 Dosage, Mode of Administration

The most advisable schedule seems to be 25 mg/kg or 500 mg t.i.d. for five consecutive days, with a maximum of 7.5 g (5 × 1.5 g). The drug is administered orally.

1.2.9.4 Side Effects

Side effects are frequent and serious, more so in the heavy infections, with a tendency toward allergic reactions: fever, edema, eruptions, myalgia, myocarditis, aphthous stomatitis, and hemorrhagic syndrome. These appear besides the usual weakness and dizziness, headache, nausea, vomiting, abdominal discomfort, urination urge, xanthopsia, and loss of hair.

1.2.9.5 Conclusions

Due to the many untoward effects and the availability of drugs with a better tolerance, tiabendazole is no longer the drug of choice in the treatment of trichinosis.

III. Comments

A number of the newer drugs, which are etiotopically active in animals, show a reassuring activity in human infections.

However, the main difficulty remains the assessment of their efficacy in early infections. Even a muscular biopsy is no guarantee at the time of migration of the larvae and their invasion of the muscles. The majority of the available results are only backed up by clinical improvement or disappearance of symptoms without specificity. Their interpretation needs caution.

Nevertheless mebendazole 200–400 mg t.i.d. for 3 days, followed by 400 mg t.i.d. for 10 days and tiabendazole 25 mg/kg t.i.d. for 5–7 days are certainly advisable drugs in trichinosis.

N. Trichostrongyliasis

I. Introduction

Whenever man is living in close contact with ruminants hosting Trichostrongyloidea (wireworms) the small intestine may become infected, as the life cycle does not involve intermediate hosts. The prevalence will vary with the habits of the community concerned.

1. Parasite

Adult *Trichostrongylus* spp. Looss 1905 are reddish-brown, slender, small strongylate worms; they are 5–10 mm in length, the males being slightly smaller. The head is very small and has no buccal capsule, and the mouth is rudimentary with three small lips; the cephalic papillae are never setose, and the excretory pore is situated in a conspicuous ventral notch near the anterior extremity.

The male has a well-developed copulatory bursa with a reduced dorsal lobe and large lateral lobe supported by stout rays. The structure of the brown, short, spoon-shaped, and equal spicules is useful for differentiating the eight species[20] which have been recovered from man. An elongated boat-shaped gubernaculum is present. The female is obviously bigger and the vulva is in the posterior half of the body and lacks an anterior flap.

The adults live with their heads embedded in the mucosa of the small intestine. The eggs, eliminated in the feces, are similar to those of the hookworm, but longer, narrower, and with more pointed ends (75–100/30–50 μm). The embryonation is more advanced and reaches the morula-type segmentation when leaving the host.

Life Cycle

In the soil, the rhabditiform L1 larva hatches and develops in about 3 days in the infective strongyloid L3. Infection occurs as a rule when the L3 larvae, still loosely included in the second-stage cuticle, are ingested. Although penetration by the cutaneous route and lung migration is possible, this infection mode has become exceptional and is disappearing.

The L3 larva burrows into the duodenal or jejunal mucosa, where the final molt occurs. The worm returns to the lumen, burrows its head in the mucosa and feeds. Maturity is reached in about 3 weeks and at that time eggs start to appear.

2. Host

Contamination results from the eating of vegetables soiled with eggs. This presupposes in turn close contact of man and livestock. The interrelationship "host-worm-environment" is complex: prevalence is highest near the fringes of rivers and grass pastures.

The worms produce traumatic damage by burrowing into the superficial layers of the duodenal and/or jejunal mucosa and by their feeding, which includes some blood-sucking.

Light infections will remain symptomless, with the exception of eosinophilia. In heavy infections desquamation of the invaded mucosa may occur, bringing about abdominal pain and diarrhea. Some blood loss may produce at most a very mild secondary anemia and the resorption of metabolic wastes a moderate eosinophilia. Emaciation and dryness of the skin are most unusual.

Man appears to be more susceptible to certain *Trichostrongylus* species: *T. colubriformis* is the most common, at the other extreme, resistance to *T. rugatus* is complete.

3. Diagnosis

The demonstration of the presence of the characteristic eggs in feces by the direct smear or concentration method, possibly culture of the free-living stages by the

20 *Trichostrongylus orientalis, T. colubriformis, T. vitrinus, T. axei, T. probolurus, T. instabilis, T. brevis,* and *T. skrjabini* (cattle, sheep, goats, camels)

Harada-Mori test tube filter paper method, must be supported by a careful differentiation of the ova from those of hookworms and of the larvae from both hookworm and *Strongyloides stercoralis*. The egg measure 70–100 × 30–50 μm. They resemble those of hookworms, but are longer, narrower, and more pointed at one end. Those present in the feces have reached the morula stage.

It will be remembered that other trichostrongylids and common intestinal parasites with similar life cycles such as *Haemonchus contortus, Ostertagia ostertagi,* and *Mecistocirrus digitatus* may also infect man.

4. Geographical Distribution

The distribution of trichostrongyliasis is extremely uneven. *Trichostrongylus* infection is relatively common in the Near East (Iran, Iraq, Turkey, Egypt) and the Far East (Korea, Japan), southern and Southeast Asia (India, Indonesia), Australia, some regions of the USSR (Armenia, Azerbadjan, southern Asiatic Republics), Africa (Ethiopia, Zaire, Cape Verde), and Latin America (Chile, Peru, Brazil).

5. Prevalence

In Khuzestan (Southwest Iran) *Trichostrongylus* is the dominant intestinal helminth, with a prevalence of 12%–49% (average 25%) in rural communities and 2%–24% (average 15%) in cities. Among nomads, 67% have been found infected. Along the Caspian Sea the prevalence is down to 4%–7%; in central Iran (Ispahan area) the mean prevalence is 33% (20%–46%), on the shores of the Strait of Hornuz, 47%; and in southern Iran, 10%. Korea has a prevalence of 24%, in the Seoul area it is up to 42%; Japan, 10%; India, 24%; Sao Paulo (Brazil), 0.05%; Africa, Zimbabwe (Burma Valley 0.12%; Harare, 0.04%; Inyanga, 1.9%); and Zaire, 10%.

In certain localities the prevalence may reach 60%–70% (Iran) and 50% (Korea). If Stoll's worldwide estimate (1947) of 5.5 million cases is true, not less than 7 million persons are infected in 1980. Due to the longer life span of this worm and close contact with infection sources its prevalence remains high also in the older age group.

II. Drugs

1. State of the Art

Owing to current confusion between the eggs of hookworm and those of *Trichostrongylus* the poor response of the wireworms to a series of specific anti hookworm drugs is a useful source of information.

2. Synthetic Drugs

2.1 Early Drugs

Among the older drugs, some activity has been ascribed to hexylresorcinol (Lamson and Ward 1932), TCE (Hall and Shillinger 1925 and Salem et al. 1965), and gentian violet. A CR of 70% has been attributed to bromo-β-naphthol.

2.2 Bephenium Hydroxynaphthoate

Table 66. Treatment of *Trichostrongylus* infection by bephenium hydroxynaphthoate

Efficacy	Dosage	Number treated	CR	ERR	References
≧70%	2.5 g base	75	77	–	HAHN et al. (1960)
≧60%	2.5 g base	24	67	–	SALEM et al. (1965)
≧50%	2.5 g base	50	56	11	FARAHMANDIAN et al. (1971)
	2.5 g base	34	56	11	FARAHMANDIAN et al. (1972)
<50%	2.5 g base	39	44	–	FARAHMANDIAN et al. (1971)
	2.5 g base	74	34	–	FARAHMANDIAN et al. (1977)
	2.5 g base	13	23	–	FARID and NIALE (1962)

2.3 More Recent Drugs

2.3.1 Bitoscanate

Table 67. Treatment of *Trichostrongylus* infestions by bitoscanate

Efficacy	Dosage	Number treated	CR	ERR	Reference
≧40%	100 mg × 3/36 h	71	39	–	ARFAA et al. (1976)

2.3.2 Flubendazole

Table 68. Treatment of *Trichostrongylus* infection by flubendazole

Efficacy	Dosage	Number treated	CR	ERR	References
100%	100 mg b.i.d./3 days	2	100	–	BRUMPT (1976)
≧80%	100 mg b.i.d./4 days	20	85	92	BECQUET and LABARRIÉRE (1980)

2.3.3 Levamisole

Table 69

Efficacy	Dosage	Number treated	CR	ERR	References
100%	2.5 mg/kg	27	100	–	FLEURY CORREA et al. (1970)
	2.5 mg/kg	27	100	–	CORREA et al. (1973)
≧90%	2.5 mg/kg	65	94	89	FARAHMANDIAN et al. (1974)
	2.5 mg/kg	27	98	–	FARAHMANDIAN et al. (1977)
	2.5 mg/kg	309	94	–	ARFAA and GHADIRIAN (1978)
	2.5 mg/kg	834	91	–	ARFAA et al. (1977)

2.3.4 Mebendazole

Table 70. Treatment of *Trichostrongylus* infection by mebendazole

Efficacy	Dosage	Number treated	CR	ERR	References
100%	100 mg b.i.d./3 days	1	100	–	YALCINKAYA (1977)
	200 mg b.i.d./3 days	4	100	–	BRUMPT (1973)
≧90%	100 mg b.i.d./3 days	48	96	97	SOH et al. (1975)
≧80%	100 mg b.i.d./3 days	6	83	–	BRUMPT (1973)
	200 mg/3 days	6	83	–	FOBA-PAGOU et al. (1978)
	100 mg b.i.d./3 days	54	82	91	FARAHMANDIAN et al. (1977)
	100 mg b.i.d./3 days	27	82	–	FARAHMANDIAN et al. (1977)
≧70%	100 mg b.i.d./3 days	4	75	70	JAROONVESAMA et al. (1978)

2.3.5 Pyrantel

Table 71. Treatment of *Trichostrongylus* infection by pyrantel

Efficacy	Dosage	Number treated	CR	ERR	References
≧90%	20 mg/kg	38	92	–	GHADIRIAN and SANATI (1972)
≧60%	10 mg/kg	75	60	–	FARAHMANDIAN et al. (1971)
≧50%	10 mg/kg	48	50	7	FARAHMANDIAN et al. (1977)
<50%	10 mg/kg	66	45	–	FARAHMANDIAN et al. (1972)
	10 mg/kg	648	30	–	GHADIRIAN and ARFAA (1975)

2.3.6 Pyrantel and Oxantel

Table 72. Treatment of *Trichostrongylus* infection by pyrantel and oxantel

Efficacy	Dosage	Number treated	CR	Reference
50%	10 mg/kg	30	50	GHADIRIAN and ARFAA (1975)

2.3.7 Tiabendazole

Table 73. Treatment of *Trichostrongylus* infection by tiabendazole

Efficacy	Dosage	Number treated	CR	ERR	References
100%	25 mg/kg b.i.d.	4	100	–	CAMPOS et al. (1963)
	50 mg/kg/5 days	1	100	–	ASSHAUER and MOHR (1966)
≧90%	50 mg/kg	38	95	–	FARAHMANDIAN et al. (1971)
	50 mg/kg	47	92	8	FARAHMANDIAN et al. (1977)
≧80%	50 mg/kg		87	–	BRUMPT (1976)

2.4 Conclusion

The drug providing the highest CRs and ERRs in bearers of *Trichostrongylus* spp. is obviously levamisole at its current dosage. Up to now a difference in sensitivity of the different strains has not been observed. For mass therapy in countries where trichostrongyliasis is a problem, mebendazole will be the best choice.

O. Trichuriasis

I. Introduction

Trichuris trichiura or whipworm is a very common and cosmopolitan intestinal helminth, colonizing the large intestine. It is roughly as widespread but with a more patchy distribution than *A. lumbricoides*. Both are often found together; however, with a variable relative prevalence *A. lumbricoides* may get the upper hand or the other way around.

The name Trichuridae is connected with the threadlike shape of the major part of the body, which becomes abruptly thick at the other end. The whole body is reminiscent of a whip with a handle. *Trichuris* means hairtail, however, which is nonsensical since the thread is the anterior part and not the tail. The name was then tentatively changed to Trichocephalus or threadlike head. A name, according to the rules of nomenclature, takes priority over facts so that *Trichuris* had to be retained.

Infection occurs by ingestion of embryonated ova. The larvae do not have a pulmonary migration stage. The adults inhabit the large intestine, with a predilection for the cecum. Heavy infections may produce diarrhea, abdominal pain, and other such manifestations or even rectal prolapse.

In numbers whipworm is next in importance to ascariasis and enterobiasis. The pathogenetic role of *T. trichiura* is slight to insignificant; it is mostly a harmless commensal. *T. trichiura* is an old companion of men: *T. trichiura* eggs were found in the frozen feces of an Inca child, 450 or more years old, and collected at an altitude of 5,300 m (PIZZI and SCHENONE 1951). Although *T. suis* can infect man, the role of the parasites of pigs in man is negligible.

1. Parasite

1.1 Morphology

The pinkish-gray adult worms consist of two distinct portions: the anterior slender, threadlike, longer "whip" part and the posterior broad, fusiform "handle." The anterior part is 100–150 μm in diameter. The narrow extremity carries a simple mouth without lips but which is provided with a stylet, facilitating penetration of the mucosa. The esophagus, except for its somewhat muscular anterior end, contains a simple nonmuscular tube enclosed partially or completely by a single row of glandular cells or stichocytes. Its lumen extends for about two-thirds the length of the anterior end. The anterior portion also contains a subcuticular structure composed of tall columnar cells with porelike openings, the bacillary band. The esophagus opens into the midgut.

The posterior part is 400–700 μm in diameter and contains the intestine and in both sexes the reproductive organs. The anus is located terminally or subterminally, near the tip of the tail. The cuticle is 5–10 μm thick, transversely striated, and carryies a broad longitudinal band of punctiform projections on the ventral surface of the anterior portion.

The male is 30–45 mm long. The coiled posterior end is useful for identification. The copulatory spicule is single and surrounded by a retractile spiny sheath or cirrus, which evaginates when the spicule is protruded. The testis, vas deferens, and ejaculatory duct constitute the reproductive tube, which joins the intestine to form the cloaca.

The female is 30–50 mm long. Its posterior extremity is bluntly rounded. The ovary, oviduct, uterus, vagina, vulva, and seminal receptacle constitute the reproductive tube, which ends near the esophageal-intestinal junction. The vulva opens at the anterior end of the fusiform hindpart of the body, near the junction of the esophagus and intestine. The uterus contains many lemon-shaped unembryonated eggs.[21]

The adult worms live in the cecum and the colon ascendens. In heavy infections they may be present in the terminal ileum, in the appendix, and throughout the colon. They attach themselves to the mucosa by their embedded narrow anterior end.

They produce the typical barrel-shaped eggs, which pass out in the feces some 2–3 months after infection. The longevity of *T. trichiura* varies from 3 to 10 years.

1.2 Life Cycle and Dynamics of Infection

The worm load is usually low. The majority of those infected are inapparent carriers of two to ten worms. This stage of harmless commensalism is outstripped when the number of worms attains 100–1,000. Although estimates of the mean egg output vary from 1,000 to 46,000, an output of about 2,000–10,000 eggs/day is generally accepted. The EPG may thus provide a rough assessment of the number of worms.[22]

The lemon-shaped yellowish-brown egg has two markedly protruding transparent mucoid polar plugs, possesses barrel-shaped smooth side walls with an inner thin layer and outer brownish thick shell, measures 50–58 × 22–27 μm, and is unsegmented when expelled. The embryonation takes from 2 weeks to many months, depending on the temperature: in moist and shady soil at 25–30 °C, the development will take about 21 days. The fertile eggs are ingested with contaminated unwashed salads and vegetables, grown in gardens fertilized with nightsoil. [ANUAR and RACHANDRAN (1977) found 50% of the vegetables in the Penang market contaminated.] Dirt-eating (pica) and promiscuous defecation, as occurs in institutions for mentally retarded children, is another mode of contamination (in the United Kingdom up to 36%).

21 *Trichuris suis* is morphologically identical, but slightly larger (50–68 × 21–31 μm). Experimental infection of man is possible. *T. ovis, T. vulpis* (dog and fox), and *T. muris* can also be transmitted

22 It has been generally agreed that an EPG <5,000 represents a light infection, 5,000–20,000 a moderate infection, and >20,000 a heavy infection

The L1 larvae hatch in the distal portion of the ileum or colon and penetrate the villi and the crypts of Lieberkühn, where they lie coiled up for about 1 week. The still immature worm emerges in the lumen of the cecum. With the help of its constantly probing and slashing stylet, the mouth penetrates just beneath the epithelium of the mucosa of the ileocecal area. After four molts the worm, readily feeding on the tissues of the host, attains maturity. The adult may survive up to 10 years.

2. Host

2.1 Epidemiology

Transmission is ensured by the ingestion of embryonated eggs. Their survival and development depends on a combination of humidity, temperature, and shade existing in many tropical and subtropical regions.

Whenever this is combined with very poor standards of sanitation, especially regarding the disposal of human feces, commensalism begins to fade out. Consequently, trichuriasis is more common in children, mainly mentally retarded dirt-eaters. Household transmission, particularly in institutions caring for mentally deficient patients, allied with a substantial turnover, is the main factor producing high rates of infection also in temperate zones.

The mode of infection is similar to that of *A. lumbricoides*. However, their presence in the feces is influenced by a greater sensitivity of *T. trichiura* to desiccation, direct sunlight, cold, and survival after immersion. In oases, *A. lumbricoides* eggs survive in water, but *T. trichiura* eggs are killed. This is clearly demonstrated by the prevalence of *T. trichiura* and *A. lumbricoides* in three well-defined regions of Algeria: in the coastal humid area the respective rates are 37% and 28%, in the central dry highlands 10% and 14%, and in the Sahara 7% and 38%.

The majority of the infected are inapparent carriers of a few worms. Eggs are found on the occasion of a routine stool examination. This harmless commensalism corresponds to an EPG $\leqq 5{,}000$.

It has been shown that intensive and prolonged effort to improve feces disposal and water supply does not significantly lower the prevalence of trichuriasis (BONNEFOY and ISAUTIER 1979, on the island of Réunion). Mass treatment offers better prospects in the short term, at least for reducing the worm load drastically.

2.2 Pathology

The worms, by embedding their anterior portion in the mucosa, mechanically compress the adjacent epithelial cells (HARTZ 1953) and bring about a blockage of the underlying crypts dilated with mucus and sometimes with fibrine and leukocytes. They may also cause small petechial subepithelial hemorrhages which can be followed by a chronic cellular infiltration with lymphocytes, plasma cells, and occasionally eosinophils. This infiltrate does not extend beyond the muscularis mucosae. The inflammatory reaction of the epithelium may induce bacterial, viral, and protozoal infections and even an allergic response.

Whenever limited to a few worms, the reaction will not produce symptoms. As soon as their number reaches or exceeds 200, the surface of the colon will become seeded with inflammatory lesions or even matted with adults. The inflammatory reaction of the mucosa can be marked and produce ulcerations and necrosis around the worm. Massive infection can end fatally (KOURI and VALDER DIAZ 1953).

Infections of this degree produce complaints in varying numbers and proportions: epigastric and abdominal pain, flatulence, tenesmus, anorexia, and chronic diarrhea, accompanied by loss of weight, headache, nervousness, insomnia, vomiting, dehydration, and emaciation.

Trichuris trichiura consumes blood. According to LAYRISSE et al. (1967) the daily quantity per worm is estimated at 0.005 ml. A daily loss of 4 ml blood corresponds to some 800 worms, which means a heavy infection. This can entail hypochromic anemia and blood-streaked stools. Malnutrition will be a precipitating factor.

Localization in the appendix can arouse symptoms of appendicitis following obstruction of the lumen brought about by inflammation and granulomata. On reexamination of the autopsy material collected by BRUMPT in 1909, DESPORTES (1938) identified *T. trichiura* in 5% of 369 ceca, with a maximum of 82 in one organ. In his thesis BALLAND (1910) mentions the presence of *T. trichiura* in 203 or 55% of cecoappendices.

In very heavy infections, increased peristalsis can lead to intussuception, and tenesmus to rectal prolapse. Anemia results from the consumption of blood where the worm population attains 800 or more. Hemorrhages in the colon descendens and sigmoideum can occur.

On proctosigmoidoscopy, the mucosa appears hyperemic and edematous, and enterorrhagia can be present.

2.3 Clinical Profile

Asymptomatic infection is the rule. In heavy infections – >200 worms – diarrhea, abdominal complaints, distension, tenesmus, pallor, and anemia are seen; if there are >800 worms, loss of weight, weakness, nervousness, and insommia are the symptoms. Exceptionally recurrent rectal prolapse and appendicular symptoms are present.

2.4 Immunity

Nothing is known about potential immune mechanisms. But the almost strictly intraluminar life cycle limits the importance of this factor as such.

3. Diagnosis

The *diagnosis* relies almost exclusively on stool examination. The brownish, lemon-shaped eggs with protuding hyaline polar plugs are typical and easy to identify. Concentration is needed only for light infections. EPG values are useful for the control of the efficacy of a treatment. Only in the early stages of the infection can an eosinophilia of about 25% appear. Rectocoloscopy will be restricted to the heavy infections.

4. Geographical Distribution

This cosmopolitan worm is more common in the warm, moist regions of the world.

5. Prevalence

Africa:
- Cameroun: 90%–95%
- Ethiopia: 48%
- Ivory Coast: 3%
- Nigeria: Benin State, 6%; Kwara State, 15%; Northern Province, 3%
- Tunesia (Gabès): 3%
- Zaire: Kinshasa (schoolchildren); Kimuenza, 77%; Livulu, 68%; Lower Zaire, 11%; Pygmies, 76%
- Zambia: 0.3%
- Zimbabwe: 0.2% (Burma Valley, 0.3%; Gatooma, 0.2%; Harare, 0.2%)

America:
- Latin America: Brazil: 34%–84%; Rio Grande do Norte, 58%; littoral micro-region, 66%
- Chile: general population, 25% (1948–1954), 19% (1957–1962); schoolchildren, 40% (1948–1954), 20% (1957–1962)
- Colombia (Amerindians): 30%
- Costa Rica: urban, 34% (12%–67%); rural, 40% (10%–69%)
- French Guyana: 18%
- Martinique: 37% (1980)
- Mexico: 21k (2%–79%, 1976); Chiapas, 60%; Distrito Federal, 44%; in Hospital infantil, 15%; littoral, 83%
- Suriname: 4%–45%
- Venezuela (on ± 90,000 examination): 82%, but 89%–90% in Sucre, Yaracui, los Llanos; EPG >2,000 in 57%
- United States: the southeastern States were previously infected up to 20%–25%. Nowadays, including Hawai, the Virgin Islands and Guam (16.4%), the general prevalence is about 2% but with surprisingly high figures in Alaska, Rhode Island, Pennsylvania, and New York. In North Carolina the infection rates in 1938 were 0.5% in whites and 3% in colored people, but reached 11%–25% among those living in the coastal region.

Asia: the published figures vary between 1% and 90%
- ≧90%: western Malaysia; Philippines, rural areas, 95% (up to 55 years of age) (CABRERA and SY 1978); west Java (Indonesia)
- ≧80%: Kuala Lumpur (squatters); Iran, Caspian area; Philippines; Sumatra; Taiwan; Indonesia (Djakarta)
- ≧70%: Philippines, urban areas, 76% (up to 20 years of age) (CABRERA and SY 1978)
- ≧60%: Korea, orphanage in Seoul, 63% (LIM 1978a, b)
- ≧40%: central Java; south Thailand

≧20%: India (Dehli, Dacca); Papua New Guinea; Sri Lanka; Suriname; Vietnam

≧10%: Yemen (children), 5%; Israel, 1%, but 17% in 1948; Iran, Khuzestan rural, 1%–18%; urban, 2%–12%

For Singapore, KAN and CHEAH (1970) states that in up to 60-year-olds it is the most common parasite.

Europe:

France (children), 12%; Paris, children 20%, rural 30%, 1–4 years 12%, 5–8 years 19%, 9–12 years 35%

Germany (World War II) 2%–40%; prisoners of war, Russians 43%–65%, Roumanians 72%, Berlin 0.9% (1953), of which 17% were symptomatic

Italy: north Italian children: 65%

Ireland: eastern: 43%

Poland: 36%

USSR: Kiev region, 30%; Georgia, 19%

United Kingdom: hospitals for mentally subnormal, 13%–36%

Oceania: Micronesia, Marshall Islands, 80%

The prevalence of *T. trichiura* is usually between 30% and 60%, but can be in excess of 90% or well under 10%. The ranges in prevalence vary within a given country according to the environment and the sample investigated (urban, rural, nomads, schoolchildren, general population). On the whole it is impossible to interpret the figures reported for the same country on the basis of the information provided by the authors. Trichuriasis responds faster to environment improvement than ascariasis; the number of eggs produced is much lower indeed.

Infection is more common in males. The 5- to 15-year-old age group is the most affected. The number of infected people can be estimated at some 700–750 million.

II. Drugs

For years trichuriasis has been a headache for practitioners. Although the vast majority of *T. trichiura* infections in man are without pathological significance, the discovery of a few eggs in the stools brings forth an insuperable urge, both in the bearer and in the majority of physicians, to eliminate the intruder.

1. Traditional Natural Drugs

The only drug widely recommended in all textbooks but seldom available has been *Leche de higueron*, or higueronia or higuerolatex, an extract from *Ficus laurifolia* or *F. glabrata* (Moraceae). The active ingredient ficin, a protease related to papain, was available, at least in theory, in Central and South America and only there. It is moreover unstable.

Bromelain, extracted from *Ananas sativus* (Bromeliaceae), and *chymotrypsin* have had their period of fame.

2. Synthetic Organic Drugs

2.1 Old Timers

Chemotherapy came into practice with the introduction of hexylresorcinol by JUNG (1954) and BASNUEVO et al. (1953). Its efficacy against trichuriasis was much lower than against ascariasis. Therefore its administration was converted into large retention enemata which were rather irritant on the anal mucosa or/and on the skin of perineum and thighs. By means of this method BASNUEVO et al. (1953) claimed at 100% CR. Its association with oil of chenopodium was given a trial, but the on the whole untoward effects outstripped the limited therapeutic value.

2.1.1 Bromo-β-naphthol (Wormin)

2.1.1.1 State of the Art

This halogenated derivative of β-naphthol is about 15 times less toxic than β-naphthol and possesses anthelmintic properties. Its use has been advocated by HSIEH et al. (1963).

2.1.1.2 Assessment

Table 74. Treatment of *Trichuris trichiura* infection by bromo-β-naphthol

Dosage	Number treated	CR	References
6 g–4 g at night and 2 g next morning	179	84%	JUTTIJUDATA et al. (1962)
9 g	–	64%	JUTTIJUDATA et al. (1962)

2.1.1.3 Dosage, Mode of Administration

The drug is available in tablets of 1 g, or in granules (1.5 g = 1 g base). The dosage for adults is 4–6 g, divided over two doses, the first at bedtime, the second the next morning; for children 7–12 years of age the dosage is 2 g and 12–15 years of age 3 g. (Enteral administration of 60 ml emulsion has also been recommended.)

2.1.1.4 Side Effects

Although bromo-β-naphthol crystals are mildly irritant for the mucosae, tolerance is good on the whole. Complaints are headaches, dizziness, loss of appetite, nausea, and vomiting abdominal pain.

2.1.1.5 Contraindications, Precautions

The use of bromo-β-naphthol is inadvisable in the presence of renal and hepatic dysfunction, and also in pregnancy.

2.1.1.6 Conclusion

More efficient products are now available.

2.1.2 Stilbazium Iodide (Monopar)

2.1.2.1 State of the Art

This substance belongs to the series of pyridine derivatives with broad-spectrum anthelmintic activity discovered by PHILLIPS and BURROWS (1961) and BURROWS et al. (1961).

2.1.2.2 Assessment

Table 75. Treatment of *Tricuris trichiura* infection by stilbazium iodide

Efficacy	Dosage	Number treated	CR	ERR	References
>50%	200 mg t.i.d./3 days	13	46	82	HSIEH et al. (1963)
	12.5–70 mg/kg/3 days	22	–	85	SWARTZWELDER et al. (1962)
	2.25–3 g over 3 days	24	29	76	JEFFERY et al. (1963)
	8.8 mg/kg b.i.d./3 days	23	39	89	HUANG and BROWN (1964)
	10 mg/kg/3 days	15	20	–	CAMPOS et al. (1967)
	10–15 mg/kg/3 days				
	Tablets	71	1.4	Transient	YOKOGAWA et al. (1968)
	Suppositories	40	2.5	Transient	YOKOGAWA et al. (1968)
	125–250 mg/2–3 days	145	0	90	MALDONADO (1965)

2.1.2.3 Dosage

Dosage is 10 mg/kg b. i. d. for 3 days in an enteric-coated formulation.

2.1.2.4 Side Effects

Tolerance is fairly good, but the stools are stained red. Nausea and vomiting may occur.

2.1.2.5 Conclusion

For a short period stilbazium looked promising, but due to the arrival of better drugs, it never became a current drug.

2.1.3 Diphetarsone (Bemarsal)

2.1.3.1 State of the Art

The ethylene-bis (*p*-amino phenylarsonic acid) decahydrate has been used for 20 years in the treatment of intestinal amebiasis. SCHNEIDER et al. (1960) suggested the use of this pentavalent organic arsenical compound in the treatment of trichuriasis in daily doses of 1 g for 7 days. Since the early thirties mention has been made off and on by different authors of the activity of pentavalent arsenicals, mainly Stovarsol, on trichuriasis (BRÜNING 1931; GOMES DE COSTA 1931; MARTIN 1936, KOURI 1957; AGUILAR et al. 1957). JUNOD (1965) observed the disappearance of *T. trichiura* from the stools of persons treated for amebiasis with diphetarsone and advocated its regular use in trichuriasis.

2.1.3.2 Assessment

Table 76. Treatment of *Trichuris trichiura* infections by diphetasone

Efficacy	Dosage	Number treated	CR	ERR	References
≧90%	1 g b.i.d./10 days	97	96	–	Junod (1965)[a]
	1 g b.i.d./10 days	33	91	–	Limbos et al. (1968)
	1 g b.i.d./10 days	25	96	–	Garin et al. (1970)
	1 g b.i.d./10 days	46	94	–	Nitulescu et al. (1970)
	10 years of age, 500 mg t.i.d./10 days		149	99	Lenczner (1972)[b]
≧80%	1 g b.i.d./10 days	91	83	92–99	Lynch et al. (1972)

[a] Junod (1965) recommends the following dose regimen for children: 8 years, 2 g; 5–8 years, 1 g; and 3–5 years, 0.75 g. Lynch et al. (1972) recommend calculating the dose for children from the body surface area, making use the *Catzel formula,* unless the weight is grossly abnormal

[b] Lenczer (1972) used, according to age: 5–10 years, 500 mg b.i.d. for 10 days; 3–5 years, 250 mg t.i.d. for 10 days; and 3 years, 50 mg/kg/10 days

2.1.3.3 Dosage, Mode of Administration

Dosage is 1 g twice daily in tablets of 500 mg for 10 days.

2.1.3.4 Side Effects

Side effects are exceptionally a transient rash, vomiting, and diarrhea.

2.1.3.5 Contraindications, Precautions

There are no contraindications.

2.1.3.6 Conclusion

Diphetarsone is very active, but a real disadvantage is the length of the treatment, which is only suitable for individual therapy.

2.1.4 Organophosphorous Compounds

2.1.4.1 Metrifonate and Dichlorvos

2.1.4.1.1 State of the Art

It has been known since 1962 (Schrader 1963; Cerf et al. 1962) that metrifonate has high anthelmintic activity in several human infections, including *T. trichiura.* It has also been established that dichlorvos is the active ingredient.

2.1.4.1.2 Assessment

Table 77. Treatment of *Trichuris trichiura* infection by metrifonate and dichlorvos

Efficacy	Dosage	Number treated	CR	CRR	References
100%	10 mg/kg	6	100	–	Cervoni et al. (1969)
	6 mg V_3[a]/kg	14	100	–	Cervoni et al. (1969)
≧80%	6 mg/kg	136	89	–	Cervoni et al. (1969)
	12 mg/kg	74	88	97	Peña-Chavarria et al. (1969)
	12 mg/kg	35	88	–	Cervoni et al. (1969)
	15 mg/kg	40	80	–	Cerf et al. (1962)
	6 mg/kg	22	82	83	Peña-Chavarria et al. (1969)
	3 mg/kg	83	83	–	Cervoni et al. (1969)
	8 mg/kg	10	80	–	Cervoni et al. (1969)
≧70%	12 mg V_3/kg	78	79	–	Cervoni et al. (1969)

[a] V_3, large size

2.1.4.1.3 Dosage, Mode of Administration

Metrifonate is available as 330-mg tablets. A dose of 6 mg/kg is satisfactory.

2.1.4.1.4 Side Effects

The doses used in man are followed by only a modest depression of the plasma and erythrocyte cholinesterases. If toxic effects do appear, it happens within 2–8 h, with anorexia, nausea, vomiting, sweating, salivation, urination, myosis, bradycardia, hypotension, and abdominal colics. Effects on the CNS include giddiness, restlessness, anxiety, tremulousness, and respiratory distress and cyanosis.

The antidote of this muscarinic and nicotinic action and of the acetylcholine accumulation is atropine, possibly supplemented by oximes (pralidoxime chlorhydrate).

2.1.4.1.5 Contraindications, Precautions

Metrifonate and dichlorvos should not be used in glucose-6-phosphate dehydrogenase-deficient persons.

2.1.4.1.6 Conclusion

Dichlorvos provides a good CR and ERR with a dosage of 6 mg/kg and has been successfully used in mass treatment. The reason for the loss of interest in this drug is its potent cholinesterase inhibitory activity and the risk of poisoning by accidental overdosage.

2.1.5 Dithiazanine Iodide (Telmid, Delvex)

2.1.5.1 State of the Art

This blue-violet dye of the dicarboxyanine series has shown a remarkable efficacy against trichiuriasis, and also against strongyloidiasis, both resistant to the then current anthelmintics. Dithiazanine iodide has a very low solubility in water and is absorbed in negligible amounts by a normal intestine; consequently, high levels are maintained in the intestinal lumen and disturb the metabolism of the helminths inhabiting the gut.

Unfortunately absorption of the dye can result from an unrecognized, disturbed, or irritated intestinal mucosa and can be followed by severe intolerance, intoxication, and even death. Due to such accidents this drug is no longer on the market.

It is, however, interesting to have an idea of its efficacy.

2.1.5.2 Assessment

Table 78. Treatment of *Trichuris trichiura* infection by dithiazanine iodide

Efficacy	Dosage	Number treated	CR	ERR	References
100%	20 mg/kg (max. doses)/4 days		2	100	CERF (1958)
	200 mg b.i.d./5 days	5	100	–	WAGNER et al. (1958)
	600 mg b.i.d./5 days	23	100	–	VINKE and VAN DER SAR (1959)
	600 mg/21 days	3	100	–	VASOJEVIC et al. (1962)
	600 mg/10 days	37	100	–	SWARTZWELDER et al. (1958)
≧90%	600 mg	27	93	–	SWARTZWELDER et al. (1958)
	20 mg/kg/10 days	16	94	–	BASNUEVO et al. (1959a, b)
	20 mg/kg/7–14 days	12	92	–	STOTT and JOPLING (1961)
	20 mg/kg/21 days	66	95	–	STOTT and JOPLING (1961)
	300–400 mg/21 days	88	94	–	GUIMARAES et al. (1961)
	600 mg/5 days	164	97	–	SWARTZWELDER et al. (1957)
	600 mg/5 days	12	92	–	PAINE et al. (1960)
	600 mg/5 days	32	97	99	SWARTZWELDER et al. (1957)
≧80%	600 mg/5–21 days	18	89	–	SWARTZWELDER et al. (1957)
	600 mg/21 days	27	88	–	LLOYD (1959)
	600 mg/5 days	11	87	–	FRYE et al. (1957)
	600 mg/5 days	133	86	–	VINKE and VAN DER SAR (1959)
	600 mg/5 days	6	83	–	PAINE et al. (1960)
	20 mg/kg/5–10 days	10	80	–	COUDERT et al. (1961)
	600 mg/5–10 days	30	83	–	PLOTNIKOV et al. (1962)
	10 mg/kg/10 days	?	81	–	SIMIONESCO et al. (1964)

Between 70% and 30% efficacy, a great variety of results are on record irrespective of the doses used, which tends to be the rule for all the anthelmintics.

2.1.5.3 Dosage, Mode of Administration

Dithiazanine was available as enteric-coated 100-mg tablets. Oral administration of 20 mg/kg/day with a maximum of 600 mg/day, divided over three doses, or 200 mg t. i. d., repeated on 5 days, gave satisfactory results.

2.1.5.4 Side Effects

See Sect. B.II.3.2.4.4.

2.1.5.5 Contraindications

See Sect. B.II.3.2.4.5.

2.1.5.6 Conclusion

Dithiazanine iodide is no longer in use.

2.2 Newer Drugs

2.2.1 Albendazole

2.2.1.1 State of the Art

This broad-spectrum anthelminthic, aimed specifically at mass treatment of soil-transmitted helminths, needs to be tried out against *T. trichiura.*

2.2.1.2 Assessment

Table 79. Treatment of *T. trichuris* infection by albendazole

Efficacy	Dosage	Number treated	CR	ERR	References
100%	1.25 mg/kg b.i.d./3 days	7	100	–	GARIN (1980)
≧90%	400 mg/3 days	22	91	–	CAMILO COURA et al. (1981b)
≧80%	200 mg b.i.d.	6	83	–	SCHETTINO and ORTEGA (1981)
	0.8 mg/kg/b.i.d./3 days	6	83	–	GARIN (1980)
≧70%	400 mg	14	71	–	CAMILO COURA et al. (1981a)
	400 mg	41	73	90	CAMILO COURA et al. (1981b)
	200 mg b.i.d.	14	79	92	LUMBRERAS CRUZ et al. (1981)
	400 mg	15	73	93	PENE et al. (1981)
	200 mg b.i.d.	99	72	60	ROSSIGNOL (1981a)
	4 mg/kg	8	75	–	GARIN (1980)
≧60%	200 mg/100 mg b.i.d.	6	67	36	GARIN (1980)
	100 mg b.i.d.	9	67	88	BARANSKI et al. (1981)
	100 mg b.i.d.	40	60	–	CRUZ LOPEZ (1981)
	10 mg/kg	?	60	–	RUBENS CAMPOS et al. (1982)
	400 mg	5	60	–	MAISONNEUVE et al. (1981)
	400 mg	39	62	58	PENE et al. (1982a)
	400 mg	74	65	86	PENE et al. (1981b)
	600 mg	25	61	85	RAMALINGAM et al. (1983)
≧50%	100 mg b.i.d.	2	50	–	SCHETTINO and ORTEGA (1981)
	400 mg	24	50	38	LUMBRERAS CRUZ (1981)
≧40%	200 mg b.i.d.	40	40	–	CRUZ LOPEZ (1981)
	100–200 mg	28	46	–	LUMBRERAS CRUZ et al. (1981)
	200 mg b.i.d.	34	41	–	RICHARD-LENOBLE et al. (1982)
	800 mg	28	48	72	RAMALINGAM et al. (1983)
≧40%	100 mg b.i.d.	10	20	63	LUMBRERAS CRUZ et al. (1981)
	200 mg b.i.d.	70	27	89	RICHARD-LENOBLE et al. (1982)
	400 mg	45	33	56	BASTIDAS (1982)
	400 mg	282	36	60	PENE et al. (1982b)
	400 mg	22	27	39	RAMALINGAM et al. (1983)

2.1.3 Dosage, Mode of Administration

Dosage is 400 mg on three consecutive days.

2.2.1.4 Side Effects

See Sect. B.II.3.2.1.4.

2.2.1.5 Contraindications, Precautions

See Sect. B.II.3.2.1.5.

2.2.1.6 Conclusion

The administration of 400-mg doses repeated over 3 days provides good results in the treatment of trichiuriasis. In contrast, with the simple-dose regimen, which is supposed to be the trump card of albendazole as an ideal new possibility for mass treatment, the results are unsatisfactory.

ROSSIGNOL and MAISONNEUVE (1984) summarize as follows the results on infection with *T. trichiura* after administration of a single dose of 400 mg (2 capsules or 20 ml suspension) irrespective of age: the CRs and ERRs are for light infections 73% and 81% and for moderate infections 46% and 71%. Not an overwhelming result.

2.2.2 Bephenium Hydroxynaphthoate (Alcopar)

The efficacy of this anthelmintic against *T. trichiura*, ensuring CRs between 0% and 44%, is too low to be of any significance, in both single and mixed infections.

2.2.3 Ciclobendazole

2.2.3.1 State of the Art

Ciclobendazole is active against *T. trichiura* and other intestinal nematodes.

2.2.3.2 Assessment

Table 80. Treatment of *T. trichiura* infection by ciclobendazole

Efficacy	Dosage	Number treated	CR	ERR	References
≧90%	1 g	65	98	99	STÜRCHLER et al. (1980)
	200 mg b.i.d./3 days	70	93	97	STÜRCHLER et al. (1980)
≧80%	100 mg b.i.d./3 days	44	84	–	DEGREMONT and STAHEL (1978)
	200 mg b.i.d./3 days	24	83	–	DEGREMONT and STAHEL (1978)
	600 mg	27	74	–	GUGGENMOOS et al. (1978)
	1,200 mg	24	88	–	GUGGENMOOS et al. (1978)

2.2.3.3 Dosage, Mode of Administration

Ciclobendazole is available in tablets of 100 mg. They should be administered at a dose of 200 mg b. i. d. for 3 days.

2.2.3.4 Side Effects

See Sect. B.II.3.2.1.4.

2.2.3.5 Contraindications, Precautions

See Sect. B.II.3.2.1.5.

2.2.3.6 Conclusion

A single dose of 1 g provides interesting results, which warrant investigations of a wider scope.

2.2.4 Flubendazole

2.2.4.1 State of the Art

Based on the analogy in the chemical structure, it could be forecasted that the efficacy of flubendazole against *T. trichiura* would not be grossly different from that of mebendazole. Since 1977, this has been confirmed worldwide by many authors.

2.2.4.2 Assessment

Table 81. Treatment of *T. trichiura* infection by flubendazole

Efficacy	Dosage	Number treated	CR	ERR	Reference
100%	100 mg t.i.d./2 days	6	100	–	DA SILVA (1979)
	100 mg t.i.d./3 days	5	100	–	DA SILVA (1979)
	100 mg b.i.d./3 days	51	100	–	BRUMPT (1976)
	2 g	16	100	–	NEYRINCK and V. D. KERCKHOVE (1976)
	100 mg b.i.d./3 days	20	100	–	GENTILINI (1976)
	100 mg b.i.d./4 days	20	100	–	GENTILINI (1976)
	200 mg/4 days	3	100	–	DANIS et al. (1980)
	300 mg/2 days	4	100	–	BUNNAG et al. (1980)
≧90%	200 mg/3 days	56	91	57	NOZAÏS (1978)
	200 mg t.i.d.	11	99	97	DA SILVA (1979)
	400 mg–2 g	32	94	–	BOUVIER (1976)
	500 mg t.i.d.	21	90	96	PEÑA-CHAVARRIA (1977)
	500 mg b.i.d.	23	91	95	PEÑA-CHAVARRIA (1977)
	100 mg b.i.d./3 days	25	96	99	DE OLIVEIRA GOMEZ (1979)
	100 mg b.i.d./3 days	31	93	99	WERSHING et al. (1979)
	100 mg b.i.d./3 days	28	93	–	DIOP MAR
	100 mg b.i.d./3 days	13	92	–	GENTILINI (1977)
	100 mg b.i.d./3 days	78	92	–	VASOLLO
	200 mg/3 days	13	92	–	DANIS et al. (1980)
	600 mg	62	90	89	BARBAIX (1981)
≧80%	200–300 mg/3 days	25	88	–	PENOT et al. (1978)
	200 mg/3 days	124	85	90	BECQUET and LABARRIERE (1980)
	100 mg b.i.d./3 days	19	89	99	YANGCO et al. (1981)
	100 mg t.i.d./2 days	32	81	94	KATZ (1980)
	100 mg t.i.d./3 days	36	86	98	ARFAA et al. (1979)

Table 81 (continued)

Efficacy	Dosage	Number treated	CR	ERR	Reference
	100 mg t.i.d./2 days	13	85	86	LEAO (1980)
	100 mg b.i.d./3 days	124	85	89	BECQUET (1976)
	400 mg	16	81	77	BARBAIX (1981)
	200 mg/3 days	50	82	–	SCHENONE et al. (1977)
	250 mg b.i.d./1 day	27	89	98	WERSHING et al. (1979)
	500 mg b.i.d./1 day	29	83	99	WERSHING et al. (1979)
	500 mg b.i.d./1 day	26	85	99	WERSHING et al. (1979)
	200 mg	22	82	91	BARBAIX (1981)
≧70%	100 mg b.i.d./3 days	61	77	98	BLECKMAN et al. (1982)
	600 mg b.i.d./3 days	14	79	–	BOUVIER et al. (1976)
	300 mg b.i.d.	27	74	98	BOTERO (1980b)
	300 mg	68	77	88	BARBAIX (1981)
	150 mg	30	73	91	BARBAIX (1981)
	200 mg/3 days	61	79	98	BLECHMAN et al. (1982)
≧60%	300 mg/2 days	–	67	97	KAN (1982)
	100 mg b.i.d./2 days	71	65	94	ARFAA et al. (1979)
	200 mg b.i.d./1 day	43	65	88	ARFAA et al. (1979)
	100 mg t.i.d./1 day	9	67	74	LEAO (1980)
	1 g	50	63	91	COLAERT (1976)
	200 mg t.i.d./1 day	21	62	94	DE OLIVAIRA GOMEZ (1979)
	500 mg	31	61	88	WERSHING et al. (1979)
≧50%	200 mg t.i.d./1 day	2	50	93	LEAO (1980)
	2 g	48	54	82	COLAERT (1976)
	300 mg b.i.d.	16	56	–	BUNNAG et al. (1980)
	100 mg	6	50	70	BARBAIX (1981)
<50%	300 mg/2 days	53	13	83	CABRERA et al. (1980)
	200 mg	–	17	90	KAN (1982)
	500 mg	–	16	91	KAN (1982)
	600 mg	–	19	88	KAN (1982)
	200 mg t.i.d./1 day	30	47	88	KATZ (1980)
	100 mg b.i.d./1 day	37	27	76	ARFAA et al. (1979)
	300 mg/2 days	99	15	80	MARGONO et al (1980)
	200 mg	47	19	42	LIONEL et al. (1980)
	500 mg	45	24	54	LIONEL et al. (1980)
	1 g	32	31	89	PEÑA-CHAVARRIA (1977)
	2 g	10	20	88	PEÑA-CHAVARRIA (1978)
	1 g b.i.d.	10	20	72	PEÑA-CHAVARRIA (1978)
	100 mg	41	46	86	WERSHING et al. (1979)
	500 mg (rural)	91	32	78	ISMAIL and LIONEL (1981)
	500 mg (urban)	79	23	70	ISMAIL and LIONEL (1981)

2.2.4.3 Dosage, Mode of Administration

Tablets containing 100 mg are available. For individual therapy the optimal dosage is 100 mg/b.i.d. for 3 days, while in mass treatment a single dose of 600 mg is recommended.

2.2.4.4 Side Effects

See Sect. B.II.3.2.7.4.

2.2.4.5 Contraindications, Precautions

See Sect. B.II.3.2.7.5.

2.2.4.6 Conclusion

A rational analysis of the divergent published results is an arduous task. In general a drug regimen of 100 mg b.i.d. on three consecutive days or to a lesser extent 100 mg t.i.d. for 2 days provides a consistently good efficacy. Higher dosages (300–600 mg–1 g) on three to seven consecutive days do not improve the results. Single dose trials are successful with 600 mg, while 1-g or 1-g 500-mg doses are no more efficient. On the whole the CRs are better when the EPGs are less than the 5,000 level. With nearly all of the dosages the ERR is very substantial (≧90%).

2.2.5 Levamisole

2.2.5.1 State of the Art

Tetramisole appeared to be almost inactive against trichiuriasis in man. The discovery that the levoisomer of tetramisole was more active than the racemate did not alter its rather poor efficacy against trichiuriasis.

2.2.5.2 Assessment

Table 82. Treatment of *T. trichiura* infection by levamisole

Efficacy	Dosage	Number treated	CR	ERR	References
100%	2.5 mg/kg	21	100	–	GATTI et al. (1970)
≧80%	2.5 mg/kg	89	89	–	GATTI et al. (1969)
	2.5 mg/kg	20	85	–	GATTI et al. (1969)
>60%	2.5 mg/kg	120	68	–	KABA et al. (1978)
≧50%	2.5 mg/kg	34	56	–	LAIGRET et al. (1969)
	2.5 mg/kg	8	50	89	BREEDVELD et al. (1977)
	2.5 mg/kg	105	55	–	GATTI et al. (1969) (Butare)
	50 mg/3 days + 100 mg mebendazole	34	56	81	ISEBAERT (1970)
<50%	3.5 mg/kg (children)	32	45	34	VAKIL (1969)
	3–7 mg/kg	42	38	–	BOUYER (1970)
	3.5 mg/kg	60	35	67	VAKIL (1969)
	2.5 mg/kg (adults)	222	22	–	COENE (1969)
	150 mg	45	22	35	VAN LANDUYT (1973)
	150 mg	31	16	25	DE JONCKHEERE (1975)
	300 mg	52	15	61	VAN LANDUYT (1973)
	2.5 mg/kg	39	13	–	KUZNICKI et al. (1972)
	2.5 mg/kg		12	–	WAGNER and REXINGER (1978)
	3.5 mg/kg	74	1.4	–	ASMERA (1974)

2.2.5.3 Dosage, Mode of Administration

The dosage of 2.5 mg/kg was used most frequently. Other dosages did not improve the efficacy.

2.2.5.4 Side Effects

See Sect. B.II.3.2.9.4.

2.2.5.5 Contraindications, Precautions

See Sect. B.II.3.2.9.5.

2.2.5.6 Conclusions

Levamisole is not recommended for the treatment of trichiuriasis. However, the gap between the high CRs recorded by some and the extremely low CRs recorded by others underlines a major difficulty in assessing the activity of drugs in mixed infections. Differences in methodologies are not the only origin, although some sort of basic standardization should be agreed upon by all those concerned. It is also very likely that the elimination of the bulk of the eggs by an active drug results in the visual appearance of lower-grade infections, which are usual in infections such as *T. trichiura*.

2.2.6 Mebendazole

2.2.6.1 State of the Art

Mebendazole is active against *Trichuris* and a number of other nematodes and cestodes (JANSSEN 1974).

2.2.6.2 Assessment

Table 83. Treatment of *T. trichiura* infection by mebendazole

Efficacy	Dosage	Number treated	CR	ERR	References
100%	440 mg/4 days	8	100	–	KLEIN (1971)
	200 mg b.i.d./4 days	7	100	–	CHOWDURY (1972–1974)
	100 mg b.i.d./3 days	6	100	–	GOLDSMID (1974)
	100 mg b.i.d./3 days	19	100	–	BIAGI et al. (1974)
	100 mg b.i.d./3 days	7	100	–	JAROONVESEMA et al. (1978)
	100 mg b.i.d./4 days	6	100	–	GENTILINI (1974)
	300 mg	10	100	–	MILLER et al. (1974)
	100 mg b.i.d./3 days	5	100	–	BEKHTI (1974)
	100 mg b.i.d./3 days	44	100	–	DE SOUZA et al. (1973b)
	100 mg b.i.d./3 days	43	100	–	YALCINKAYA (1977)
	100 mg b.i.d./3 days	40	100	–	PALACIOS and SANCEDO (1973a)
	100 mg b.i.d./3 days	10	100	–	DE PAULA CASTRO et al. (1973)
	100 mg b.i.d./4 days	6	100	–	LAGUNAS FLORES (1979)
	100 mg b.i.d./4 days	68	100	–	LAGUNAS FLORES (1979)
	100 mg b.i.d./3 days/×2	30	100	–	NAGALINGAM et al. (1976)
	100 mg b.i.d./3 days	105	100	–	BELTRAN-HERNANDEZ et al. (1976

Table 83 (continued)

Efficacy	Dosage	Number treated	CR	ERR	References
	100 mg b.i.d./3 days	39	100	–	THIENPONT (1972)
	100 mg b.i.d./3 days	29	100	–	PATRON et al. (1973)
	100 mg b.i.d.	26	100	–	NARMADA et al. (1974)
	100 mg b.i.d./4 days	13	100	–	MEENAKSHI-SHAH (1979)
	200 mg b.i.d./3 days	4	100	–	MEENAKSHI-SHAH (1979)
	600 mg	27	100	–	GUGGENMOOS et al. (1978)
≧90%	100 mg b.i.d./3 days	52	98	99	GATTI et al. (1972b)
	100 mg b.i.d./4 days	109	99	99	GATTI et al. (1972)
	100 mg b.i.d./4 days	109	90	99	VANDEPITTE et al. (1973)
	100 mg b.i.d./2 days	20	92	99	PEÑA CHAVARRIA et al. (1973)
	100 mg b.i.d./3 days	39	99	–	CHAIA et al. (1972)
	100 mg b.i.d./3 days	116	97	99	VANDEPITTE et al. (1972)
	100 mg b.i.d./4 days	127	95	99	GATTI and VANDEPITTE (1973)
	100 mg/3 days	63	97	–	KRUBWA et al. (1974b)
	100 mg b.i.d./3 days	100	98	–	DE SOUZA et al. (1973a, b)
	100 mg b.i.d./3 days	47	98	–	DE OLIVEIRA GOMES (1974)
	200 mg b.i.d./2 days	30	97	99	SHAFEI (1974)
	200 mg b.i.d./3 days	24	96	90	CHOWDURY (1974)
	100 mg b.i.d./3 days	33	94	–	HUTCHINSON et al. (1975)
	100 mg b.i.d./3 days	50	94	–	FERNANDES (1974)
	100 mg b.i.d./3 days	26	94	–	NGOY and KALOMBO (1975)
	100 mg b.i.d./3 days	12	95	–	MONTERO and SANCHEZ (1975)
	100 mg b.i.d./3 days	126	96	–	DEGRÉMONT and BAUMGARTNER (1975)
	100 mg b.i.d./3 days	42	94	94	CHONGSUPHAJAISIDDHI et al. (1978)
	100 mg b.i.d./3 days	22	95	–	BERTI et al. (1976)
	100 mg b.i.d./3 days	60	98	–	OTERO et al. (1977)
	200 mg	14	93	–	MUTTALIB et al. (1981)
	100 mg b.i.d./3 days	96	91	–	KROTOSKI et al. (1979)
	100 mg b.i.d./3 days	96	90	–	WELLENS and THIENPONT (1978)
	100 mg b.i.d./3 days	54	94	–	HUDSON (1976)
	100 mg b.i.d./3 days	104	96	–	ASPÖCK et al. (1977)
	100 mg b.i.d./3 days	29	99	–	MARTINS and GABURRI (1974)
	100 mg b.i.d./3 days	47	98	–	DE OLIVEIRA-GOMES (1974)
	100 mg b.i.d./3 days	34	91	–	SCHENONE et al. (1974)
	200 mg b.i.d./4 days	76	97	–	CHAIA ans DA CUNHA (1971a)
	100 mg b.i.d./3 days	131	98	–	CHANCO and VIDAD (1978)
	100 mg b.i.d./3 days	50	96	–	MAQBOOL et al. (1975)
	100 mg b.i.d./3 days	10	90	100	PAUL and ZAMAN (1975)
	100 mg b.i.d./3 days	131	98	–	CHANCO and ATIENZA (1973)
	100 mg b.i.d./3 days	131	90	–	BARRETT-CONNER (1975)
	100 mg b.i.d./5 days	20	95	–	PEREIRA et al. (1979)
≧80%	100 mg b.i.d./3 days	51	88	96	JUWONO and TANTULAR (1973)
	100 mg b.i.d./4 days	27	89	99	PENA-CHAVARRIA et al. (1973)
	100 mg b.i.d./3 days	91	80	92	LOUZADA et al. (1973)
	100 mg b.i.d./4 days	20	85	–	BRUMPT (1973)
	75 mg/2 days	22	86	91	GATTI and VANDEPITTE (1973)
	100 mg b.i.d./3 days	52	88	99	GATTI and VANDEPITTE (1973)
	100 mg/3 days	37	84	87	GATTI and VANDEPITTE (1973)
	200 mg/3 days	31	84	–	RUAS (1973)

Table 83 (ontinued)

Efficacy	Dosage	Number treated	CR	ERR	References
	100 mg b.i.d./3 days	163	86	99	ABADI (1974)
	100 mg b.i.d./3 days	247	85	97	SOH et al. (1974)
	100 mg b.i.d./3 days	43	86	99	SEAH (1976)
	100 mg b.i.d./3 days	12	83	–	FOBA-PAGOU et al. (1978)
	100 mg b.i.d./3 days	91	84	–	RICHARD LENOBLE et al. (1981)
	100 mg b.i.d./3 days	473	84	–	DE SAEDELEER (1975)
	200 mg b.i.d./2 days	43	88	–	CHAIA and DA CUNHA (1971a)
	100 mg b.i.d./6 days	25	88	–	SCRAGG and PROCTOR (1978)
	100 mg b.i.d./3 days	69	80	–	STEINRÜCH et al. (1976)
	100 mg b.i.d./3 days	30	83	–	RODRIGUEZ PAVON (1973)
	100 mg b.i.d./4 days	30	88	–	BARRETT-CONNER (1975)
	100 mg b.i.d./4 days	63	84	–	AGUILAR et al. (1973)
	100 mg b.i.d./4 days	28	89	96	SARGENT et al. (1975)
	50 mg b.i.d./4 days	31	81	–	MEENAKSHI SHAH (1979)
	75 mg b.i.d./4 days	7	86	–	MEENAKSHI SHAH (1979)
	100 mg b.i.d./3 days	49	82	87	BLECHMAN (1975)
	100 mg b.i.d./3 days (urban)	57	86	96	ISMAIL and LIONEL (1981)
≧70%	200 mg	70	70	98	PEÑA-CHAVARRIA (1973)
	100 mg b.i.d./3 days	28	75	–	PEÑA-CHAVARRIA (1973)
	100 mg b.i.d./3 days	8	75	99	BRUMPT (1973)
	200 mg b.i.d./2 days	16	75	–	BRUMPT (1973)
	200 mg b.i.d./4 days	18	78	–	BRUMPT (1973)
	100 mg/3 days	271	79	–	LORIA-CORTES et al. (1974)
	100 mg/3 days	147	77	–	PARTONO et al. (1974)
	100 mg b.i.d./3 days	30	73	95	SHAFEI (1974)
	100 mg b.i.d./3 days	113	79	96	BOTERO and PEREZ (1976)
	100 mg b.i.d./3 days	42	71	–	ISLAM and CHOWDURY (1976)
	100 mg b.i.d./3 days	24	75	95	AGUILAR et al. (1977)
	100 mg b.i.d./3 days	113	75	–	CARRIÉ et al. (1978)
	100 mg b.i.d./4 days	48	75	99	MUSGRAVE et al. (1979)
	100 mg b.i.d./3 days	69	78	–	PADELT et al. (1977)
	100 mg b.i.d./3 days	26	76	–	LAGUNAS-FLORES (1979)
	100 mg b.i.d./3 days	170	74	–	SHIRATSUCHI et al. (1975)
	25 mg b.i.d./4 days	4	75	–	MERDIVENCI et al. (1977)
	100 mg b.i.d./3 days	28	75	90	PEREIRO et al. (1979)
	100 mg b.i.d./3 days	28	75	–	BARRETT-CONNER (1975)
	100 mg b.i.d./3 days (rural)	71	79	95	ISMAIL and LIONEL (1981)
≧60%	100 mg b.i.d./3 days	15	67	–	GENTILINI (1974)
	100 mg b.i.d./3 days	100	64	–	HUGGINS (1976)
	100 mg b.i.d./3 days	143	65	–	RICHARD-LENOBLE (1980)
	100 mg b.i.d./3 days	35	69	–	MILLER et al. (1974)
	300 mg	107	68	98	WOLFE and WERSHING (1974)
	100 mg b.i.d./3 days	29	64	87	SARGENT et al. (1974)
	100 mg/4 days	21	67	96	SARGENT et al. (1974)
	100 mg × 2 (48-h interval)	61	64	–	CHAIA and DA CUNHA (1971b)
	200 mg b.i.d.	50	68	–	CHAIA and DA CUNHA (1971b)
	50–100 or 200 mg	78	64	–	KARNAUKOV et al. (1978)
	100 mg b.i.d./3 days	23	64	87	SARGENT et al. (1974)

Table 83 (continued)

Efficacy	Dosage	Number treated	CR	ERR	References
	100 mg b.i.d./4 days	21	67	96	SARGENT et al. (1974)
	100 mg b.i.d./3 days	32	66	69	SARGENT et al. (1975)
	600 mg	41	63	–	RICHARD LENOBLE et al. (1981)
≧50%	100 mg b.i.d./3 days	54	59	–	AMATO NETO et al. (1973)
	100 mg b.i.d./3 days	54	56	76	BUNNAG (1976)
	100 mg b.i.d./3 days	25	52	91	DISSANAIKE (1978)
	100 mg b.i.d./4 days	63	59	79	CIMMERMAN et al. (1980)
	100 mg b.i.d./2 days	22	53	95	SARGENT et al. (1974)
	100 mg b.i.d./3 days	90	58	–	LENGYEL et al. (1975)
	600 mg (EPG ≦5,000)	26	58	85	KAN (1983b)
<50%	300 mg × 1	18	44	96	PEÑA-CHAVARRIA (1973)
	100 mg/3 days	52	37	76	GATTI and VANDEPITTE (1973)
	100 mg	50	12	24	GATTI and VANDEPITTE (1973)
	200 mg	49	4	62	GATTI and VANDEPITTE (1973)
	200 mg	41	12	83	CABRERA (1980)
	400 mg	17	12	84	CABRERA (1980)
	600 mg	22	27	91	CABRERA (1980)
	40 mg	27	19	–	CHAIA and DA CUNHA (1971)
	100 mg × 2	54	17	–	CHAIA and DA CUNHA (1971)
	110 mg b.i.d./2 days	81	46	–	CHAIA and DA CUNHA (1971)
	100 mg b.i.d./3 days	68	27	–	LAGUNO-FLORES (1979)
	100 mg b.i.d./3 days × 2	50	48	–	LAGUNO-FLORES (1979)
	100 mg b.i.d./3 days	6	16	71	YOKOGAWA et al. (1976)
	100 mg b.i.d./3 days	30	17	–	NAGALINGAM et al. (1976)
	100 mg b.i.d./3 days	19	42	88	MARTINEZ and MAYA UGALDE (1973)
	100 mg b.i.d./4 days	15	40	87	PARAMAESEWARAN and LUNG (1976)
	100 mg b.i.d./3 days	14	0	76	DAVISON (1979)
	100 mg b.i.d./4 days	21	10	90	DAVISON (1979)
	100 mg b.i.d./4 days	25	20	–	DAVISON (1979)
	600 mg (EPG 22,000)	14	7	89	KAN (1983b)

2.2.6.3 Dosage, Mode of Administration

The usual dose of 100 mg b. i. d. on three consecutive days provides excellent CRs and ERRs. However, KAN (1983 b) states that a single dose of 600 mg in very light to very heavy infections provides ERRs and CRs similar to those obtained with the recommended multiple-dose regime. RICHARD-LENOBLE et al. (1982) estimate the loss at 10%–15% of the efficacy.

2.2.6.4 Side Effects

See Sect. B.II.3.2.10.4. In mixed infections erratic migration of *Ascaris* can occur (CHANCO and VIDAD 1978; PĔNA-CHAVARRIA et al. 1973; PARTONO et al. 1974; MUTTALIB et al. 1981; KAN 1983 b).

2.2.6.5 Contraindications, Precautions

See Sect. B.II.3.2.10.5.

2.2.6.6 Conclusions

Mebendazole emerges as the drug of choice against *T. trichiura*. With a total dose of 600 mg, on a drug regimen of 100 mg twice a day for three consecutive days, the CR falls only exceptionally under 75%–80%, but often reaches 100%. Attempts with a longer-lasting schedule (4–5 days) or by redoubling the dose do not improve results. For individual therapy 100 mg b.i.d. for three days is an excellent standard dosage, which also provides a reliable efficacy in mass treatment.

However, for community-wide treatment, single doses are more indicated. Within this option prospects with single doses of 600 mg are fairly good and deserve closer attention. It should be kept in mind that after mebendazole therapy the morphology of the eggs evacuated with the stools is clearly altered. These eggs are no longer viable, and thus the infectivity potential is reduced.

Easy to administer, well accepted, well tolerated, less expensive, and possessing a broad-spectrum effect, mebendazole is of considerable importance to public health.

2.2.7 Oxantel

2.2.7.1 State of the Art

Oxantel has been known since 1972 to be active against whipworm in mice and dogs. It was tried out by LIM in humans in 1974, and the administration of a single dose of 10 mg/kg produced a CR of 91% and an ERR of 98%. Moreover, 10 mg/kg b.i.d. for 3 days relieved the symptoms in severe clinical trichiuriasis in children. This compound is, however, ineffective against ascariasis.

2.2.7.2 Assessment

Table 84. Treatment of *T. trichiura* infections by oxantel

Efficacy	Dosage	Number treated	CR	ERR	References
100%	20 mg/kg	15	100	–	LEE et al. (1976)
	20 mg/kg	10	100	–	GARCIA (1976)
≧90%	10 mg/kg	46	91	98	LIM (1974)
	15 mg/kg (syrup)	50	90	91	LIM (1978)
	20 mg/kg (syrup)	15	93	99	LIM (1978)
	15 mg/kg (syrup)	17	94	98	RIM et al. (1976)
	15 mg/kg	25	92	87	GARCIA (1976)
≧80%	15 mg/kg	33	88	90	LEE et al. (1976)
	10–15 mg/kg	171	83	97	RIM et al. (1976)
	10 mg/kg b.i.d./4 days	7	88	88	PAUL and ZAMAN (197(
	10–15 mg/kg	193	84	97	LIM (1978)
≧70%	25 mg/kg	12	75	96	LIM (1978)
	10 mg/kg	26	77	72	GARCIA (1976)
≧60%	10 mg/kg	70	63	92	LIM (1973)
	10 mg/kg b.i.d./3 days	25	68	–	LEE et al. (1975)
≧50% (underpriviliged children)					
	10 mg/kg	70	57	92	PARK et al. (1973)
	10 mg/kg	122	57	90	LEE et al. (1976)
	10 mg/kg	28	57	91	RIM et al. (1976)

2.2.7.3 Dosage, Mode of Administration

Oxantel pamoate is available as a suspension with 50 mg oxantel base per milliliter. A single oral dose of 15 mg/kg body weight is already efficient.

2.2.7.4 Side Effects

Side effects are mild, transitory, and occur within the first 24 h in about one in four cases, e.g., headache, nausea, abdominal pain, and diarrhea. Biochemical tests in blood and urine show no significant differences between pre- and post-treatment samples. The compound is well tolerated and suitable for use on an outpatient basis.

2.2.7.5 Contraindications, Precautions

Oxantel has no known contraindications.

2.2.7.6 Conclusions

Oxantel is one of the reliable drugs against *T. trichiura*. Single doses of 10–25 mg/kg are effective only in light infections, with an indication that 15-mg or higher doses, repeated on two consecutive days, provide the best results. The investigations of LEE et al. (1975) underline the necessity of an administration sustained over several days, with a possible repeat.

The treatment of symptomatic trichiuriasis can be achieved with this drug.

2.2.8 Oxantel and Pyrantel (Quantrel)

2.2.8.1 State of the Art

Pyrantel is effective in a single dose against ascariasis (BELL and NASSIF 1971) AND ENTEROBIASIS (BUMBALO et al. 1969) and on a 3-day regimen against hookworm (BOTERO and CASTANO 1973), but is ineffective against *T. trichiura* (CERVONI and OLIVER-GONZALES 1971). Since its analogue oxantel is effective against the latter, it was rational to try to cover a wider spectrum of activity with a combination of both drugs. This possibility has been offered by a mixture of oxantel and pyrantel.

2.2.8.2 Assessment

Table 85. Treatment of *T. trichiura* infections by oxantel and pyrantel

Efficacy	Dosage	Number treated	CR	ERR	Refernces
100%	20 mg/kg/2 days[a]	10	100	–	LEE (1978)
≧90%	20 mg/kg/2 days	50	98	93	KALE (1977)
	15 mg/kg/2 days	10	90	92	LEE (1978)
	15 mg/kg	10	90	99	LIM (1978)
	15 mg/kg b.i.d.	34	94	99	CABRERA and CRUZ (1980b)

Table 85 (continued)

Efficacy	Dosage	Number treated	CR	ERR	Refernces
≧80%	15–20 mg/kg/3 days	32	84	–	GARCIA (1978)
	15 mg/kg b.i.d.	37	89	–	CABRERA and SY (1978)
	20 mg/kg	37	84	95	CABRERA and CRUZ (1980b)
	15–20 mg/kg	32	84	79–95	CHANCO and VIDAD (1981)
≧70%	10 mg/kg	56	73	92	RIM et al. (1975)
	10 mg/kg	24	75	88	GARCIA (1975)
	10 mg/kg	75	77	81	LIM (1978)
	20 mg/kg/2 days	45	71	–	CABRERA and SY (1978)
	15–20 mg/kg	19	76	98	CHANCO and VIDAD (1978)
≧50%	15–20 mg/kg/3 days	24	67	95	DISSANAIKE (1978)
	15 mg/kg (rural)	193	53	–	CABRERA and SY (1978)
<50%	20 mg/kg	90	41	–	CABRERA and SY (1978)
	15–20 mg/kg	17	29	97	DISSANAIKE (1978)

[a] 20 mg each of oxantel and pyrantel

2.2.8.3 Dosage, Mode of Administration

Oxantel and pyrantel is available as an oral suspension containing 50 mg pyrantel and 50 mg oxantel/ml. The recommended dose is 10 mg/kg of each constituent without exceeding 20 mg/kg of each, especially in children. This means that below 6–7 kg body weight not more than 2.5 ml should be administered.

2.2.8.4 Side Effects

Side effects are rare and mainly limited to gastrointestinal complaints. See Sect. B.II.3.2.12.4.

2.2.8.5 Contraindications

See Sect. B.II.3.2.12.5.

2.2.8.6 Conclusions

The results of this combination are on the whole satisfactory. A broadening of the anthelmintic spectrum has indeed been achieved. Single doses produce, however, generally less satisfactory CRs than dosages repeated for 2 or 3 days, at least at a dosage of 10 mg/kg. But even an increase to 15 or 20 mg/kg body weight does not improve the efficacy of the single-dose regime (CABRERA and SY 1978).

2.2.9 Piperazine

This safe anthelmintic is effective against roundworms and threadworms but has no significant effect on whipworms. CAVIER and BELLON (1960), confirming unpublished observations made by SAVATON-PILLET (1957), state that at least *piperazine sebacate* (Nematorazine), renowned for its good tolerance, produces a CR of 70%, provided that the administration is prolonged and repeated (four courses). This compound is mentioned for the sake of completeness.

2.2.10 Pyrantel Pamoate (Combantrin)

2.2.10.1 State of the Art

This broad-spectrum neuro-blocking anthelmintic, successfully tried out in the treatment of various helminths in man, has, according to DESOWITZ et al. (1970), virtually no effect against trichiuriasis. This inefficiency has been confirmed by the majority of the reported experiments.

2.2.10.2 Assessment

Table 86. Treatment of *T. trichiura* infections by pyrantel pamoate

Efficacy	Dosage	Number treated	CR	ERR	References
≧90%	10 mg/kg	172	96%	99%	STRÜCKLER et al. (1980)
≦50%	20 mg/kg/2 days	13	46%	–	KATZ et al. (1972)
	20 mg/kg/3 days	7	43%		KATZ et al. (1972)
<10%	11 mg/kg	69	–	10%	CERVONI-GONZALES (1971)
	11 mg/kg	52 (adults)	2%	–	PITTS-MIGLIARDI (1974)
	11 mg/kg	159 (children)	0.6%	–	PITTS and MIGLIARDI (1974)
	11 mg/kg	23	4%	11%	WERSHING et al. (1975)

2.2.10.3 Dosage, Mode of Administration

Pyrantel pamoate is available in chewing tablets of 250 mg and an oral suspension of 250 mg/5 ml. See Sect. B.II.3.2.11.3.

2.2.10.4 Side Effects

See Sect. B.II.3.2.11.4.

2.2.10.5 Contraindications, Precautions

See Sect. B.II.3.2.11.5.

2.2.10.6 Conclusion

An obvious explanation for these contradictory results is not at hand. In any case the manufacturing pharmaceutical industry has agreed on limited efficacy and therefore combined pyrantel with the more efficient oxantel.

2.2.11 Pyrvinium Pamoate (Vanquin)

2.2.11.1 State of the Art

This red cyanine dye is effective in a single dose of 5 mg/kg in *E. vermicularis* infections. It has been tried out by VILELA et al. (1964) against whipworm.

2.2.11.2 Assessment

Table 87. Treatment of *T. trichiura* infection by pyrvinium pamoate

Efficacy	Dosage	Number treated	CR	ERR	References
	10 mg/kg/3 days	28	46		VILELA et al. (1964)

2.2.11.3 Dosage, Mode of Administration

Ten milligrams per kilogram is an unusually high dose. See Sect. E.II.3.2.8.3.

2.2.11.4 Side Effects

See Sect. E.II.3.2.8.4.

2.2.11.5 Contraindications, Precautions

See Sect. E.II.3.2.8.5.

2.2.11.6 Conclusion

Overall efficacy is poor. Since pyrvinium is less active on immature worms, its use would imply an administration lasting several days or a repetition of the treatment. This drug, which stains stools and clothes, has been displaced by the newer anthelmintics.

2.2.12 Tiabendazole (Mintezol)

2.2.12.1 State of the Art

While treating strongyloidiasis with tiabendazole, VILELA et al. (1962) noted that this drug had some action against *T. trichiura*. As tiabendazole has a rather broad anthelmintic spectrum in addition to a valuable efficacy, it was a matter of common sense to investigate this possibility.

2.2.12.2 Assessment

Table 88. Treatment of *T. trichiura* infection by tiabendazole

Efficacy	Dosage	Number treated	CR	ERR	References
≧50%	1 g 500 mg	8	62	–	IWATA et al. (1963a, b)
	30 mg/kg/3 days	50	58	–	ZUCATO and VILELA (1964)
≧40%	25 mg/kg	29	48	–	CHANCO and PAGUIO (1964)
	25 mg/kg	34	44	–	FRANZ et al. (1965)

Table 88 (continued)

Efficacy	Dosage	Number treated	CR	ERR	References
	1 g/3 days	26	42	–	Ishizaki et al. (1963)
	1 g 250 b.i.d.	7	42	–	Vakil et al. (1965)
≧30%	25 mg/kg/2 days	101	55	55	Escobar (1964)
	50 mg/kg	313	38	72	Escobar (1964)
	25 mg/kg		32	–	Chanco and Tagama (1965)
	25 mg/kg/5 days	46	33	47	Escobar (1964)
	1 250 mg	8	38	–	Vakil et al. (1965)
	1 g 250 mg b.i.d	16	31	–	Vakil et al. (1965)
<30%	2 g 500 mg	11	27	–	Salunke et al. (1964)
	2 g 500 mg	11	27	–	Vakil et al. (1965)
	1 g 250 mg	8	25	–	Salunke et al. (1964)
	1 g	10	20	–	Iwata et al. (1963)
	25 mg/kg	234	13	43	Escobar (1964)

2.2.12.3 Dosage, Mode of Administration

See Sect. B.II.3.2.13.3.

2.2.12.4 Side Effects

See Sect. B.II.3.2.13.4.

2.2.12.5 Contraindications, Precautions

See Sect. B.II.3.2.13.5.

2.2.12.6 Conclusion

Results have been disappointing. The CR varies between 0% and 62% with doses of 15–50 mg/kg for 1–3 days. An increase in dose and in number of treatment days might improve the CR, but will also augment the side effects. This drug is almost useless against trichuriasis.

III. Drug Combinations

Tiabendazole and Pyrvinium Pamoate

1. State of the Art

As tiabendazole and pyrvinium are chemically unrelated, their anthelmintic activity might act through a different mechanism. This has been the reason for checking a possible synergistic action.

2. Assessment

Table 89. Treatment of *T. trichiura* infection by a combination of tiabendazole and pyrvinium pamoate

Dosage	Number treated	CR	ERR	References
Tiabendazole and pyrvinium				
30 mg/kg + 10 mg/kg/3 days	50	92		VILLELA et al. (1968)
30 mg/kg + 10 mg/kg/3 days	28	21	–	AMATO-NETO and DE MOURA-V. (1968)
25 mg/kg + 15 mg/kg/6 days or 12.5 mg/kg + 7.5 mg/kg/12 days	50	86	–	ATRA et al. (1965)

3. Conclusion

The association of both drugs, whether the expected synergism is present or not, is more effective than either drug alone and the activity extends to *A. lumbricoides* and *S. stercoralis*. Nevertheless this association has been displaced by the new generation of anthelmintics.

References

Abadi K (1974) Mebendazole (R 17635) in the treatment of intestinal helminthiasis in low socio-economic group in Ujung Pandang, South Sulawesi. Janssen Pharmaceutica Clin Res Report, N 8250

Abadie DH, Samuels M (1965) A fatality associated with dithiazanine iodide therapy. J Am Med Assoc 192:326–327

Abdallah A (1959) Epidemiology of ancylostomiasis. J Min Health 1:4–12

Abdallah A, Saif M (1963) The efficacy of single-dose treatment of ancylostomiasis with bephenium hydroxynaphtoate. J Trop Med Hyg 66:45–47

Adam W, Janssens PG (1965) L'Ankylostomiase. Rev Hyg Mines 20:101–125

Adiao AC, Mejia SS, Mundo F Del (1961) Clinical observations on the use of pyrvinium pamoate in enterobiasis. J Philipp Med Assoc 37:485–488

Aguilar FJ (1959) The polyanthelmintic action of dithiazanine iodide. Am J Trop Med Hyg 8:305–306

Aguilar FJ (1981) Helminthiasis humanas transmitidas a travès del suelo en Guatemala. Bol Chil Parasitol 36:6–9

Aguilar FJ, Tanchez G, Cifuentes CE, Folgar M (1973) Trichuriasis: tratamiento con mebendazole. Rev Coleg Medico 24:182–184

Aguilar FJ, Cifuentes CE, Samayoa A (1977) Comparative clinical study: Oxantel-pyrantel, mebendazole in uncinariasis, trichuriasis and ascariasis. 4th Congr latino americano San José, Costa-Rica (1976). Parasitologia 28:101–118

Ahmad N, Ghulam R (1959) Bephenium hydroxynaphtoate against hookworm in West Pakistan. J Trop Med Hyg 12:284

Ahmad N, Rasool G (1959) Bephenium hydroxynaphtoate against hookworm in West-Pakistan. J Trop Med Hyg 62:284–285

Ahmad N, Keeling JED, Wahid A (1964) A clinical trial of two bephenium hydroxynaphtoate preparations against hookworm and roundworm in West-Pakistan. Am J Trop Med Hyg 13:693–697

Akagi K (1973) *Enterobius vermicularis* and enterobiasis. In: Marishita et al. (eds) Progress of medical parasitology in Japan, vol 5. pp 229–279

Albos Martinez J, Arce L (1956) La piperacina en el tratamiento de las helminthiasis intestinales. Med Clin 27:350–354

Alekseeva MI, Pucenko AY (1980) Comparative effectiveness and tolerance in the Vanquin, Combatrin and Vermox treatments of enterobiasis. Med Parazitol 49:34–38

Alexander F, Drijkoningen G, Flahaut J, Raveschot H (1970) Comparative study of the therapeutic efficacy and tolerance of pyrvinium pamoate and pyrantel pamoate in *Enterobius vermicularis* infections (in Dutch). Tijdschr Geneeskd 26:333–335

Alicata JE, Jindrak K (1970) Angiostrongylosis in the Pacific and Southeast Asia. Thomas, Springfield

Al-Issa TB, Wahab HA (1971) Comparative trial of pyrantel, levamisole and bephenium in the treatment of intestinal worms in Iraq. Bull Endem Dis 18:109–115

Al-Saffar G, Al-Saleem M, Bakhous IJ (1971) L-Tetramisole in the treatment of ancylostomiasis. Trans R Soc Trop Med Hyg 65:836–837

Amato-Neto V (1969) Sintomatologia atribuivel a enterobiasis. Rev Inst Med Trop Sao Paulo 11:343–347

Amato-Neto V (1970) Oxantel-pyrantel. Rev Inst Med Trop Sao Paulo 12:207–210

Amato-Neto V, Correa M (1956) Tratamento da ascaridiase pelo hydrato de piperazina. O Hospital 49:103–107

Amato-Neto V, Moura-Vasconcellos AT De (1965) Tratamento da trichocefaliase pelo associaço de Tiabendazole é pamoato de pirvinio. O Hospital 68:1413–1418

Amato-Neto V, Wanderley RA, Correa MOA (1967) Traitement des porteurs d'*Ascaris* par le tetramisole dans une zone rurale. O Hospital 72:585–591

Amato-Neto V, Levi GC, Vilela E, Oliveira Gomes MC De, Campos R (1969a) Sintomatologia atribuivel à enterobiase, analisada entre crianças residentes em habitacao coletiva. Rev Inst Med Trop Sao Paulo 11:343–347

Amato-Neto V, Levi GC, Aly J, Correa MOA (1969b) Observacoes sobre a atividade curativa da forma levogyra do tetramisole (RO 8299.L) en relaçao a ascaridase. O Hospital 75:171–176

Amato-Neto V, Levi GC, Stefani NV, Konichi SR, Dias JCP, Oliveira LR, Campos LL (1973) Nossas primeiras observacoes sobre a acao terapeutica de mebendazole novo medicamento anti-helmintico dotado de amplo espectro de atividade. Rev Inst Med Trop Sao Paulo 15:34–37

Amato-Neto V, Sinto T, Pedro RJ, Levi GC, Tsukumo MKK, Moraes VMC, Correa LL (1978) Nossas observacoas iniciais sobre a efficacia do cambendazole no tratamento da estrongiloidiase. Rev Inst Med Trop Sao Paulo 20:161–163

Amato-Neto V, Mareira AA, Campos R, Lazarro ES, Chiaramelli MC, Castillo VL, Gomes AE, Pinto PL (1983) Tratamento da ancilostomiase por meio da albendazol. Rev Inst Med Trop Sao Paulo 25:42–46

Ambre S, Mak JW (1981) The effect of mebendazole and flubendazole on *Angiostrongylus malaysiensis* infections in rats. Southeast Asian J Trop Med Public Health 12:228–280

Andrade Freire D, Oetting A Jr, Machado Freire E, Cubero Ruano A, Amato-Neto V (1969) Tratamento da ascaridiase por meio do levamisole-base. O Hospital 76:1715–1719

Anthony PP, McAdam IWJ (1972) Helminthic pseudotumours of the bowel: thirty-four cases of helminthoma. Gut 13:8–16

Anuar A Kh, Ramachandran CP (1977) A study on the prevalence of soil transmitted helminths among lettuce leaves sold in local markets in Penang (Malaysia). Med J Malaysia 31:262–265

Apt W, Hisamoto T, Llorens P, Alcaino H (1980) Anisakiasis gastrica in Chile. Rev Med Chil 108:825–827

Arada III EV, Augustin EC, Bagasao MG, Chung EO, Diadula HM, Ibarra AN, Libarnes RL, Lim AC, Padilla EP, Tan ES (1978) A double blind comparative study of the efficacy of mebendazole and flubendazole in the treatment of enterobiasis. J Manila Med Soc 16:39–46

Arfaa F, Farahmandian I (1976) Progress achieved in the chemotherapy of soil-transmitted helminths. In: Williams JD, Geddes AM (eds) Chemotherapy 6:11–22

Arfaa F, Ghadirian E (1977) Epidemiology and mass-treatment of ascariasis in six rural communitees in central Iran. Am J Trop Med Hyg 26:866–867
Arfaa F, Ghadirian E (1978) The effect of mass-treatment in the control of helminthiasis in Ispahan, central Iran. Iran J Public Health 7:100–114
Arfaa F, Sahba GH, Farahnandian I, Jalali H (1977) Evaluation of the effect of different methods of control of soil-transmitted helminths in Khuzestan, southwest Iran. Am J Trop Med Hyg 26:230–233
Arfaa F, Farahmandian I, Miller MJ (1979) Flubendazole in the treatment of hookworm disease complicated or not by trichuriasis and/or ascariasis. Janssen Pharmaceutica, Clin Res Report, N 17494
Arguedas JA, Villarejos VM, Swartzwelder JC, Chavarria AP, Zeledon R, Kotcher E (1975) Community control of *Strongyloides stercoralis* by thiabendazole. Tex Rep Biol Med 33:265–268
Asami KT, Watanuki H, Sakai H, Smano H, Okamoto R (1963) Two cases of stomach granuloma caused by *Anisakis*-like larval nematodes in Japan. Am J Trop Med Hyg 14:119–123
Asford RW, Hall AJ, Babona D (1981) Distribution and abundance of intestinal helminths in man in Western Papua New Guinea with special reference to strongyloides. Ann Trop Med Parasitol 75:269–279
Asmera J (1974) Decaris Janssen – evaluation of clinical trials. Janssen Pharmaceutica, Clin Res Rep N 5166
Aspöck H, Flamm H, Picher O, Wiedermann G (1977) Mebendazol – Ein polyvalentes Antihelminthicum für die ambulante Entwurmung. Wien Med Wochenschr 127:88–91
Asshauer E, Mohr W (1966) Thiabendazol in der Behandlung von Wurminfektionen. Arzneimittelforsch 16:428–431
Aswapoker N, Saravich S (1978) Mebendazole, a new broad spectrum anthelminthic. J Med Assoc Thai 61:675–680
Atchley FO, Wysham DN, Hemphill EC (1956) Mass treatment of Ascariasis with a single dose of piperazine citrate. Am J Trop Med Hyg 5:881–887
Atra E, Vilela MP de, Zucas AW (1965) Therapeutica da trichocephaliase. Resultados obtidas com una nova associaçao medicamentosa em adultos. O Hospital 61:217–224
Avery JL (1956) Treatment of enterobiasis with one oral dose of promethazine hydrochloride. JAMA 161:681–683
Ayad El-Masry N, Trabolsi B, Bassily S, Farid Z (1983) Albendazole in the treatment of *Ancylostoma duodenale* and *Ascaris lumbricoides* infections. Trans R Soc Trop Med Hyg 77:160–161
Bächlin A, Degremont A (1979) Oxyuren Befall in Basler Kindergärten. Schweiz Rundschau Med 68:1183–1185
Baer JG (1951) Ecology of animal parasites. University of Illinois Press, Urbana
Baker NF, Walters CT (1971) Antihelmintic efficacy of cambendazole in cattle. Am J Vet Res 32:29–33
Balagopal R (1974) Study of oxyuriasis in families. Inst Child Health, Madras
Baldez D, Conti LMZ, Sette PC, Sette H, Silva LC Da, Saez-Alquezar A (1978) Flubendazole no tratamento das parasitoses intestinais: comparacao entre dois esquemas posologicas. Ann XIV congresso Soc Brasiliera de Med Trop, Joao Pessoa
Bannerjee D, Prakash O, Kaliyugaperumal V (1972a) A clinical trial of mebendazole (R 17635) in cases of hookworm infection. Indian J Med Res 60:562–566
Bannerjee D, Kaliyugaperumal V, Prakash O (1972b) Tetramisole in hookworm infections. Indian J Med Res 60:834–839
Banzon TC, Singson CN, Cross JH (1976) Mebendazole treatment for intestinal nematodes in a Philippine Barrio. A preliminary report. J Philipp Med Assoc 52:7–8
Baranski MC, Silva AF Da, Kotaka PI, Gomes NR, Giovannoni M, Telles JEQ (1978) Tratamento da estrongiloidiase humana com novo antihelmintica, o cambendazole. Estudo Duplo cego. Rev Inst Med Trop Sao Paulo 20:213–218
Baranski MC, Fontoura A da, Guimaraes LM (1981) Tratamiento de las helminthiasis intestinales con Albendazol, un nuevo antihelmintico del grupo de los benzimidazoles. Estudio doble ciego. Compendium Invest Clin latino americanos [Suppl] 1:82–89

Barbaix E (1981) Flubendazole in the treatment of trichuriasis, ascariasis and hookworm disease. Janssen Pharmaceutica, Clin Res Report, N 24062

Barrett-Connor E (1975) Recent advances in the treatment of common intestinal helminths. Am J Gastroenterol 63:105–116

Basnuevo JG, Kowin A (1959) Accion antihelminthia del Yoduro de Ditiazanina. Rev Kuba Med Trop 15:27–36

Basnuevo JG, Delgado FS, Fontao JA (1953) La mezcla hexilresorecinol – tetracloroetileno sustituye ventajosamente al helecho macho en el tratamiento de la taeniaisis. Rev Kuba Med Trop 9:48–50

Basnuevo JG, Rodrigues JJ, Borbolla L (1959a) Tratamiento de la strongyloidiasis con ditiazanina. Rev Kuba Med Trop 15:5–8

Basnuevo JG, Rodrigues JJ, Borges F (1959b) Tratamiento de lo trichocefaliasis con ditiazanine. Rev Kuba Med Trop 15:15–19

Bastidas GrJ (1982) Albendazol a dosis unica en nematodiasis intestinales multiples. Invest Med Intern 9:308–312

Batzinger RP, Bueding E, Crawford K, Bruce J (1979) Prevention of the mutagenic activation of antischistosomal isothiocyanate in primates by an antibiotic. Environ Mutagen 1:353–360

Bawa YS, Chopra JS, Sharma TD (1965) Comparative study of bephenium hydroxynaphtoate and tetrachlorethylene in hookworm disease. Indian J Med Sci 19:605–608

Beck JW (1964) Treatment of pinworm infections with reduced single dose of pyrvinium pamoate. JAMA 189:511

Beck JW (1966) The treatment of *Ascaris lumbricoides* and *Enterobius vermicularis* with combination drug composed of Pyrvinium pamoate and piperazine. Acta Med Costaricense 9:9–11

Beck JW, Saavedra D, Antell GJ, Tefeiro B (1959) The treatment of pinworm infections in humans with pyrvinium chloride and pyrvinium pamoate. Am J Trop Med Hyg 8:349–352

Becquet R (1963) Traitement de l'ankylostomose par l'hydroxynaphtoate de bephenium. J Sci Méd (Lille) 81:316–321

Becquet R (1976) Expertise clinique – flubendazole comprimés. Janssen Pharmaceutica, Clin Res Report R 17889/G, N 12249

Becquet R, Labarriere F (1980) Le flubendazole dans le traitement des nématodoses digestives. Méd Actuelle 7:4

Behar RR (1971) Eratamiento de la estrongiloidiasis en la infancia. Rev Cubana Med Trop 23:141–150

Beheyt P, Lebrun A, Cerf J, Dierick J, Groote V De (1961) Toxicity for man of an organophosphorus insecticide. Bull WHO 24:465–473

Bekhti A (1974) Un nouvel anthelminthique, le mebendazole. Acta Gastroenterol Belg 37:302–306

Bell WJ, Gould GC (1971) Preliminary report on pyrantel pamoate in the treatment of human hookworm infection. East Afr Med J 48:143–151

Bell WJ, Nassif S (1971) Comparison of pyrantel pamoate and piperazine phosphate in the treatment of ascariasis. Am J Trop Med Hyg 20:584–588

Bellani L, Mantovani A, Pampiglione S, Filippini I (1978) Observations on an outbreak of human trichinellosis in Northern Italy. In: Kim ChW, Pawlowski ZP (eds) Trichinellosis. University Press of New England. Hannover, New Hampshire, pp 535–539

Beltran-Hernandez F, Sanchez-Carrillo C, Caballero-Guerrero C (1976) Control de las helminthiasis transmitidas por el suelo (HTS) con Mebendazole, en una communidad de la Selva Lacandona (Mexico). 4th congr latino americano de parasitol, San Jose, Costa Rica

Berti JJ, Silva H, Simonovis A De (1976) Evaluacion del mebendazol y de la combinacion oxantel-pyrantel en el tratamiento de helminthiases intestinales. 4th Congr Latino americano de parasitol, San José, Costa Rica

Bettecken F (1957) Über EEG-Veränderungen durch Piperazin im Kindesalter. Z Kinderheilk 80:225–231

Bezjak Br (1968) A clinical trial of thiabendazole in strongyloidiasis. Am J Trop Med Hyg 17:733–736
Bhaibulaya M, Indra-Ngarm S (1979) *Amaurornis phoenicurus* and *Ardeola bacchus* as experimental definitive hosts for *Capillaria philippinensis* in Thailand. Int J Parasitol 9:321–322
Bhaibulaya M, Punnavutti V, Yamput S (1975) Mass treatment of hookworm infection with a single dose of pyrantel pamoate. J Med Assoc Thai 59:347–350
Bhaibulaya M, Benjapong W, Noeypatimanond S (1977) Infection of *Capillaria philippinensis* in man from Phetchabun Province, northern Thailand: a report of the fifth case. J Med Assoc Thai 69:507–509
Bhaibulaya M, Indra-Ngarm S, Anathapruti M (1979) Freshwater fishes of Thailand as experimental intermediate hosts for *Capillaria philippinensis*. Int J Parasitol 9:105–108
Bhandari B, Shrimali LN (1969) Clinical evaluation of phenylene di-isothiocyanate (Jonit ®) in paediatric patients with hookworm disease. J Trop Med Hyg 72:164–166
Bhandari B, Singhi SV (1969) Phenylene di-isothicocyanate in the treatment of adult patients infected with hookworm. Ann Trop Med Parasitol 63:177–180
Bhandari B, Singhi A (1980) Fenbendazole (Hoe 881) in enterobiasis. Trans R Soc Trop Med Hyg 74:691
Biagi F (1980) Levamisol en el tratmiento de la ascariasis. Janssen Pharmaceutica, Int Clin Res Report, N 19198
Biagi F, Rodrigues O (1960) A study of ascariasis eradication by repeated mass treatment. Am J Trop Med Hyg 9:274–276
Biagi F, Zavala J, Malagon F (1969) Accion antiparasitaria del connuesto 16842 en la uncinariaris y trichocefalosis. Rev Inst Med Trop Sao Paulo 11:444–448
Biagi F, Smyth J, Gonzalez C (1974) Mebendazole en helminthiasis intestinales. La Prensa Med Mexicana 39:3–5
Bicalho SA, Leao OJ, Pena Q Jr (1983) Cambendazole in the treatment of human strongyloidiasis. Am J Trop Med Hyg 32:1181–1183
Biguet J, Deblock S, Capron A, Machez JM (1952) La cure éclair de l'oxyurose par le pamoate de pyrroviniquinium. Presse Méd 67:1739–1740
Biguet J, Coutelen F, Deblock S, Doby JM, Mullet S (1953) Etude de l'activité de la pipérazine dans l'oxyurose. Bull Soc Pathol Exot Filiales 48:40–46
Bijkerk H (1969) Haringwormziekte (Anisakiasis). Ned Tijdschr Geneeskd 113:906–907
Bijkerk H (1970) Haringwormziekte. Ned Tjdschr Geneeskd 114:856
Bijkerk H (1971) Haringwormziekte (Anisakiasis). Ned Tijdschr Geneeskd 115:763
Bina JC, Figueiredo JFM, Barreto Ailho A, Carvalho F (1977) Tratamento en massa, por meio do mebendazol das helminthiases intestinais mas comuns en meio rural, con estudo dos indices de reinfestacao. Rev Inst Med Trop Sao Paulo 19:47–51
Blechman MG (1975) Clinical effectiveness of mebendazole in the treatment of trichuriasis. Curr Ther Res 18:800–803
Blechman MG, Pena-Chavarria A, Diermissen AG (1982) Double-blind study of flubendazole in the treatment of *Trichuris trichiura* infection. Clin Res Rev 2:115–120
Bogojawlenski NA, Demidova AJ (1928) Sur la présence dans la mucus nasal de l'homme des oeufs de vers parasites. Russian J Trop Med 6:153–156 (in Russian, French summary)
Bonnefoy X, Isautier H (1978) Variations de l'incidence des helminthiases à la réunion en fonction de differents paramètres. Bull Soc Pathol Exot Filiales 71:70–78
Borda CE, Rea MJ, Borda RW (1976) Accion antiparasitaria del mebendazole en la Anquilostomiasis. Prensa Med Argent 63:55–58
Borda CE, Dho MC, Rea MJF, Borda RW (1978) Eficacia del mebendazol en la uncinariasis por *Ancylostoma duodenale*. Bol Chil Parasitol 33:57–61
Botero D (1964) Report on clinical investigations with thiabendazole. Tribuna Medica 3:1–8
Botero D (1965) Treatment of human intestinal helminthiases with thiabendazole. Am J Trop Med Hyg 14:618–621
Botero D (1922) Possibilities of controlling soil transmitted helminths by mass treatment. Bol Chil Parasitol 34:39–43

Botero D (1975) Epidemiology and public health importance of intestinal nematode infections in Latin America. Fortschr Arzneimittelforsch 19:28–43

Botero D (1980a) Human intestinal *Angiostrongylus* WHO mimeogr. Int Parasitol SG/WP/80-25

Botero D (1980b) Treatment on intestinal helminthiasis with flubendazole. Janssen Pharmaceutica, Clin Res Report N 20710

Botero RD, Castano GA (1972) Tratamiento comparativo de uncinariasis y ascariasis com pamoato de Pirantel, hidroxynaftoato de befenio y tetracloretileno. Antioquia Medica 22:581–591

Botero D, Castano A (1973) Comparative study of pyrantel pamoate, bephenium hydroxynaphtoate and tetrachlorethylene in the treatment of *Necator americanus* infections. Am J Trop Med Hyg 22:45–52

Botero D, Perez CA (1970) Clinical evaluation of a new drug for the treatment of ancylostomiasis. Am J Trop Med Hyg 19:471–475

Botero D, Perez AC (1976) Tratamiento de helminthiasis intestinales con mebendazole. Tribuna Medica 54:30–32

Botero D, Orozco HI, Perez A (1966) Ensayo de una mezcla de piperacina y pirvinio en el tratamiento de ascaridiasis y oxyuriasis. Bol Chil Parasitol 21:111–114

Botero-Ramos D (1974) Helmintiasis intestinales. Tratamiento en masa con pamoato de pirantel. Tribuna Medica 50:5, A21–126

Bourderioux C, Chevalier C (1982) Traitement par l'albendazole à Dakar de 85 sujets atteints d'ankylostomose, de trichocéphalose isolée ou d'une association ankylostomose-trichocéphalose, ascaridiose-trichocéphalose. Med Afr Noire 29:23–26

Bouree P, Kouchner G, Gascon A (1976) A propos d'une épidemie de Trichinose dans la banlieu parisienne. Bull Soc Pathol Exot Filiales 69:177–181

Bouree P, Cazin A, Kouchner G (1978) Le fluoromebendazole: nouvel antihelminthique à large spectre. Short communications D_3-26. 4th int congress of parasitology. Polish Scientific Publishers, Warszawa

Bouree P, Bouvier JB, Passeron J, Galanaud P, Dormont J (1979) Outbreak of trichinosis near Paris. Br Med J 1:1047–1049

Bouree P, Thulliez Ph, Kouchner G, Gascon A (1982) Liquid fluorobendazole effectiveness against nematodes. In: Müller M, Gutteridge W, Köhler P (eds) Molecular and biochemical parasitology. Elsevier Biomedical, Amsterdam pp 528

Bouvier JB (1976) Expertise clinique flubendazole compr. Janssen Pharmaceutica, Clin Res Report, N 12247

Bouyer C (1970) Traitement des parasitoses intestinales par le levamisole. Bull Soc Pathol Exot Filiales 63:255–264

Breedveld PH, Geus A De, Jong-Stoelinga MHFM De (1977) Intestinale worminfecties bij migranten uit Suriname. Ned Tijdschr Geneeskd 121:1126–1130

Brock N, Erhardt A, Wilmanns H (1952) Zur Behandlung der Oxyuriasis mit Atrimon. Dtsch Med Wochenschr 77:240–242

Brown HW (1954) The treatment of *Ascaris lumbricoides* infections with piperazine. J Pediatr 45:419–424

Brown HW (1969) Anthelmintics, new and old. Clin Pharmacol Ther 10:5–21

Brown HW, Chan KF (1955) Treatment of *Enterobius vermicularis* infections with piperazine. Am J Trop Med Hyg 4:321–325

Brown HW, Cort WW (1927) The egg production of *Ascaris lumbricoides*. J. Parasitol 14:88–90

Brown HW, Sterman MM (1958) Chemotherapy of strongyloidiasis with pyrrovinylquinium (Vanquin). Am J Trop Med Hyg 7:255–256

Brown HW, Chan KF, Yolken H (1956a) Efficacy of promethazine and pyrathiazine against enterobiasis. JAMA 162:1049–1051

Brown HW, Chan KF, Hussey KL (1956b) Treatment of enterobiasis and ascariasis with piperazine. JAMA 161:515–520

Browne DC, Contacos PG, Welch GE, McHardy G (1957) Treatment of *Strongyloides stercoralis* infection with intravenous gentian violet. Am J Trop Med Hyg 6:1066–1067

Bruch K, Haas J (1976) Effectiveness of single doses of fenbendazole (Hoe 881) against *Ascaris*, hookworm and *Trichuris* in man. Ann Trop Med Parasitol 70:205–211

Brudastov AN, Lemelev VR, Kholmukhamedov SK, Krasnosos LN (1971) Clinical picture of the migration phase of ascariasis in self-infection. Med Parazitol 40:165–168

Brugmans JP, Thienpont DC, Wijngaarden I Van, Parijs OF Van, Schuermans VL, Lauwers HL (1971) Mebendazole in enterobiasis. Radiochemical and pilot clinical study in 1,278 subjects. JAMA 217:313–316

Brumpt E (1949) Précês de parasitologie. Masson, Paris

Brumpt L (1973) Etude de l'activité du mebendazole dans diverses parasitoses. Janssen Pharmaceutica, Clin Res Report N 7229

Brumpt L (1976) Expertise clinique – flubendazole comprimés –. Intern Clin Report, Janssen Pharmaceutica 12.248

Brumpt L, Ho-Thi-Sang (1953) Le traitement des ankylostomoses graves par le tétrachloréthylène. Bull Soc Pathol Exot Filiales 46:1024–1037

Brumpt L, Ho-Thi-Sang (1954) Traitement de l'ascaridose et de l'oxyurose par les dérivés de piperazine. Bull Soc Pathol Exot Filiales 47:817–822

Brumpt L, Ho-Thi-Sang (1959) La dithiazanine, nouveau vermifuge polyvalent. Presse Mèd 67:289–290

Budzhe MM, Bljuger AF, Dakhovker SF, Ladyznja BS (1959) Comparative study of diverse patterns of ascariasis treatment with piperazine salts. Med Parazitol 28:436–438

Bueding E, Swartzwelder C (1957) Anthelmintics. Pharmacol Rev 9:329–365

Bueding E, Batzinger R, Petterson G (1976) Antischistosomal and some toxicological properties of a nitrodiphenylamino-isothiocyanate (C 9333-90/CGP 4540). Experientia 32:604–606

Bui-Quoc-Huong, Buu-Hoi, Tran-Lu-Y, Tang-Nhiep, Nguyen-Van-Dick, Vu-Dingh-Minh (1962) Activité anthelminthique du 2(4'-thiazolyl) benzimidazole chez l'homme. Chemotherapia 5:326–331

Bumbalo TS, Geist H (1964) The treatment of pinworm infection in a school for the mentally retarded. Am J Trop Med Hyg 13:822–825

Bumbalo TS, Plummer LJ (1957) Piperazine (Antepar) in the treatment of pinworm and roundworm infections. Med Clin North Am 43:575–585

Bumbalo TS, Gustinia FJ, Oleksiak RE (1953) The treatment of pinworm infection (enterobiasis). J Pediat 44:386–391

Bumbalo TS, Plummer LJ, Warner JR (1957) Treatment of enterobiasis with one oral dose of promethazine hydrochloride. JAMA 164:1651–1653

Bumbalo TS, Plummer LJ, Warner JR (1958) The treatment of enterobiasis in children. A comparative study of piperazine (Antepar) and pyrvinium chloride (Vanquin). Am J Trop Med Hyg 7:212–214

Bumbalo TS, Fugazzotto DJ, Wyczalek JV (1969) Treatment of enterobiasis with pyrantel pamoate. Am J Trop Med Hyg 18:50–52

Bunnag D (1976) Clinical trial of mebendazole (Vermox) on whipworm, hookworm and *Ascaris*. Janssen Pharmaceutica Clin Res Rep N 11281

Bunnag D, Harinasuta T, Vasuvat C, Visuthikosol Y, Vidhyanonth C, Chulajata N (1978) Clinical trial of mebendázole (Fugacar) on whipworm and hookworm. 4th int congress of parasitology. Polish Scientific Publishers, Warszawa, D 44

Bunnag D, Harinasuta Tr, Viravan Ch, Jarupakorn V, Chindanond D, Desakorn V (1980) Clinical field trial of flubendazole on hookworm, *Trichuris* and *Ascaris* infection. Southeast Asian J Trop Med Public Health 11:363–366

Burriel LM, Fernandes Aguado P, Gomez HO, Bachiller L (1969) Preliminary clinical trial with a new drug (pyrantel) in the treatment of intestinal parasitism by oxyurus. Med Klin (Span. edit) 96:63–67

Burriel LM, Fernandes Aguado P, Gomez Hernandes O, Bachiller L (1973) El problema del diagnostico de la oxiuriasis en pediatrica. Estudio epidemiologico y su tratamiento con el pamoate de pyzantel. Acta Paediatr Espan 31:67–72

Burrows RB, Hunt GR, Lillis WG (1961) A new series of pyridines with anthelminthic activity. J Parasitol [Suppl] 47:35–36

Cabrera BD (1980) Results of clinical trial of mebendazole on soil-transmitted helminthiasis in Cabusao, Naga City, Philippines. A single-dose study comparing 200–400 and 600 mg. Janssen Pharmaceutica, Clin Res Report, N 19698

Cabrera BD, Cruz AC (1980a) Clinical trial of mebendazole on soil-transmitted helminthiasis in rural communities. Acta Med Philipp 16:55–57

Cabrera BD, Cruz AC (1980b) Clinical trial of oxantel-pyrantel (Quantrel) against trichuriasis. Acta Med Philipp 16:97–102

Cabrera BD, Sy Fr S (1978) Oxantel-pyrantel in various regimens for the treatment of soil transmitted helminthiasis in rural and urban communities. Drugs [Suppl] 15:16–24

Cabrera BD, Garcia EG, Cruz TA, Jueco NL (1960) Treatment of ascariasis with piperazine. J Philipp Med Assoc 36:904–908

Cabrera BD, Canlas B Jr, Danz U (1967) Human intestinal capillariasis III, Parasitological features and management. Acta Med Philipp 4:92–103

Cabrera BD, Juego NL, Cruz TA (1971) Clinical evaluation of levamisole in ascariasis during an intestinal survey at Victoria, Laguna. Janssen Pharmaceutica, Clin Res Rep, N 5167

Cabrera BD, Arambulo III PV, Portillo GP (1975) Ascariasis control and/or eradication in a rural community in the Philippines. Southeast Asian J Trop Med Public Health 6:510–518

Cabrera BD, Valdez EV, Go T (1980) Clinical field trials of broad spectrum anthelminthics against soil-transmitted helminthiasis. Southeast Asian J Trop Med Public Health 11:502–506

Cahill KM (1967) Thiabendazole in massive strongyloidiasis. Am J Trop Med Hyg 16:451–453

Cain GD, Raj RK (1980) Anisakis, Phocanema, Contracaecum and Sulcascarius spp, electrophoresis and thermostability of alcohol and molate dehydrogenases from larvae. Exp Parasitol 49:56–67

Camilo-Coura L, Velho Soli A De S, Lima N Dos Santos, Castro Peixoto TH De, Willcox HPF (1981a) Tratamiento de las helminthiasis intestinales con Albendazol, un derivado benzimidazolico nuevo – estudio doble ciego. Compendium de investigaciones clinicos Latino-Americanas. In: Simp Latino-Americano geohelminthiasis y albendazol. Cancun, Mexico, pp 67–74

Camilo-Coura L, Velho Soli A De S, Willcox HPF (1981b) Ensayo con Albendazol en el tratamiento de las helminthiasis intestinales de los ninos. Symp. latino americano Geohelminthiasis y Albendazol. In: Compendium de Investigaciones clinicos latino americanos. Cancun, Mexico, pp 75–81

Campbell WC (1961) Effect of thiabendazole upon infections of *Trichinella spiralis* in mice and upon certain other helminthiases. J Parasitol [Suppl] 47:37

Campbell WC, Blair LS (1974) Chemotherapy of *Trichinella spiralis* infections (a review). Exp Parasitol 35:304–334

Campbell WC, Cuckler AC (1964) Effect of thiabendazole upon the enteral and parenteral phases of trichinosis in mice. J Parasitol 50:481–488

Campbell WC, Cuckler A (1969) Thiabendazole in the treatment and control of parasitic infections in man. Tex Rep Biol Med [Suppl 2] 27:665–695

Campbell WC, Hartman RK (1968) Changes in the efficacy of three anti-helminthics during the maturation of a nematode (*Trichinella spiralis*). J Parasitol 54:112–116

Campos R, Croce J, Amato-Neto V (1963) Tratamento da Trichostrongiliase humana pelo thiabendazol. O Hospital 64:261–264

Campos R, Amato-Neto V, Vasconcellos AT de M, Wanderley RA (1967) Tratamento da ascaridiase e da trichocefaliase pelo iodeto de estilbasio. O Hospital 71:703–709

Campos R, Kusninsky N, Scheinberg MA, Pereira W Jr, Inacio V, Paschoalotti MD (1968) Tratamento da ascaridiase com novo derivado piperazinico (di-glicosyl-piperazine) em dosa unica. O Hospital 73:23–26

Canese A, Canese J, Vargas H De, Galeano A, Moleon A, Alsina P (1978) Accion del flubendazol en algunas parasitosis intestinales. Rev Paraguaya Microbiol 13:31–33

Canzonieri CJ (1980) Results obtained in ascariasis with massive periodic treatments with pyrantel pamoate. Prensa Med Argent 67:924–925

Canzonieri CJ, Rodrigues RR, Castillo HE, Ibanez De Ballela C, Lucena M (1977) Ensayos therapeuticos con praziquantel in *Taenia saginata* e *Hymenolepis nana*. Bol Chil Parasitol 32:41–42

Carney DE, O'Reilly BJ, Tweddell ED (1971) Pyrantel embonate in the treatment of enterobiasis. Med J Aust 2:254–256

Carr HR, Pichardo Sardo ME, Nunes NA (1954) Anthelmintic treatment of uncinariasis. Am J Trop Med Hyg 3:495–503

Carrie J (1968) Activité du thiabendazole dans le traitement de la strongiloidose. In: 8e Conf techn OCCGE, Bamako, Haute Volta pp 424–428

Carrie J (1978) Activité du mebendazole sur trois parasitoses intestinales. 12e conf techn OCEAC, Yaounde, Cameroun

Carrie J, Ravinet, Durand B (1978) Essai de controle des helminthiases intestinales. Résultats obtenus par traitement systématique par le mebendazole. 12th conf techn OCEAC, Yaounde

Carter FS (1949) Plasma cell hyperplasia and hyperglobulinemia in trichinosis. The duration of larviposition. Am J Pathol 25:309–323

Carter FS (1953) Cerebral cysticercosis. East Afr Med J 30:295–301

Castro LP de, Cunha AS, Ribeiro TC de, Resende HP (1973) Estudo farmacoclinico e terapeutico de um novo anti-helmintico, o Mebendazole (R 17635), em criancas poliparasitadas. Rev Assoc Med Bras 19:441–446

Cavier R (1963) Recherches sur les proprietés anthelminthiques de l'hydroxy-1-phenothiazine et des associations phénothiazines + hydrate de pipérazine. Bull Soc Pathol Exot Filiales 56:1049–1055

Cavier R (1973) Chemotherapy of intestinal nematodes. In: Radouco Thomas C (ed) International encyclopedia of pharmacology and therapeutics. Pergamon, Oxford, pp 215–436 (Chemotherapy of helminthiasis, section 64, vol 1, chapter 4)

Cavier R, Bellon R (1960) Essai de traitement de la trichocephalose par le sébacate de pipérazine. Bull Soc Pathol Exot Filiales 53:626–629

Cavier R, Gaulin J (1951) Recherches sur les proprietés anthelminthiques de la piperazine et de quelques uns de ses dérivés. Tunis Med 39:902–905

Cavier R, Hawking F (1973) Chemotherapy of helminthiasis vol I. In: Radouco Thomas C (ed) International encyclopedia of pharmacology and therapeutics. Pergamon, Press Oxford

Cavier R, Rossignol JF (1980) Etude comparative des propriétés oxyuricides de l'albendazole, du mebendazole, du pamoate de pyrantel et du praziquantel chez la souris expérimentalement infectée. Ann Pharm Fr 40:55–60

Cerf J (1958) Traitement de la strongyloidose par la dithiazanine. Ann Soc Belg Med Trop 38:1027–1030

Cerf J, Lebrun A, Dierickx J (1962) A new approach to helminthiasis control: the use of an organophosphorous compound. Am J Trop Med Hyg 11:514–517

Cervoni W, Oliver-Gonzales J (1971) Clinical evaluation of pyrantel pamoate in helminthiasis. Am J Trop Med Hyg 20:589–591

Cervoni WA, Oliver-Gonzales J (1975) Single oral doses of levamisole and pyrantel pamoate in the treatment of ascariasis: a placebo-controlled comparison for cure and reinfestation rates and for mean egg reduction. Janssen Pharmaceutica, Clin Res Report, N 10240

Cervoni WA, Oliver-Gonzales J, Kaye S, Slomka MB (1969) Dichlorvos as a single dose intestinal anthelminthic therapy for man. Am J Trop Med Hyg 18:912–919

Cespedes R, Salas J, Mekbel S, Troper L, Müllner F, Morera P (1967) Granulomas entericas y limfaticos con intensa eosinofilia tissular, producidos par un estrongilidea (Strongylata). Acta Med Costarric 10:235–255

Chabaud AG (1972) Description de *Stefanskostrongylus dubosti* n. sp. parasite du potomajole et essai de classification des nématodes Angiostrongylinae. Ann Parasitol Hum Comp 47:735–744

Chabaud AG, Lariviere M (1958) Sur les oesophagostomes parasites de l'homme. Bull Soc Pathol Exot Filiales 51:384–393

Chai J-Yi, Hong S-T, Lec S-Hy, Seo By-S (1981) Fluctuation of the egg production amounts according to worm burden and length of *Ascaris lumbricoides*. Kor J Parasitol 19:38–44

Chaia G, Cunha AS Da (1966) Terapeutica experimentel com o tiabendazol na estrongiloidiase. Rev Inst Med Trop Sao Paulo 8:173–176

Chaia G, Cunha AS Da (1971 a) Therapeutic action of mebendazole (R 17635) against human helminthiasis. Folha Med 63:67–76

Chaia G, Cunha S Da (1971 b) Therapeutic action of mebendazole (R 17635) against human helminthiasis. Folha Med 63:843–852

Chaia G, Metene F, Chiari L, Araujo S de M, Abreu IB De (1972) Mebendazole – un novo antihelminthico de acao terapeutica polivalente. Folha Med 64:139–145

Chanco PP, Atienza MR (1973) Trichuriasis – incidence, hazards and treatment with mebendazole (R 17635). Preliminary report. Philipp J Microb Infect Dis 2:27–38

Chanco PP, Paguio A (1964) Thiabendazole, a new broad spectrum anthelminthic. J Philipp Med Assoc 40:561–569

Chanco PP, Tagama R (1965) Thiabendazole pamoate chewable tablets and plain thiabendazole chewable tablets. Int Med 3:33–40

Chanco PP, Vidad JY (1978) A review of trichuriasis, its incidence, pathogenicity and treatment. Drugs [Suppl 1] 15:87–93

Chanco PP, Vidad JY (1981) Review of trichiuriasis and its treatment with reference to the use of a single dose of oxantel/pyrantel suspension. Pfizer forum on common parasitic diseases

Chanco PP Jr, Talag-Padero J, Coo-Barcelona L, Vidad JY (1972) A new drug for the treatment of ancylostomiasis and necatoriasis: a preliminary report on Jonit. Asian J Med 8:152–157

Chandra RK (1977) Nutritional deficiency and susceptibility to infection. Bull WHO 57:167–177

Chandrasoma PT, Mendis KN (1977) *Enterobius vermicularis* in ectopic sites. Am J Trop Med Hyg 26:644–649

Chappel LH (1980) Physiology of parasites. Blackie, Glasgow

Chaptal J, Jean R, Labauge R, Bonnet H, Aghai E (1963) Myoclonies oppositionnelles par intoxication à la pipérazine. Arch Fr Pediatr 20:17–23

Chege SW, Gitoko F, Wanene GSN, Mwega VJ, Rees PH, Kinyanjui H (1974) Single dose treatment of hookworm in Meerang'a District. East Afr Med J 51:60–62

Chernyshenko AI, Frolova AA, Chilikin MM, Bezuglov DA, Voevodina AI (1980) Combantrin effectiveness and tolerance in the mass treatment of enterobiasis, ascariasis, trichocephaliasis. Med Parazitol 49:66–68

Chitanondh H, Rosen L (1960) Fatal eosinophilic encephalitis caused by the nematode *Gnathostoma spinigerum*. Am J Trop Med Hyg 16:638–645

Chitrathorn S, Acalabol M, Thongkong M, Kamolsin C (1972) A single dose of phenylene-di-isothiocyanate (1,4) Jonit in the treatment of adult patients with hookworm infection in Sawan – pracharate hospital, Thailand. Southeast Asian. J Trop Med Public Health 3:103–105

Chitwood MB, Velasquez C, Salazar NP (1964) Physiological changes in a species of *Capillaria* (Trichuroidea) causing a fatal case of human intestinal capillariasis. In: Proc int congress parasit. Roma, Sept 21–26, vol 2. Pergamon, Oxford, pp 797–798

Chitwood MB, Velasquez C, Salazar NP (1968) *Capillaria philippinensis* sp. n. (Nematoda: *Trichinellida*) from the intestine of man in the Philippines. J Parasitol 54:368–371

Cho SY (1976) Anthelminthic efficacy of combined preparation of pyrantel pamoate and oxantel pamoate on human intestinal nematodes. Kor J Pharmacol 12:69–73

Cho SY (1977) Study on the quantitative evaluation of reinfection of *Ascaris lumbricoides*. Kor J Parasitol 15:17–29

Cho SY (1980) A case of human anisakiasis in Korea. Seoul J Med 21:203–208

Cho SY, Ahn Yo-R, Ryang Yo-S, Seo By-Se (1977) Evaluation of anthelminthic treatment on *Enterobius vermicularis* infection in a highly endemic population by prolonged observation. Kor J Parasitol 15:100–107

Chobanov RE, Safieva LA, Sadykhov IA, Koleshichenko ML (1981) New data on *Trichostrongylus* parasitism in man. Med Parazitol 50:17–18
Chongsuphajaisiddhi T, Sabcharoen A, Attanath P, Panasoponkul C, Radomyos P (1978) Treatment of soil-transmitted nematode infections in children with mebendazole. Ann Trop Med Parasitol 72:59–63
Chowdury AB (1971) Ascariasis – a health hazard. J Indian Med Assoc 57:294–296
Chowdury AB (1972–1974) Open trial of mebendazole in *Trichuris trichiura* and hookworm infection. Janssen Pharmaceutica, Clin Res Report, N 5722/N 8113
Chowdury AB (1974) Clinical trials with mebendazole. Status Report, Ethnor
Chowdury AB, Bandyopadhyay AK, Banerjee M (1964) Preliminary observations on the clinical trial of thiabendazole against human helminthiasis. Bull Calcutta Sch Trop Med 12:124–125
Chu WG, Chen PM, Huang CC, Hsu CT (1972) Neonatal ascariasis. J Pediatr 81:783–785
Cimerman B, Pereira Fernandes M de F, Hernandes N, Campos Neto J, Campos Neto M (1980) Mebendazole – esquemas terapeuticos na practica clinica. Folha Med 4:80
Cobbold R (1864) Entozoa: an introduction to the study of helminthology. Groombridge, London
Cobbold R (1879) Parasites: a treatise on the entozoa of man and animals, including some account of entozoa. Churchill, London
Coene A (1969) Rapport sur le traitement des helminthiases par le levo-tetramisole chez les malades hospitalisés à l'hôpital général de Bukavu. Janssen Pharmaceutica, Clin Res Rep N 522
Colaert J (1976) Essai thérapeutique avec le flubendazole dans une école primaire à Kinshasa résultats préliminaires, remarques, critiques. Janssen Pharmaceutica, Clin Res Report N 11303
Combescot Ch, Duong TH (1980) Action du fluoromebendazole (flubendazole) sur les helminthiases digestives. Méd Mal Infect 10:735–738
Commey JOO, Haddock DRW (1970) Probable resistance to bephenium in *Necator americanus* infection. Ghana Med J 9:94–97
Constazo S (1975) Evaluacion de un nuevo antiparasitario Mebendazol (R 17635). Prensa Med Argent 62:12–13
Conte VP, Zaterka S, Costa FAB, Bettarello A (1974) Pirantel versus mebendazol no tratamento de ancilostomiase. Estudo comparetivo em 40 casos. Arq Gastoenterol 11:143–149
Cornwell L, Jones RM (1968) Anthelmintic activity of pyrantel pamoate against *Ancylostoma caninum* in dogs. J Trop Med Hyg 71:165–166
Correa MOA (1958) Estudo da açao terapeutica da thiazanina na estrongiloidose e na tricocefalose humana. Rev Inst Adolfo Lutz 18:123–131
Correa MOA, Correa Fleury G, Lacerda Correo L De (1973) Terapeutica anthelminthica pelo levamisol em patientes pordadores de trichostrongilideos. Rev Inst Adolfo Lutz 33:45–47
Cort WW, Stoll NR (1931) Studies on *Ascaris lumbricoides* and *Trichuris trichiura* in China. Am J Hyg 14:655–689
Costa FV, Dos Santos CNR, Garcia CP de (1966) Contribucao as estudio comparativo de açao entre o hidroxinaftoato de befeno e o tetrachloretilenico. Açoa sobre a ancylostomiase e avaliaçao secundaria sobre a ascaridiase e tricocefaliase. Rev Bras Med 23:111–118
Costanzo S (1975) Evaluacion de un nuevo antiparasitario, mebendazol (R 17635) Prensa Med Argent 62:12–13
Coudert J, Garin JP, Battesti MR, Estienne J (1961) La dithiazanine, premier anthelminthique actif sur le trichocéphale. J Med Lyon 37:389–406
Coulaud JP, Rossignol JF (1982) Albendazole: a new single dose anthelmintic. Study of 1,455 patients. Acta Trop 41:87–90
Coulaud JP, Deluol AM, Cenac J, Rossignol JF (1982a) L'albendazole dans le traitement de la strongyloidose. A propos de 66 observations. Bull Soc Pathol Exot Filiales 75:530–533

Coulaud JP, Duchatelle C, Rouvillois A, Deluol AM (1982b) Le Zentel ® dans le traitement des helminthiases intestinales, au Niger, en Guinée et à Paris. Med Afr Noire 29:41–52

Coutelen F, Biguet J, Capron A, Deblock S, Mine L (1956) Contrôle de l'action de quelques antihistaminiques dans le traitement de l'oxyurose. Thérapie 11:1119–1124

Cram EB (1943) Studies on oxyuriasis XXVIII – Summary and conclusions. Am J Dis Child 65:46–59

Croce JR, Campos V, Amato-Neto V, Dias De Avila Pires C, Campos Martins AC, Laurenti R, Mello e Albuquerque FJM (1963) Tratamento da estrongyloidiase pelo tiabendazol. Rev Inst Med Trop Sao Paulo 5:194–197

Croll NA, Ghadirian E (1981) Wormy persons: contributions to the nature and patterns of overdispersion with *A. lumbricoides, A. duodenale, N. Americanus* and *T. trichiura*. Trop Geog Med 33:241–248

Cross JH, Banzon TC, Clarke MD, Basaca-Servilla V, Watten RH, Dixon J (1972) Studies on experimental transmission of Capillaria philippinensis in monkeys. Trans R Soc Trop Med Hyg 66:819–827

Cross JH, Banzon TC, Singson C (1978) Further studies on *Capillaria philippinensis:* development of the parasite in the Mongolian gerbil. J Parasitol 64:208–213

Cross JH, Singson CN, Battad S, Basaca-Sevilla V (1980) Intestinal capillariasis: epidemiology, parasitology and treatment. In: Health policies in developing countries. Intern congress and symposium series. R Soc Medicine, London, pp 81–87

Cruz Lopez A (1981) Estudio en poblacion abierta con albendazol. Sinp. latino americano Geohelminthiasis y albendazol. In: Compendium de invest clin Latino Americanas. Cancun, Mexico, pp 99–103

Cruz Lopez O, Alcantrara R (1980) Estudio abierto de levamisole en el tratamiento de la ascariasis. Janssen Pharmaceutica, Clin Res Report, N 19199

Cuckler AC (1961) Thiabendazole. J Parasitol [Suppl] 47:36–37

Cuckler AC, Mezey KC (1966) The therapeutic efficacy of thiabendazole for helminthic infections in man. Arzneimittelforsch 16:411–428

Cuckler AC, Egerton JR, Alicota JE (1965) Therapeutic effect of thiabendazole on *Angiostiongylus cantonensis* infections in rats. J Parasitol 51:392–396

Da Cruz Ferreira FS, Cunha CAL Da, Guedes De Carvalho RF (1960) Ensaios terapeuticos com o „Bayer 2349" na ancilostomiase. An Inst Hig Med Trop 17:655–668

Daensvang S (1968) Further observations on the experimental transmission of *Gnathostomum spinigerum*. Ann Trop Med Parasitol 62:88–94

Dan V, Senghor G, Niang I (1973) Utilisation en médecine de masse des anthelminthiques (helminthes intestinaux). Med Afr Noire 20:997–1006

Dancescu P, Toma L (1978) Some characters of a strain of *Strongyloides stercoralis* peculiar from Luzopa, sect C1, 6. ICOPA IV, Warsawa

Danis M, Datry A, Meunier Y, Gentilini M (1980) Un nouvel anthelminthique à large spectre: le flubendazole. A propos de 125 observations. Gaz Méd Fr 87:5444–5446

D'Antoni JS, Sawitz W (1941) The treatment of oxyuriasis. Am J Trop Med 20:377–383

Da Silva G (1979) Flubendazole in the treatment of hookworm disease and trichuriasis: a dose range study. Janssen Pharmaceutica, Clin Res Report, N 18075

Da Silva JR, Courra LC, Carvalho HT de, Lopes PFD (1963) Tratamento do estrongilidiase. O Hospital 63:1247–1264

Davis A (1973) Drug treatment in intestinal helminthiasis. World Health Organisation, Geneva

Davis JH (1965) Thiabendazole in pinworm infestations. Am J Dis Child 109:567–570

Davis JH (1966) Thiabendazole in pinworm infestations. Am J Dis Child 112:49–51

Davis JH (1969) Pinworm infestations. Therapy with Thiabendazole. Tex Rep Biol Med [Suppl 2] 27:623–628

Davis MJ, Cilo M, Plaitakis A, Yahr MD (1976) Trichinosis: severe myopathic involvement with recovery. Neurology 26:37–40

Davison RP (1979) Evaluation of mebendazole for the treatment of trichuriasis. Med J Aust 1:401–403

Degremont A, Baumgartner MW (1975) Le traitement des helminthiases intestinales au mebendazole: a propos de 294 patients traités. Schweiz Med Wochenschr 105:1830–1832
Degremont A, Stahel E (1978) Klinische Bewertung von Ciclobendazol (C-C 2481) bei der Behandlung von Wurmerkrankungen des Darmes. Schweiz Med Wochenschr 108:1430–1433
De Jonckheere U (1975) Single oral doses of levamisole in the treatment of ascariasis. Janssen Pharmaceutica, Clin Res Report, R 12564/26, N 9707
Deme J, Sagnet H (1961) Traitement de l'ankylostomose par l'hydroxynaphtoate de béphenium. Méd Trop 21:393–395
Demoen P, Aelst C Van, Loomans J, Verhaegen H, Cree J De, Verbruggen F, Ringoir S (1973) The absorption and urinary excretion of mebendazole after oral administration. Janssen Pharmaceutica, Clin Res Report, R 17635/36
De Oliveira Gomez MC (1974) Tratamento das parasitoses intestinais com mebendazole suspensao. Folha Med 68:541–543
De Oliveira Gomez MC (1977) Tratamento da estrongiloidiase pelo cambendazole. Folha Med 74:535–537
De Oliveira Gomez MC (1979) Flubendazole in the treatment of trichiuriasis: a dose range study. Janssen Pharmaceutica, Clin Res Report, N 17495
De Oliveira Gomez MC, Zangari CLM (1979) Treatment of intestinal parasitosis with flubendazole. Janssen Pharmaceutica Clin Res Report N 21273
De Oliveira MC, Souza DWC De, Castro A De, Neves J (1971) O tetramisole levogiro na terapeutica da ascaridiase. Folha Med 62:59–63
De Paulo Castro L, Pereira Rezende H, Carvalho MF De (1970) Tratamento de ascaridiase com o levamisole. Analise de 200 casos. Rev da Assoc Med de Minas Gerais 21:165–167
De Paulo Castro L, Pereira Rezende H, Carvalho MF De, Horizonte B (1971) Estudo Comparativo, pelo metodo duple-cego, entre o'tetramisole' e o 'levamisole' na terapeutica da ascaridiase. Rev Assoc Med Brasil 17:237–240
De Paulo Castro L, Cunha SA Da, Ribeiro de CT, Resende PH (1973) Estudo farmacoclinico e terapeutico de un novo anti-helmintico, o mebendazole (R 17635), em criancas poliparasitadas. Rev Assoc Med Brasil 19:441–446
De Saedeleer G (1975) Mebendazole, traitement efficace de la trichocéphalose. Louvain Med 94:41–48
Desai AS (1962) Single dose treatment of oxyuriasis with pyrvinium embonate. Br Med J 2:1583–1585
Deschiens R (1943) Sur les proprietés anthelminthiques des dérivés du triphénylméthane. CR Séances Acad Sci 217:513–515
Deschiens R (1946) L'action anthelminthique de la phénothiazine (Thiodiphenylamine) et de ses dérivés. Presse Mèd 54:53–54
Deschiens R, Benex J (1957) Essais experimentaux et cliniques de traitement de l'anguillulose intestinale par le sous-nitrate et par le carbonate de bismuth. Bull Soc Pathol Exot Filiales 50:70–74
Deschiens R, Poirier M, Lamy L (1954) Sur l'action anthelminthique des dérivés de l'ethylenediamine et de la piperazine. Bull Soc Pathol Exot Filiales 47:83–86
De Souza DWC, Neves J, Lemos MS De (1972) Estudo comparativo entre a efficacia terapeutica do pamoate de pirantel e do levamisole na ascaridiase. Rev Inst Med Trop Sao Paulo 14:67–72
De Souza CDW, Lemos Souza MS De, Neves J (1973 a) Açao terapeutica do mebendazole (R 17635) em pacientes poliparestidaos. Resultados preliminares. Rev Inst Med Trop Sao Paulo 15:30–35
De Souza DW, Lemos Souza S De, Neves J (1973 b) Açao terapeutica do mebendazole (R 17635) em patientes poliparasitados. Resultados finais. Rev Soc Brasil Med 7:237–241
Desowitz RS, Bell Th, Williams J, Cardines R, Tamarua M (1970) Anthelminthic activity of pyrantel pamoate. Am J Trop Med Hyg 19:775–778
Dessakorn V (1980) Clinical field trial of flubendazole on hookworm, *Trichuris* and *Ascaris* infection. Janssen Pharmaceutica, Clin Res Report, N 17449

Detels R, Gutman L, Jaramillo J, Zerrudo E, Banzon T, Valera J, Murrell KD, Cross J, Dizon JJ (1969) An epidemic of intestinal capillariasis in man. Am J Trop Med Hyg 18:676–682

De Wulf MD (1975) Flubendazole in the treatment of enterobiasis: a double-blind placebo-controlled study. Janssen Pharmaceutica, Clin Res Report, R 17889/5

Digues La Tonche DM (1962) Bephenium compared with tetrachlorethylene in mass treatment of hookworm. J Trop Med Hyg 65:107–111

Dissanaike AS (1978) A comparative trial of oxantel-pyrantel and mebendazole in multiple helminth infection in school children. Drugs [Suppl] 15:11–15

Dizon JJ, Watten RH (1969) Preliminary observations on a new disease in man: intestinal capillariasis. J Philippine Med Assoc 45:5–20

Domart A, Gentilini M, Therizol M, Carbon C (1967) Traitement de la strongyloidose par le thiabendazole (à propos de 100 cas). Bull Mém Soc Méd Hop 118:1047–1050

Do Nascimento OB, Halsman M, Oria H, Martins Campos JV (1966) Clinical study of the therapeutic value of single oral doses of a new anthelminthic tetramisole (R 8299) against ascariasis. Rev Inst Med Trop Sao Paulo 8:143–147

Donoso F, Atias A (1961) Tratamiento de la oxyuriosis con pamoate de la pyrvinium pamoate (Poquil). Bol Chil Parasitol 16:88–90

Doshi JC, Vaidya AB, Sen HG, Mankodi NA, Nair CN, Greural RS (1977) Clinical trials of a new anthelmintic 4-isothiocyanato-4-nitrodiphenylamine for the cure of hookworm infection. Am J Trop Med Hyg 26:636–639

Dudley BW, Lease EJ (1973) Intestinal helminths in children in coastal South Carolina: follow-up report. South Med J 66:1100

Dürr JM (1969) Résultats des essais thérapeutiques du dérivé levogyre du tetramisole dans les helminthiases humaines. Thèse, Paris

Dufek M, Kalivoda R (1973a) Levamizol a mebendazol – nova anthelmintika. Cas Lek Cesk 112:633

Dufek M, Kalidova R (1973b) Treatment of intestinal parasitic infections with levamisole and mebendazole. Bull Inst Marit Med Gdansk 24:325–327

Dutta JK (1970) Treatment of ankylostomiasis with combined therapy of bephenium hydroxynaphtoate and tetrachlorethylene. J Indian Med Assoc 54:150–152

Egerton JR, Campell WC (1970) The efficacy of 5-isopropoxycarbonylamino-2-(4-thiazolyl)-benzimidazole against helminths in sheep. Res Vet Sci 11:193–195

Eliachar E, Pavlotski D, Tassy R (1960) Incidents neurologiques après l'utilisation de piperazine comme vermifuge. Arch Fr Pédiatr 17:797–803

El-Mosry NA, Trabolsi B, Bassily S, Farid Z (1983) Albendazole in the treatment of *Ancylostoma duodenale* and *Ascaris lumbricoides* infections. Trans R Soc Trop Med Hyg 77:160–161

Ericksen V (1964) Treatment of oxyuriasis with pyrvinpamoate. Acta Paediatr 53:489–491

Escobar AJJ (1964) Tiabendazol, un nuevo antihelmintico de amplio espectro. Antioquia Med 14:369–387

Evdokimov V, Ntibarutaye J (1970) Ascaridiose et son traitement par levo-tetramisole (Decaris) au Burundi. Rev Méd Burundi 2:15–21

Excler JL, Mojon M, Petavy AF, Cadi-Soussi M (1981) Foyer d'ankylostomiase dans une plantation de jasmin. Essai thérapeutique par l'albendazole, mené en double aveugle. Bull Soc Pathol Exot Filiales 75:349–355

Farahmandian I, Sahba GH, Sadeghi E (1971) Prevalence of helminthiasis in a village of the derful area and comparison of therapeutic effect of alcopar and mintezol. J Gen Med Teheran Univ 9:305–307

Farahmandian J, Sahba GH, Arfar F, Jabali H (1972) A comparative evaluation of the therapeutic effect of pyrantel pamoate and bephenium hydroxynaphtoate on *Ancylostoma duodenale* and other intestinal helminths. J Trop Med Hyg 75:205–207

Farahmandian I, Arfaa F, Sahba GH, Jalali H (1974) Preliminary trial on the effect of laevo-tetramisole on various intestinal helminthiases in Iran. Iran J Public Health 3:92–96

Farahmandian I, Arfaa F, Jalali H, Reza M (1977) Comparative studies on the evaluation of the effects of new antihelminthics on various helminthiases in Iran. Chemotherapy 23:98–105

Farid Z (1963) Treatment of oxyuriasis. Br Med J 1:330

Farid Z (1964) Treatment of multiple helminthic infections in Egypt with dithiazanine. J Trop Med Hyg 67:200–203

Farid Z, Miale A Jr (1962) Treatment of hookworm infection in Egypt with bephenium hydroxynaphtoate and the relationship between iron deficiency, anemia and intensity of infection. Am J Trop Med Hyg 11:497–505

Farid Z, Bassily S, Wissa J, Omar MS (1966) Single-dose treatment for ascaris infection with piperazine citrate, with a study of the egg-parasite ratio. Am J Trop Med Hyg 15:516–519

Farid Z, Bassily S, Young SW, Hassan A (1973) Tetramisole in the treatment of *Ancylostoma duodenale* and *Ascaris lumbricoides* infections in Egyptian farmers. Trans R Soc Trop Med Hyg 67:425–426

Farid Z, Bassily S, Miner WF, Hassan A, Laughlin AW (1977) Comparative single dose treatment of hookworm and roundworm infections with levamisole, pyrantel and bephenium. J Trop Med Hyg 80:107–108

Fayard C (1949) Ascaridase et piperazine. Thése Méd., no. 889, Paris

Feldmeyer H, Bienzle U, Dömring E, Dietrich M (1982) Flubendazole versus mebendazole in intestinal helminthic infections. Acta Trop 39:185–189

Feng DCH, Mao SH-G, Liv ERHS (1960) Research on parasitic diseases in new China. Chin Med J 80:1–20

Fernandes JL, Garcia E (1976) Atividade terapeutica da associaçao piperazina-tiabendazol em escolares portodores des verminose. Rev Soc Bras Med Trop 5:155–158

Fernandes P (1974) A importenzia do mebendazole no combate as helmintiases das populacoes rurais. Folha Med 69:301–302

Fernandez Ortega F (1982) Albendazol a dosis unica, en parasitosis indestinales en ninos. Informe de 100 cases. Invest Med Int (Mexico) 9:124–126

Fernando MA, Balasuriya S (1977) Control of *Ascariasis* by mass treatment with piperazine citrate. Ceylon Med J 22:120–128

Ferreira FSC da, Cunha CAL Da, Carvalho RF (1960) Ensaios terapeuticos com o Bayer 2349 na ancilostomiase. An Inst Hig Med Trop 17:655–668

Fierlafijn E (1971) L'oxyurose: traitement ancien et actuel. Brux Méd 51:605–608

Fierlafijn E, Parijs OF Van (1973) Mebendazole in enterobiasis. Trop Geogr Med 25:242–244

Figuerredo-Mendes T, Fonesca EE, Guedes R, Salun N, Garrido I (1962) Treatment of penitentiary inmates for intestinal parasites in Rio de Janeiro. Am J Trop Med Hyg 11:631–632

Filho FF, Duarté GG, Teruel JR, Franco AR (1971) Estudo de uma attociaçãs antihelmintica em parasitoses intestinais multiplas. Rev Soc Bras Med Trop 5:209–212

Fleury Correa G, Correa AMO, Amato-Neto V (1970) Identificacao do *Trichostrongylus colubriformis* coma parasita do homem. Rev Inst Med Trop Sao Paulo 12:288–292

Foba-Pagou R, Carrie J, Ripert C (1978) Traitement des helminthiases humaines: teniase, ascaridose, necatorose, trichocephalose, strongyloidose par le mébendazole. 12e Conf techn OCEAC, Yaounde

Forrester ATT, Nelson GS, Sander G (1961) The first record of an outbreak of trichinosis in Africa south of the Sahara. Trans R Soc Trop Med Hyg 55:503–513

Franz KH (1963) Clinical trials with thiabendazole against human strongyloidiasis. Am J Trop Med Hyg 12:211–214

Franz KH (1965) Clinical trials with thiabendazole against intestinal nematodes infecting humans. Am J Trop Med Hyg 14:383–386

Franz KH, Schneider WJ, Pohlman MH (1965) Clinical trials with thiabendazole against intestinal nematodes infecting humans. Am J Trop Med Hyg 14:383–386

Freire DA, Oetting GA Jr, Freire EM, Ruano AC, Amato Neto V (1969) Tratamento da ascaridiase por meio do levamisole-base. O Hospital 76:1715–1719

Fritz L (1965) Ein Beitrag zur Ein-Dosis Behandlung der *Oxyuris vermicularis* mit pyrvinium pamoate. Wien Med Wochenschr 115:122–124

Fry GF, Moore JG (1969) *Enterobius vermicularis:* 10,000-year-old human infection. Science 166:1620

Frye WW, Swartzwelder C, Lampert R, Abadie SH, Carson CB (1957) An effective trichuricide suitable for oral administration. Am J Trop Med Hyg 6:890–893

Gaitonde BB, Kamat RA, Kulkarni HJ, Vakil BJ (1969) Clinical evaluation of a new anthelminthic; phenylene di-isothyocyanate (bitoscanate) in hookworm and roundworm infestation. J Trop Med Hyg 72:253–258

Gamboa JA, Eduarte CA, Marin RM, Migliardi JR, Villarejos VM (1969) Pyrantel Pamoate: un nueva antihelminthico. 37th congresso med nac de San Jose, November 1969, Costa Rica

Garcia EG (1976) Treatment of trichuriasis with oxantel. Am J Trop Med Hyg 25:914–915

Garcia EG (1978) Treatment of multiple intestinal helminthiasis with oxantel and pyrantel. Drugs [Suppl 1] 15:70–72

Garin JP (1962) Traitement de l'oxyurose de l'enfant de moins de 10 ans par une dose unique d'embonate de pyrvinium (Povanyl). Pédiatrie 17:551–552

Garin JP (1980) L'Albendazole dans l'oxyurose. Int Clin Res Report Smith Kline French, Lyon, France

Garin JP (1981) L'Albendazole dans la trichocéphalose et dans l'ankylostomose. Int Clin Res Rep Smith Kline French

Garin JP, Mojon M (1980) Albendazole in the treatment of intestinal helminthiasis. A double blind controlled multicenter clinical trial. Congress, Marseille, November 1980

Garin JP, Despeigne J, Tasseau M (1965) L'Anguillulose et son traitement. J Med Lyon 46:1071–1088

Garin JP, Despeignes J, Woehrle R, Ambroise-Thomas P (1970) La diphetarsone, médicament actuel de la trichocephalose. Bull Soc Pathol Exot Filiales 63:94–100

Garin JP, Mojon M, Piens MA, Rossignol JF (1980a) Albendazole efficacy on a long term follow up in patients with intestinal helminthiasis. In: 10th international congress of tropic medicine malaria, Manila, abstract 235. Printing, Quezon City, p 148

Garin JP, Mojon M, Piens MA, Rossignol JF (1980b) Albendazole in the treatment of intestinal helminthiasis: a Euro-African double blind controlled multicenter clinical trial. In: 10th Int congress trop med malaria, Manila, abstract 236. Printing Quezon City, p 148

Gatherer A (1977) The prevalence, diagnosis and treatment of threadworm infestation. Practioner 219:871–875

Gatti F, Vandepitte J (1973) The efficacy of various dosages of mebendazole for the treatment of major intestinal roundworm parasites. Janssen Pharmaceutica, Clin Res Report, N 7320

Gatti F, Vanderick F, Parent M, Bulihereme S, Vandepitte J (1969) Treatment of roundworm infection in African children with a single dose of tetramisole (R 8299). Ann Soc Belg Méd Trop 49:51–62

Gatti F, Krubwa F, Vandepitte J, Thienpont D (1970) Antinematodal effect of the trimestrial administration of a single dose of levamisole to Congolese schoolchildren. 5th intern congress infect diseases, Aug 31–Sept 5 1970, Vienna

Gatti F, Krubwa F, Vandepitte J, Thienpont D (1972a) Control of intestinal nematodes in African schoolchildren by the trimestrial administration of levamisole. Ann Soc Belg Méd Trop 52:19–32

Gatti F, Krubwa F, Lontie M, Vandepitte J, Thienpont D (1972b) Clinical experience with mebendazole, a new broad-spectrum anthelminthic. Advances in antimicrobial and antineoplastic chemotherapy. Urban, Schwarzenberg

Gelpi MC, Mustafa A (1967) Seasonal pneumonitis with eosinophilia. A study of larval ascariasis in Saudi Arabia. Am J Trop Med Hyg 16:646–657

Gelpi MC, Mustafa A (1968) *Ascaris pneumonia.* Am J Med 44:377–389

Gentilini M (1974) Expertise clinique du mebendazol. Janssen Pharmaceutica, Clin Res Report N 8247

Gentilini M (1976) Expertise clinique – flubendazole comprimés. Janssen Pharmaceutica, Clin Res Report N 12250
Gentilini M, Robineau M, Durr JM, Domart A (1970) Résultats des essais thérapeutiques dans les helminthiases traitées par le L-tetramisole. Bull Soc Pathol Exot Filiales 63:52–61
Gentilini M, Danis M, Dürr JM, Garabiol B (1971) Traitement de l'ankylostomiase par l'association thiabendazole-lévamisol. Bull Soc Pathol Exot Filiales 64:891–900
Gentilini M, Danis M, Dournovo P (1976) Activité et tolerance du pamoate de pyrantel dans les nématodoses intestinales. La Vie Médicale 10:603–604
Ghadirian E (1978) Human infection with *Trichostrongylus lerouxi* in Iran. Am J Trop Med Hyg 26:1212–1213
Ghadirian E, Arfaa F (1975) Present status of trichostrongyliasis in Iran. Am J Trop Med Hyg 24:935–941
Ghadirian E, Sanati A (1972) Preliminary studies on the treatment of hookworm with pyrantel pamoate in Iran. J Trop Med Hyg 75:199–201
Ghadirian E, Sanati A, Misaghian G, Yossefi A (1972) Treatment of ascariasis with pyrantel pamoate in Iran. J Trop Med Hyg 75:195–197
Ghyssels G, Sartiaux P (1959) Le traitement de l'ankylostomiase par l'hydroxynaphtoate de bephenium. Ann Soc Belg Méd Trop 39:637–642
Goeters W (1955a) Die Behandlung der Oxyuriasis mit Terramycin (Oxytetracyclin). Arzneimittelforsch 5:517–519
Goeters W (1955b) Zur Behandlung der Oxyuriasis im Kindesalter. Dtsch Med Wochenschr 80:312–313
Goldsmid JM (1972a) Tiabendazole in the treatment of human infections with *Ternidens deminutus* (nematoda). S Afr Med J 46:1046–1047
Goldsmid JM (1972b) *Ternidens deminutus* and hookworm in Rhodesia and a review of the treatment of human infections with *T. deminutus*. Cent Afr J Med [Suppl] 18:1–14
Goldsmid JM (1973) The use of mebendazole as a broad spectrum anthelminthic in Rhodesia. S Afr Med J 48:2265–2266
Goldsmid JM (1974) The use of mebendazole as a broad spectrum anthelminthic in Rhodesia. S Afr Med J 48:2265–2266
Goldsmid JM, MacCabe RJ (1972) Preliminary studies on the use of phenylene-di-isothiocyanete (1,4) in the treatment of hookworm and *Ternidens deminutus* infections in Rhodesia. Cent Afr J Med 18:227–229
Goldsmid JM, Saunders CR (1972) Preliminary trial using pyrantel pamoate for the treatment of human infections with *Ternidens deminutus*. Trans R Soc Trop Med Hyg 66:375
Goldsmid JM, Saunders RC (1973) Pyrantel pamoate for human hookworm infection. S Afr Med J 47:25–26
Gomez-Ferrar W (1963) Tratamento da estrongiloidiase e da ascaridiase com thiabenazol. O Hospital 64:1381–1388
Goodwin LG, Standen OD (1954) Treatment of roundworm with piperazine citrate "Antepar." Br Med J 2:1332–1333
Goodwin LG, Standen OD (1958) Treatment of ascariasis with various salts of piperazine. Br Med J 1:131
Goodwin LG, Jayewardene LG, Standen OD (1958) Clinical trials with bephenium hydroxynaphtoate ("Alcopar") against hookworm in Ceylon. Br Med J 2:1572–1576
Gordon JA, Ross CM, Affleck H (1969) Abdominal emergency due to an oesophagostome. Ann Trop Med Parasitol 63:161–164
Gorodner JO, Gorodner AM, Navarro E (1977) Accion therapeutica del mebendazole (R 17635) en uncinariasis y enterobiasis. Medicina 37:389–392
Gould SE (1945) Trichinosis in man and animals. Thomas, Springfield
Gould SE (1971) The story of trichinosis. Am J Clin Pathol 55:2–11
Graham CF (1941) A device for diagnosis of *Enterobius* infection. Am J Hyg 21:159–161
Grove DI (1982) Treatment of strongyloidiasis with thiabendazole: an analysis of toxicity and effectiveness. Trans R Soc Trop Med Hyg 76:114–118

Guarniera D, Leonardi G, Ceccarelli G (1969) Pyrantel pamoate in the therapy of infestations from *E. vermicularis*. Ped Int

Guerrero L, Holguin J, Botero D (1960) The use of dithiazanine as a mass treatment for intestinal helminthiasis. Am J Trop Med Hyg 9:37–38

Guggenmoos R, Akhtaruzzaman KM, Rosenkaimer F, Gaus W, Bienzle U, Dietrich M (1978) Comparative trial of therapeutic effectiveness of the new anthelminthic drug: ciclobendazole. Tropenmed Parasitol 29:423–426

Guilhon J (1977) Origine des récentes épidemies de trichinose humaine observées en France. Bull Acad Natl Méd 161:174–178

Guimaraes JX, Ferraz WPG, Adura M, Villela M de P, Pucei H, Soares MA, Lopes ER (1961) O emprego do iodeto de ditiazanina na estrongiloidose. Rev Paul Med 58:389–394

Guimaraes VMA, Penha Sobrinho OA, Marcondes Silva C (1971) O levamisole na tratmento da ascaridiase en pacientes internados. Folha Med 63:129–134

Guiness Book of Records (1977) Guiness Superlatives, London

Gunders AE (1962) Dithiazanine in the treatment of intestinal nematodes. Parasite infections in the tropics. West Afr Med J 11:74–76

Gupta MC, Basu AK, Tandon BN (1974) Gastrointestinal protein loss in hookworm and roundworm infections. Am J Clin Nutr 27:1386–1389

Gupta MC, Mithal S, Tandon BN (1976) Use of tetramisole for mass deworming in a community with heavy *Ascaris* infection. J Indian Med Assoc 67:180–182

Gupta MC, Mithal S, Arora KL, Tandon BN (1977) Effect of periodic deworming on nutritional status of ascaris-infected preschool children receiving supplementary food. Lancet 2:108–110

Gupta PS, Gambhir DS, Oswal S, Kumar N (1979) 4-nitro-4-isothiocyanediphenylamin. A new anthelmintic in hookworm infestation. J Trop Med Hyg 82:117–119

Haaf E, Soest AH Van (1964) Oesophagostomiasis in man in North Ghana. Trop Geogr Med 16:49–53

Hahn SS, Kang HY, Hahn YS (1960) The anthelminthic effect of bephenium hydroxynaphtoate on intestinal helminths. J Trop Med Hyg 63:180–184

Haleem MA, Lari FA, Rahimtoola RJ (1971) Comparative efficacy and toxicity of pyrantel pamoate and piperazine citrate in paediatric ascariasis. J Pakist Med Assoc 22:276–282

Hall MC (1921) Carbon tetrachloride for the removal of parasitic worms, especially hookworms. J Agric Res 21:157–175

Hall MC, Shillinger J (1925) Tetrachlorethylene, a new anthelminthic. Am J Trop Med 5:229–237

Hall SA, Joseph MM, Saggar SN, Wood CH, Gleisner E (1970) A trial of ketrax (the laevo-isomer of tetramisole) in the treatment of ascariasis. East Afr Med J 47:424–433

Hanna M, Shehata A (1955) Treatment of ascariasis in children with piperazine adipate. Br Med J 2:417–418

Harada Y, Mori O (1953) A new method for culturing hookworm. Yonago Act Med 1:177–179 [in: Trop Dis Bull 53:343 (1956)]

Harfouche JK, Abi-Yaghi MJ, Karam M, Isawi F (1974) Single oral dose of combantrin (pyrantel pamoate) in the treatment of enterobiasis and ascariasis. Leban Med J 27;159–168

Hartz PH (1953) Histopathology of the colon in massive trichocephaliasis in children. Doc Med Geogr Trop 5:303–323

Harwood PD, Jerstad AC, Swanson LE (1938) The efficacy of phenothiazine for removal of ascarids from swine. J Parasitol [Suppl] 24:16–17

Hatchuel W, Isaacson M, Villiers DJ De (1973) Pyrantel pamoate in round worm infestation. A comparative trial with piperazine citrate given in a single dose. S Afr Med J 47:91–93

Hayashi S (1980) A model for the evaluation and assessment of the effect of control of soil transmitted helminthiases. In: Collected papers on the control of soil-transmitted helminthiases. Asian Parasite Control Organization 1:265–273

Hayashi S, Wakai R, Motoyoshi K, Mori Y, Isozaki A (1976) The efficacy of a newly developed tablet of pyrvinium pamoate against pinworm. Jpn J Parasit 25:100–108 (in Japanese)

Hewitt RI, White E, Wallace WS, Stewart HW, Kushner S, Subba Row Y (1947) Experimental chemotherapy of filariasis. II. Effect of piperazine derivatives against naturally acquired filarial infections in cotton rats and dogs. J Lab Clin Med 32:1304–1313

Hewitt R, Wyeth W, White E, Subrarow Y (1948) The treatment of ascariasis in dogs with 1-diethyl-carbamyl-4 methylpiperazine hydrochloride. J Parasitol 34:237–239

Hoekenga MT (1955) Treatment of multiple intestinal worm infections with piperazine citrate. Am J Trop Med Hyg 4:1088–1090

Hoeppli R (1959) Parasites and parasitic infections in early medcine and science. University of Malaya Press, Singapore

Hoff DR, Fisher MH, Bochis BJ, Lusi A, Waksmunski F, Egerton JR, Yakstis JJ, Cuckler AC, Campell WC (1970) A new broad-spectrum anthelminthic 2-(4-thiazolil)-5-isopropylcarbonylamino-benzimidazole. Experientia 26:550–551

Holtz J, Adhman D, Gunardi AT, Murat S, Sadeli OR, Wuisan JO (1972) A single dose of Jonit in the treatment of human ancylostomiasis. Southeast J Trop Med Public Health 3:99–102

Howes HL Jr (1972) Trans-1,4,5,6-tetrahydro-2-(3-hydroxystyryl)-1- methyl pyrimidine (CP-14445) a new antiwhipworm agent. Proc Soc Exp Biol Med 139:394–398

Howes HL, Lynch JE (1967) Anthelmintic studies with pyrantel; therapeutic and prophylactic efficacy against the enteral stages of various helminths in mice and dogs. J Parasitol 53:1085–1091

Howie VM (1955) Ten-day treatment of pinworm infection with piperazine. Am J Child Dis 89:202–203

Hsieh Hs-Ch, Chen EN-R (1970) Evaluation of anthelmintic activity of pyrantel pamoate (Combantrin) against *Ascaris* and hookworm. Chin J Microb 3:126–130

Hsieh HC, Chow LP, Shih CC (1960a) Mass treatment of hookworm infections with tetrachlorethylene and 1-bromo-naphtol 2 at two rural villages in southern Taiwan. J Formosan Med Assoc 59:53–59

Hsieh HC, Brown HW, Fite M, Chow LP, Cheng CS, Hsu CC (1960b) The treatment of hookworm, *Ascaris* and *Trichuris* infections with bephenium hydroxynaphtoate. Am J Trop Med Hyg 9:496–499

Hsieh HC, Kuo M, Chow LP, Cheng CS, Chen CY, Chang CR (1961) A combined dose of bephenium hydroxynaphtoate and tetrachlorethylene against mixed infection of *A. duodenale* and *N. americanus*. J Formosan Med Assoc 60:926–936

Hsieh HC, Brown HW, Chen ER, Chen CY, Shih CC (1963) Treatment of *Fasciolopsis buski, Ancylostoma duodenale, Ascaris lumbricoides, Trichuris trichiura* and *Enterobius vermicularis* infections with stilbazium iodide. J Parasitol 49:425–427

Hsieh Hs-Ch, Chen Ch-Y, Yi CH-Y, Chen M-Hs, Hong J-M (1970) The therapeutic efficacy of phenylene-di-isothiocyanate (1,4) against *A. duodenale* and *N. americanus* in Taiwan. Chi J Microbiol 69:13–17

Hsieh Hs-Ch, Chen EN-R, Shih CC (1971) Treatment of *Enterobius vermicularis* infections with pyrantel pamoate in Taiwan. Chin J Microbiol 4:247–253

Huang WH, Brown HW (1963) The efficacy of thiabendazole against hookworm and ascariasis in man. J Parasitol 49:1014–1018

Huang WH, Brown HW (1964) Clinical trials of stilbazium iodide (Monopar) in the treatment of *Trichuris* and *Ascaris* infections. Am J Trop Med Hyg 13:54–56

Hudson B (1976) Clinical summary: phase IV study-Vermox-Ortho Aug. Clin Res Rep Ortho Pharmaceutical Corporation, RD, Raritan, New Jersey 08869

Huggins D (1970) Ensaio terapeutico com o levamisole (composto R 8299) na ascariase. O Hospital 78:247–251

Huggins DW (1976) Ensaio clinico com mebendazole no tratamento das helminthiases intestinais. IV congr. Latino Americano de parasitologia, San Jose. D. A. 10, p 121

Huggins D (1977–1978) Terapeutica das helmintiases intestinais com an nova associaçao medicamentosa: cambendazol + mebendazol. An Inst Hig Med Trop 5:409–419

Huggins DW (1979a) Ensaio clinico com nova Associaçao: tinidazol + flubendazol, para o tratamento das enteroparasitoses. Rev Bras Med 36:581–583

Huggins DW (1979b) Cambendazole – nova substancia para o tratamento da estrongiloidiase. Folha Med 34:373–375 [GEN 33:301–305 (1979)]

Huggins DW (1979–1980a) Tratamento das enteroparasitoses com a associaçao tinidazol + mebendazol + cambendazol. An Inst Hig Med Trop 6:1–4, 45–48

Huggins DW (1979–1980b) Essaio clinico com nova associaçao: tinidazol + flubendazol para o tratamento das enteroparasitoses. An Inst Hig Med Trop 6:41–43

Huggings D, Ferreira RP, Xavier CC (1958) Dose unica do hydrato de piperazine na erradicaçao da ascariase. Rev Soc Brasil Med Trop 2:255–257

Hutchinson JGP, Johnston NM, Plevey MVP, Thangkhiew I, Aidney C (1975) A clinical trial of mebendazole. A broad-spectrum anti-helminthic. Br Med J 1:309–310

Hutton PW, Somers K (1961) A comparison of bephenium hydroxynaphtoate with tetrachlorethylene in hookworm infestation. Trans R Soc Trop Med Hyg 55:431–434

Huys J, Kayihigi J, Freyens P, Vandenberghe G (1973) Treatment of *Ascaris* infection with levamisole. Medikon 2:15–17

Huys J, Vandenberghe G, Freyens P, Kayihige J (1976) Treatment of ankylostomiasis with levamisole. Afr J Med Sci 5:75–77

Isebaert A (1970) Essai thérapeutique avec le R 17635 et son association avec le lévamisole. Janssen Pharmaceutica, Clin Res Report, N 4694

Ishizaki T, Kitsumi H, Yasurakoa K, Hosaka Y (1963) The anthelmintic effects of thiabendazole against *Ascaris*, whipworm and hookworm infections in man. Jpn J Parasitol 12:182–185

Islam N, Chowdury NA (1976) Mebendazole and pyrantel pamoate as broad spectrum anthelminthics. Southeast Asian. J Trop Med Public Health 7:81–84

Ismail MM, Lionel NDW (1981) A comparative trial of flubendazole, flubendazole with levamisole, and mebendazole for mass anthelminthic treatment and an assessment of re-infection rates. JOICFP Research Project, Sri Lanka

Iswariah V, Naryana-Rao MS (1964) Thiabendazole: a new broad spectrum anthelminthic. J Assoc Physicians India 12:305–308

Iwata S, Araki T, Ueda G, Kida A, Wada T, Kawata S (1963a) Notes on the treatment of human *ascaris, trichuris*, and *enterobius* infections with T. E. D. 3 as a broad spectrum anthelminthic. Jpn J Parasitol 12:174–181

Iwata S, Araki T, Ueda G, Wada T, Kida A (1963b) Treatment of intestinal parasitosis with MK 360. Bull Osaka Med Sch 9:23–30

Jancloes M, Jancloes-Diepart M (1981) Campagnes périodiques d'assainissement et de chimiothérapie de masse contre les nématodes intestinaux appliqués isolément et en combinaison au Bas Zaïre. Ann Soc Belg Med Trop 111–118

Jancloes MF, Cornet P, Thienpont D (1979) Mass control of ascariasis with single oral doses of levamisole. Trop Geogr Med 31:111–112

Janssen PAJ (1974) Recent advances in the treatment of parasitic infection in man. In: Jukker E (ed) Fortschritte der Arzneimittelforschung, vol 18. Birkhäuser, Basel, pp 191–203

Janssens PG (1948) De AEX concentratie methode voor wormeieren. Ann Soc Belg Med Trop 28:213–220

Janssens PG (1965) Les symptômes de la strongyloïdose. Ann Soc Belg Med Trop 45:131–150

Janssens PG (1971) Anguillulose – aspects cliniques et therapeutiques. Acta Gastroenterol Belg 34:301–321

Janssens PG, Muynck A De, d'Arenberg St (1966) Thiabendazole, a sensational new anthelmintic agent (in Dutch). Ann Soc Belg Méd Trop 46:397–420

Jaroonvesama N, Charoenlarp K, Muangmanee L, Saravich S, Aswapokee N, Saravich S (1978) Mebendazole, a new broad spectrum anthelminthic. J Med Assoc Thai 61:675–680
Jayewardane LG, Ismail MM, Wijayaratnam Y (1960) Bephenium hydroxynaphtoate in the treatment of ascariasis. Br Med J 2:268–271
Jeffery GM, Rondeau EA, Harrison AJ, Phifer KO (1963) Effects of stilbazium iodide on *Enterobius vermicularis* and other intestinal helminths. J Parasitol 49:639–641
Johnson SC (1971) A comparative study of bitoscanate (jonit), bephenium hydroxynaphtoate and tetrachlorethylene in hookworm infection. J Trop Med Hyg 74:133–136
Jorge J, Barbosa W (1964) Tratamento da estrongiloidose pelo tiabendazol. Rev Goiana Med 10:135–140
Jung RC (1954) Use of hexylresorcinol tablet in enema treatment of whipworm infection. Am J Trop Med Hyg 3:918–921
Jung RC, MacCroan JE (1960) Efficacy of bephenium and tetrachlorethylene in mass treatment of hookworm infection. Am J Trop Med Hyg 9:492–495
Junod Ch (1965) Essai de traitement de la trichocephalose par la diphétarsone. Bull Soc Pathol Exot Filiales 58:653–660
Juttijudata P, Guptavanij P, Harinasuta C (1962) A comparison of the efficacy of anthelminthic drugs in the treatment of hookworm infection. Jpn J Med Sci Biol 15:61–65
Juwono R, Tantular K (1973) Clinical experience with mebendazole, a new broad spectrum anthelminthic. Janssen Pharmaceutica, Clin. Res. Report, N 5723
Kaba AS, Luvwezo M, Nzuzi K, Thienpont D (1978) Le traitement anthelminthique périodique d'enfants d'âge scolaire au Zaire. Ann Soc Belg Med Trop 58:241–249
Kadio A, Moreau J, Gazin J, Gaudet M (1982) L'Albendazole (Zentel®) dans le traitement de l'ankylostomiase en Côte d'Ivoire. Méd Afr Noire 29:27–28
Kahn AA (1966) Practical aspects of the treatment of hookworm infection in Kampala children. Trans R Soc Trop Med Hyg 60:322–324
Kale OO (1977) The anthelminthic efficacy of a mixture of pyrantel pamoate and oxantel pamoate. Curr Ther Res 22:802–806
Kaminsky RG, Ndinya-Achola JO (1977) *Oesophagostomum* sp. from Kenya. Identification through tissue sections. East Afr Med J 54:296–297
Kaminsky RG, Zimmerman RR (1977) *Trichinella spiralis:* incidental finding. East Afr Med J 54:643–646
Kan SP (1979) Atypical nematode ova in a patient treated with pyrantel pamoate. Ann Trop Med Parasitol 73:397–398
Kan SP (1982) Soil-transmitted helminthiasis in Selangor, Malaysia. Med J Malaysia 37:180–190
Kan SP (1983a) The antihelminthic effects of flubendazole on *Trichuris trichiura* and *Ascaris lumbricoides*. Trans R Soc Trop Med Hyg 77:668–670
Kan SP (1983b) The efficacy of single doses of flubendazole plus levamisole in the treatment of *Trichuris* and *Ascaris* infections. In: Yokogawa et al. (eds) Collected papers on the control of soil-transmitted helminthiases, vol 2. Asian Parasite Control Organisation, Tokyo, pp 145–149
Kan SP (1983c) Efficacy of single doses of mebendazole in the treatment of *Trichuris trichiura* infection. Am J Trop Med Hyg 32:118–122
Kan SP, Cheah JS (1970) Prevalence and intensity of helminthic infections in adults among the ethnic groups in Singapore. Singapore Med J 11:283–296
Karnaukov VK, Ozeretskovskaya NN, Linewitch OM, Scherbakow AM, Djakomara AM, Drozdova TI, Laskovenko AI (1978) Clinical study of vermox (mebendazole) in trichocephalosis and other helminthiases. Janssen Pharmaceutica, Clin Res Report, N 14277
Kato K, Miura M (1954) Comparative examinations. Jpn J Parasitol 3:35 (in Japanese)
Katz M (1977) Anthelmintics. Drugs 13:124–136
Katz N (1980) Dose-range study of flubendazole in the treatment of hookworm disease and trichiuriasis. Janssen Pharmaceutica, Clin Res Report, R 17889/19
Katz N, Zicker F, Chaves A, Antunes CMF (1972) Clinical trials with pyrantel pamoate in intestinal parasitoses. Rev Inst Med Trop São Paulo 14:212–221

Kean BH, Hoskin DW (1964) Treatment of trichinosis with thiabendazole. A preliminary report. JAMA 190:852–853

Keller AE, Leathers WS (1936) The incidence and distribution of *Ascaris lumbricoides, Trichuris trichiura, Hymenolepis nana* and *Hymenolepis diminuta* in 36 counties in Kentucky. Am J Hyg 23:216–230

Kilala CP (1971) *Ternidens deminutus* infecting man in southern Tanzania. East Afr Med J 48:636–645

Kilala CP, Chimbe A, Zikambona A (1970) Clinical trial of a new anti-hookworm drug: Jonit. In: Health and disease in Africa. East Afr Literature Bureau, Nairobi

Kilpatrick ME, Trabolsi B, Farid Z (1981) Levamisole compared to mebendazole in the treatment of *Ancylostoma duodenale* in Egypt. Trans R Soc Trop Med Hyg 75:578–579

Klein E (1971) Single blind study in trichuriasis and ancylostomiasis. Janssen Pharmaceutica, Clin Res Report, N 5 500

Klein J, Zakharenko DF, Dolgina LE, Braginetz WR, Linko IA (1981) Etiotropic therapy and prophylaxis of trichinellosis. In: Kim ChW, Ruitenberg EJ, Teppema JS (eds) Proc 5th intern conf trich. pp 291–296

Kliks MM (1983) Anisakiasis in the Western United States: four new case reports from California. Am J Trop Med Hyg 32:526–532

Kobayashi A (1970) Anthelminthic effect of pyrantel pamoate (Combantrin) against ascariasis (in Japanese). Jpn J Parasitol 19:296–300

Kobayashi A (1971) Anthelmintic effect of pyrantel pamoate against hookworm infection. Jpn J Parasitol 20:52–57

Kobayashi A (1980) Theory and practice applied in Japan for the eradication of *Ascaris* infection. In: Yokogawa M et al. (eds) Collected papers on the control of soil-transmitted helminthiases. Asian Parasite Control Organization 1:232–242

Koino S (1923) Infection experiments of ascariasis in human body. Jpn Med World 4:46–47

Komiya Y, Kobayashi A, Ogawa H, Kumada M (1960a) Mass treatment of oxyuriasis with pyrvinium pamoate (Povan). Jpn J Parasitol 9:551–555

Komiya Y, Kobayashi A, Kutsumi H, Kojima K, Kumada M, Ogawa H (1960b) On the mass treatment of hookworm infection. 4. The comparative study of the enthelmintic effect of 4-iodo-thymol and 1-bromonaphtol. Jpn J Parasitol 9:195–198

Komiya Y, Mori Y, Yamauchi K (1962) Anthelminthic effect of pyrvinium pamoate (Poquil) on pinworm with the administration in its smaller quantity. Jpn J Parasitol 11:390–392

Kosin E (1973) Clinical trial with mebendazole (R 17635) in schoolchildren. Janssen Pharmaceutica, Clin Res Report, N 6683

Kouri P, Valdez Dias R (1953) Concepto actual sobre el papel patogeno del *Trichocefalo dispar* (*Trichuris trichiura*). Sintomatologia gastro-intestinal particularmente ceco-apendicular y recto-sigmoideana. Rev Kuba Med Trop Parasitol 8:37–41

Krasa E, Kaupeny M (1977) Anthelmintika – Therapie mit Mebendazole bei Kindern mit bronchopulmonalen Erkrankungen. Paediatr Paedol 12:73–75

Krotoski WA, Knudsen K, Cogswell FB, Conard R (1979) Efficacy of mebendazole against the helminth parasites of a Pacific Island population. 75th Annual meeting Tucson, November, Am Soc Trop Med Hyg

Krubwa F, Gatti F, Lontie M, Vandepitte J, Thienpont D (1974a) Community-wide periodic anthelminthic treatment with levamisole. Ann Soc Belg Med Trop 54:167–176

Krubwa F, Gatti F, Lontie M, Nguete K, Vandepitte J, Thienpont D (1974b) Administration trimestrielle de mebendazole en milieu scolaire suburbain. Med Trop 34:679–687

Kuzmicki R, Gajda-Kazikowa E, Jozwiak S (1972) The results of treatment of helminthiasis with levatetramisole. Wiad Parazytol 18:73–77

Kuzmicki R, Jozwiak SC, Gajda-Kazikowa E, Savrasewicz B (1979) Mebendazole treatment for human ascariasis. Janssen Pharmaceutica Clin Res Report N 17518

Kwo H, Jürsuf MA (1973) Efficacy of pyrantel pamoate (Combantrin) in the mass treatment of ascariasis and hookworm infections. Yonsei Rep Trop med 4:163–165

Kwo EH, Kosman ML (1973) Treatment of intestinal parasites with mebendazole (R 17 635). Yonsei Rep Trop Med 4:166–167

Labarriere F, Labarriere-Pollet E (1979) Contribution à l'étude de l'action antihelminthique du flubendazole à propos de 339 observations. Thése, Lille
Lacan A (1978) Considerations pratiques sur les présentations et les modalités d'utilisation des agents thérapeutiques en campagnes de masse. In: Marois M (ed) Development of chemotherapeutic agents for parasitic diseases. Elsevier, Amsterdam, pp 126–131
Laengsvang S (1968) Further observations on the experimental transmission of *Gnathostoma spinigerum*. Ann Trop Med Parasitol 62:88–94
Lagunas Flores A (1979) Efectividad terapeutica del mebendazole en la trichocefalosis masiva. Salud Publica Mex 21:83–87
Laigret J, Tourres M, Boschi S (1969) Action antihelminthique de l'isomère lévogyre du tetramisole. Bull Soc Pathol Exot Filiales 62:734–740
Lambotte C, Bayoka S, Mulunda LE, Bosilo P (1960) L'Hydroxynaphtoate de bephenium dans l'ankylostomose du nourrisson et de l'enfant. Ann Soc Belg Méd Trop 40:771–781
Lamina J (1980) Larva-migrans-visceralis-Infektionen durch *Toxocara*-Arten. Dtsch Med Wochenschr 105:796–797
Lamson PD, Ward CB (1932) The chemotherapy of helminth infestations. J Parasitol 18:173–199
Larivière M, Aziz MA, Diallo S, Diop Mar I, Porta M (1982) Efficacité et tolérance de l'ivermectine (MK 933) dans l'Onchocercose humaine. In: Coulaud JP, Gaxotte Ph (eds) Ophtalmologie tropicale. Onchocercose. La Francaise d'Edition et d'Imprimerie, Paris, pp 227–233
Latonio AA (1973) Blind studies on three drugs in treatment of mixed nematodal infections. Philipp J Microbiol Infect Dis 2:59–69
Latonio AA, Gonzales FA (1973) Open study of mebendazole in mixed nematodal infections. Philipp J Microbiol Infect Dis 2:47–58
Layrisse M, Aparcedo L, Martinez-Torres C, Roche M (1967) Blood loss due to infection with *Trichuris trichiura*. Am J Trop Med Hyg 16:613–619
Leao RN (1980) Dose-range study of flubendazole in the treatment of hookworm disease and trichiuriasis complicated or not by ascariasis . Janssen Pharmaceutica, Clin Res Report N 21 274
Lechat MF, Jancloes MF, Galambos FG, Cornet P, Thienpont D (1974) Control by levamisole of ascariasis and ancylostomiasis in rural areas. Trop Geogr Med 26:441–445
Lecomte-Ramioul S (1975) Traitement de l'oxyurase par le mébendazole. Schémas therapeutiques applicables à une communauté d'enfants. Rev Méd Liége 30:733–736
Lee En-L, Lyngkaran N, Gruve AW, Robinson MJ, Dissanaike AS (1975) Therapeutic evaluation of oxantel pamoate in severe *Trichuris trichiura* infection. Am J Trop Med Hyg 25:563–567
Lee SH, Lim JK (1978) A comparative study of the effect of oxantel-pyrantel suspension and mebendazole in mixed infections with *Ascaris* and *Trichuris*. Drugs [Suppl 1] 15:94–98
Lee SH, Seo BS, Cho SY, Kang SY (1976) Clinical trial of oxantel pamoate (CP-14445) on *Trichocephalus trichiurus* infection. Kor J Parasitol 14:25–31
Leikina ES, Poletaeva OG (1980) Immunology of ascariasis. Intestinal Parasites S. G./WP/ 80, 15. WHO
Lenczner MM (1972) Treatment of trichiuriasis. Correspondence. Trans R Soc Trop Med Hyg 66:510–511
Lengyel A, Rove J, Balle T, Lehoczky I (1973) New experiences in the therapy of ascariasis in children. Janssen Pharmaceutica, Clin Res Report, N 7280
Lengyel A, Levai J, Rovo JT (1975) L'importance du mebendazole dans le traitement des infestations dues au *Trichuris trichiura*. Ther Hung 23:64–67
Lengyel A, Albi I, Rovo TJ (1978) Mebendazole (Vermox) in the treatment of enterobiasis. Ther Hung 26:64–66
Lepercq G (1974) Expertise clinique du mebendazole. Janssen Pharmaceutica, Clin Res Report, 8248
Levai J, Lengyel A, Bank IG (1972) The first experiences with a new anthelminthic in Hungary. Janssen Pharmaceutica, Clin Res Report N 7987

Levi GC, Neto VA, Konichi SR, Stefani HNV (1972) Tratamento da ascaridiase em zona rural: estudo comparativo entre as actavidades de doses unicas de hexahidrato de piperazina, tetramisole e pamoate de pirantel. Rev Inst Med Trop Sao Paulo 14:392–396

Levin ML (1983) Treatment of trichinosis with mebendazole. Am J Trop Med Hyg 32:980–983

Lian WN, Zi ZY (1981) Observations on the prevalence and therapy of *enterobius vermicularis* infection among kindergarten children. Chin J Prevent Med 15:81 (abstract, WHO 82.5/10)

Lie Kian Joe (1940) Helminthiasis of the intestinal wall caused by *Oesophagostomum apiostomum* (Willach, 1891). Raillet and Henry 1905. Doc Neerl et Indones Trop 1:75–80

Lim JK (1973) Anthelminthic effect of trans-1,4,5,6-tetrahydro-2-(3-hydroxystyryl)-1-methyl pyrimidine on *Trichocephalus trichuris*. Seoul J Med 14:228–232

Lim JK (1974) Anthelminthic effect of oxantel pamoate against *Trichocephalus trichiuris* infection. Kor J Pharmacol 10:25–28

Lim JK (1978 a) Anthelminthic effect of multiple intestinal helminthiasis with oxantel and pyrantel. Drugs [Suppl 1] 15:70–72

Lim JK (1978 b) Anthelminthic effect of oxantel and oxantel-pyrantel in intestinal nematode infections. Drugs [Suppl 1] 15:99–103

Limbos P, Muynck A De, Janssens PG (1968) Traitement de la trichocephalose par la diphetarsone. Acta Gastroenterol. Belg 31:492–496

Lionel NDW, Mirando EH, Nanayakkara JC, Soysa PE (1969) Levamisole in the treatment of ascariasis in children. Br Med J 1:340–341

Lionel NDW, Rafapakre L, Soysa P, Aiyathurai JEJ (1975) Mebendazole in the treatment of intestinal helminthiasis with special reference to whipworm infections. J Trop Med Hyg 78:75–77

Lionel NDW, Silva DGH Da, Jayatilleka SMO (1980) Flubendazole in the treatment of intestinal helminthiasis. A comparative study using single dosage regimens. Janssen Pharmaceutica, Clin Res Report N 22 140

Lloyd EL (1959) Struggles with *Strongyloides*. Practitioner 182:740

Lopez Montero E, Calzada Sanchez JA (1975) Mebendazole en el tratiemento de las poliparasitosis intestinales. Janssen Pharmaceutica, Clin Res Report, N 9411

Lorenz WA, Henglein A, Schrader G (1955) The new insecticide o,o-dimethyl 2,2,2-trichloro-1-hydroxy-ethyl-phosphonate. J Am Chem Soc 77:2554–2556

Loria-Cortez R, Lobo-Sanahuja JF (1980) Clinical abdominal angiostrongylosis. A study of 116 children with intestinal eosinophilic granuloma caused by *Angiostrongylus costaricensis*. Am J Trop Med Hyg 29:538–544

Loria-Cortez R, Lizano C, Chavarria AO, Villavicencio N, Calzada Castro LD (1974) Experience with mebendazole in children with multiple intestinal helminthiasis. Janssen Pharmaceutica, Clin Res Report, N 7327

Lormans JAG, Wesel AJT, Parijs OF Van (1975) Mebendazole (R 17635) in enterobiasis. Chemotherapy 21:255–260

Loughlin EH, Mullin WG (1955) The treatment of enterobiasis with cristalline oxytetracycline. Antibiot Med 1:145–150

Loughlin EH, Rappaport I, Mullin WG, Wells HS, Shookhof HB (1951) The treatment of enterobiasis with Terramycin base. Antibiot Chemother 1:588–593

Louw JH (1974) Biliary ascariasis in childhood. S Afr J Surg 12:219–225

Louzada GZ, Louzada JLZ, Becker MdL, Louzada FZ, Agra HNC, Garcia PR, Garcia PC, Vasconcelos N (1973) Experimentacao clinica com mebendazole. Doenças infectiosas e parasitarias. Folha Med 66:317–334

Lucas AO, Oduntan SO (1972) Treatment of hookworm infection and other intestinal parasites with L-tetramisole (Ketrax). Ann Trop Med Parasitol 66:391–398

Luengo J, Barriga O (1966) Efecto del thiabendazole sobre differentes fases de la triquinosis experimental de la rata. Bol Chil Parasitol 27:2–11

Lumbreras H, Guerra H, Ortiz-Valqui R, Tello R, Vega O (1974) Enterobiasis y ascariasis en un orfanatorio de Lima – tratamiento massivo con dosis unica de pamoate de pyrantel. Acta Med Peru 3:185–190

Lumbreras Cruz H, Tello R, Antunez A, Mayolo A De, Campos M, Guerra H, Soto J (1981) Ensayo terapeutico controlado de albendazol en helminthiasis intestinal. Compendium de Invest Clin Latino Americanas, I Simposio Latino americano Geohelminthiasis y albendazol. Cancun Mexico 1:104–109
Lynch DM, Green EA, McFadzean JA, Pugh IM (1972) *Trichuris trichiura* infestations in the United Kingdom and treatment with difetarsone. Br Med J IV:73–76
Lyndoh E, Barua P, Dutta S (1962) Bephenium hydroxynaphtoate in hookworm and other helminthic infestations. J Indian Med Assoc 39:350–353
Maccowen M, Callender ME, Lawlis JF, Brandt MC (1953) The effect of erythromycin against certain parasitic organisms. Am J Trop Med Hyg 2:212–218
Maccowen MC, Callender ME, Brandt MC (1957) The anthelminthic effect of dithiazanine in experimental animals. Am J Trop Med Hyg 6:894–897
Mackay DM, Ahmed T, Ali S (1979) Pyrantel in the mass eradication of roundworm and hookworm. Health Hyg 2:123–125
Mackerras MJ (1961) A promising new drug for the elimination of hookworms. Med J Aust 2:261–263
Maisonneuve H, Piens MA, Mojon M, Garin JP (1981) L'albendazole. Evaluation de la tolérance et de l'efficacité dans l'oxyurose, la trichocephalose, l'ankylostomose, l'ascaridiose, l'anguillulose. Bull Soc Pathol Exot Filiales 75:434–444
Maka G (1963) Un oxyuricide des temps modernes: le pamoate de pyrvinium. Thése Méd, Lyon, no 118
Maldonado JF (1965) Stilbazium iodide (monopar) in the treatment of human trichiuriasis. Bol Asoc Med PR 57:57–66
Mandour AM, Oman LAM (1976) Efficiency of levamisole "Ketrax" on some nematode infections in Assiat province. In: Proceedings of the 9th international congress of chemotherapy, July 1975, London, vol 6. Parasites, fungi, viruses. Plenum, New York, pp 97–104
Manson-Bahr Gh (1940) Phenothiazine as an anthelminthic. Lancet 2:808–809
Mantovani A, Filippini I, Sachetti A, Bergomi S, Cavrini C, Marastoni G (1976) Observations sur un foyer de trichinose humaine en Italie. Bull Acad Vet Fr 49:213–217
Maqbool S, Lawrence D, Katz M (1975) Treatment of trichuriasis with a new drug, mebendazole. J Pediatr 86:463–465
Margono S, Mahfudin H, Abidin AN, Rasad R, Rasidi R (1980) Flubendazole and oxantel-pyrantel pamoate in the treatment of soil-transmitted helminths. Janssen Pharmaceutica Clin Res Report N 22 139
Markell EK (1968) Pseudohookworm infection – trichostrongyliasis. N Engl J Med 278:831–833
Marroud J, Arfaa F, Jalali H, Keyvan S (1980) Prevalence of intestinal helminths in Khuzestan, S. W. Iran 1977. Am J Trop Med Hyg 29:389–392
Martins NA, Gaburri DP (1974) Ensaio clinico com um novo anti-helmintico polivalente – o mebendazole. Folha Med 68:33–35
Martirani I, Rodrigues LD (1976) Ensaio clinico com o cambendazole, uma nova droga na terapeutica anti-helmintica (nota previa). Rev Inst Med Trop Sao Paulo 18:71–75
Martirani I, Soares W, Rodrigues LD, Ferreira LE, Ayres N, Aguiar Filho E (1976) Cambendazole – um nova antelmintico. Estuerdos de biovaliabilidade. Folha Med 73:11–14
Marx R, Tonthanien (1961) Essais de traitement de l'ankylostomose en Viet-Nam par l'hydroxynaphtoate de bephenium. Bull Soc Pathol Exot Filiales 54:844–850
Mathies AW (1961) *Enterobius vermicularis* infection. Certain aspects of host-parasite relationship. Am J Dis Child 101:174–177
Mathies AW (1969) Thiabendazole in the treatment of *Enterobius vermicularis*. Tex Rep Biol Med [Suppl 2] 27:611–614
Mathies AW (1973) The efficacy of mebendazole in the treatment of *Enterobius*. Janssen Pharmaceutica, Clin Res Rep N 7331
Meenakshi Shah (1979) Clinical evaluation of mebendazole in trichuriasis in children. Indian Pediatr 16:267–270
Mehrez R (1947) Les nouveaux traitements de l'oxyurose. Thése Méd no 546, Paris

Mehrotra MP, Malaviya VS (1963) Single dose treatment of hookworm disease with bephenium hydroxynaphtoate. Indian J Med Sci 17:930–933
Meira DA, Neto VA, Campos R (1961) Tratamento da estrongiloidiase pelo pamoate de pirvinio. O Hospital 59:1135–1138
Mejia R, Biagi F (1959) El ioduro de dithiazanina en algunas helminthiasis. Med Mex 39:346–348
Merdivenci A, Samasti M, Baturalp I (1977) Trihuriyazin mebendazole ile iyiletimi uzerine arastirnalar. Turk Microbiol Cem Derg 7:45–53
Migasena S, Suntharasamai P, Harinasuta T (1978) Mebendazole, tetrachlorethylene and pyrantel pamoate in the treatment of hookworm infection. Ann Trop Med Parasitol 72:199–200
Miller JH, Anthony SO, Swarzwelder JC, Frye WW, Lampert R (1958) Treatment of enterobiasis with dithiazanine. Am J Digest Dis 3:229–231
Miller MJ (1976) Protozoan and helminth parasites – A review of current treatment. In: Jucker E (ed) Progress in drug research. Birkhaeuser, Basel, pp 433–464
Miller MJ (1980) Use of levamisole in parasitic infections. Drugs 19:122–130
Miller MJ, Arfaa F (1975) Levamisole compared with piperazine citrate in the treatment of schoolchildren with ascariasis. Janssen Pharmaceutica Clin Res Report N 10443
Miller MJ, Katz N (1975) Single oral doses of levamisole and of piperazine citrate in the treatment of children with ascariasis. Janssen Pharmaceutica, Clin Res Report, N 10 444
Miller MJ, Krupp IM, Little MD, Santos C (1974) Mebendazole, an effective anthelminthic for trichuriasis and enterobiasis. JAMA 230:1412–1414
Miller MJ, Krupp IM, Little MD (1976) Placebo-controlled comparison of levamisole with pyrantel pamoate in the treatment of ascariasis in children. Janssen Pharmaceutica, Clin Res Report, N 10543
Miller MJ, Farahmandian I, Arfaa F, Katz N, Winsor E, Bennett E (1978) An evaluation of levamisole for treatment of ascariasis. South Med J 71:137–140
Misra SS, Misra RN, Soleja MZ (1965) A trial of bephenium hydroxynaphtoate in ankylostomiasis. J Assoc Physicians India 13:199–204
Misra A, Visen PKS, Katiyar JC (1981) Comparative efficacy of standard antihookworm drugs against various test nematodes. J Helminth 55:273–278
Mittermayer T, Spaldonova R (1981) The use of mebendazole in the treatment of trichinellosis in man. Folia Parasitol 28:235–242
Mittermayer T, Chroust K, Dedina L, Simunova M (1978) Clinical and therapeutical experience of trichinosis treated with thiabendazole and mebendazole. Cas Lek Ces 117:1053–1056
Mittermayer T, Cisarova A, Carnicka A, Magyar B, Maloveska M, Schreter I (1979) Acute trichinellosis with neurological and mental manifestations treated with mebendazole and corticoids. Cas Lék Ces 118:1175–1179
Miyazaki I (1960) On the genus *Gnathostoma* and human gnathostomiasis, with special reference to Japan. Exp Parasitol 9:337–370
Miyazaki I (1966) *Gnathostoma* and gnathostomiasis in Japan. In: Progress of medical parasitology in Japan. Meguro Parasitological Museum, Tokyo
Miyazaki L (1968) On the genus *Gnathostoma* and human gnathostomiasis, with special reference to Japan. Exp Parasitol 62:88–94
Moens M, Dom J, Burke WE, Schlossberg S, Schuermans V (1978) Levamisole in ascariasis – A multicenter controlled evaluation. Am J Trop Med Hyg 27:897–904
Mojon M, Piens MA (1982) L'Albendazole et anguillulose. Méd Afr Noire 29:9–14
Mojon M, Melet V, Durand-Peyre F, Jacquet M (1981) Anguillulose et albendazole. Lyon Med 245:99–104
Mojon M, Cadi-Soussi M, Excler JL (1982) Efficacité de l'albendazole en prise unique dans le traitement de l'ankylostomiase. Essai thérapeutique mené en double aveugle. Méd Afr Noire 29:5–8
Molina Pasquel Cl, Diaz Muñoz A (1959) Effectividad del tetradoretileno emulsionado en el tratamiento de la uncinariasis. Rev Inst Salubr Enferm Trop (Mexico) 19:11–14

Montero LE, Sanchez CJA (1975) Mebendazole en el tratamento de las poliparasitosis intestinales. Janssen Pharmaceutica Clin Res Rep N 9411

Moreau JP, Lagraulet J (1972) Survie „in vitro" des larves de troisième stade *d'Angiostrongylus cantonensis*. Ann Parasitol Hum Comp 47:525–529

Morera P (1979) Life histroy and redescription of *Angiostrongylus costaricensis* Morera and Cespedes. Am J Trop Med Hyg 22:613–622

Morera P, Cespedes R (1971) Angiostrongilosis abdominal. Una nueva parasitosis humana. Acta Med Cost 14:159–173

Morera P, Perez FR, Mora F, Castro L (1982) Visceral larva migrans-like syndrome caused by *Angiostrongylus costaricensis*. Am J Trop Med Hyg 31:67–70

Moser RH (1974) From Bismark to Polar bears. JAMA 228:735–737

Most H (1963) Treatment of the more common worm infections. JAMA 185:874–877

Most H, Yoeli M, Champbell WC, Cuckler C (1965) The treatment of *Strongyloides* and *Enterobius* infections with thiabendazole. Am J Trop Med Hyg 14:379–382

Mouriquand G, Roman E, Coisnard J (1951) Essai de traitement de l'oxyurose par la pipérazine. J Med Lyon 32:189–195

Mouriquand G, Roman E, Coisnard G (1953) Traitement de l'oxyurose infantile par le pipérazine. Rev Kuba Med Trop Parasitol 9:37–38

Müller G (1953) Untersuchungen über die Lebensdauer von Ascarideneiern in Gartenerde. Z Bakteriol Parasitol Infektionskrankheiten Hyg Orig 159:377–379

Müller RW (1949) Über die Allergie und Immunität bei der *Ascaris* Infektion des Menschen. Z Hyg Inf Krank 130:28–35

Mullin WG, Imperato P (1969) Treatment of oxyuriasis with thiabendazole. Tex Rep Biol Med [Suppl 2] 27:615–621

Musgrave IA, Hawes RB, Jameson JL, Sloane RA, Quayle PA (1979) Mebendazole: evaluation of a new antihelminthic for trichiuriasis, hookworm and strongyloidiasis. Med J Aust 1:403–405

Mutalik GS, Gulati RB (1969) Clinical trial of bitoscanate (jonit) in hookworm disease. Clin Pharmacol Ther 10:635–637

Mutalik GS, Gulati RB (1972) Comparative clinical trial of bitoscanate, bephenium hydroxynaphtoate and tetrachlorethylene in hookworm infection. Indian J Med Sci 26:718–722

Mutalik GS, Balwani JH, Pal VR, Joglekar GV (1964) *4*-Iodothymol (thymolan) in the treatment of ankylostomiasis. J Trop Med Hyg 67:75–76

Mutalik GS, Gulati RB, Iqbal AK (1970) Evaluation of phenylene 1,4-di-isothiocyanate (bitoscanate: Jonit®) in intestinal parasitic infection: a field study. Ann Trop Med Parasitol 64:79–85

Muttalib UA, Kahn MV, Hacq JA (1981) Single dose regime of mebendazole in the treatment of polyparasitism in children. J Trop Med Hyg 84:159–160

Nagalingam I, Lam LE, Robinson MJ, Dissanaike AS (1976) Mebendazole in treatment of severe *Trichuris trichiura* infection in Malaysian children. Am J Trop Med Hyg 25:568–572

Nagaty HF, Rifaat MA (1959) Clinical trials with bephenium hydroxynaphtoate against *Ancylostoma duodenale* and other helminthic infestations. J Trop Med Hyg 62:255–258

Nagaty HF, Mohajeri M, Elahi R (1978) Clinical trial of levamisole in the treatment of ascariasis in Khorasan, Iran. J Trop Med Hyg 81:195–197

Nakasato H (1974) Immunoglobulin levels in helminthic infections: ancylostomiasis, ascariasis, and trichiuriasis. Jpn J Parasitol 23:325–334

Narmada R, Jagadesewara RM, Adinaraynan P, Balagopal Raju V (1974) Study on oxyuriasis and trichuriasis in children and evaluation of mebendazole. Indian Pediatr 11:417–419

Narmada R, Jagadeeswara RM, Balagopal RV (1977) Study of oxyuriasis in families. Janssen Pharmaceutica, Clin Res Report, N 13712

Nassif S, Bell WJ, Prescott JEG (1974) Comparison of pyrantel pamoate syrup and pyrvinium pamoate syrup in the treatment of enterobiasis in Egypt. J Trop Med Hyg 77:270–271

Nauenberg W, Edelman MH, Spingarn CI (1970) Observations on the treatment of strongyloidiasis with thiabendazole in New York City. Mt Sinai J Med 37:607–611
Navarro-Hildago A, Uribe J de R (1962) Ensayos sobre tratamientos colectivos de la helminthiasis intestinal en la edad escobar. Rev Invest Bol Univ (Guadalajara) 2:253–260
Nelson GS, Richman R, Pester FRN (1961) Feral trichinosis in Africa. Trans R Soc Trop Med Hyg 55:514–517
Neyrinck B, Kerckhove N Van de (1976) Flubendazole. Single oral doses in adult patients which ascariasis, trichiuriasis and for hookworm. Janssen Pharmaceutica Clin Res Report N 11655
Ngoy K, Kalombo M (1975) Therapeutical effectiveness and safety of 2% mebendazole syrup in various helminthiasis. Janssen Pharmaceutica, Clin Res Report N 9537
Ninane G, Poffe F (1959) Essai clinique de l'hydroxynaphtoate de bephenium dans l'ankylostomiase. Ann Soc Belg Méd Trop 39:887–892
Ninane G, Brakel J, Coster P De (1957) A propos de l'emploi de l'adipate de piperazine pour le traitement de masse de l'ascaridiose. Ann Soc Belg Méd Trop 37:279–284
Nishimura T, Okumara T, Sakaguchi H, Maeyama T, Takahashi N (1965) Pinworm infection in children and its mass treatment with a small dose of pyrvinium pamoate. Jpn J Parasitol 14:204–212
Nitzulescu V (1971) Traitement de l'ascaridiose par le chlorhydrate de L-tretramisole (Decaris). Janssen Pharmaceutica, Clin Res Report N 5617
Nitzulescu V, Simionescu O, Lucian O, Corijescu V, Brinzei A, Juvara AM (1970) Le traitement de la trichocéphalose par le Bemarsal. Bull Soc Pathol Exot Filiales 63:251–255
Nozais JP (1978) Etude de l'activité du fluoromebendazole (flubendazole) sur *Ascaris lumbricöides, Necator americanus* et *Trichuris trichiura* en pays d'endémie. Méd Afr Noire 25:473–475
O'Holohan DR, Hugoe-Matthews J (1972) Single dose regimens of phenylene-di-isothiocyanata (1,4), Jonit, in the treatment of hookworm infestation in Malaysia. Southeast Asian. J Trop Med Public Health 3:403–410
Oishi K, Nagano K, Suzuki M (1974) Pathogenic capacity of anisakinae larvae from cod/ and Alaska pollack. Proc 3rd int congr Parasitol, München G2 (22), Facta Publication, H Egermann, A1170 Vienna, p 1626
Ora M, Klein I, Cohen S, Meital Z (1976) Comparative efficacy of levamisole and piperazine in ascariasis. Janssens Pharmaceutic Clin Res Report N 10594
Orban A (1972) Mass treatment of a Congolese population with a single oral dose of levamisole. Janssen Pharmaceutica, Clin Res Report N 5898
Oshima T (1972) Anisakis and anisakiasis in Japan and adjacent area (1). In: Morishita K, Komiya Y, Matsubayashi H (eds) Progr Med Parasitol in Japan, vol 4, pp 303–393
Otero DR, Galvez OM, Estevez CB (1977) Primer ensayo clinico-terapeutico en Cuba con mebendazol en algunas helminthiasis. Rev Cubana Med Trop 29:13–16
Owings RS (1955) Pinworms and oxytetracycline. Some of the symptoms before treatment. Antibiot Med 1:280–282
Ozeretskovskaya NN (1968) The clinical and epidemiological peculiarities of trichinellosis originating from the different geographical regions of the USSR. Med Parazitol 34:387–397
Ozeretskovskaya NN, Pereverzeva EV, Tumolskaya NI, Bronshtein AM, Morenez TM, Imamkuliev KD (1976) Benzimidazoles in the treatment and prophylaxis of synanthropic and sylvatic trichinellosis. In: Kim Chw, Pawlowsky ZS (eds) Proc 4th int conf trich University Press of New England, Hannover, New Hampshire, pp 381–393
Ozeretskovskaya NN, Morenetz TM, Pereverzeva EV, Bronstein AM, Veretennikova NL, Kolosova MO, Poverenny AM, Podgorodnichenko VK, Kagorodin DA (1981) Therapeutical properties of benzimidazoles in trichinellosis and the side effects of the treatment. In: Kim ChW, Ruitenberg EJ, Teppema JS (eds) Trichinellosis. Proceedings of the 5th international conference on trichinellosis. Reedbooks, Chertsey, Surrey
Padelt H, Hölzer E, Steinrück M (1977) Neue Aspekte in der Therapie des Wurmbefalls. Janssen Pharmaceutica, Clin Res Report N 13276
Paine DHD, Lower ES, Cooper TV (1960) Treatment of trichuriasis with dithiazanine in a hospital for mental defectives. Br Med J 1:770–774

Palacios y Saucedo (1973 a) Estudio pediatrico (40 casos) de un antihelmintico de amplio spectro. Janssen Pharmaceutica, Clin Res Report N 7575
Palacios y Saucedo J (1973 b) Estudio pediatrico (40 casos) de un antihelmintico de amplio spectro. Status Report, Mexico
Palmer ED (1950) A note on the treatment of strongyloidiasis with intravenous gentian violet. Am J Trop Med 30:91–92
Pampinglione S, Ricciardi ML (1971) The presence of *Strongyloides fülleborni* von Linstow 1905, in man in central and east Africa. Parasitologia 13:257–269
Pampiglione S, Baldelli R, Corsini C, Mari S, Mantovani A (1978) Infezione Sperimentale del Cavallo con Larve di *Trichina*. Parasitologia 20:183–193
Pandey KN, Saratchandra S, Sarin G, Ajmani NK, Chuttani HK (1971) Pyrantel pamoate in treatment of hookworm infestation. Br Med J 4:399–400
Papasarathorn T, Chularenk U, Tongkoom B (1964) Studies on therapeutic effects of thiabendazole (MK 360) against ascariasis, trichuriasis, strongyloidiasis and hookworm infections in man. Jpn J Med Sci Biol 17:217–221
Paramaeswaran H, Lung TK (1979) Mebendazole in the treatment of symptomatic trichuriasis. A preliminary efficiency report. Janssen Pharmaceutica, Clin Res Report N 7,223
Park C-W, Lim J-K, Shim S-J, Kim M-S, Chung M-H (1973) Anthelmintic effect of trans-1, 4, 5, 6, tetrahydro-2-(3-hydroxystyryl)-1 methyl pyrimidine (CP 14445) on *Trichocephalus trichiuris*. Seoul J Med 14:228–232
Partono F, Purnomo, Tangkilisan A (1974) The use of mebendazole in the treatment of polyparasitism. Southeast Asian J Trop Med Public Health 5:258–264
Pascual J, Bouli RP, Aguiar H (1981) Eosinophilic meningoencephalitis in Cuba, caused by *Angiostrongylus cantonensis*. Am J Trop Med Hyg 30:960–962
Patel KM, Olweny CLM (1972) Comparison of bitoscanate ("Jonit") and tetrochlorethylene in treatment of *N. americanus* infection. East Afr Med J 49:270–272
Patron F, Zavala J, Carranza J (1973) Evaluacion del efecto antitrichocefalosica del mebendazole. Rev Coleg Medicos Yucatan 2:12–19
Paugrain J, Delavat A (1970) Bilan de l'action anthelminthique de l'isomère levogyre du tetramisole en Polynésie Française. Bull Soc Pathol Exot Filiales 63:507–513
Paul FM, Zaman V (1975) A trial of mebendazole in trichuriasis (whipworm) infestation in Singapore children. Singapore Med J 16:11–18
Paul FrM, Zaman V (1976) A trial of oxantel in trichiuriasis. Singapore Med J 17:219–224
Paviot JJ, Nioguy C (1960) Essais d'un nouvel anthelminthique sel de bephenium. Bull Soc Pathol Exot Filiales 53:806–809
Pawlowski ZS (1981) Control of trichinellosis. In: Kim ChW, Ruitenberg EJ, Teppema JS (eds) Proc 5th int congr trich. Reedbooks, Chertsey, Surrey, England, pp 7–20
Pawlowski Z, Chodera L (1975) Mebendazol – Nowy Lek Przeciw Robaczycom. Pol Tyg Lek 30:1035–1037
Peña-Chavarria A (1977) Efficacy of one to two grams of flubendazole in the treatment of trichuriasis. Janssen Pharmaceutica, Clin Res Report N 12865
Peña-Chavarria A, Villarejos VM (1975) Cure, egg reduction and reinfestation rates in children with ascariasis after single oral doses of anthelminthics: a placebo-controlled comparison of levamisole with pyrantel pamoate. Janssen Pharmaceutica, Clin Res Report N 10384
Peña-Chavarria A, Lizano C, Courtney KO, Thompson PE (1963) The effect of trichlorfenol piperazine in patients parasitized by hookworms, ascarids, or trichurids. Am J Trop Med Hyg 12:378–382
Peña-Chavarria A, Swartzwelder JC, Villarejos VM, Kotcher E, Arguedas J (1969) Dichlorvos, an effective broad spectrum anthelminthic. Am J Trop Med Hyg 18:907–911
Peña-Chavarria A, Swartzwelder JC, Villarejos VM, Zeledon R (1973) Mebendazole, an affective broad-spectrum anthelminthic. Am J Trop Med Hyg 22:592–595
Pene P, Ngembi N'Bina C, Vincentelli JM, Bourderioux CH, Rossignol JF (1981 a) El Albendazol en ninos. In: 1st simp latino-americano geohelminthiasis y albendazol. Comp de Invest Clin Latino-americanas, Cancun, pp 114–116

Pene P, Vicentelli JM, Soula G, Bourderioux CH, Rossignol JF (1981 b) Le zentel (albendazole) dans le traitement des nématodoses intestinales. Etude multicentrique en Afrique de l'Ouest. A propos de 390 observations. Med Afr Noire 28:483–485

Pene P, Mojon M, Garin JP, Coulaud JP, Rossignol JF (1982 a) Albendazole: a new broad spectrum anthelminthic. Double blind multicenter clinical trial. Am J Trop Med Hyg 31:263–266

Pene P, Coulaud JP, Soula G, Rossignol JF, Monges P, Chaudet H (1982 b) Le zentel® dans le traitement des helminthiases intestinales en Afrique de l'Ouest. Med Afr Noire 29:43–48

Penot C, Picot H, Lavarde V (1978) Essai thérapeutique d'un nouvel anti-helminthique en Amazonie columbienne: le flubendazole. Bull Soc Pathol Exot Filiales 71:370–375

Pereira JFV, Ghosh HK, Conklin S, Ryan S (1979) Mebendazole therapy of whipworm infestation. Med J Aust 1:134–135

Phillips AP, Burrows RB (1961) Pyridine derivatives with anthelminthic activity. Nature 191:707–708

Phills JA, Harrold AJ, Whitman GV, Perelmutter L (1972) Pulmonary infiltrates, asthma and eosinophilia due to *Ascaris suum* infestation in man. N Engl J Med 286:965–975

Piekarski G (1975) Medizinische Parasitologie in Tafeln. Springer, Berlin Heidelberg New York

Pigott J, Hansburger EA Jr, Heafie RC (1970) Human ascariasis. Am J Clin Pathol 53:223–234

Pitts NE, Migliardi JR (1974) Antiminth (pyrantel pamoate). The clinical evaluation of a new broad-spectrum anthelminthic. Clin Pediatr 13:87–94

Pizzi TE, Schenone H (1951) Haltazgo de huevos de *Trichuris trichiura* en contenido intestinal de un cuerpo arqueologico incaico. Bol Chil Parasitol 9:73–75

Plotnikow NN, Ozeretskovskaya NN, Ananina NO (1962) Therapeutic efficacy of dithiazanine and degree of its tolerance in trichuriasis. Med Parazitol 31:515–521 (in Russian)

Pobee JOM, Amissah JK (1970) Clinical trial of a new anti-hookworm drug phenylene diisothiocyanate (1,4) Jonit®. Ghana Med J 9:98–101

Polak MF, Kapmelmacher EH (1967) Haringwormziekte in 1965 en in de voorgaande jaren. Versl Meded Volksgezondh 12:344

Pond HS, Bokat RB, Johnson JP, Knight JL, Healy GR, Gleason NN, Hall ER (1970) Mass treatment for ascariasis: value of prophylactic use of piperazine in groups heavily infected with *Ascaris lumbricoides*. South Med J 62:599–602

Pradatsundarasar A, Pecharanon K, Chintanawongs C, Ungthavorn P (1973) The first case of intestinal capillariasis in Thailand. Southeast Asian J Trop Med Public Health 4:131–134

Prakash O, Banerjee D, Sama SK (1970) A clinical trial of tetramisole (R 8299) in cases of ascariasis. Indian J Med Res 58:1578–1583

Purnomo, Partono F, Soewarta A (1980) Human intestinal parasites in Karakuak, West Flores, Indonesia, and the effect of treatment with mebendazole and pyrantel pamoate. Southeast Asian J Trop Med Public Health 11:324–331

Rachelson MH, Ferguson WR (1955) Piperazine in the treatment of enterobiasis. Am J Dis Child 89:346–349

Radoev V (1974) The efficacy and tolerance of L-tetramisol (Decaris) in the treatment of nematode infections. Probl Zaraz Paraz Boleste 2:261–271

Ramalingham Sh, Sinniah B, Krishnan U (1983) Albendazole, an effective single dose, broad spectrum anthelmintic drug. Am J Trop Med Hyg 32:984–989

Ramirez Martinez J, Maya Ugalde R (1973) Tricocefalosis: valoracion clinica de un neuevo antihelmintico. El Medico de Mexico 9:59–62

Ranque PH, Soula G, Espieu C, Kessalis N (1982) Traitement de l'ankylostomose au Mali par l'albendazole (Zentel®). A propos de 137 observations. Méd Afr Noire 29:19–22

Ricci M, Corbo S (1956) Sull'azione dell'idrato di piperazina verso *Enterobius vermicularis*. Recon Inst Sup Sanita 19:230–239

Ricci M, Corbo S (1957) Sull'azione dell'adipato di piperazina verso *e. vermicularis* e *a. lumbricoides*. Reon Ist Super Sanita 20:258–260

Ricci M, Frederico A (1972) Experimento di lotta contro l'ascaridiasi nel comune di parenti (Cosenza). Riv Parasitol 38:209–218

Richard-Lenoble D, Gentilini M (1980) Nematodoses intestinales au Gabon et et mebendazole (vermox). Janssen Pharmaceutica, Clin Res Report N 18928

Richard-Lenoble D, Kombila M, Maganga ML, Gentilini M (1981) Mebendazole et nematodoses intestinales au Gabon. Bull Soc Pathol Exot Filiales 74:444–450

Richard-Lenoble D, Kombila M, Gassita F, Coniquet C (1982) L'Albendazole (Zentel®): traitement des nématodoses intestinales au Gabon. Méd Afr Noire 29:37–39

Rim HJ, Lim JK (1972) Treatment of enterobiasis and ascariasis with Combantrin (pyrantel pamoate). Trans R Soc Trop Med Hyg 66:170–175

Rim HJ, Lim JK, Seo BS (1975) Anthelminthic effect of Combantrin (pyrantel pamoate) against intestinal nematodes in Korea. Proc 10th SEAMEO TROPMED Seminar. Korean J Parasitol 13:97–101

Rim H-J, Chang Yu-Sh, Ha JHw, Lim J-K (1976) Anthelmintic effect of oxantel pamoate (CP 14445) against trichuriasis. Kor Un Med J 13:205–211

Rim H-J, Joo K-H, Kim Y-Y, Lee JS, Song S-D (1980) Anthelminthic effect of Amidantel (Bay d 8815) against *Ancylostoma duodenale* infection. Korean J Parasitol 18:24–36

Rim H-J, Lee J-S, Joo Ky-Hw, Kim Yu-Sh (1981) Anthelminthic effects of fenbendazole and oxantel-pyrantel pamoate to the intestinal-nematodes. Korean J Parasitol 13:97–101

Rizzotti G (1952) Risultati della cura con violetto de genziana per via orale nella infestazione de *Strongyloides stercoralis*. Riv Parasitol 13:315–320

Rodrigues LD, Vilela M de P, Capell JI (1966) Novo anti-helminthics [ciclamato de 2,3,5,6-tetrahidro-6-penilimidazo-(2,1-B/Tiazol)] na ascariase humana. Rev Bras Med 23:861–866

Rodrigues LD, Vilela M de P, Capell JI (1967 a) O tratamento da ascariase e de outras parasiteses intestinais humanes pelo ciclamato de tetramisol. O Hospital 71:1757–1770

Rodrigues LD, Vilela M de P, Capell JI, Mello E De BF, Reibscheid S (1967 b) Tratamento da ascaridiase com dosa unica de fumarato de piperazina. Rev Brasil Med 24:442–446

Rodrigues LD, Martirani I, Cabeca M, Soares W, Brandao JA (1977) Cambendazol novo anti-helmintico na terapeutica da estrongiloidiase humana. Experimentacao clinica. Rev Inst Med Trop Sao Paulo 19:57–67

Rodrigues YT, Pecego GF, Coura LC, Negrisoli D, Galvao-Pereira FA, Rodriguez da Silva J (1960) Tratamento da oxiurase com dosa unica de pamoate de pirvinio. J Pediatr 25:324–330

Rodrigues de Curet H, Valiaga MP, del Pilar (1968) Dithiazanine intoxication, a case report. Bol Ass Med P Rico 55:469–472

Rodrigues Pavon A (1973) Estudio de la accion del mebendazole en la trichocefalosis. Status Report, Mexico

Rodriguez da Silva J, Camillo-Coura L, Tinoco de Carvalho H, Almeida-Lopes PF (1968) Tratamento da estrongylioidase. Resultados preliminares da ensaio com un novo entihelmintico o thiabendazol. O Hospital 63:247–264

Roels-Broadhurst D, Mayer EM De (1957) Le phosphate de pipérazine comme moyen de traitement de l'ascaridiose en milieu coutumier. Ann Soc Belge Méd Trop 37:925–931

Rombaut N, Scheijgrond H, Parijs O Van (1975) Flubendazole in enterobiasis. A placebo-controlled study. Janssen Pharmaceutica, Clin Res Report N 9986

Rossi MA, Bisson FW (1983) Fatal case of multiple liver abscesses caused by adult *Ascaris lumbricoides*. Am J Trop Med Hyg 32:523–525

Rossignol JF (1981) Albendazol: estudios clinicos realizados en Francia y Africa Occidental. Informe sobre 1,034 casos. Comp de Invert Clin I Simp, vol 1, Latino Americanos Geohelminthiasis y albendazol. Cancun, pp 117–125

Rossignol JF, Coulaud JP (1983) Evaluation of albendazole in Europe, West Africa and Asia as a single dose anthelmintic. Report on 1,455 patients. R Soc Med Int Congress and Symp Ser 57:19–27

Rowland HAK (1966) A comparison of tetrachlorethylene and bephenium hydroxynaphtoate in ancylostomiasis. Trans R Soc Trop Med Hyg 60:313–321

Royer A (1956) Preliminary report on a new antioxyuritic. Can Med Assoc J 74:297–299
Royer A, Baronikoff K (1962) Pinworm infestation in children: the problem and its treatment. Can Med Assoc J 86:60–65
Ruas AO (1973) Mebendazole in the treatment of worm infections. Janssen Pharmaceutica, Clin Res Report, N 7516
Rubens Campos (1982) Tratamento da ascariase e da tricuriase or meio do albendazol. 18e Congr soc Brasil med trop E15
Rubens Campos, Croce J, Amato Neto V (1963) Tratamento da trichostrongiliase humana pelo Tiabendazol. O Hospital 64:261–264
Ruitenberg EJ (1970) Anisakiasis: pathogenesis, serodiagnosis and prevention. Thesis, University of Utrecht, p 139
Ruitenberg EJ, Sluiten JF (1974) Trichinella spiralis infections in the Netherlands. In: Kim W (de) Trichinellosis. Proceedings of the 3rd international conference on Trichinellosis. Intext, New York
Sabharwal DV, Tikare SK, Gupta PS, Chuttani HK (1966) Thiabendazole in hookworm infection. Trans R Soc Trop Med Hyg 60:490–492
Sadun EH, Vajrathira S (1954) The effect of maklua (diospyros mollis) in the treatment of human hookworm. J Parasitol 40:49–53
Sadun EH, Melvin DM, Brooke MM, Carter CH (1956) Evaluation of promethazine hydrochloride R 02-5655/3, phtalylsulfathiazole and piperazine hexahydrate in the treatment of enterobiasis in a mental institution. Am J Trop Med Hyg 5:382–383
Saif M, Bell WJ, Taha A, Abdel-Meguid M, Abdallah A (1971) Comparison of pyrantel pamoate and bephenium hydroxynaphtoate in the treatment of *Ancylostoma duodenale* infection. J Egypt Med Assoc 54:791–797
Salazar Schettino PM, Haro Ortega (1981) Ensayo clinico doble ciego con Albendazol in Mexico. In: I. Simp latino americano geohelminthiasis y albendazol. Comp de Invest clin Latino americanas, Cancun, pp 90–95
Salem HH, Sherif AF, Abd. Rabbou H, Morcos W, El Niny H (1961) A single dose treatment of enterobiasis by pyrvinium pamoate. J Egypt Public Health Assoc 36:225–234
Salem HH, Hayattee ZG, Awaness AM (1962) Clinical trials with thiabendazole in the treatment of human intestinal helminthiasis. J Trop Med Hyg 11:268–272
Salem HH, Morcos WW, El Niny HM (1965) Clinical trials with bephenium hydroxynaphtoate against *A. duodenale* and other intestinal helminths. J Trop Med Hyg 68:21–25
Salem HH, Hayatee ZG, Awaness AM, Al-Allaf G (1968) Evaluation of the anthelmintic activity of thiabendazole in man. J Trop Med Hyg 71:11–17
Salunkhe DS, Gaitonde BB, Vakil R (1964) Clinical evaluation of a new anthelminthic thiabendazole [2-(4′thiazolyl) benzimidazole]. Am J Trop Med Hyg 13:412–416
Sanati A, Ghadirian EG (1971) Treatment of enterobiasis with pyrantel pamoate in Iran. J Trop Med Hyg 74:160–161
Sanchez-Carillo CMC, Beltran-Hernandez F (1977) Efectividad terapeutica del fenbendazol (Hoe. 881) en las helminthiasis transmitidas por el suelo en el Estado de Chiapas, Mexico. Salud Publica Mex 19:691–700
Sanders A, Hall W (1960) Comparison of dithiazanine iodide and pyrvinium pamoate in the treatment of enterobiasis. J Lab Clin Med 56:413–416
Sandground JH (1929) *Ternidens deminutus* (Raillet and Henry) as a parasite of man in southern Rhodesia; together with observations and experimental studies on an unidentified nematode parasite of man. Ann Trop Med Parasitol 22:23–29
Sandground JH (1931) Studies on the life-history of *Ternidens deminutus*, a nematode parasite of man, with observations on its incidence in certain regions of southern Africa. Ann Trop Med Parasitol 25:147–184
San Juan F (1962) A violeta de genciana e o iodeto de ditiazanina na estrongyloidose. Bol Centro Estudos Hosp Servidores Estato 14:195–203
Sanpakit S, Suksungvol S, Bhaibulaya M (1974) Intestinal capillariasis from Sarburi Province, Thailand: report of a second case. J Med Assoc Thai 57:458–460
Sargent RC, Chambers JC (1976) Controlled study comparing levamisole with piperazine citrate and pyrantel pamoate in the treatment of ascariasis. Janssen Pharmaceutica, Clin Res Report N 10542

Sargent RG, Dudley BW, Fox AS, Lease EJ (1972) Intestinal helminths in children in coastal South Carolina: a problem in southern United States. South Med J 65:294–298
Sargent RG, Savory AM, Mina A, Lee PR (1974) A clinical evaluation of mebendazole in the treatment of trichuriasis. Am J Trop Med Hyg 23:375–377
Sargent RG, Dotterer TD, Savory AM, Lee PR (1975) A clinical evaluation of the efficacy of mebendazole in the treatment of trichuriasis. South Med J 68:38–40
Sauerbrey M (1977) A precipitin test for the diagnosis of human abdominal angiostrongyliasis. Am J Trop Med Hyg 26:1156–1158
Saugrain J, Delavat A (1970) Bilan de l'action anthelminthique de l'isomère levogyre du Tetramisol en Polynésie Française. Bull Soc Pathol Exot Filiales 63:507–513
Savaton-Pillet J (1957) Personal communication. In: Cavier R (1973) Chemotherapy of intestinal hematodes, chapter 4. Chemotherapy of helmintheasis. Pergamon, Oxford
Sawitz WG, Karpinski FE (1956) Treatment of oxyuriasis with pyrroviquinium chloride (Poquil.) Am J Trop Med Hyg 5:538–543
Schenone H, Orfali A, Goldames M, Doren G, Inzunza E, Jimenez M, Romero E, Pinto CG, Anrique B (1974) Tratamiento de las helminthiasis intestinales humanas con mebendazole. Bol. Chil Parasitol 29:2–5
Schenone H, Goldames M, Inzunza E, Jimenez M, Romero E, Bloomfield R (1977) Flubendazol en el tratamiento de infecciones por nematodes intestinales en ninos. Bol Chil Parasitol 32:85–86
Schettino SPM, Ortega I de H (1981) Ensayo clinico doble ciego con albendazol en México. Comp Invest Clin Latino Am [Suppl 1] 1:90–95
Schmitz D, Knackfuss BAL (1971) Levamisole na tratamento da ascaridiase en pacientes de grupo etario comprendido entre 1 e 15 anos. Folha Med 63:149–151
Schneider J, Biguet J, Machez JM (1960) Traitement de l'oxyurose par le diphétarsone – spiramycine et le diphetarsone. Thérapie 15:648–654
Schrader G (1963) Die Entwicklung neuer insectizider Phosphorsäureester. Verlag Chemie, Weinheim
Schreiber W (1959) Intraduodenal therapy for *Taenia*, hookworm and *Strongyloides* infection. Gastroenterology 37:346–349
Scragg JN, Proctor EM (1978) Further experience with mebendazole in the treatment of symptomatic trichuriasis in children. Am J Trop Med Hyg 27:255–257
Seah SKK (1976) Mebendazole in the treatment of helminthiasis. Can Med Assoc J 115:777–779
Sen HG (1976) 4-isothiocyanato-4-nitrodiphenylamine (C 9333-90/CGP 4540) a new anthelminthic with potent antihookworm activity. Acta Trop 33:101–102
Sen HG, Joshi BS, Parthasarathy FC, Kamat VN (1974) Anthelminthic efficacy of diospyrol and its derivatives. Arzneimittelforsch 24:2000–2003
Sentilhes L, Carrie J (1982) Contribution à l'étude l'efficacité et de la tolérance de l'albendazole dans le traitement des helminthiases intestinales. Méd Afr Noire 29:33–36
Seo BS (1981) Ascariasis and its control problems in Korea. Seoul J Med 22:323–341
Seo BS, Cho SY, Chai SY (1978) Reduced single dose of mebendazole in treatment of *Ascaris lumbricoides* infection. Korean J Parasitol 16:21–25
Seung Yu-Ch (1977) Study on the quantitative evaluation of reinfection of *Ascaris lumbricoides*. Kor J Parasitol 15:17–29
Sezi CL (1974) The efficacy of levamisole in hookworm disease. Uganda Med J 3:73–77
Shafei AZ (1955) Piperazine as anthelmintic. Lancet II:827–828
Shafei AZ (1973) Clinical trials on mebendazole in the treatment of intestinal nematodes. Janssen Pharmaceutica, Clin Res Report N 7229
Shafei AZ (1974) Clinical trials on mebendazole in the treatment of intestinal nematodes. Janssen Pharmaceutica, Clin Res Report M 8165
Shafei AZ (1976) Clinical trials of mebendazole in the treatment of strongyloidiasis. Janssen Pharmaceutica, Clin Res Report N 10494
Shafei AZ, Abaza HH, Hammouda N, Elgohary Y (1971) Clinical trials with compound L 6842, a new anthelminthic agent. J Egypt Med Assoc 54:361–375
Shah KS, Zaman S (1964) Clinical trials with thiabendazole against human helminths. Pakist J Med Res 2:69–105

Shigeo Iwata, Goro-Ueda, Isueneji-Araki, Koichi-Taki, and Takashi-Kageyama (1962) Treatment of ancylostomiasis with bephenium salts in Japan. J Trop Med Hyg 65:9–11
Shiratsuchi MS, Levi GC, Amato Neto V, Avila CA De, Stefani HNV, Mosterio L, Tsukumo MKK, Konichi SR, Correa L de L (1975) Tratamento da tricocefaliase pelo mebendazole. Rev Inst Med Trop Sao Paulo 17:206–209
Simionesco O, Lucian O, Ghelber A (1964) Tratamental tricocefalozei en Telmid. Mirco. Parazitol Epidemiol 9:267–271
Singh DS, Bala-Subramanian R, Bhatia VN, Vasantha Kumar, Chandrasekar S (1981) Study of the efficacy of compound 90.9333 (Ciba-Geigy) in hookworm infestation Chemotherapy 27:220–223
Singhal KC, Gupta MC; Saxena PN (1975) A clinical trial with mebendazole in ascariasis and ankylostomiasis. J Assoc Physicians India 23:903–907
Singson CN (1969) Human intestinal capillariasis. Philip J Int Med 7:189–200
Singson CN (1974) Recurrences in human intestinal capillariasis. Philipp J Microbiol Infect Dis 31:7–13
Singson CN, Banzon TC (1969) A preliminary report on levo-tetramisole: a new drug for intestinal capillariasis. J Philipp Med Assoc 45:627–632
Singson CN, Banzon TC, Cross JH (1974) The treatment of human intestinal capillariasis. Janssen Pharmaceutica Clin Res Report N 8542
Singson CN, Banzon TC, Cross JH (1975) Mebendazole in the treatment of intestinal capillariasis. Am J Trop Med Hyg 24:932–934
Singson CN, Banzon TC, Cross JH (1977) Short term mebendazole treatment for *Capillariasis philippensis*. J Philipp Med Assoc 53:31–33
Sinniah B, Sinniah D (1981) The anthelmintic effects of pyrantel pamoate, oxantel-pyrantel pamoate, levamisole and mebendazole in the treatment of intestinal nematodes. Ann Trop Med Parasitol 75:315–321
Sinniah B, Sinniah D, Dissanaike AS (1980) Single dose treatment of intestinal nematodes with oxantel-pyrantel pamoate plus mebendazole. Ann Trop Med Parasitol 74:619–623
Soh Ch-Th, Lee BO-H, Min D-Y, Lee JH (1975) Clinical trial of Vermox (mebendazole), a new broad spectrum anthelminthic. Janssen Pharmaceutica Clin Res Report N 8842
Sonnet JJ, Thienpont D (1977) The treatment of trichinosis with mebendazole. Acta Clin Belg 32:297–302
Soprunova N, Soprunov FF, Lur'e AA (1973) Nachweis von helminthen Metaboliten im Harn des Wirtes als ein diagnostischer Test für Helminthiases. Angew. Parasitol 14:11–17
Sornwell RL, Jones RM (1968) Anthelminthic activity of pyrantel pamoate against *Ancylostoma caninum* in dogs. J Trop Med Hyg 71:165–166
Soula G, Siopathis RM (1982) Le zentel dans le traitement des nématodoses en République Centreafricaine. Méd Afr Noire 29:29–32
Spaeth GL, Adams RE, Soffe AH (1964) Treatment of trichinosis. Case report. Arch Ophthalmol 71:359–363
Standen OD (1953) Experimental chemotherapy of oxyuriasis. Br Med J II:757–758
Steele JH, Schultz MG (1978) Trichinellosis. A review of the current problem. In: Kim CW, Pawlowski ZS (eds) Trichinellosis. New England University Press, Hannover, pp 45–75
Steinrück M, Basener G, Hölzer E (1976) Klinische Erprobung von Vermox' (mebendazole). Janssen Pharmaceutica Clin Res Report N 19915
Stemmerman GN, Nakasone N (1980) *Strongyloides stercoralis* infestation: malabsorption defect with reaction to dithiazanine iodide. JAMA 174:1250–1253
Stewart DF (1955) Self-cure in nematode infestations of sheep. Nature 176:1273–1274
Stoll NR (1923) Investigations on the control of hookworm disease. XV. An effective method of counting hookworm eggs in feces. Am J Hyg 3:59–70
Stoll NR (1947) This wormy world. J Parasitol 33:1–18
Stoll NR (1962) On endemic hookworm. Where do we stand to-day? Exp. Parasitol. 12:241–252
Stoll NR, Hauscher WC (1926) Accuracy in the dilution egg counting method. Am J Hyg [Suppl] 6:80–133, 134–145

Stone OJ, Mullins JF (1963) First use of thiabendazole in creeping eruption. Tex Rep Biol Med 21:422–424
Stone OJ, Stone ChT Jr, Mullins FFr (1964) Thiabenazole – probable cure of trichinosis. JAMA 187:536–538
Stott GJ, Jopling WH (1961) Dithiazanine in strongyloidiasis and trichiuriasis. J Trop Med Hyg 64:73–74
Striebel HP (1976) 4-isothiocyanato-4-nitrodiphenylamine (C 9 333-90/CGP 4 540), an anthelmintic with an unusual spectrum of activity against intestinal nematodes, filarias and schistosomes. Experientia 32:457–458
Stürchler D, Stahel E, Saladin K, Saladin B (1980) Intestinal parasitoses in eight Liberian settlements: prevalences and community anthelminthic chemotherapy. Tropen med Parasitol 31:87–93
Sun SC, Cross JH, Berg HS, Kau SL, Singson CN, Banzon TC, Watten RH (1974) Ultrastructural studies of intestinal capillariasis. *Capillaria philippinensis* in human and gerbil hosts. Southeast Asian J Trop Med Public Health 5:524–533
Suzuki R, Yamauchi K, Kobayashi A (1961) Mass treatment of enterobiasis with pyrvinium pamoate (poquil.). Jpn J Parasitol 10:298–301
Swartzwelder JC, Miller JH, Sappenfield RW (1955) The treatment of cases of ascariasis with piperazine citrate. Am J Trop Med Hyg 4:326–331
Swartzwelder JC, Miller JH, Sappenfield RW (1957a) The effective use of piperazine for the treatment of human helminthiases. Gastroentrology 33:87–96
Swartzwelder JC, Frye WW, Mühleisen JP, Miller JH, Lampert R, Peña-Chavarria AA, Abadie SH, Anthony SO, Sappenfield RW (1957b) Dithiazanine, an effective broad spectrum anthelmintic. JAMA 165:2063–2067
Swartzwelder JC, Lampert R, Miller JH, Sappenfield RW (1958) Therapy of trichuriasis and ascariasis with dithiazanine. Am J Trop Med Hyg 7:329–333
Swartzwelder JC, Miller JH, Lampert R, Peña-Chavarria A, Abadie SH, Frye WW, Muhleisen P, Lizano C (1962) Anthelmintic activity of stilbazium iodide (Monopar) against intestinal nematodes in man. J Parasitol 48:29–30
Swartzwelder JC, Abadie SH, Miller JH, Sappenfield RW (1963) Stilbazium iodide (Monopar). An effective, single dose anthelminthic for treatment of *Enterobius vermicularis* infection. Clin Pediatr 2:701–702
Swellengrebel NH, Sterman MM (1961) Animal parasites in man. D. van Nostrand Co, Princeton, NJ
Symmers XStC (1950) Pathology of oxyuriasis. Arch Pathol 50:475
Szorady I, Brosody A, Natusovits L (1976) Experiences in the treatment of childhood oxyuriasis with mebendazole (Vermox). Janssen Pharmaceutica, Clin Res Report N 11 118
Takamura S (1963) Fundamental studies on anthelminthics-XV. Jpn J Parasitol 12:147–150
Takata I (1951) Experimental infections of man with *Ascaris* of man and the pig. Kitasato Arch Exp Med 23:49–50
Talaat SM (1964) Dipterex: an oral therapeutic agent in the treatment of schistosomiasis and other intestinal parasites. J Egypt Med Assoc 47:589–593
Tanaka H, Shiroma Y, Kumada W, Fukamine K, Kwawamitsu H (1960) An efficacious application of gentian violet to the treatment of human strongyloidiasis. Bull Tokyo Med Dental Univ 7:137–150
Tanaka H, Shiroma Y, Mitsui G (1965) Studies on the treatment of human strongylidiasis with pyrvinium pamoate suspension. Jpn J Parasitol 14:20–26
Tesh RB, Ackerman LJ, Dietz WM, Williams JA (1973) *Angiostrongylus costaricensis* in Panama. Prevalence and pathologic findings in wild rodents infected with the parasite. Am J Trop Med Hyg 22:348–356
Theodorides VJ, Gyurik RJ, Kingsbury WD, Parisk RC (1976) Anthelmintic activity of albendazole against liver flukes, tapeworms, lung and gastrointestinal roundworms. Experientia 32:702
Thienpont D (1972) Le traitement actuel de la trichocephalose. Acta Gastroenterol Belg 35:439–443
Thienpont D (1976) Le traitement de la trichinose. Nouv Presse Méd 5:1759–1760

Thienpont D, Parijs OFJ van, Raeymaekers AHM, Vandenberk J, Demoen PJA, Allewijn FTN, Marsboom RPH, Niemegeers CJE, Schellekens KHL, Janssen PAJ (1966) Tetramisole (R 8299), a new, potent broad spectrum anthelminthic. Nature 209:1084–1085

Thienpont D, Brugmans J, Abadi K, Tanamal S (1969) Tetramisole in the treatment of nematode infections in man. Am J Trop Med Hyg 18:520–525

Thienpont D, Parijs O van, Niemezeers C, Marsboom R (1978) Biological and pharmacological properties of flubendazole. Arzneimittelforsch 28:605–612

Thomas HW (1910) The pathological report of a case of oesophagostomiasis in man. Ann Trop Med Hyg 5:57–88

Tidball JS, Aguas JP, Aldis JW (1978) A new concentration of human intestinal capillariasis on western Luzon. Southeast Asian J Trop Med Public Health 9:33–40

Toma L, Danescu P (1977) Certain aspects of strongyloidiosis in Europe. 1st Med Conf on Parasitology, october, Izmir

Torhoudt L (1974) Efficacy of flubendazole in enterobiasis. Janssen Pharmaceutica, Clin Res Report N 9292

Uchida A, Nozue S, Kaneko IK, Tanaka A, Kondo T, Saito M, Uchida F, Araki T, Karube F (1964) Field trials on mass treatment of hookworm infection with bephenium hydroxynaphtoate. Jpn J Parasitol 13:464–471

Ulyangco C. Reys VM, Cabilong VP, Camacho RC (1968) Capillariasis. J Philip Med Assoc 44:743–757

Undeutsch K, Stumpf J, Landgraf H (1981) Some aspects in the treatment of 25 patients with trichinellosis in Ebermanstadt. In: Kim ChW, Ruitenberg EJ, Teppema JC (eds) Trichinellosis. Reedbooks, Surrey, pp 283–285

Vaidya AB, Sen HG, Mankodi NA, Paul T, Sheth UK (1977) Phase 1, tolerability and searching dose studies with 4-isothiocyanato-4-nitrodiphenylamine (C 9333-90/CGP 4540), a new anthelminthic. Br J Pharmacol 4:463–467

Vaidya AB, Mankodi NA, Taiwalker Sh, Kale NA, Doshi JC, Paul T, Sheth UK (1981) Cardiovascular function in chronic hookworm anaemie before and after a new anthelmintic-4-isothiocyanato-4-nitrodiphenylamin. J Assoc Phys Ind 29:279–283

Vakil BJ (1969) Clinical trials with L-tetramisole on school children. Janssen Pharmaceutica, Clin Res Report N 521

Vakil BJ, Dalah NJ (1975) Comparative efficacy of newer anthelminthics. Prog Drug Res 19:166–175

Vakil BJ, Bandisode MS, Gaitonde BB, Salunkhe DS, Kulkarni HJ (1965) Clinical trials with a new anthelminthic: thiabendazole. J Trop Med Hyg 68:287–295

Vakil BJ, Dahal NJ, Gangrade RR, Bhise KB (1972) Clinical trial with L-tetramisole in roundworm and hookworm infection. Trans R Soc Trop Med Hyg 66:250–254

Vakil BJ, Dalal NJ, Enjetti E (1975) Clinical trials with mebendazole, a new broad spectrum anthelminthic. J Trop Med Hyg 78:154–158

Vakil BJ, Dalal NJ, Shah PN (1977) Clinical evaluation of a new anthelmintic (9333-90/CGP 4540) in human hookworm infection. Trans R Soc Trop Med Hyg 71:247–250

Vandepitte J, Gatti F, Lontie M, Krubwa F, Nguete M, Thienpont D (1973) Le mebendazole, un nouvel anthelminthique à large spectre très actif contre le trichocéphale. Bull Soc Pathol Exot Filiales 66:165–178

Donckt J Van der, Verbruggen F, Heylen G, Parijs O van, Scheygrond H (1975) Double blind comparison of flubendazole and placebo in the treatment of enterobiasis. Janssen Pharmaceutica Clin Res Report R 17889/4

Van Landuyt H (1973) Levamisole and hookworm in Kinshasa (in Dutch). Janssen Pharmaceutica Clin Res Report N 5483

Van Landuyt H (1974) Decaris in hookworm disease, ascariasis, trichuriasis and strongyloidiasis. Janssen Pharmaceutica Clin Res Report N 5483

Vanneste JAL, Ansink BJJ, Snijders CJ, Hölscher JFM (1975) Neurologische bijwerkingen van piperazine. Ned Tijdschr Geneeskd 119:1899–1901

Van Olphen AHF, Nabben FAE (1974) Mebendazole (R 17635) in the treatment of enterobiasis in children. A double blind placebo-controlled study. Janssen Pharmaceutica, Clin Res Report LMD 6668

Van Thiel PH (1962) Anisakiasis. Parasitology 52:16–17

Van Thiel PH (1976) The present state of anisakiasis and its causative worms. Trop Geogr Med 28:75–85
Van Thiel PH, Bakker PM (1981) Gastric worm granulomas in the Netherlands and Japan. Ned Tijdschr Geneeskd 125:1365–1370
Van Thiel PH, Kuipers FC, Roskam RTh (1960) A nematode parasitic to herring, causing acute abdominal syndromes in man. Trop Geogr Med 2:97–113
Vasojevic S, Jevtic M, Suvakovic V (1962) Observations personnelles préliminaires relatives au traitement des strongyloidoses par la dithiazanine. Srpki Arch Celokup lekarst 90:191–195
Venkatachelam PS, Patwardhan VN (1953) The role of *Ascaris lumbricoides* in the nutrition of the host. Effect of ascariasis on digestion of protein. Trans R Soc Trop Med Hyg 47:169–175
Verwilghen NM (1974) Mebendazole in single and mixed worm infections. Janssen Pharmaceutica, Clin Res Report 1:40
Vik R (1964) Anisakis larvae in Norwegian food fishes. In: Corradetti A (ed) Proc 1st int congr parasitol, Roma. Pergamon, Oxford, pp 568–569
Villarejos VM, Saldana J (1959) Mass deparasitization experiment with dithiazine iodide. Antibiot Med Clin Therapy 6:718–723
Villarejos VM, Arguedas-Gamboa JA, Eduarte E, Swartzwelder JC (1971) Experiences with the anthelminthic pyrantel pamoate. Am J Trop Med Hyg 20:842–845
Villela MP, Rodrigues LD, Capell JI, Brandao JA, Martirani I, Zucato M (1962) O emprigo do thiabendazol no tratamento da estrongiloidiase e de outras parasitosis humanas. O Hospital 62:691–710
Villela MP, Zucato M, Nascimento SR (1964) Tratamento da tricocefaliase intestinal pelo pamoate de pirvino. O Hospital 66:151–153
Villela MP, Zucas AW, Iglesias J (1968) The therapy of trichiuriasis with a combination of thiabendazole and pyrvinium pamoate. O Hospital 68:1413–1418
Vinke B, Sar A Van der (1959) Dithiazanine, a new anthelmintic. Trop Geogr Med 11:335–338
Vujosevic M, Kostic A, Lalic R, Zerjav S (1979) Mebendazole (Vermox) in the treatment of *Trichinella spiralis* infections. In: 3rd Congr Yugoslav. Infectiologists, pp 213–215
Wagner ED (1963) Pyrvinium pamoate in the treatment of strongyloidiasis. Am J Trop Med Hyg 12:60–61
Wagner ED, Rexinger DD (1978) *In vivo* effects of mebendazole und levamisole in the treatment of trichuriasis and ascariasis. Am J Trop Med Hyg 27:203–205
Wagner ED, Lemon FR, Burnett HS (1958) The use of dithiazanine in the treatment of helminthiasis in Mexican farm labourers. Am J Trop Med Hyg 7:600–602
Walfe MJ, Wershing JM (1974) Mebendazole treatment of trichuriasis and ascariasis in Bahamian children. JAMA 230:1408–1411
Wang CC, Galli GA (1965) Strongyloidiasis treated with pyrvinium pamoate. JAMA 193:847–848
Wang Ch-I, Hu Hs-J, Wang H-Hs, Peng YF (1964) The anthelminthic effects of bephenium hydroxynaphtoate on hookworm and other nematode infections of the intestinal tract. Chin Med J 83:1–10
Watson JM (1960) Medical helminthology. Baillière Tindall Cox, London
Watten RH, Beckner WM, Cross JH, Cunning J-J, Jarimillo J (1972) Clinical studies on *Capillariasis philippinensis*. Trans R Soc Trop Med Hyg 66:828–834
Webb JL (1937) The helminth of the intestinal canal in man in Mauritius; and a first record of *Trichostrongylus axei* locally. Parasitology 29:469–476
Wellens D, Thienpont D (1978) Mebendazole (Vermox) for chemotherapy of intestinal helminths. Med Digest 4:23–27
Weng L-Ch, Mao Sh-G, Liu Er-Hs (1960) Research on parasitic diseases in New China. Chin Med J 80:1–20
Wershing JM, Wolfe MS, Burke FG (1975) Placebo-controlled comparison of levamisole, pyrantel pamoate, thiabendazole, piperazine citrate and various dosages of mebendazole in the treatment of ascariasis and trichuriasis in children. Janssen Pharmaceutica, Clin Res Report N 10422

Wershing JM, Burke FG, Wolfe MS (1979) Dose range study of flubendazole in children with *Ascaris lumbricoides* and/or *Trichuris trichiura* infections. Janssen Pharmaceutica, Clin Res Report R 17889/14

Whalen GE, Strickland GT, Cross JH, Uylangco C, Rosenberg EB, Gutman RA, Watten RH, Dizon JJ (1969) Intestinal capillariasis – a new disease in man. Lancet 1:13–16

Whalen GE, Rosenberg EG, Gutman RA, Cross JH, Fresh JW, Strickland T, Uylangco S (1971) Treatment of intestinal capillariasis with thiabendazole, bithionol and bephenium. Am J Trop Med Hyg 20:95–100

White RHR, Scopes JW (1960) A single dose treatment of threadworm in children. Lancet 278:256–257

White RHR, Standen OD (1953) Piperazine in the treatment of threadworms in children. Br Med J 755–757

WHO (1964) Soil transmitted helminths. WHO Tech Rep Ser 277

WHO (1967) Control of ascariasis. WHO Tech Rep Ser 379

Winsor EL, Totten JC (1976) Controlled study comparing levamisole with piperazine citrate in the treatment of ascariasis in children. Janssen Pharmaceutica, Clin Res Report N 10571

Wolfe MS, Wershing JM (1974) Mebendazole: treatment of trichuriasis and ascariasis in Bahamian Children. JAMA 230:1408–1411

Wollweber H, Niemers E, Flucke W, Andrews P, Schulz HP, Thomas H (1979) Amidantel, a potent anthelminthic from a new chemical class. Arzneimittelforsch 29:31–32

Wright WH, Brady FJ (1938) Studies on oxyuriasis. A preliminary note on therapy with gentian violet. Proc Helminthol Soc 5:5–7

Wright WH, Brady FJ (1940) Studies on oxyuriasis. JAMA 114:861–866

Yalcinkaya F (1977) A polivalent anthelminthic "mebendazole." In: 1st Med conf on parasitol. Izmyr, october 5–10, p 122

Yanagisawa T (1957) Rinsko shokakibyogaku 5:41–42 (in Japanese)

Yangco B, Klein T (1980) Single-blind comparison of flubendazole with mebendazole in the treatment of trichuriasis and hookworm disease. Janssen Pharmaceutica, Clin Res Report N 21275

Yangco BG, Klein TRW, Deresinski SC, Vickery AC, Graig ChP (1981) Flubendazole and mebendazole in the treatment of trichuriasis and other helminthiasis. Clin Ther 4:285–290

Yoeli M, Most H, Beruan HH, Tesse BI (1963) The problems of strongyloidiasis among the mentally retarded in institutions. Trans R Soc Trop Med Hyg 57:336–345

Yokogawa M, Yosmimura H (1967) Clinicopathologic studies on larval anisakiasis in Japan. Am J Trop Med Hyg 16:723–728

Yokogawa M, Yoshimura H, Sano M, Araki K, Koyama H, Furusawa H (1968) Mass treatment of human trichuriasis with stilbasium iodide. Jpn J Parasitol 17:27–35

Yokogawa M, Araki K, Kojima S, Niimura M, Ogawa K (1970) Clinical evaluation of a new antihelmintic, pyrantel pamoate in hookworm infection. Jpn J Parasitol 19:301–306

Yokogawa M, Sano M, Saito K (1976) Anthelminthic efficacy of mebendazole for trichuriasis. Jpn J Parasitol 25:16–18

Yoshida Y, Nakanishi Y, Shimatani T, Matuo K (1960) Comparative studies on the anthelminthic effect of bephenium hydroxynaphtoate, tetrachlorethylene, 1-bromo-β-naphtol and 4-iodothymol against human hookworm. Jpn J Parasitol 9:620–628

Young MD, Freed JE (1956) The effect of puromycin against *E. histolytica* and other intestinal parasites. South Med J 49:537–538

Young MD, Jeffery GM, Freed JE, Morehouse WG (1958) Bephenium a new active drug against human hookworm. J Parasitol 44:611–612

Young MD, Jeffery GM, Morehouse WG, Freed JE, Johnson RS (1960) The comparative efficacy of bephenium hydroxynaphtoate and tetrachlorethylene against hookworm and other parasites. Am J Trop Med Hyg 9:488–490

Zahedi M, Oothuman P, Sabapathy NN, Bakar NA (1980) Intestinal nematode infections and efficacy study of oxantel-pyrantel pamoate among plantation workers. Med J Malaysia 35:31–37

Zakine J, Zakine Cl (1960) Essais thérapeutiques dans l'ankylostomose en Tunisie par un dérivé quaternaire de l'ammonium. Bull Soc Pathol Exot Filiales 53:314–321
Zaman V, Loh YP (1974) Clinical trial of pyrantel embonate, levotetramisol and bephenium hydroxynaphtoate against *Necator americanus*. Singapore Med J 15:147–148
Zimmermann WJ, Zinter DE (1971) The prevalence of trichuriasis in swine in the United States, 1966–1970. Health Serv Rep 86:937–943
Zimmermann WJ, Steele JH, Kagan IG (1973) Trichuriasis in the US population 1966–1970, prevalence epidemologic factors. Health Serv Rep 88:606–623
Zucato M, Vilela MP (1964) Tratamento da tricocefaliose intestinal pelo tiabendazol. J Bras Med 8:1219

CHAPTER 6

Chemotherapy of Gastrointestinal Nematodiasis in Ruminants

J. H. BOERSEMA

A. Introduction

Effective control of gastrointestinal nematodes in ruminants must be based on a thorough knowledge of the epidemiology of these parasites. In some instances gastrointestinal nematodes can be controlled by good pasture management (BORGSTEEDE and KLOOSTERMAN 1977; EYSKER and HENDRIKX 1977). Other systems depend on frequent treatments with short intervals. Most control systems, however, are based on both pasture management and strategic or tactical treatments (see Chap. 3, this volume).

B. Factors and Circumstances Influencing the Choice of Anthelmintic

I. Diagnosis

In ruminants with clinical signs of a gastrointestinal nematode infection lesions are almost always caused by a variety of different species. Thus it is important to use an anthelmintic effective against the whole range of species. Most anthelmintics used in practice nowadays are effective against nearly all these parasites. Some even have a broader spectrum, being also effective against lungworms, cestodes, and trematodes. Problems with these parasites, however, seldom occur at the same time. An anthelmintic with such a broad spectrum will therefore seldom be necessary. Anthelmintics are given to animals not only with clinical signs of a parasitic infection. In England 88% of all anthelmintic doses given to cattle are given prophylactically (MICHEL et al. 1981).

Prophylactic treatments are given either to prevent disease in the animal (e.g., ostertagiasis type II) or to prevent pasture contamination. To prevent ostertagiasis type II it is necessary to use an anthelmintic effective against inhibited larvae of *Ostertagia ostertagi*. Whether this anthelmintic is effective against other trichostrongylids, lungworms, cestodes, and trematodes is of no interest.

The occurrence of multiple resistance against broad-spectrum anthelmintics, as already reported from Australia (SANGSTER et al. 1979), can limit the choice to narrow-spectrum anthelmintics. Such anthelmintics, e.g., closantel and disophenol, have already been tested, with good result against a resistant *Haemonchus contortus* strain (HALL et al. 1981 a).

II. Toxicity at the Therapeutic Dose and Drug Interactions

With the development of modern anthelmintics, efficacy has increased and the spectrum has become larger. Simultaneously the toxicity of these anthelmintics has decreased. The margin between the therapeutic and toxic dose in modern anthelmintics is so wide that toxic reactions hardly occur. The majority of cases of toxic reactions in trials are due to poor equipment, overestimation of body weight, or poor reading of the manufacturer's instructions. Anthelmintics with a very wide safety margin are the benzimidazoles. However, some of them have appeared to be very toxic under certain circumstances. LAPRAS et al. (1973) were the first to describe an embryotoxic effect of parbendazole. Given at the therapeutic dose between the 9th and 21th day of gestation to ewes this anthelmintic caused malformations in 25% of the lambs born. This embryotoxic effect of parbendazole was repeated in other parts of the world (MIDDLETON et al. 1974; SAUNDERS et al. 1974; SHONE et al. 1979; SZABO et al. 1974). Not only a teratogenetic but also an embryolethal effect was found by MIDDLETON et al. (1974). At high doses of 180 mg/kg given in the 2nd month of pregnancy, brain lesions causing paralysis were seen in lambs (PROZESKY et al. 1981).

Other benzimidazoles have proved to be embryotoxic in early pregnancy in sheep. An embryotoxic effect of cambendazole was found by DELATOUR et al. (1974). An embryolethal but no teratogenic effect was found in sheep treated with oxibendazole at 4.5 times the therapeutic dose (DELATOUR et al. 1976). This effect was not found at three times the therapeutic dose (THEODORIDES et al. 1977). Oxfendazole at a dose of 22.5 mg/kg was both embryolethal and teratogenic (DELATOUR et al. 1977). Fenbendazole, however, which is extensively metabolized into oxfendazole (MARRINER and BOGAN 1981), was found to have no embryotoxic effects (TIEFENBACH 1975; DELATOUR et al. 1977). Mebendazole was not embryotoxic in sheep, but in rats it is embryotoxic at a dose of 10 mg/kg (DELATOUR et al. 1974). Albendazole has proven to be embryotoxic in rats (DELATOUR et al. 1981) and sheep (JOHNS and PHILIP 1977). Further details are given in Chap. 4, this volume. The embryotoxic effect of these benzimidazoles has been proven to be an antimitotic effect (DELATOUR et al. 1975).

At a dose of three times the recommended dose, cambendazole caused toxic effects in calves. Three out of eight animals died. In these animals the thoracic cavity contained large amounts of a clear yellow fluid which clotted at exposure to air. The bronchi contained froth, the lungs were edematous, and the interlobular septa were dilated. Ecchymoses were present on the epicardium (MAIN and VASS 1980). Lung disorders after treatment with cambendazole were also seen in calves by STOYE et al. (1971) and in sheep (ANON 1978). There seems to be a connection with feeding concentrates.

Lung disorders were also seen in calves infected with lungworms and treated with fenbendazole (MCEWAN et al. 1979; JARETT et al. 1980; URQUHART et al. 1981). The pulmonary lesions resemble those seen in fog fever. The etiology is so far unknown but an allergic reaction caused by the release of antigen from dead lungworms is suggested.

The margin between the therapeutic and the toxic dose of levamisole is rather small. In ruminants nervous symptoms are the most obvious manifestations of toxicity. Because levamisole has nicotine-like activities, toxic effects may be blocked by atropine sulfate (0.5 mg/kg body weight, one-third of this dose intraveneously, two-thirds subcutaneously every 4–6 h with a maximum of 6 mg/kg body weight).

On theoretical grounds combinations of levamisole with pyrantel, morantel, metyridine, bephenium, and organic phosphorus compounds are less recommendable. HSU (1980), however, showed that the combination of levamisole and dichlorvos did not lower that LD_{50} of levamisole.

The organic phosphorus compounds are a group of anthelmintics with a narrow margin between the toxic and therapeutic dose, especially in young animals. Toxic symptoms consist of salivation, frequent urination, diarrhea, colic, bradycardy, and muscle fibrillation followed by paralysis and dyspnea. Atropine sulfate can be used as an antidote at a dose of 0.5 mg/kg body weight, given as above. This can be combinded with oxim compounds, e.g., the cholinesterase reactivator, pralidoxim at a maximum dose of 100 mg/kg body weight, or obidoxim at a dose of 3 mg/kg body weight.

Combination of organic phosphorus compounds with pyrantel, morantel, levamisole, metyridine, and bephenium is less recommendable on theoretical grounds (however, see HSU 1980).

Phenothiazine at the therapeutic dose can bring about photosensitization in sheep and cattle. This is caused by its metabolite, phenothiazine sulfoxide. This metabolite can reach the chamber fluid of the eye. The clinical symptoms consist of lacrimation, photophobia, and corneal opacity. The blindness is mostly temporary but ulcerations with perforation can cause permanent blindness. Photosensitization of white parts of the body in cattle and unwooled parts (ears, nose) in sheep have also been seen. Animals with photosensitization can best be kept indoors or at least in the shadow.

III. Formulation

Many formulations are in use to treat parasites in ruminants. The choice of the formulation depends mostly on personal preference and the availability of different formulations. Most of them are given orally as a drench, paste, or bolus, or in the feed or drinking water. Important differences in efficacy between drench, paste, and bolus have not been recorded. Given as a food additive at the therapeutic dose insufficient efficacy may be the results of differences in intake by the individual animals (BAKER et al. 1978).

A particular method of parenteral treatment is the dermal administration of levamisole as a pour-on formulation. Levamisole is formulated at a concentration of 10% in a solvent system promoting dermal absorbtion. The drug is administered to cattle, at a dose of 10 mg/kg body weight, by means of a measuring cylinder on both sides of the spine. The efficacy obtained with this formulation is about the same as that obtained by levamisole administered orally or subcutaneously (CURR 1977; ROWLANDS and BERGER 1977; DORCHIES et al. 1981).

In sheep the levamisole pour-on formulation, at a dose of 7.5 mg/kg body weight, was very effective against *Haemonchus* and *Trichostrongylus* (BROOKER and GOOSE 1975).

Low dose level administration of anthelmintics has been used from the beginnings of anthelmintic treatment. Especially phenothiazine was used in this way in South Africa in lick blocks. Recently, renewed attention has been given to the low-dose administration. It was found that inhibited larvae, which are in general less susceptible than the adult parasites, could be killed when they were exposed for a longer time to a benzimidazole. The lower energy demand of inhibited larvae may enable them to withstand a short period of exposure to these anthelmintics. The long persistence in the host of oxfendazole and fenbendazole, however, is probably responsible for the high efficacy of these anthelmintics against inhibited larvae (PRICHARD et al. 1978). Trials with fenbendazole at a low dose rate administrated in feed blocks for about 1 week gave a high efficacy in sheep and cattle (MCBEATH et al. 1977, GAENSSLER et al. 1978; THOMAS 1978; MCBEATH et al. 1979).

The disadvantage of this method is that it is not an individual treatment. THOMAS (1978) showed that the efficacy in sheep taking 0.25 mg/kg/day fenbendazole for 14 days or less was insufficient.

In every flock or herd there may be some animals which do not take enough food for sufficient treatment. These animals will miss the beneficial effect of the anthelmintic and will continue shedding eggs, so the other animals can be reinfected in a short time. Another disadvantage of a low dose is that it may select more for resistance. This is especially important when efficacy is low.

A particular form of low dose level administration for cattle was described by ANDERSON and LABY (1979). A special-shaped syringe containing a spring, plunger, and matrix with oxfendazole is orally administered into the reticulum. In the reticulum the shape changes, thus preventing regurgitation and the matrix is slowly released in about 5 days. The efficacy against adult *O. ostertagi* was high and against developing larvae and inhibited larvae of this nematode moderate.

In sheep a similar capsule with an average effective life of 41 days was very effective against adults developing larvae and inhibited larvae of *O. circumcinta.* In a field experiment the egg output was zero during the effective life, thus reducing the level of pasture contamination (ANDERSON et al. 1980). LEJAMBRE et al. (1981) showed that this formulation was also very effective against *H. contortus* and *Trichostrongylus colubriformis* and against benzimidazole-resistant strains of *H. contortus, O. circumcincta,* and *T. colubriformis.*

Another method of low-level administration is the sustained release bolus designed to release morantel tartrate continuously for about 60 days in calves. The stainless steel cylinder containing morantel tartrate in a matrix is orally administered by an applicator into the reticulum. Because of its weight the bolus cannot be regurgitated. The bolus is administered just before turnout of the calves. Overwintered infective larvae picked up by these calves are killed by the drug. In the first 2 months of the grazing season no gastrointestinal nematodes will mature in these animals. As result the mid-summer increase in pasture larval counts is prevented. Good results with this method have been obtained by ARMOUR et al. (1981), JONES (1981 a), JACOBS et al. (1981), BORGSTEEDE (1981), and BÜRGER et al. (1981). Treatment of calves with the sustained release bolus containing morantel tartrate in the first months of the grazing season does not affect their susceptibility to parasite infections as yearlings in the following grazing season (JONES

1981 b). The use of this bolus does not influence the effect of a lungworm vaccination (GRIMSHAW et al. 1981). The disadvantage of this method is again, as in other low-dose administrations, the possibility of the development of resistant strains. JONES and BLISS (1981), however, were not able to demonstrate any change in susceptibility of *Ostertagia* after the use of morantel tartrate in this formulation in cattle during three consecutive grazing seasons on the same farm.

IV. Presence of Inhibited Larvae

Many nematodes conditioned by stimulants such as temperature and moisture can undergo inhibition in their hosts. It is an excellent adaptation of the parasite for overcoming cold or dry seasons. After the cold or dry season the larvae resume their development. The emergence of the larvae out of the mucosa has some important consequences. In cattle the resumed development of inhibited larvae of *O. ostertagi* can lead to extensive damage of the abomasal mucosa. The disease caused by this damage is known by the name ostertagiasis type II.

In sheep particular trichostrongylids pass the winter or dry season mainly as inhibited larvae. In lactating ewes these larvae develop to adult parasites, through which the postparturient egg rise occurs. This egg rise may have far-reaching consequences for the lambs. So, for cattle it is important to have an anthelmintic effective against inhibited larvae to prevent ostertagiasis type II. For sheep the treatment of inhibited larvae is important to prevent disease in the lambs. The first anthelmintic with a high efficacy against inhibited larvae at a therapeutic dose was fenbendazole (DUNCAN et al. 1976). After this publication other reports of high efficacy were recorded (MCBEATH et al. 1977; CALLINAN and CUMMINS 1979). However, moderate, low, or variable efficacy has also been reported (SEARSON and DOUGHTY 1977; ELLIOT 1977; LANCASTER and HONG 1977; INDERBITZIN and ECKERT 1978; CRAIG and BELL 1978; WILLIAMS et al. 1981 b). The cause of these differences is so far unknown but some speculations have been made. A possible variation in the depth of inhibition in the course of the inhibition period has been suggested. DUNCAN et al. (1978), however, showed that there is hardly any difference in efficacy between a treatment in November and January. Another suggestion is the closure of the esophageal groove when the anthelmintic is given as a suspension. Experiments carried out by KELLY et al. (1977) prove that the route of administration has influence on the efficacy of the anthelmintic. Intra-abomasal administration was less effective than intraruminal administration. The difference, however, was only seen in resistant strains of *H. contortus* and *T. colubriformis*.

In susceptible strains there was no difference between the two administration routes. Nevertheless in cases where resistance is present the route of administration or the eventual closure of the esophageal groove may play a role in the efficacy. WILLIAMS et al. (1981 b) suggest that the time between treatment and slaughter in critical tests may cause differences in the results. Large numbers of dead inhibited larvae were seen in aliquots and tissue from animals treated with fenbendazole and slaughtered 1 week later. When the animals were slaughtered between 12 and 20 days after treatment no dead or degenerated larvae were found.

In two papers recording good efficacy against inhibited larvae with fenbendazole the interval between treatment and slaughter was 10 days (Duncan et al.; McBeath et al. 1977). In other papers recording high efficacy of fenbendazole, however, the interval between treatment and slaughter was 7 days (Callinan and Cummins 1979; Thomas and Reid 1980).

With oxfendazole high efficacy against inhibited larvae has been recorded by Chalmers (1978), Armour et al. (1978), Ogunsusi (1979), and Thomas and Reid (1980).

Good results of albendazole against inhibited larvae of *O. ostertagi* were obtained by Williams et al. (1979b) and Downey (1978). Low efficacy of albendazole against inhibited larvae of *O. ostertagi* was found by Williams et al. (1979a) and Williams et al. (1981a).

The probenzimidazole thiophanate was very effective against inhibited larvae of *O. ostertagi* and *Cooperia spp.* after five daily doses of 20 mg/kg body weight (Duncan et al. 1979).

Ivermectin, a compound with high efficacy against various nematodes, is also effective against inhibited larvae of *O. ostertagi* in cattle (Armour et al. 1980; Elliot and Julian 1981; Williams 1981c).

V. Ovicidal Effect

After anthelmintic treatment of ruminants, nematode eggs can be found in the feces for about 2 or 3 days. If these animals are moved to a clean pasture immediately after treatment this pasture will be contaminated with these eggs.

Besides their activity against adult nematodes, developing stages, and, in some of them, inhibited larvae, the benzimidazoles have an ovicidal effect. This ovicidal effect is achieved about 8 h after treatment. Ruminants treated with a benzimidazole will shed eggs for 2 or 3 days, but only the eggs shed in the first 8 h after treatment can develop into infective larvae. For this reason it is advisable to keep animals yarded for 8 h after treatment. Yarding the animals during this time may, however, be a problem of place and time. Kingsbury and Rowlands (1981) showed that sheep treated with oxfendazole could stay in the infested pasture safely during 24 h. Infective larvae picked up during this time did not mature. This effect will probably be the same with other benzimidazoles.

VI. Resistance

The number of reports on resistance against anthelmintics in nematodes has increased dramatically. So far cases of resistance have been found in nematodes in sheep, goats, and horses.

In sheep resistance was found in *H. contortus* (Drudge et al. 1957), *T. colubriformis* (Sangster et al. 1979), and *O. circumcincta* (Hall et al. 1979). In goats resistance was found in *H. contortus* (I. H. Boersema 1981, unpublished data) and *Trichostrongylus* spp. (Hall et al. 1981b). Many more articles about resistance against anthelmintics have been published. Resistance in sheep has been found for all the benzimidazoles commercially available; tiabendazole (Drudge et al. 1964), parbendazole (Hotson et al. 1970), cambendazole (Colglazier et al. 1974), mebendazole (Hall et al. 1978), fenbendazole (Hogarth-Scott et al.

1976), oxibendazole (HALL et al. 1978), oxfendazole (WEBB and MCCULLY 1979), and albendazole (VLASSOFF and KETTLE 1980).

Resistance against the probenzimidazole thiophanate was found by EDWARDS and DE CHANEET (1980). Resistance was recorded against levamisole and morantel, drugs with a similar mode, of action, by SANGSTER et al. (1979). Resistance has also been proved against some compounds with a narrow spectrum: rafoxanide (VAN WIJK and GERBER 1980) and naftalofos (GREEN et al. 1981). Resistance against phenothiazine was recorded in 1957 by DRUDGE et al.

Resistance of trichostrongylids in cattle has not been reported to date. The reason for this is not known but it may be caused by differences in treating strategies between cattle and sheep. Some evidence of resistance, however, may have been found by WILLIAMS et al. (1979 a) and LYONS et al. (1981 b, c).

Resistance against anthelmintics has been reported mainly from countries where anthelmintics have been used at a high frequency, such as Australia, South Africa, and New Zealand.

C. The Anthelmintics

The more important findings about the activity of the anthelmintics against gastrointestinal nematodes are summarized here for cattle, sheep, and goats. There are few reports about the efficacy of anthelmintics in goats. It is supposed that the activity in goats will be the same as in sheep. There are, however, indications that this is not true in all cases (HALL et al. 1981 b). The results under the headings "Sheep and Goats" are based on trials with sheep. In trials with goats, this host is mentioned. The efficacies of the anthelmintics discussed in this chapter are summarized in Tables 1–7.

I. Phenothiazine

The efficacy of phenothiazine was reviewed by WERKGROEP WORMMIDDELEN (1973 a). Good efficacy was found against *Haemonchus, Trichostrongylus, Chabertia,* and *Oesophagostomum.* Efficacy is variable against *Ostertagia,* low against *Cooperia, Nematodirus,* and *Bunostomum,* and almost nil against *Strongyloides papillosus* and *Trichuris.* Toxic effects at the therapeutic dose consist principally of photosensitization caused by phenothiazine sulfoxide. This shows mainly as keratitis and seldomly as eczema solare. Resistance against phenothiazine was found in *H. contortus* in DRUDGE et al. (1957) and others.

II. Bephenium

The results of efficacy trials with bephenium are conflicting. The only trichostrongylids against which a high efficacy was found in all tests were *Nematodirus* spp., both in cattle and in sheep at doses of 200 and 250 mg/kg body weight respectively (WERKGROEP WORMMIDDELEN 1973 b).

Table 1. Efficacy of the anthelmintics against the most important adult gastrointestinal nematodes in cattle

Classification	Anthelmintics	Dosage in mg/kg body weight (oral)	Abomasum			Small intestine					Large intestine
			Ostertagia	Haemonchus	Trichostrongylus	Trichostrongylus	Cooperia	Nematodirus	Bunostomum	Strongyloides	Oesophagostomum
I.	Phenothiazine	400	++	+++	+++	+++	+	+	+	–	+++
II.	Bephenium	200	–	–	–	–	–	+++	–	–	–
III.1.	Coumafos	2[a]	++	+++	+++	+++	+++	–	–	–	–
2.	Fenclofos	100	–	+++	–	–	–	–	–	–	–
3.	Haloxon	50	–	+++	–	–	+++	–	–	–	–
4.	Naftalofos	50	–	+++	–	–	+++	–	–	–	–
5.	Trichlorphon	60	–	+++	–	–	–	–	–	–	–
IV.	Metyridine	200	+	+	+	++	++	++	–	–	–
V.2.	Nitroxynil	10	–	+++	–	–	–	–	+++	–	+++
VI.1.	Tiabendazole	100	+++	+++	+++	+++	+++	+++	+++	+++	+++
2.	Parbendazole	30	+++	+++	+++	+++	+++	+++	–	+++	+++
5.	Fenbendazole	7.5	+++	+++	+++	+++	+++	+++	+++	++	+++
6.	Oxibendazole	10	+++	++	+++	+++	+++	++	+++	+++	+++
7.	Oxfendazole	2.5	+++	+++	+++	+++	+++	+++	+++	+++	+++
8.	Albendazole	7.5	+++	+++	+++	+++	+++	+++	+++	+++	+++
VII.2.	Rafoxanide	7.5	–	+++	–	–	–	–	+++	–	+++
VIII.1.	Pyrantel	25	+++	+++	–	–	+++	+++	–	–	–
2.	Morantel	10	++	+++	+++	+++	+++	+++	+++	–	+++
IX.	Levamisole	Oral 7.5 s.c. and i.m. 5	+++	+++	+++	+++	+++	+++	+++	–	+++
X.1.	Thiophanate	50	+++	+++	+++	+++	+++	++	–	–	–
2.	Febantel	7.5	+++	+++	+++	–	+++	–	–	–	–
XI.	Ivermectin	0.2	+++	+++	+++	+++	+++	++	–	–	+++

Classification of efficacy: +++, 95%–100%; ++, 80%–100%; +, 0%–100%; –, not effective or insufficient data

[a] Daily for 1 week

Table 2. Efficacy of the anthelmintics against the most important adult gastrointestinal nematodes in sheep and goats

Classification	Anthelmintics	Dosage in mg/kg body weight (oral)	Abomasum			Small intestine						Large intestine	
			Haemonchus	Ostertagia	Trichostrongylus	Trichostrongylus	Cooperia	Nematodirus	Bunostomum	Gaigeria	Strongyloides	Oesophagostomum	Chabertia
I.	Phenothiazine	600	+++	++	+++	+++	+	+	+	–	–	+++	+++
II.	Bephenium	250	–	–	–	–	–	+++	–	–	–	–	–
III.2.	Fenclofos	100	+++	–	–	–	–	–	–	–	–	–	–
3.	Haloxon	50	+++	–	–	–	+++	–	–	–	–	–	–
4.	Naftalofos	50	+++	–	–	–	+++	–	–	–	–	–	–
5.	Trichlorophon	60	+++	–	–	–	–	–	–	–	–	–	–
IV.	Metyridine	200	–	–	–	++	++	++	–	–	–	–	–
V.1.	Disophenol	10	+++	–	–	–	–	–	–	–	–	–	–
2.	Nitroxynil	10	+++	–	–	–	–	–	+++	–	–	+++	–
VI.1.	Tiabendazole	75	+++	+++	+++	+++	+++	+++	+++	+++	+++	+++	+++
2.	Parbendazole	30	+++	+++	+++	+++	+++	++	+++	–	++	+++	+++
4.	Mebendazole	15	+++	+++	+++	+++	+++	++	+++	+++	+	++	+++
5.	Fenbendazole	5	+++	+++	+++	+++	+++	+++	++	+++	++	+++	+++
6.	Oxibendazole	10	+++	+++	+++	+++	+++	+++	+++	–	+++	+++	+++
7.	Oxfendazole	5	+++	+++	+++	+++	+++	+++	+++	+++	++	+++	+++
8.	Albendazole	5	+++	+++	+++	+++	+++	+++	–	+++	–	+++	+++
VII.1.	Clioxanide	20	+++	–	–	–	–	–	–	–	–	–	–
2.	Rafoxanide	7.5	+++	–	–	–	–	–	–	+++	–	–	++
3.	Bromoxanide	5	+++	–	–	–	–	–	–	–	–	–	–
4.	Closantel	5	+++	–	–	–	–	–	–	–	–	–	–
VIII.1.	Pyrantel	25	+++	+++	+++	++	–	+++	+++	+++	–	–	+++
2.	Morantel	10	+++	+++	–	+++	–	+++	–	+++	–	+++	+++
IX.	Levamisole	Oral 7.5 s.c. and i.m.5	+++	+++	+++	+++	+++	+++	+++	–	++	+++	+++
X.1.	Thiophanate	50	+++	+++	+++	+++	+++	++	–	–	–	–	+++
2.	Febantel	5	+++	+++	+++	+++	+++	++	+++	–	++	+++	–
XI.	Ivermectin	0.2	+++	+++	+++	+++	+++	–	–	–	–	+++	–

Classification of efficacy: +++, 95%–100%; ++, 80%–100%; +, 0%–100%; –, not effective or insufficient data

Table 3. Efficacy of the anthelmintics against developing larvae of the most important gastrointestinal nematodes in cattle

Classi-fica-tion	Anthelmintics	Dosage in mg/kg body weight (oral)	Abomasum			Small intestine					Large intestine
			Ostertagia	Haemon-chus	Tricho-stron-gylus	Tricho-stron-gylus	Cooperia	Nemato-dirus	Buno-stomum	Strongy-loides	Oesopha-gosto-mum
VI.2.	Parbendazole	30	++	+++	+++	+++	+++	–	–	+++	–
5.	Fenbendazole	7.5	+++	+++	+++	+++	+++	+++	+++	–	+++
6.	Oxibendazole	10	+	++	++	+++	+++	–	–	–	–
7.	Oxfendazole	2.5	+++	+++	+++	+++	+++	++	–	–	–
8.	Albendazole	7.5	+++	+++	+++	+++	+++	–	+++	+++	–
VII.2.	Rafoxanide	7.5	++	–	–	–	–	–	–	–	++
IX.	Levamisole	Oral 17.5 s.c. and i.m. 5	++	+++	++	++	+++	+++	–	–	–
X.1.	Thiophanate	50	+++	+++	+++	+++	–	–	–	–	+++
2.	Febantel	7.5	–	+++	+++	–	–	–	–	–	–
XI.	Ivermectin	0.2	+++	+++	+++	+++	+++	–	–	–	+++

Classification of efficacy: +++, 95%–100%; ++, 80%–100%; +, 0%–100%; –, not effective or insufficient data

Table 4. Efficacy of the anthelmintics against developing larvae of the most important gastrointestinal nematodes in sheep and goats

Classi-fica-tion	Anthelmintics	Dosage in mg/kg body weight (oral)	Abomasum			Small intestine						Large intestine	
			Hae-mon-chus	Oster-tagia	Tricho-stron-gylus	Tricho-stron-gylus	Co-operia	Nemato-dirus	Buno-stomum	Gaigeria	Strongy-loides	Oeso-phago-stomum	Cha-ber-tia
V.2.	Nitroxynil	10	+++	–	–	–	–	–	–	–	–	–	–
VI.2.	Parbendazole	30	+++	+++	+++	+++	+++	–	+++	–	–	+++	+++
5.	Fenbendazole	5	+++	+++	+++	+++	+++	+++	+++	+++	–	++	++
6.	Oxibendazole	10	+++	+++	+++	–	+++	+++	+++	–	+++	+++	+++
7.	Oxfendazole	5	+++	+++	+++	+++	+++	+++	–	+++	–	+++	+++
8.	Albendazole	5	+++	+++	+++	+++	–	+++	–	+++	–	++	+++
VII.1.	Clioxanide	20	++	–	–	–	–	–	–	–	–	–	–
VIII.1.	Pyrantel	25	+++	–	–	++	–	+++	–	–	–	–	–
2.	Morantel	10	+++	–	–	+++	–	+++	–	–	–	–	–
IX.	Levamisole	Oral 7.5, s.c. and i.m. 5	+	+++	+++	+++	++	+	–	–	–	–	–
X.1.	Thiophanate	50	+++	+++	+++	+++	–	–	–	–	–	–	–
2.	Febantel	5	+++	+++	+++	+++	–	–	+++	–	–	+++	–
XI.	Ivermectin	0.2	–	+++	–	–	–	–	–	–	–	–	–

Classiffication of efficacy: +++, 95%–100%; ++, 80%–100%; +, 0%–100%; –, not effective or insufficient data

Table 5. Anthelmintics effective against inhibited larvae of *Ostertagia ostertagi* in cattle

Classification	Anthelmintics	Dosage in mg/kg body weight	Efficacy
VI.5.	Fenbendazole	7.5	+−+++
		1/day for 10 days	+−+++
7.	Oxfendazole	2.5	++
		5	
8.	Albendazole	7.5	+−+++
IX.	Levamisole	7.5 s.c.	+
X.1.	Thiophanate	132	+
		20/day for 5 days	+++
XI.	Ivermectin	0.2	+++

Classification of efficacy: +++, 95%–100%; ++, 80%–100%; +, 0%–100%

Table 6. Anthelmintics effective against inhibited larvae of gastrointestinal nematodes in sheep

Classification	Anthelmintics	Dosage in mg/kg body weight	Haemonchus	Ostertagia	Trichostrongylus	Nematodirus
VI.5.	Fenbendazole	1.4/day for 4 days	+++	+++	+++	+++
		0.8/day for 7 days	+++	+++	+++	+++
		0.4/day for 14 days	+++	+++	+++	+++
7.	Oxfendazole	5	+++	+++	+++	+++

Classification of efficacy: +++, 95%–100%

III. Organic Phosphorus Compounds

1. Coumafos

In cattle coumafos has been tested mainly as a food additive administered over about a week or more. At a dose of 2 mg/kg body weight given daily for 6 days high efficacy was found against *H. placei, Trichostrongylus*, and *Cooperia*. Efficacy against *O. ostertagi, Oesophagostomum*, and *Trichuris* was moderate (CIORDIA 1972; ZEAKES et al. 1976).

In sheep toxic symptoms or even death can occur at doses below the therapeutic dose (GORDON 1958).

2. Fenclofos

Results in both cattle and sheep are conflicting. At a dose of 100 mg/kg body weight it is probably only effective against adult *Haemonchus* (GIBSON 1975).

3. Haloxon

Results in both cattle and sheep are conflicting. At a dose of 50 mg/kg body weight it is probably only effective against adult *Haemonchus* and *Cooperia* (GIB-

Table 7. Anthelmintics effective against gastrointestinal nematodes in ruminants

Classification	Generic name	Suppliers	Product names	Formulations
I.	Phenothiazine	Various	Various	Powder
II.	Bephenium	Burroughs Wellcome	Alcopar	
III.1.	Coumafos	Bayer, Chemagro	Baymix, Co-Ral	Grumbles
2.	Fenclofos	Dow	Ectoral, Ronnel	
3.	Haloxon	Cooper	Halox, Loxon, Verloxon	Suspension
4.	Naftalofos	Bayer	Maretin, Rametin	Powder, bolus
5.	Trichlorphon	Bayer	Neguvon	Powder
IV.	Metyridine	ICI	Mintic, Promintic	Solution, injectable solution
V.1.	Disophenol	Cyanamid	Ancylol	Injectable solution
2.	Nitroxynil	May & Baker, Specia	Dovenix, Trodax	Injectable solution
VI.1.	Tiabendazole	MSD	Thibenzole, Omnizole	Paste, suspension Bolus, premix, powder
2.	Parbendazole	Smith Kline	Helmatac, Worm Guard	Bolus, premix, powder
4.	Mebendazole	Janssen Pharmaceutica	Ovitelmin, Multispec	Bolus
5.	Fenbendazole	Hoechst	Panacur, Axilur	Paste, suspension, bolus, granules, powder
6.	Oxibendazole	Smith Kline	Neplon 100, Loditac	Suspension, premix Powder
7.	Oxfendazole	Syntex, Wellcome	Synanthic, Systamex	Suspension, bolus
8.	Albendazole	Smith Kline	Valbazen	Paste, suspension bolus
VII.1.	Clioxanide	Parke Davis	Tremarad	
2.	Rafoxanide	MSD	Ranide	Suspension, bolus
3.	Bromoxanide	Smith Kline		Suspension
4.	Closantel	Janssen Pharmaceutica		Injectable solution
VIII.1.	Pyrantel	Pfizer	Banminth, Exhelm	Bolus, powder, premix
2.	Morantel	Pfizer	Banminth II, Bovhelm, Expar Glylox, Ibantic Nematel, Ovithelm, Paratect	Bolus, powder, premix, Sustained release bolus
IX.	Levamisole	Janssen Pharmaceutica	Anthelsol, Nemisol, Nilverm GL, Pagliderm, L-Tramisol, L-Ripercol, L-Ripercol drench	Injectable solution, oral solution, granules, pour-on formulation
X.1.	Thiophanate	May & Baker	Nemafax	Suspension, bolus
2.	Febantel	Bayer	Rintal	Suspension, bolus, granules
XI.	Ivermectin	MSD	Ivomec	Injectable solution

son 1975). Toxic effects at the therapeutic dose were found in sheep by Williams et al. (1976).

4. Naftalofos

Results in both cattle and sheep are conflicting. At a dose of 50 mg/kg body weight it is probably only effective against adult *Haemonchus* and *Cooperia* (Gibson 1975).

5. Trichlorphon

At a dose of 60 mg/kg body weight, given orally, trichlorphon was effective against *Haemonchus* in both cattle and sheep (Gibson 1975). High efficacy against *H. placei* in cattle was found after a subcutaneous dose of 11 mg/kg.

IV. Metyridine

The results of efficacy trials with metyridine are conflicting. In both cattle and sheep, efficacy against trichostrongylids in the abomasum is in general low and efficacy against trichostrongylids in the small intestine moderate at a dose of 200 mg/kg body weight given subcutaneously, intraperitoneally, or orally (Werkgroep Wormmiddelen 1973 c).

V. Nitrophenols

1. Disophenol

Disophenol is an anthelmintic with prolonged activity against blood-consuming parasites. At a dose of 10 mg/kg body weight given subcutaneously it was capable of preventing infection with *H. contortus* in sheep during a period of 90 days or more. It had no effect against other trichostrongylids, strongylids, and inhibited larvae (Gordon 1974). Disophenol given to sheep at a dose of 7.5 mg/kg subcutaneously every 3 months protected them against haemonchaisis during the whole treatment period. There was no effect against *Trichostrongylus* and *Oesophagostomum* (Soetedjo et al. 1980). Reinecke et al. (1981) found a high degree of protection for 2 months after a dose of 10 mg/kg. Less good results were obtained by Hall et al. (1981 a), who found that disophenol at a subcutaneous dose of 10 mg/kg was prophylactic against *H. contortus* in sheep when infected 30 days after treatment. When sheep were infected 60 days after treatment efficacy was 54%. Infection 90 days after treatment resulted in an efficacy of only 7%.

2. Nitroxynil

Nitroxynil at a dose of 10 mg/kg body weight given subcutaneously was very effective against *H. placei* and *Bunostomum phlebotomum* in cattle. Efficacy against *O. radiatum* was moderate. There was no effect against *Cooperia* (Wellington 1978). A subcutaneous dose of 20 mg/kg given to cattle was effective against adult *H. contortus, B. phlebotomum,* and *O. radiatum* (Guilhon et al. 1970). A dose of

10 mg/kg given subcutaneously was very effective against adults and developing stages of *H. contortus*. When given intraruminally no effect was found (LUCAS 1971).

VI. Benzimidazoles

1. Tiabendazole

a) Cattle

Tiabendazole at a dose of 100 mg/kg was very effective against *Ostertagia* and *Trichostrongylus*, but against *Cooperia* efficacy was moderate (BAKER and DOUGLAS 1962). High efficacy against *O. ostertagi* and moderate efficacy against *Cooperia oncophora* at a dose of 100 mg/kg was also found by AMES et al. (1963). Moderate efficacy against *Cooperia* spp. was also found by RUBIN et al. (1965) and LANGELER (1966). BENZ (1973), however, found high efficacy against *C. pectinata* and *C. punctata* at a dose of 83 mg/kg in a paste formulation. Efficacy against *H. placei, O. ostertagi, T. axei,* and *B. phlebotomum* was also high, but was low against *Trichuris* spp. and developing larvae of *Ostertagia* sp. High efficacy at a dose of 100 mg/kg was found against *S. papillosus* by RESTANI and BORELLI (1968). AMES et al. (1966) reported high efficacy at a dose of 110 mg/kg against *O. ostertagi, H. placei, Cooperia* spp., and *Oesophagostomum radiatum*. At a dose of 67 mg/kg efficacy against *Cooperia* spp. and *O. radiatum* was moderate, but high against the other mentioned nematodes. Administered in feed blocks over a period of 3 days, 3,3% tiabendazole was very effective against *Haemonchus* spp., *Ostertagia* sp., *Nematodirus* sp., and *Oesophagostomum* sp.; efficacy against *Trichostrongylus* spp. and *Cooperia* spp. was moderate. The estimated daily uptake of tiabendazole was about 37 mg/kg (AMES and HUTCHINSON 1973).

b) Sheep and Goats

At a dose of 50 mg/kg body weight high efficacy was found against *T. axei, T. vitrinus, T. colubriformis,* and *Oesophagostomum* sp. and moderate efficacy against *Ostertagia* sp., *H. contortus,* and *Nematodirus* spp. (HEBDEN 1961).

A high efficacy at a dose of 50 mg/kg against *H. contortus* and *T. axei* was found by SNIJDERS and LOUW (1966). At a dose of 75 mg/kg they found a high efficacy against *H. contortus, Ostertagia* sp., *Trichostrongylus* spp., *Gaigeria pachyscelis, B. phlebotomum, C. ovina,* and *O. venulosum*.

LYONS et al. (1967) reported a high efficacy against *H. contortus, Ostertagia* sp., *Trichostrongylus* spp., *Cooperia* spp., and *Nematodirus* spp. at a dose of 50 mg/kg. Against *Strongyloides papillosus* high efficacy was found by CAIRNS (1961) and HORAK et al. (1970). Resistance of trichostrongylids against tiabendazole was shown among others by DRUDGE et al. (1964), HOTSON et al. (1970), and HALL et al. (1979).

2. Parbendazole

a) Cattle

A dose of 20 mg/kg body weight given as a drench was very effective against adult *Ostertagia, T. axei,* and *Cooperia*. Given as a food additive the same effect was obtained. A dose of 30 mg/kg body weight was necessary for high efficacy against developing stages of these species (RUBIN 1968).

The same effect with the same dose and administration route was obtained against *H. placei*, *N. fillicollis*, and *O. radiatum* (RUBIN 1969). BORGSTEEDE (1974) found high efficacy against adults and developing stages of *C. oncophora*, *C. punctata*, *Trichostrongylus* spp., *H. contortus*, and *S. papillosus* with a dose of 30 mg/kg given as a drench. High efficacy against adult *O. ostertagia* was also found but efficacy was moderate against developing stages. A similar result was reported by ROSS (1970).

b) Sheep and Goats

High efficacy was obtained by ROSS (1968) at a dose of 15 mg/kg body weight against adult and developing stages of *Haemonchus* and *Trichostrongylus*. High efficacy against adult *Ostertagia* was also recorded, but against *N. battus* efficacy was low. LYONS et al. (1974) found high efficacy against adults and developing stages of *Haemonchus*, *Ostertagia*, *Trichostrongylus*, *Cooperia*, *Bunostomun*, *Chabertia*, and *Oesophagostomum* after a drench at a dose of 15 mg/kg. The effect against *Strongyloides* was moderate. Little effect was found against *Nematodirus*, *Trichuris*, and *Capillaria*. A 3% pellet formulation was comparatively less effective against *Haemonchus*. Moderate activity at a dose of 20 mg/kg was found against *N. spathiger* by COLGLAZIER et al. (1971 b).

Toxic effects after a therapeutic dose have been seen in ewes treated within 1 month after mating. LAPRAS et al. (1973) was the first who recorded malformations in lambs when ewes were treated about 3 weeks after mating. These malformations consisted of anophthalmia, cyclopia, atresia ani, and skeletal deformations.

These observations were confirmed by SAUNDERS et al. (1974), SHONE et al. (1979), and SZABO et al. (1974). An embryolethal effect was recorded by MIDDLETON et al. (1974). For this reason parbendazole is not suitable for the treatment of ewes in the 1st month of pregnancy.

Resistance of trichostrongylids against parbendazole was found in 1970 by HOTSON et al. (1970).

3. Cambendazole

Because of its toxicity in ruminants this anthelmintic was withdrawn in 1980 by the manufacturer. Toxicity of cambendazole has been shown in sheep (ANON 1978) and cattle (STOYE et al. 1971; MAIN and VASS 1980). Lesions are characterized by lung edema and follicular necrosis of the pulmonary lymph nodes. This seems to be associated with feeding concentrates. An embryotoxic effect of cambendazole in pregnant ewes was recorded by DELATOUR et al. (1974).

4. Mebendazole

Given at a dose of 10–15 mg/kg, mebendazole was effective against trichostrongylids in sheep (GUILHON et al. 1972; VARGA and JANISH 1975; KELLY et al. 1975 a; WALLNÖFER 1977) and goats (RIBBECK and WINTER 1977). It should be noted that these studies were based on egg counts only.

5. Fenbendazole

a) Cattle

A high efficacy of fenbendazole against *Ostertagia, Trichostrongylus, Cooperia, Nematodirus,* and *Bunostomum* was found at a dose of 7.5 mg/kg body weight given as a 10% suspension (ENIGK et al. 1975). Efficacy against strongylids was moderate (CHROUST and DIJK 1975). Administrated in a gelatin capsule at a dose of 7.5 mg/kg fenbendazole showed high efficacy against *Haemonchus, Ostertagia,* and *Cooperia* (TODD et al. 1976). The effect against *Nematodirus helvetianus* was tested by PFEIFFER and SUPPERER (1976). A 10% suspension administered by stomach tube at a dose of 7.5 mg/kg was very effective against adults and developing larvae. Effectivity against inhibited larvae was low. When administered at a dose of 0.25 mg/kg daily in the food for 5 days fenbendazole was very effective against *Ostertagia, Trichostrongylus, Cooperia,* and *Oesophagostomum.* To obtain the same efficacy against *Haemonchus* 1 mg/kg body weight daily was necessary (CROWLEY et al. 1977).

Administered in a feed block at a total dose of 10 mg/kg for 5 days fenbendazole was very effective against adult *O. ostertagi* and developing larvae of *Cooperia* spp. and *O. radiatum* (GAENSSLER et al. 1978). It was also very effective against inhibited larvae of *O. ostertagi* when administered in a feed block (840 ppm fenbendazole) and offered with unrestricted access for 10 days. The daily dose was about 1 mg/kg (MCBEATH et al. 1977).

After the publication of DUNCAN et al. (1976) on the efficacy of a single therapeutic dose of fenbendazole against inhibited larvae of *O. ostertagi,* much research on this subject was carried out. However, there have been important differences between the efficacies against inhibited larvae of *O. ostertagi* found by different researchers. Very good results were recorded by DUNCAN et al. (1976), MCBEATH et al. (1977), CALLINAN and CUMMINS (1979), and WILLIAMS et al. (1979 b); moderate, variable, or low efficacy was found by SEARSON and DOUGHTY (1977), ELLIOT (1977), LANCASTER and HONG (1977), CRAIG and BELL (1978), INDERBITZIN and ECKERT (1978), and WILLIAMS et al. (1981 b). Many reasons have been suggested for these differences. They are discussed in Sect. B.IV. The effect of fenbendazole on semen quality of bulls was studied by KRAUSE et al. (1975). Three oral doses of 10 mg/kg with a 4-week interval had no demonstrably harmful effect on semen quality.

b) Sheep and Goats

Fenbendazole at an oral dose of 5 mg/kg body weight was very effective against *Haemonchus, Ostertagia, Cooperia, Nematodirus, Oesophagostomum,* and *Chabertia* (KELLY et al. 1975 b; KENNEDY and TODD 1975). A dose 3.5 mg/kg body weight given as a 2.5% suspension was very effective against *Haemonchus, Trichostrongylus, Cooperia, Nematodirus, Oesophagostomum,* and *Chabertia.* The effect against *Ostertagia* and *Bunostomum* was moderate. A dose of 5 mg/kg body weight was necessary for the same effect against these nematodes. The effect against *Trichuris* was low (CHROUST and DIJK 1975).

Efficacy against *Strongyloides* at a dose of 5 mg/kg body weight was moderate (BEHRENS and MATSCHULLAT 1975; GRIMBEEK and TERBLANCHE 1980). High efficacy against developing larvae of *H. contortus, O. circumcincta, T. colubriformis*, and *Nematodirus battus* was found at a dose of 5 mg/kg (ROSS 1975).

The effect against inhibited larvae was tested by THOMAS (1978b). Fenbendazole was given in feed blocks (840 ppm). The doses tested were 1.4 mg/kg for 4 days, 0.8 mg/kg/day for 7 days, and 0.4 mg/kg/day for 14 days. All doses had a high efficacy against inhibited larvae of *Haemonchus, Ostertagia, Trichostrongylus*, and *Nematodirus*. Doses of 0.25 mg/kg/day for 14 days or less were less effective.

Resistance of trichostrongylids against fenbendazole was recorded by HOGARTH-SCOTT et al. (1976).

6. Oxibendazole

a) Cattle

Oxibendazole administered at a dose of 5 mg/kg body weight was very effective against *O. ostertagi, T. axei, T. colubriformis*, and *O. radiatum*. The effect against *H. contortus* and *C. oncophora* was moderate. High efficacy against these parasites was obtained at a dose of 10 mg/kg. At this dose high efficacy was found against developing larvae of *T. colubriformis* and *C. oncophora*. The effect on developing larvae of *H. contortus* and *T. axei* was moderate and low against developing larvae of *O. ostertagi* (HERLICH 1975). THEODORIDES et al. (1976a) found a high efficacy at a dose of 10 mg/kg against adults of *O. ostertagi, T. axei, C. oncophora, T. colubriformis, S. papillosus*, and *O. radiatum*. The effect against *H. contortus* was moderate. In another trial the efficacy of 15 mg/kg given as a premix was moderate against *Ostertagia, Nematodirus, Bunostomum*, and *Strongyloides*. Efficacy against developing stages of *Ostertagia* was low.

WILLIAMS et al. (1978) found oxibendazole given as a feed premix at a dose of 15 mg/kg to be very effective against *Haemonchus, Trichostrongylus, Cooperia, Bunostomum*, and *Oesophagostomum*. Efficacy against *Ostertagia* was 96%. Efficacy against *Trichuris* was moderate.

Moderate efficacy against developing larvae of *Ostertagia* and *Haemonchus* was found at a dose of 15 mg/kg given as a feed premix (CROWLEY et al. 1976).

b) Sheep and Goats

In a preliminary study THEODORIDES et al. (1973) found, after an oral dose of 5, 7, 5, and 10 mg/kg body weight, an efficacy of 90%–100% against immature and adult stages of *Haemonchus, Ostertagia, Trichostrongylus, Nematodirus, Cooperia, Bunostomum, Chabertia, Oesophagostomum*, and *Strongyloides*.

The embryotoxic effect of oxibendazole was studied by DELATOUR et al. (1976). At a dose of 15 mg/kg given twice at day 14 and day 21 after mating there was no embryotoxic effect. Doses of 45 mg/kg on the same days or 150 mg/kg at day 21 caused embryolethality. THEODORIDES et al. (1977) found no embryotoxic effect when oxibendazole was given to ewes eight times in early pregnancy at a dose of 30 mg/kg.

7. Oxfendazole

a) Cattle

At a dose of 2.5 mg/kg body weight oxfendazole showed high efficacy against adults and developing larvae of *Ostertagia* and *Cooperia* and against adult *Haemonchus, Trichostrongylus,* and *Nematodirus.* Efficacy against *Trichuris* was moderate. At a dose of 5 mg/kg high efficacy was found against *Trichuris* (DOWNEY 1976).

BORGSTEEDE (1977) found high efficacy at a dose of 2.5 mg/kg given as a drench against *Ostertagia, Haemonchus, Cooperia,* and *Trichostrongylus.* The effect against *Strongyloides* was moderate. Given at a dose of 2.5 mg/kg as a 2.265% suspension it had a high efficacy against adult *Ostertagia, Trichostrongylus, Cooperia, Chabertia,* and *Oesophagostomum.* There was also a high efficacy against developing larvae of *Trichostrongylus* and *Cooperia* but efficacy against developing larvae of *Ostertagia* and *Nematodirus* was moderate. A paste and bolus formulation gave the same results. A pelleted feed additive given as a top dressing gave nonuniform efficacy as result of the differences in intake by the individual calves (BAKER et al. 1978).

TODD and MANSFIELD (1979) found high efficacy against *Haemonchus, Ostertagia, Trichostrongylus, Cooperia, Bunostomum,* and *Oesophagostomum* at a dose of 2.5 mg/kg. At a dose of 5 mg/kg the efficacy was 95%. High efficacy against inhibited larvae of *Ostertagia* was found by KISTNER et al. (1979).

A special intraruminal capsule releasing 0.48 mg/kg oxfendazole/day for 5 days was very effective against adults and inhibited larvae of *Ostertagia* (ANDERSON and LABY 1979).

b) Sheep and Goats

Oxfendazole at a dose of 5 mg/kg body weight administered as a 2.265% suspension was very effective against *Haemonchus, Ostertagia, Cooperia, Trichostrongylus,* and *N. battus* (LEIMBACHER et al. 1976). CHALMERS (1977) found high efficacy at a dose of 5 mg/kg against developing stages and adults of *Haemonchus, Ostertagia, Trichostrongylus, Nematodirus, Cooperia, Oesophagostomum,* and *Chabertia.* The effect against *Trichuris* and *Strongyloides* was moderate.

A moderate effect against *Strongyloides* was also found by BORGSTEEDE et al. (1981) and BERGER (1980). BERGER (1980) recorded high efficacy against adults and developing larvae of *Gaigeria* at a dose of 5 mg/kg.

The efficacy against inhibited larvae was tested by DOWNEY (1977). Oxfendazole given to ewes at about parturition at a dose of 5 mg/kg gave a large reduction in egg output. The predominant genus was not determined but was probably *Ostertagia.* OGUNSUSI (1979) found a high efficacy at a dose of 4.53 mg/kg against inhibited larvae of *Haemonchus.*

THOMAS and REID (1980) found high efficacy against inhibited larvae of *Haemonchus, Ostertagia, Trichostrongylus,* and *Nematodirus* at a dose of 5 mg/kg.

No differences in efficacy between drench and bolus formulation were found by THOMAS and REID (1980) and BORGSTEEDE et al. (1981). A special intraruminal capsule releasing oxfendazole over 41 days was very effective against adults, developing larvae, and inhibited larvae of *O. circumcincta* (ANDERSON et al. 1980).

LE JAMBRE et al. (1981) showed that this formulation was also very effective against *H. contortus* and *T. colubriformis* and against benzimidazole-resistant strains of *H. contortus, O. circumcincta*, and *T. colubriformis*. In goats oxfendazole at a dose of 4.5 mg/kg body weight was very effective against adults and developing stages of *Haemonchus, Trichostrongylus, Ostertagia, Cooperia, Bunostomum*, and *Chabertia* (MICHAEL et al. 1979).

An embryotoxic effect of oxfendazole given to sheep about 3 weeks after the introduction of rams at a dose of 22.5 mg/kg body weight was recorded by DELATOUR et al. (1977). A dose of 7.5 mg/kg body weight produced no embryotoxic effect. PIERCY et al. (1979) showed that a dose of 15 mg/kg body weight had no embryotoxic effect when given to ewes in early pregnancy. There was no harmful effect on fertility in rams. High efficacy at the therapeutic dose against benzimidazole-resistant *Haemonchus* strains was found by KISTNER and WYSE (1978) and WEBB et al. (1979). However, BERGER (1980) found a moderate efficacy of oxfendazole against a benzimidazole-resistant *Haemonchus* strain. Resistance in a field strain of *Haemonchus* against oxfendazole was found by WEBB and MCCULLY (1979).

8. Albendazole

a) Cattle

Albendazole given as a 10% suspension at a dose of 5.0–7.5 mg/kg body weight was very effective against adult *O. ostertagi, T. axei, Cooperia punctata*, and *C. oncophora*. At a dose of 2.5 mg/kg the activity against *C. oncophora* was reduced. At all doses the efficacy against *H. contortus* was low. A possible reason for this low efficacy may be resistance against benzimidazoles, because in this trial *H. contortus* of sheep was used (BENZ and ERNST 1977). Similar results have been obtained by HERLICH (1977). At a dose of 10 mg/kg albendazole given as a 10% suspension was very effective against adult *O. ostertagi, T. colubriformis*, and *C. oncophora*. Activity against adult *H. contortus* was low in this experiment, in which a known cambendazole-resistant *H. contortus* strain was used.

THEODORIDES et al. (1976c) found a high efficacy at a dose of 5 mg/kg against adults and developing stages of *O. ostertagi, H. contortus, T. axei, C. oncophora, T. colubriformis, B. phlebotomum*, and *S. papillosus*. An efficacy of 92% and 86% against developing larvae in the abomasum and small intestine respectively was found after a dose of 5 mg/kg by WILLIAMS et al. (1977a). Given as a bolus at a dose of 8 mg/kg albendazole showed a high efficacy against *Ostertagia, Trichostrongylus, Cooperia*, and *Nematodirus* (WESCOTT et al. 1979).

The results of trials with albendazole against inhibited larvae of *O. ostertagi* vary. DOWNEY (1978) found an efficacy of 90% at a dose of 7.5 mg/kg. Roughly the same effect was obtained in trials by BORGSTEEDE (1979) and WILLIAMS et al. (1977b) with activities of 85% and 84% respectively, both using doses of 7.5 mg/kg. Low activity of albendazole against inhibited larvae of *O. ostertagi* at a dose of 7.5 mg/kg was found by WILLIAMS et al. (1979a, 1981a). The reason for these differences is not known but is discussed in Sect. B.IV.

The influence of albendazole on male reproduction was studied by BERNDTSON et al. (1980). A dose of 22.5 mg/kg did not influence the reproductive function of bulls.

b) Sheep and Goats

Albendazole given as an oral suspension at a dose of 5 mg/kg body weight was very effective against *H. contortus*. Efficacy against *N. spathiger* was 100% (THEODORIDES et al. 1976b). ROSS et al. (1978) found a high efficacy against *O. circumcincta* and *T. colubriformis* at a dose of 3.8 mg/kg.

VAN SCHALKWIJK et al. (1979) reported a high efficacy against adults and developing larvae of *H. contortus, O. circumcincta T. colubriformis, N. spathiger, G. pachyscelis, Cooperia* ssp., and *Chabertia ovina* at a dose of 2.5 mg/kg. High efficacy against adults, but moderate against developing larvae, of *O. columbianum* was found.

Resistance against albendazole was found by VLASSOFF and KETTLE (1980).

VII. Salicyclanilides

1. Clioxanide

Clioxanide at a dose of 20 mg/kg body weight given orally was very effective against adult *H. contortus* in sheep. Efficacy against developing larvae of *H. contortus* was moderate (PEARSON et al. 1970).

2. Rafoxanide

a) Cattle

Rafoxanide at a dose of 7.5 mg/kg body weight given intraruminally reduced adults and developing larvae of *H. placei* by 90% (SNIJDERS et al. 1971). SNIJDERS and HORAK (1975) found a moderate efficacy against developing larvae of *H. placei* at a dose of 7.5 mg/kg. Adult *B. phlebotomum* was highly sensitive. A 5% injectable formulation given subcutaneously at a dose of 3 mg/kg was very effective against adult *H. placei, B. phlebotomum,* and *O. radiatum,* whereas efficacy against developing larvae of *H. placei* and *O. radiatum* was moderate. At 5 mg/kg high efficacy against developing larvae of *H. placei* was found (SCHRÖDER et al. 1977).

b) Sheep and Goats

Rafoxanide at a dose of 10 mg/kg body weight given as a drench was very effective against adults and developing stages of *H. contortus*. The *Haemonchus* strain used in this test was resistant against tiabendazole (EGERTON et al. 1970).

Given at a dose of 5 mg/kg intraruminally rafoxanide was very effective against adult benzimidazole-resistant *H. contortus* (CAMPBELL and HOTSON 1971). At a dose of 7.5 mg/kg high efficacy against *H. contortus was also found by* HORAK et al. (1972) and LE JAMBRE and BARGER (1979). No effect against inhibited larvae of *H. contortus* was found (SNIJDERS et al. 1973; LE JAMBRE and BARGER 1979). HORAK et al. (1972) found high efficacy against adult *G. pachyscelis* at a dose of 7.5 mg/kg. The effect against *Chabertia ovina* was moderate.

Blindness in sheep treated with rafoxanide was described in one study (PROZESKY and PIENAAR 1977).

Resistance against rafoxanide in a *H. contortus* strain was found by VAN WIJK and GERBER (1980).

3. Bromoxanide

Bromoxanide at a dose of 5 mg/kg body weight given orally was very effective against adult *H. contortus* in sheep (THEODORIDES et al. 1974).

4. Closantel

Closantel at a dose of 2.5 mg/kg body weight given intraruminally by injection was very effective against adult benzimidazole-resistant *H. contortus*. A dose of 5 mg/kg was necessary to obtain a high efficacy against developing larvae of *H. contortus*. There was no effect against *T. colubriformis* (HALL et al. 1980).

An intraruminal injection with closantel at a dose of 10 mg/kg 30 days before an artificial infection with a tiabendazole-resistant *H. contortus* strain reduced the infection almost entirely (HALL et al. 1981 a).

VIII. Tetrahydropyrimidines

1. Pyrantel

a) Cattle

Pyrantel tartrate at a dose of 25 mg/kg body weight was very effective against adult *O. ostertagi* and *Cooperia*. The efficacy against developing stages of *O. ostertagia* was low (CORNWELL and JONES 1970a.) A high efficacy based on egg counts against *Ostertagia, Haemonchus, Cooperia,* and *Nematodirus* at a dose of 25 mg/kg was found by RAYNAUD (1968).

b) Sheep and Goats

Pyrantel tartrate at a dose of 20 mg/kg body weight given intraruminally was very effective against *H. contortus, O. circumcincta, O. trifurcata, T. colubriformis, N. spathiger, G. pachyscelis,* and *Chabertia ovina* (ANDERSON 1968). CORNWELL (1966) found a high efficacy against adults and developing larvae of *N. battus* after a dose of 25 mg/kg.

The efficacy against adults and developing larvae of *H. contortus* was very high after a dose of 25 mg/kg (GIBSON and PARFITT 1968). In the same trial a moderate effect was found against adult and developing stages of *T. colubriformis*. COLGLAZIER et al. (1971 a) also found a moderate effect against *T. colubriformis* after a dose of 25 mg/kg. However, this dose was very effective against adults and developing larvae of *T. axei*. High efficacy against *B. trigonocephalum* was found by STOIMENOFF and STEPHANOFF (1975) at a dose of 25 mg/kg. In the same trial high efficacy against *H. contortus* and *Nematodirus* was also found.

2. Morantel

a) Cattle

Morantel tartrate administered as a bolus at a dose level of 10.5–11.5 mg/kg body weight was very effective against *H. placei*, *T. axei*, *Cooperia*, and *T. colubriformis*. The effect against *O. ostertagi* was moderate (CIORDIA and MCCAMPBELL 1973). CONWAY et al. (1973) found a high efficacy against *Haemonchus*, *Cooperia*, and *Oesophagostomum*. The effect against *O. ostertagi* and *T. axei* was moderate. A high efficacy at a dose of 5 mg/kg was found against *H. placei*, *Cooperia*, *Bunostomum*, and *Oesophagostomum*, but the efficacy against *O. ostertagi* was low (ANDERSON and MARAIS 1975).

In cattle infected daily with infective larvae of *O. ostertagi* and treated daily with 1.25 mg/kg morantel tartrate, an efficacy of 87% was found (JONES et al. 1978). Morantel tartrate given to cattle in the feed at a dose of 1.5 mg/kg daily during the first months of the grazing season reduced pasture contamination by 85% in the second half of the grazing season (POTT et al. 1979).

A special sustained release bolus[1] was designed for the continuous release of morantel tartrate over 2 months. The bolus is administered with a special bolus gun into the reticulum of calves just prior to turning out in their first grazing season. Overwintered infective larvae picked up by these animals do not mature during the first 2 months. As a result the mid-summer increase in pasture larvae is prevented. Good results with this system have been found by ARMOUR et al. (1981), JONES (1981 a), JACOBS et al. (1981), BORGSTEEDE et al. (1981), and BÜRGER et al. (1981).

b) Sheep and Goats

Morantel tartrate at a dose of 10 mg/kg body weight was very effective against *Ostertagia*, *T. colubriformis*, *N. spathiger*, *G. pachyscelis*, *Chabertia ovina*, and *O. columbianum* in sheep and goats (ANDERSON and MARAIS 1972). High efficacy was found against adult and developing stages of *H. contortus*, *T. colubriformis*, and *N. battus* (CORNWELL and JONES 1970 b).

A small daily dose of 1.25 mg/kg for 28 days had an efficacy of 92% against *T. colubriformis* (JONES et al. 1978).

Side resistance of morantel tartrate was found in a levamisole-resistant *Ostertagia* strain (LE JAMBRE and MARTIN 1979).

IX. Imidazothiazoles

Levamisole

a) Cattle

Levamisole at a dose of 1.5 mg/kg body weight given subcutaneously was very effective against *Haemonchus*, *Trichostrongylus*, *Cooperia*, *Nematodirus*, and *Oesophagostomum*. Efficacy against *Ostertagia* and *T. axei* was moderate. The

1 More information on the morantel-sustained release bolus can be found in a special issue of Veterinary Parasitology (12:215–353, 1983)

same results were obtained with 7.5 mg/kg given orally. To obtain a high efficacy against *T. axei* a dose of 7.5 mg/kg given subcutaneously was necessary (HART et al. 1969).

LYONS et al. (1972) showed that 8 mg/kg given as bolus or drench was very effective against adult *Haemonchus, O. ostertagi, C. oncophora, C. punctata, O. radiatum*, and *Trichuris*. Efficacy against *T. axei* was moderate. High efficacy against *T. axei* and *T. vitrinus* was found after a dose of 8 mg/kg given orally (BAKER and FISK 1972). In this trial high efficacy against *Cooperia* and *N. helvetianus* was also recorded. Efficacy against *O. ostertagi* was 95%. A subcutaneous dose of 8 mg/kg had a moderate efficacy against adult *O. ostertagi* and a low activity against developing stages of this nematode (LYONS et al. 1975). In the same trial high efficacy was found against *T. axei, T. colubriformis, C. oncophora, C. punctata*, and *O. radiatum*. A high efficacy against *Bunostomum* was found after a dose of 3.3 mg/kg given subcutaneously (FORSYTH 1968). A moderate effect against adult *O. ostertagi* was reported by ANDERSON (1977) and ANDERSON and LORD (1979). A low efficacy against *O. ostertagi* was found by LYONS et al. (1981 b, c). Resistance is a possible explanation for these findings.

The effect against inhibited larvae of *O. ostertagi* at the therapeutic dose is low (ANDERSON 1977; DOWNEY 1978; ANDERSON and LORD 1979; CUMMINS and CALLINAN 1979). A dose of 10 mg/kg given subcutaneously three times with 10- to 14-days intervals gave a good clinical response in cattle suffering from ostertagiasis type II (FORSYTH and SHEPERD 1977).

The dermal administration of levamisole is discussed in Sect. B.III.

b) Sheep and Goats

Levamisole given orally at a dose of 5 mg/kg body weight had a high efficacy against *Haemonchus, Trichostrongylus, Nematodirus, Oesophagostomum*, and *Chabertia*. Activity against developing larvae of *T. axei* and *Trichuris* was moderate. For a high efficacy against *Ostertagia* 7.5 mg/kg was necessary (HART et al. 1969). At an oral dose of 8 mg/kg high activity was found against *Ostertagia, Trichostrongylus, Nematodirus* (including *N. battus*), *Chabertia* (DOWNEY 1977), adult *O. circumcincta, T. axei*, and *T. vitrinus* (CALLINAN and BARTON 1979). In the same trial high efficacy against developing larvae of *O. circumcincta* was also found. Against *H. contortus* high efficacy was found at an oral dose of 7.5 mg/kg (CRAIG and SHEPERD 1980). A moderate efficacy against *Strongyloides* was found after a dose of 8 mg/kg given subcutaneously (KISTNER and WYSE 1975). Eight milligrams per kilogram gave excellent results against inhibited larvae of *H. contortus* (MCKENNA 1974). High efficacy against larvae of *Ostertagia* was found after an oral dose of 5.5–6.0 mg/kg (REID et al. 1976). FORSYTH and GIBBON (1980) found a high efficacy of levamisole at a dose of 2.7 mg/kg given orally or subcutaneously against a benzimidazole-resistant *H. contortus* strain. Levamisole did not affect *Trichuris* (DOWNEY 1977). Resistance against levamisole was found in *T. colubriformis* and *O. circumcincta* (SANGSTER et al. 1979).

A levamisole-resistant *O. circumcincta* strain was susceptible to tiabendazole, oxfendazole, and albendazole (LE JAMBRE 1979). The dermal administration of levamisole is discussed in Sect. B.III.

X. Probenzimidazoles

1. Thiophanate

a) Cattle

Thiophanate at a dose of 50 mg/kg body weight was very effective against adults and developing stages of *O. ostertagi, T. axei, H. contortus,* and *T. colubriformis.* The effect against *C. oncophora* and *N. helvetianus* was moderate. A dose of 100 mg/kg had an efficacy of 96% and 93% against *C. oncophora* and *N. helvetianus* respectively (EICHLER 1973).

FABIVI et al. (1979) tested the effect against *H. placei, C. punctata,* and *C. pectinata.* Based on egg counts they found a high efficacy against adult *Haemonchus* and *Cooperia* but not against inhibited stages of these parasites.

At a dose of 50–70 mg/kg thiophanate was very effective against adult *Haemonchus, Ostertagia, Trichostrongylus,* and *Cooperia* (BAINES and BELL 1980). DUNCAN et al. (1979) found an efficacy of 68% against inhibited larvae of *O. ostertagi* at a dose of 132 mg/kg. The effect against inhibited larvae of *Cooperia* was 100%. At a dose of 20 mg/kg daily administered in a feed block over 5 days the efficacy against inhibited stages of *O. ostertagi* and *Cooperia* was 97% and 100% respectively.

b) Sheep and Goats

Thiophanate at a dose of 50 mg/kg body weight was very effective against adults and developing stages of *H. contortus, O. circumcincta, T. axei, T. colubriformis,* and *Chabertia ovina.* The effect against *N. spathiger* was low and against *N. battus* moderate (EICHLER 1973). BAINES and BELL (1980) found a high efficacy against *T. axei, Ostertagia, Trichostrongylus, Cooperia,* and *Chabertia ovina* at a dose rate of 43–71 mg/kg. The efficacy against *N. filicollis* and *N. spathiger* was 96%. The efficacy against *Trichuris* was low. Small daily doses of 8.5–15.3 mg/kg during 14 weeks given to sheep grazing infested pasture had a moderate effect against trichostrongylids. During the treatment egg output was suppressed for the first 10 weeks. This suggests the development of a resistant population (DALTON 1978).

No embryotoxic effect was found after the treatment of ewes with 150 mg/kg body weight at 2, 3, and 4 weeks after the introduction of rams to the flock (BAINES and COLEGRAVE 1977).

2. Febantel

a) Cattle

Febantel at a dose of 5 mg/kg body weight given as a 5% suspension was very effective against adult and developing larvae of *H. contortus, T. axei,* and *Cooperia oncophora.* The effect against *O. ostertagi* was moderate. At a dose of 7.5 mg/kg it was fully effective against *O. ostertagi* (GRELCK et al. 1980).

b) Sheep and Goats

Febantel at a dose of 2.5 mg/kg body weight was very effective against adults and developing larvae of *Haemonchus, Ostertagia, Trichostrongylus,* and *Oesophago-*

stomum (THOMAS 1978a). The same effect was found at doses of 5 and 7.5 mg/kg against *H. contortus, O. circumcincta, T. colubriformis,* and *B. trigonocephalum* (BÜRGER 1978). High efficacy was also found against these nematodes by HOPKINS and RAFFERTY (1978). They found an efficacy of 95% against *N. spathiger.* The efficacy against tiabendazole-resistant strains of *H. contortus* and *T. colubriformis* was low, suggesting side resistance (HOPKINS and RAFFERTY 1978). The efficacy at a dose of 5 mg/kg against *S. papillosus* was 85% (GRIMBEEK and TERBLANCHE 1980). In rams a dose of 10 mg/kg given five times at 3-week intervals had no adverse effect on semen quality (TERBLANCHE 1978).

XI. Avermectins

Ivermectin

a) Cattle

Ivermectin given orally at a dose of 0.1 mg/kg was very effective against adult *H. placei, O. ostertagi, T. axei, C. oncophora, C. punctata,* and *O. radiatum.* Efficacy against *T. colubriformis* was moderate. High efficacy against the developing stages of these nematodes was found at a dose of 0.2 mg/kg (EGERTON et al. 1981).

BENZ and ERNST (1981) found, at an oral dose of 0.2 mg/kg, a high efficacy against adult *O. ostertagi, T. colubriformis,* and *C. punctata.* Efficacy against *T. axei, C. oncophora,* and *O. radiatum* was moderate.

Given subcutaneously at a dose of 0.2 mg/kg it was very effective against adult *O. ostertagi, T. axei, T. colubriformis, C. oncophora,* and *C. punctata.* Efficacy against *O. radiatum* was moderate (BENZ and ERNST 1981). EGERTON et al. (1981) found a high efficacy after a subcutaneous dose of 0.2 mg/kg against adults and developing stages of *H. placei, O. ostertagi, T. axei, C. oncophora, C. punctata,* and *O. radiatum.* Efficacy against *T. colubriformis* was moderate. Ivermectin has a high efficacy against adults and developing stages of *O. ostertagi* and *T. axei* (LYONS et al. 1981); efficacy against *Nematodirus* is moderate (ARMOUR et al. 1980; LYONS et al. 1981a).

Efficacy against inhibited larvae of *O. ostertagi* at a dose of 0.2 mg/kg given subcutaneously is very high (ARMOUR et al. 1980; WILLIAMS et al. 1981c; ELLIOTT and JULIAN 1981).

b) Sheep and Goats

Ivermectin at a dose of 0.1 mg/kg given orally was very effective against *H. contortus, O. circumcincta, T. axei, T. colubriformis, C. curticei, O. columbianum,* and inhibited larvae of *Cooperia.* A dose of 0.2 mg/kg was necessary for a high efficacy against developing and inhibited larvae of *O. circumcincta.* The *H. contortus* and *T. colubriformis* strains used in this test were benzimidazole resistant (EGERTON et al. 1980). Given subcutaneously at a dose of 0.2 mg/kg ivermectin was very effective against adult *H. contortus, O. circumcincta, Marshallagia marshalli, T. axei, T. colubriformis,* and *C. curticei.* Efficacy against *Nematodirus* spp. was moderate. The *Haemonchus* strain was benzimidazole resistant (WESCOTT and LEAMASTER 1982).

A high efficacy of 0.1 mg/kg administered by intraruminal injection was found against *Haemonchus, Ostertagia,* and *Trichostrongylus* in goats (HALL et al. 1981b). The *Trichostrongylus* strain used in this test was resistant against oxfendazole and levamisole.

References

Ames ER, Hutchinson HD (1973) Safety and efficacy of thiabendazole (TBZ) in protein blocks. Vet Med Small Anim Clin 68:1376–1381

Ames ER, Cheney JM, Rubin R (1963) The efficacy of thiabendazole and bephenium hydroxynaphthoate against *Ostertagia ostertagi* and *Cooperia oncophora* in experimentally infected calves. Am J Vet Res 24:295–299

Ames ER, Rubin R, Cheney JM (1966) A critical evaluation of the efficacy of thiabendazole against important helminths of cattle. Vet Med Small Anim Clin 61:66–70

Anderson N (1977) The efficiency of levamisole, thiabendazole and fenbendazole against naturally acquired infections of *Ostertagia ostertagi* in cattle. Res Vet Sci 23:298–302

Anderson N, Laby RH (1979) Activity against *Ostertagia ostertagi* of low doses of oxfendazole continuously released from intraruminal capsules in cattle. Aust Vet J 55:244–246

Anderson N, Lord V (1979) Anthelmintic efficiency of oxfendazole, fenbendazole and levamisole against naturally acquired infections of *Ostertagia ostertagi* and *Trichostrongylus axei* in cattle. Aust Vet J 55:158–162

Anderson N, Laby RH, Prichard RK, Hennessy D (1980) Controlled release of anthelmintic drugs: a new concept for prevention of helminthosis in sheep. Res Vet Sci 29:333–341

Anderson PJS (1968) The anthelmintic efficacy of pyrantel tartrate. JS Afr Vet Med Assoc 39:47–54

Anderson PJS, Marais TS (1972) The anthelmintic efficacy of morantel tartrate in sheep and goats. JS Afr Vet Assoc 43:271–285

Anderson PJS, Marais FS (1975) The control of adult parasitic nematodes of cattle with morantel tartrate. JS Afr Vet Assoc 46:325–329

Anonymous (1978) Cambendazole poisoning. Vet Rec 103:219

Armour J, Duncan JL, Reid JFS (1978) Activity of oxfendazole against inhibited larvae of *Ostertagia ostertagi* and *Cooperia oncophora.* Vet Rec 102:263–264

Armour J, Bairden K, Preston JM (1980) Anthelmintic efficiency of ivermectin against naturally acquired bovine gastrointestinal nematodes. Vet Rec 107:226–227

Armour J, Bairden K, Duncan JL, Jones RM, Bliss DH (1981) Studies on the control of bovine ostertagiasis using a morantel sustained release bolus. Vet Rec 108:532–535

Baines DM, Bell PDM (1980) The efficacy of thiophanate in natural nematode infestations of sheep and cattle. Aust Vet J 56:350–351

Baines DM, Colegrave AJ (1977) Field trials in sheep with the anthelmintic thiophanate. Vet Rec 100:217–219

Baker NF, Douglas JR (1962) Critical trials with thiabendazole as an anthelmintic in the gastrointestinal tract of cattle and sheep. Am J Vet Res 23:1219–1223

Baker NF, Fisk RA (1972) Levamisole as an anthelmintic in calves. Am J Vet Res 33:1121–1125

Baker NF, Fisk RA, Miller JE (1978) Anthelmintic efficacy of oxfendazole in calves. Am J Vet Res 39:1258–1261

Behrens H, Matschullat G (1975) Prüfung des Anthelminthikums Fenbendazole bei natürlich infizierten Schafen. Dtsch Tierärztl Wochenschr 82:58–63

Benz GW (1973) Evaluation of paste form of cambendazole and thiabendazole for administration of calves. Am J Vet Res 34:35–37

Benz GW, Ernst JV (1977) Anthelmintic activity of albendazole against gastrointestinal nematodes in calves. Am J Vet Res 38:1425–1426

Benz GW, Ernst JV (1981) Anthelmintic efficacy of 22,23 dihydroavermectin B_1 against gastrointestinal nematodes in calves. Am J Vet Res 42:1409–1411

Berger J (1980) Oxfendazole: anthelmintic activity in sheep artificially infected with nematodes. Results of trials against nine species including benzimidazole resistant *Haemonchus contortus*. JS Afr Vet Assoc 51:51–58

Berndtson WE, Chenoweth PJ, Olar TT, Pickett BW, Seidel GE (1980) Influence of albendazole on reproductive function of bulls. Am J Vet Res 41:640–644

Borgsteede FHM (1974) Activity of parbendazole against gastrointestinal nematodes in calves (in Dutch). Tijdschr Diergeneeskd 99:991–995

Borgsteede FHM (1977) A field trial with a new anthelmintic oxfendazole in naturally infected calves. Tijdschr Diergeneeskd 102:801–804

Borgsteede FHM (1979) The activity of albendazole against adult and larval gastrointestinal nematodes in naturally infected calves in the Netherlands. Vet Q 1:181–188

Borgsteede FHM (1981) The efficacy of oxfendazole administered as a bolus compared with a drench formulation. Vet Q 3:101–103

Borgsteede FHM, Kloosterman A (1977) Epidemiologie en profylaxe van trichostrongylose bij het rund. Tijdschr Diergeneeskd 102:1428–1436

Borgsteede FHM, Oostendorp D, Burg WPJ Van den, Harmsen HE, Tarrij H Van (1981) Profylaxe van maagdarmworminfecties door middel van het Paratect bolus systeem. Tijdschr Diergeneeskd 106:1255–1264

Brooker PJ, Goose J (1975) Dermal application of levamisole to sheep and cattle. Vet Rec 96:249–250

Bürger HJ (1978) Efficacy of febantel in sheep experimentally infected with five species of gastrointestinal nematodes. Vet Rec 103:572–574

Bürger HJ, Jones RM, Bliss DH (1981) Mehrmonatige Meta- und Prophylaxe der parasitären Gastroenteritis bei Kälbern durch Gabe eines Paratect – Langzeitbolus vor dem Austrieb. Berl Münch Tierärztl Wochenschr 94:311–319

Cairns GC (1961) The efficacy of thiabendazole (MK 360) as an anthelmintic in sheep. NZ Vet J 9:147–152

Callinan APL, Barton NJ (1979) Efficacies of thiabendazole and levamisole against sheep nematodes in Western Victoria. Aust Vet J 55:255

Callinan APL, Cummins LJ (1979) Efficacy of anthelmintics against cattle nematodes. Aust Vet J 55:370–373

Campbell NJ, Hotson JK (1971) The anthelmintic efficiency of clioxanide and rafoxanide against *Fasciola hepatica* and *Haemonchus contortus* in sheep. Aust Vet J 47:5–8

Chalmers K (1977) The efficacy of oxfendazole against natural infections of nematodes and cestodes in sheep. NZ Vet J 25:266–269

Chalmers K (1978) The efficacy of oxfendazole against natural infections of nematodes in cattle. NZ Vet J 26:162–164

Chroust K, Dyk V (1975) Zur Wirksamkeit von Fenbendazole, Thiabendazole und Tetramisole auf Magen- und Darmnematoden der Wiederkäuer. Dtsch Tierärztl Wochenschr 82:487–490

Ciordia H (1972) Activity of a feed premix and crumbles containing coumaphos in the control of gastrointestinal parasites of cattle. Am J Vet Res 33:623–626

Ciordia H, McCampbell HC (1973) Anthelmintic activity of morantel tartrate in calves. Am J Vet Res 34:619–620

Colglazier ML, Kates KC, Enzie FD (1971 a) Activity of levamisole pyrantel tartrate and rafoxanide against two thiabendazole-tolerant isolates of *Haemonchus contortus* and two species of *Trichostrongylus* in sheep. Proc Helm Soc Wash 38:203–205

Colglazier ML, Kates KC, Enzie FD, Lindahl JL, Samuelson G (1971 b) Comparative activity of pyrantel tartrate, parbendazole and levamisole at two dose levels against naturally acquired helminth infections in sheep. J Parasitol 57:1078–1082

Colglazier ML, Kates KC, Enzie FD (1974) Cambendazole-resistant *Haemonchus contortus* strain in sheep: further experimental development. J Parasitol 60:289–292

Conway DP, De Goosh C, Arakawa A (1973) Anthelmintic efficacy of morantel tartrate in cattle. Am J Vet Res 34:621–622

Cornwell RL (1966) Controlled laboratory trials in sheep with the anthelmintic pyrantel tartrate. Vet Rec 79:590–595

Cornwell RL, Jones RM (1970a) Controlled laboratory trials with pyrantel tartrate in cattle. Br Vet J 126:134–141
Cornwell RL, Jones RM (1970b) Controlled laboratory trials in sheep with the anthelmintic morantel. Br Vet J 126:142–148
Craig TM, Bell RR (1978) Evaluation of fenbendazole as an anthelmintic for gastrointestinal nematodes of cattle. Am J Vet Res 39:1037–1038
Craig TM, Shepherd E (1980) Efficacy of albendazole and levamisole in sheep against *Thysanosoma actinioides* and *Haemonchus contortus* from the Edwards Plateau, Texas. Am J Vet Res 41:425–426
Crowley JW, Todd AC, Bliss DH, Kennedy TJ (1976) Efficacy of oxibendazole against adult and larval nematodes of cattle. Am J Vet Res 37:1285–1286
Crowley JW, Foreyt WJ, Bliss DH, Todd AC (1977) Further controlled evaluations of fenbendazole as a bovine anthelmintic. Am J Vet Res 38:689–692
Cummins LJ, Callinan APL (1979) Effects of levamisole and human chorionic gonadotrophin on ostertagiasis in western Victoria, Australia. Vet Rec 104:77–78
Curr C (1977) The effect of dermally applied levamisole against the parasitic nematodes of cattle. Aust Vet J 53:425–428
Dalton SE (1978) Thiophanate as a low daily dosage anthelmintic in sheep. Vet Rec 130:131–134
Delatour P, Lorgue G, Lapras M, Deschanel JP (1974) Propriétés embryotoxiques (rat) et résidus (ovins, bovins) de trois anthelminthiques dérivés du benzimidazole. Bull Soc Sci Vet Med Comp 76:147–154
Delatour P, Lorgue G, Lapras M, Richard Y, Nain, Cantenot G (1975) Mise en évidence des propriétés antimitotiques du cambendazole. Bull Soc Vét Méd Comp Lyon 77:185–194
Delatour P, Lorgue G, Courtot D, Lapras M (1976) Tolérance embryonnaire de l'oxibendazole chez le rat et le mouton. Rec Méd Vét 152:467–470
Delatour P, Debroye J, Lorgue G, Courtot D (1977) Embryotoxicité expérimentale de l'oxfendazole chez le rat et le mouton. Rec Méd Vét 153:639–645
Delatour P, Parish RC, Guyrik RJ (1981) Albendazole: a comparison of relay embryotoxicity with embryotoxicity of individual metabolites. Ann Rech Vét 12:159–167
Dorchies PO, Ducos De Lahitte J, France M (1981) Contrôle de l'activité anthelminthique du levamisole administré par voie transcutanée aux bovins. Rev Méd Vét 132:341–347
Downey NE (1976) Evaluation of oxfendazole against natural infections of gastrointestinal nematodes and lung-worms in calves. Vet Rec 99:267–270
Downey NE (1977) Controlled trials of the anthelmintic oxfendazole in ewes and lambs naturally infected with gastrointestinal nematodes. Vet Rec 101:260–263
Downey NE (1978) Action of albendazole on gastrointestinal nematodes in naturally infected calves. Vet Rec 103:427–428
Drudge JH, Leland SE, Wyant ZN (1957) Strain variation in the response of sheep nematodes to the action of phenothiazine. I Studies of mixed infections in experimental animals. Am J Vet Res 18:133–141
Drudge JH, Szanto J, Wyant ZN, Elam G (1964) Field studies on parasite control in sheep: comparison of thiabendazole, ruelene and phenothiazine. Am J Vet Res 25:1512–1518
Duncan JL, Armour J, Bairden K, Jennings FW, Urquhart GM (1976) The successful removal of inhibited fourth stage *Ostertagia ostertagi* larvae by fenbendazole. Vet Rec 98:342
Duncan JL, Armour J, Bairden K (1978) Autumn and winter fenbendazole treatment against inhibited 4th stage *Ostertagia ostertagi* larvae in cattle. Vet Rec 103:211–212
Duncan JL, Armour J, Bairden K (1979) The efficacy of thiophanate against gastrointestinal nematodes of cattle including inhibited larvae of *Ostertagia ostertagi*. Vet Rec 105:444–445
Edwards JR, De Chaneet G (1980) Resistance of *Haemonchus contortus* to thiophanate. Res Vet Sci 29:370–372
Egerton JR, Yakstis J, Campbell WC (1970) The efficacy of rafoxanide (3,5-diiodo-3-chloro-4-(*p*-chlorophenoxy) salicylanilide) against *Haemonchus contortus* in sheep. Res Vet Sci 11:382–384

Egerton JR, Birnbaum J, Blair LS, Chabala JC, Conroy J, Fisher MH, Mrozik H, Ostlind DA, Wilkins CA, Campbell WC (1980) 22,23-Dihydroavermectin B1, a new broad-spectrum antiparasitic agent. Br Vet J 136:88–97

Egerton JR, Eary CH, Suhayda D (1981) The anthelmintic efficacy of ivermectin in experimentally infected cattle. Vet Parasitol 8:59–70

Eichler DA (1973) The anthelmintic activity of thiophanate in sheep and cattle. Br Vet J 129:533–543

Elliot DC (1977) The effect of fenbendazole in removing inhibited early-fourth-stage *Ostertagia ostertagi* from yearling cattle. NZ Vet J 25:145–147

Elliot DC, Julian AF (1981) The removal of inhibited early fourth stage *Ostertagia ostertagi* from yearling cattle by MK 933, an ivermectin formulation. NZ Vet J 29:68–69

Enigk K, Dey-Hazra A, Batke J (1975) Zur Wirksamkeit von Fenbendazole auf den Magen-Darmstrongyliden- und Lungenwurmbefall des Rindes. Dtsch Tierärztl Wochenschr 82:137–139

Eysker M, Hendrikx WML (1977) Epidemiologie van trichostrongyliden infecties en profylaxe van trichostrongylose bij het schaap in Nederland. Tijdschr Diergeneeskd 102:1441–1449

Fabiyi JP, Oluyede DA, Negedu JO (1979) Thiophanate in the treatment of *Cooperia punctata, C. pectinata* and *Haemonchus contortus*. Vet Rec 105:375

Forsyth BA (1968) The anthelmintic activity of the optical isomers of tetramisole in sheep and cattle. Aust Vet 44:395–397

Forsyth BA, Gibbon AJ (1980) The anthelmintic efficacy of half-dose rates of levamisole against benzimidazole resistant *Haemonchus contortus*. Aust Vet J 56:203–204

Forsyth BA, Sheperd GE (1977) The clinical assessment of levamisole and fenbendazole in the treatment of type II ostertagiasis. Aust Vet J 53:598–599

Gaenssler JG, Wilkins CA, O'Donnovan WM (1978) The divided dosage/low dosage concept using fenbendazole. JS Afr Vet Assoc 49:345–349

Gibson TE (1975) Veterinary anthelmintic medication, 3rd edn. Commonwealth Institute of Helminthology, St. Albans

Gibson TE, Parfitt JW (1968) An evaluation of the anthelmintic pyrantel tartrate using the improved controlled test. Br Vet J 124:69–71

Gordon HMcL (1958) Studies on anthelmintics for sheep. Some organic phosphorus compounds. Aust Vet J 34:104–110

Gordon HMcL (1974) Disophenol (2,6-diiodo-4-nitrophenol) a remarkable anthelmintic. Proc Third Int Congr Parasitol 3:1392–1393

Green PE, Forsyth BA, Rowan KJ, Payne G (1981) The isolation of a field stain of *Haemonchus contortus* in Queensland showing multiple anthelmintic resistance. Aust Vet J 57:79–84

Grelck H, Hörchner F, Wöhrl H (1980) Zur Wirkung von Rintal gegen Lungen- und Magendarmwürmer des Rindes. Vet Med Nachr No 2:154–159

Grimbeek P, Terblanche HJJ (1980) A re-assessment of the efficacy of febantel (Rintal) and fenbendazole (Panacur) against *Strongyloides papillosus* in sheep and goats. JS Afr Vet Assoc 51:49

Grimshaw WTR, Bonnazi E, Armour J (1981) Studies on the interaction between immunity to *Dictyocaulus viviparus* and a morantel slow release rumen device. Proc 9th Int Conf WAAVP, Budapest, pp 63

Guilhon J, Graber M, Birgi E (1970) Action du nitroxynil sur divers parasites du Zebu en Afrique Central. Rev Elev Méd Vét Pays Trop 23:347–359

Guilhon J, Caillier R, Hubert J (1972) Action d'un nouveau dérivé de l'imidazole sur les nématodes parasites du tube digestif du mouton. Bull Acad Vet France 45:445–452

Hall CA, Kelly JD, Campbell NJ, Whitlock HV, Martin ICA (1978) The dose response of several benzimidazole anthelmintics against resistant strain of *Haemonchus contortus* and *Trichostrongylus colubriformis* selected with thiabendazole. Res Vet Sci 25:364–367

Hall CA, Campbell NJ, Carrol SN (1979) Resistance to thiabendazole in a field population of *Ostertagia circumcincta* from sheep. Aust Vet J 55:229–231

Hall CA, Graham MJ, McDonell PA (1980) Anthelmintic activity of closantel against benzimidazole resistant strains of *Haemonchus contortus* and *Trichostrongylus colubriformis* in sheep. Aust Vet J 56:461–462

Hall CA, Kelly JD, Whitlock HV, Ritchie L (1981a) Prolonged anthelmintic effect of closantel and disophenol against a thiabendazole selected resistant strain of *Haemonchus contortus* in sheep. Res Vet Sci 31:104–106

Hall CA, Ritchie L, McDonell PA (1981b) Investigations for anthelmintic resistance in gastrointestinal nematodes from goats. Res Vet Sci 31:116–119

Hart JA, James PS, Curr C (1969) The anthelmintic efficiency of laevo-tetramisolehydrochloride against nematode parasites of sheep and cattle. Aust Vet J 45:73–77

Hebden SP (1961) The anthelmintic activity of thiabendazole (MK 360) Aust Vet J 37:264–269

Herlich H (1975) Efficacy of oxibendazole as an anthelmintic in cattle. Proc Helm Soc Wash 42:135–137

Herlich H (1977) Anthelmintic efficacy of albendazole in cattle: comparison of critical and controlled test. Am J Vet Res 38:1247–1248

Hogarth-Scott RS, Kelly JD, Whitlock HV, Ng BKY, Thompson HG (1976) The anthelmintic efficacy of fenbendazole against thiabendazole resistant strains of *Haemonchus contortus* and *Trichostrongylus colubriformis* in sheep. Res Vet Sci 21:232–237

Hopkins TJ, Rafferty M (1978) Die anthelminthische Wirksamkeit von Febantel gegen Magendarmwürmer beim Schaf. Vet Med Nachr No. 2:154–159

Horak JG, Louw JP, Raymond SM, Snijders AJ (1970) The anthelmintic efficacy of feed mash or pellets medicated with thiabendazole. JS Afr Vet Med Assoc 41:307–312

Horak IG, Snijders AJ, Louw JP (1972) Trials with rafoxanide 5. Efficacy studies against *Fasciola hepatica, Fasciola gigantica, Paramphistomum microbothrium* and various nematodes in sheep. JS Afr Vet Assoc 43:397–403

Hotson K, Campbell NJ, Smeal MG (1970) Anthelmintic resistance in *Trichostrongylus colubriformis*. Aust Vet J 46:356–360

Hsu WH (1980) Toxicity and drug interactions of levamisole. J Am Vet Med Assoc 176:1166–1169

Inderbitzin F, Eckert J (1978) Die Wirkung von Fenbendazole (Panacur) gegen gehemmte Stadien von *Dictyocaulus viviparus* und *Ostertagia ostertagi* bei Kälbern. Berl Munch Tierarztl Wochenschr 91:395–399

Jacobs DE, Fox MT, Walker MJ, Jones RM, Bliss DH (1981) Field evaluation of a new method for the prophylaxis of parasitic gastroenteritis in calves. Vet Rec 108:274–276

Jarret WFH, Urquhart GM, Bairden K (1980) Treatment of bovine parasitic bronchitis. Vet Rec 106:135

Jones RM (1981a) A field study of the morantel sustained release bolus in the seasonal control of parasitic gastroenteritis in grazing calves. Vet Parasitol 8:237–251

Jones RM (1981b) The effect of the use of the Paratect bolus on host immunity. Pfizer Congress, Budapest

Jones RM, Bliss DH (1981) The effect of repeated use of the morantel sustained release bolus (MSRB) on the susceptibility of *Ostertagia ostertagi* to morantel. Proc 9th Int Conf WAAVP Budapest, p 59

Jones RM, Pott JM, Cornwell RL (1978) Low level feed administration of morantel tartrate in prophylaxis of experimental nematode infections in lamb and calves. Br Vet J 134:166–170

Johns and Philip (1977) Albendazole: Safety in sheep. Abstr 8th conference of the WVAAP, Sydney

Keith RK (1964) Subcutaneous injection of an organic phosphorus compound as an anthelmintic procedure for cattle. Aust Vet J 40:402–405

Kelly JD, Chevis RAF, Whitlock HV (1975a) The anthelmintic efficacy of mebendazole against *Fasciola hepatica* and a concurrent mixed nematode infection in sheep. NZ Vet J 23:81–84

Kelly JD, Whitlock HV, Hogarth-Scott RS, Mears FA (1975b) The anthelmintic efficacy of fenbendazole against a mixed nematode infection in sheep. Res Vet Sci 19:105–107

Kelly JD, Hall CA, Whitlock HV, Thompson HG, Campbell NJ, Martin ICA (1977) The effect of route of administration on the anthelmintic efficacy of benzimidazole anthelmintics in sheep infected with strains of *Haemonchus contortus* and *Trichostrongylus colubriformis* resistant or susceptible to thiabendazole. Res Vet Sci 22:161–168

Kennedy TJ, Todd AC (1975) Efficacy of fenbendazole against gastrointestinal parasites of sheep. Am J Vet Res 36:1465–1467

Kingsbury PA, Rowlands DT (1981) Persistence of anthelmintic activity after administration of oxfendazole and levamisole hydrochloride to lambs. Vet Rec 109:104

Kistner TP, Wyse D (1975) Anthelmintic efficacy of injectable levamisole in sheep. Proc Helm Soc Wash 42:93–97

Kistner TP, Wyse D (1978) Efficacy of oxfendazole against an ovine isolate of benzimidazole resistant *Haemonchus contortus*. Aust Vet J 54:469–470

Kistner TP, Wyse D, Averkin E (1979) Efficacy of oxfendazole against inhibited *Ostertagia ostertagi* in naturally infected cattle. Aust Vet J 55:232–235

Krause D, Reinhard HJ, Köhler W, Tiefenbach B (1975) Untersuchungen über die Wirkung des Anthelminthikums Fenbendazol auf die Spermaqualität von Besamungsbullen. Dtsch Tierarztl Wochenschr 82:231–233

Lancaster MB, Hong C (1977) Action of fenbendazole on arrested fourth stage larvae of *Ostertagia ostertagi*. Vet Res 101:81–82

Langeler JET (1966) The action of methyridine ("Mintic" ICI) and thiabendazole ("Thibenzole", MSD) on *Cooperia* in calves (in Dutch) Tijdschr Diergeneeskd 91:658–673

Lapras M, Deschanel JP, Delatour P, Gastellu J, Lombard M (1973) Accidents tératologiques chez le mouton après administration de parbendazole. Bull Soc Sci Vét Méd Comp 75:53–61

Leimbacher F, Nicolas JA, Delahaye J (1976) Expérimentation dans les conditions d'élevage de l'oxfendazole un nouvel anthelminthique pour lutter contre les „strongyloses" gastro-intestinales des agneaux à l'herbe. Rev Méd Vét 127:941–957

Le Jambre LF (1979) Effectiveness of anthelmintic treatments against levamisole-resistant *Ostertagia*. Aust Vet J 55:65–67

Le Jambre LF, Barger JA (1979) Efficiency of rafoxanide and naphthalophos against inhibited *Haemonchus contortus*. Aust Vet J 55:346–347

Le Jambre LF, Martin PJ (1979) Effectiveness of morantel tartrate and naphthalophos against levamisole resistant *Ostertagia* in sheep. Vet Sci Comm 3:153–158

Le Jambre LF, Prichard RK, Hennessy DR, Laby RH (1981) Efficiency of oxfendazole administered as a single dose or in a controlled release capsule against benzimidazole-resistant *Haemonchus contortus*, *Ostertagia circumcincta* and *Trichostrongylus colubriformis*. Res Vet Sci 31:289–294

Lucas JMS (1971) The anthelmintic activity of nitroxynil (4-hydroxy-3-iodo-5-nitrobenzonitrite) against parasitic nematodes in ruminants. Res Vet Sci 12:500–502

Lyons ET, Drudge JH, Knapp FW (1967) Controlled test of anthelmintic activity of trichlorfon and thiabendazole in lambs with observations on *Oestrus ovis*. Am J Vet Res 28:1111–1116

Lyons ET, Drudge JH, La Bore DE, Tolliver SC (1972) Field and controlled test evaluations of levamisole against natural infections of gastrointestinal nematodes and lungworms in calves. Am J Vet Res 33:65–71

Lyons ET, Drudge JH, Tolliver SC (1974) Controlled test of parbendazole and thiabendazole against natural infections of gastrointestinal helminths of lambs. Am J Vet Res 35:1065–1070

Lyons ET, Drudge JH, La Bore DE, Tolliver SC (1975) Controlled test of activity of levamisole administered to calves via drinking water, subcutaneous injection or alfalfa pellet premix. Am J Vet Res 36:777–780

Lyons ET, Tolliver SC, Drudge JH, La Bore DE, (1981a) Ivermectin: controlled test of anthelmintic activity in dairy calves with emphasis on *Dictyocaulus viviparus*. Am J Vet Res 42:1225–1227

Lyons ET, Tolliver SC, Drudge JH, Hemken RW, Buttons FS (1981 b) Efficacy of levamisole against abomasal nematodes and lungworms in dairy calves: preliminary test indicating reduced activity for *Ostertagia ostertagi*. Am J Vet Res 42:1228–1230

Lyons ET, Tolliver SC, Drudge JH, Hemken RW, Button FS (1981 c) Reduced activity of levamisole against *Ostertagia ostertagi* in dairy calves. Mod Vet Pract 62:847–850

Main DC, Vass DE (1980) Cambendazole toxicity in calves. Aust Vet J 56:237–238

Marriner SE, Bogan JA (1981) Pharmacokinetics of fenbendazole in sheep. Am J Vet Res 42:1146–1148

McBeath DG, Best JMJ, Preston NK (1977) The treatment of ostertagiasis type II in cattle using fenbendazole in feed blocks. Vet Rec 101:285

McBeath DG, Preston NK, Thompson F (1979) Studies in sheep on the efficacy of fenbendazole administered via a feed-block carrier. Br Vet J 135:271–278

McEwan AD, Oakley GA, Robinson M (1979) Effect of anthelmintics on the pathology of *Dictyocaulus viviparus* infection in cattle. Vet Rec 105:15–16

McKenna PB (1974) The anthelmintic efficacy of thiabendazole and levamisole against inhibited *Haemonchus contortus* larvae in sheep. NZ Vet J 22:163–167

Michael SA, Higgins AJ, Refajj AH El (1979) Oxfendazole-anthelmintic activity in Egyptian goats artificially infected with gastrointestinal nematodes. Trop Anim Health Prod 11:63–68

Michel JF, Latham JO, Church BM, Leech PK (1981) Use of anthelmintics for cattle in England and Wales during 1978. Vet Rec 108:252–258

Middleton HD, Plant JW, Walker CE, Dixon ET, Johns DR (1974) The effect of methyl-5(6) butyl-2-benzimidazole carbamate (parbendazole) on the reproduction in sheep and other animals. Teratological study in ewes in Australia. Cornell Vet 64:56–68

Ogunsusi RA (1979) The anthelmintic efficacy of oxfendazole and haloxon against arrested *Haemonchus contortus* larvae in sheep. Res Vet Sci 27:131–132

Pearson JG, Whitlock HV, Goosh CP De, Farrington KJ, Jones RC, Haigh JA (1970) Clioxanide a new anthelmintic against *Fasciola hepatica* and *Haemonchus contortus* in sheep. Aust Vet J 46:480–484

Pfeiffer H, Supperer R (1976) Zur Wirksamkeit von Fenbendazole gegen *Nematodirus helvetianus* des Rindes. Berl Munch Tierarztl Wochenschr 89:249–252

Piercy DWT, Reynolds J, Brown PRM (1979) Reproductive safety studies of oxfendazole in sheep and cattle. Br Vet J 135:405–410

Pott JM, Jones RM, Cornwell RL (1979) Observations on parasitic gastroenteritis and bronchitis in grazing calves: effect of low level feed incorporation of morantel in early season. Int J Parasitol 9:153–157

Prichard RK, Donald AD, Dash KM, Hennessy DR (1978) Factors involved in the relative anthelmintic tolerance of arrested 4th stage larvae of *Ostertagia ostertagi*. Vet Rec 102:382

Prozesky L, Pienaar JG (1977) Amaurosis in sheep resulting from treatment with rafoxanide, Onderstepoort. J Vet Res 44:257–260

Prozesky L, Joubert JPJ, Ekron MD (1981) Paralysis in lambs caused by overdosing with parbendazole, Onderstepoort. J Vet Res 48:159–167

Raynaud JP (1968) Strongylose digestive des bovins. Essais d'efficacité du pyrantel réalisés en France dans les strongyloses mixtes. Rec Méd Vét 144:963–982

Reid JFS, Duncan JL, Bairden K (1976) Efficacy of levamisole against inhibited larvae of *Ostertagia* spp. in sheep. Vet Rec 98:426–427

Reinecke RK, Bruckner C, Villiers IL De (1981) A residual anthelmintic 2,6-diiodo-4-nitrophenol (disophenol): methods of testing its anthelmintic efficacy. JS Afr Vet Assoc 52:195–200

Restani R, Borelli D (1968) Richerche sulla attiva del tiabendazole nella infestazione sperimentale da *Strongyloides papillosus* dei vitelli. Atti Soc Ital Sci Vet 22:722–725

Ribbeck R, Winter J (1977) Ziegen als Versuchstiere – Untersuchungen zur Magen-Darm-Nematoden. Bekämpfung mit Mebendazole. Monath Veterinärmed 33:706–707

Ross DB (1968) Parbendazole. Effect on *Haemonchus contortus, Ostertagia circumcincta, Trichostrongylus colubriformis* and *Nematodirus battus* in experimentally-infected lambs. Vet Rec 82:731–735

Ross DB (1970) The effect of oral parbendazole against *Ostertagia ostertagi* and *Cooperia punctata* in experimentally infected calves. Vet Rec 86:60–61
Ross DB (1975) The effect of fenbendazole on nematode parasites in experimentally infected lambs. Vet Rec 96:357–359
Ross DB, Eichler DA, Cameron D (1978) The effect of albendazole on nematode parasites in experimentally infected lambs. Vet Rec 102:556–557
Rowlands DT, Berger J (1977) Levamisole: anthelmintic activity in calves following dermal application. JS Afr Vet Assoc 48:85–93
Rubin R (1968) Efficacy of parbendazole against *Ostertagia, Trichostrongylus* and *Cooperia* spp. in cattle. Am J Vet Res 29:1385–1389
Rubin R (1969) Treatment of gastrointestinal parasitism of cattle with parbendazole. J Am Vet Med Assoc 154:177–180
Rubin R, Ames ER, Cheney JM (1965) The efficacy of thiabendazole against *Cooperia oncophora, Cooperia punctata* and *Ostertagia ostertagi* in cattle. Am J Vet Res 26:668–672
Sangster NC, Whitlock HV, Russ JG, Gunawan M, Griffin DL, Kelly JD (1979) *Trichostrongylus colubriformis* and *Ostertagia circumcincta* resistant to levamisole, morantel tartrate and thiabendazole: occurrence in a field strain. Res Vet Sci 27:106–110
Saunders LZ, Shone DK, Philip JR, Birkhead HA (1974) The effect of methyl-5(6) butyl-2-benzimidazole carbamate (parbendazole) on the reproduction in sheep and other animals. Malformations in newborn lambs. Cornell Vet 64:7–10
Schröder J, Honer MR, Louw JP (1977) Trials with rafoxanide 8. Efficacy of an injectable solution against trematodes and nematodes in cattle. JS Afr Vet Assoc 48:95–97
Searson JE, Doughty FR (1977) The efficiency of fenbendazole in the treatment of naturally acquired nematode infections in cattle. Aust Vet J 53:456–457
Shone K, Philip JR, Fricker JM (1979) The effect of methyl-5(6) butyl-2-benzimidazole carbamate (parbendazole) on the reproduction in sheep and other animals. Teratological study in ewes in South Africa. Cornell Vet 64:69–76
Snijders AJ, Horak JG (1975) Trials with rafoxanide 7. Efficacy against *Fasciola hepatica, Haemonchus placei* and *Bunostomum phlebotomum* in cattle. JS Afr Vet Assoc 46:265–267
Snijders AJ, Louw JP (1966) A comparison of anthelmintics administered intraruminally in sheep. JS Afr Vet Med Assoc 37:121–131
Snijders AJ, Horak JG, Louw JP (1971) Trial with rafoxanide 2. Efficacy against *Fasciola gigantica* in cattle. JS Afr Vet Med Assoc 42:253–257
Snijders AJ, Horak JG, Louw JP (1973) Trials with rafoxanide 6. The effect of repeated and single treatments with rafoxanide against *Haemonchus contortus* and *Oestrus ovis* in sheep. JS Afr Vet Assoc 44:251–263
Soetedjo R, Beriajaya D, Henderson AWK, Kelly JD (1980) Use of disophenol for the control of *Haemonchus contortus* in sheep in West Java, Indonesia. Trop Anim Health Prod 12:198–202
Stoimenoff K, Stephanoff S (1975) Wirksamkeit von Pyranteltartrat auf den Hakenwurmbefall des Schafes. Prakt Tierarzt 56:288–289
Stoye M, Enigk K, Bürger HJ (1971) Die Wirkung von Cambendazole bei experimentellen *Ostertagia*- und *Cooperia*-Infektionen des Rindes. Tierärztl Umschau 26:108–110
Szabo KT, Miller CR, Scott GC (1974) The effect of methyl-5(6) butyl-2-benzimidazole carbamate (parbendazole) on the reproduction in sheep and other animals. Teratological study of ewes in the USA. Cornell Vet 64:41–55
Terblanche HJJ (1978) Versuche mit Rintal (Febantel) Wirkung auf die Fruchtbarkeit von Schafböcken. Vet Med Nachr No. 2:180–185
Theodorides VJ, Chang J, DiCullo CJ, Grass GM (1973) Oxibendazole, a new broad spectrum anthelmintic effective against gastrointestinal nematodes of domestic animals. Br Vet J 129:XCVII–XCVIII
Theodorides VJ, Parish RC, Fuchsman CH, Lee RM (1974) Bromoxanide, a new anthelmintic. Vet Rec 95:84–85
Theodorides VJ, Nawalinski T, Freeman JF, Murphy JR (1976 a) Efficacy of oxibendazole against gastrointestinal nematodes of cattle. Am J Vet Res 37:1207–1209

Theodorides VJ, Nawalinski T, Chang J (1976b) Efficacy of albendazole against *Haemonchus, Nematodirus, Dictyocaulus* and *Moniezia* of sheep. Am J Vet Res 37:1515–1516
Theodorides VJ, Nawalinski T, Murphy J, Freeman J (1976c) Efficacy of albendazole against gastrointestinal nematodes of cattle. Am J Vet Res 37:1517–1518
Theodorides VJ, DiCuollo CJ, Nawalinski T, Miller CR, Murphy JR, Freeman JF, Killeen JC, Rapp WR (1977) Toxicologic and teratologic studies of oxibendazole in ruminants and laboratory animals. Am J Vet Res 38:809–814
Thomas H (1978 a) The efficacy of febantel on gastrointestinal nematodes in sheep. Res Vet Sci 25:290–293
Thomas RJ (1978 b) The efficacy of in-feed medication with fenbendazole against gastrointestinal nematodes of sheep, with particular reference to inhibited larvae. Vet Rec 102:394–397
Thomas RJ, Reid JFS (1980) Efficacy of oxfendazole against *Nematodirus battus* and inhibited stages of sheep nematodes. Res Vet Sci 28:134–136
Tiefenbach B (1975) Fenbendazole [Methyl (5-(phenyl-thio)-benzimidazole-2-carbamat) Prüfung der Teratogenität an Schafen in Feldversuchen. 20th World Vet Congr vol 1, Thessaloniki, p 172
Todd AC, Bliss D, Scholl P, Crowley JW (1976) Controlled evaluation of fenbendazole as a bovine anthelmintic. Am J Vet Res 37:439–441
Todd KS, Mansfield ME (1979) Evaluation of four forms of oxfendazole against nematodes of cattle. Am J Vet Res 40:423–424
Urquhart GM, Jarret WFH, Bairden K, Bonazzi EF (1981) Control of parasitic bronchitis in calves: vaccination or treatment? Vet Rec 108:180–182
Van Schalkwijk PC, Geyser TL, Récio M, Erasmus FPG (1979) The anthelmintic efficacy of albendazole against gastrointestinal roundworms, lungworms and liverflukes in sheep. JS Afr Vet Assoc 50:31–35
Van Wijk JA, Gerber HM (1980) A field strain of *Haemonchus contortus* showing slight resistance to rafoxanide, Onderstepoort. Am J Vet Res 47:137–142
Varga J, Janisch M (1975) Anthelmintic efficacy of mebendazole against gastrointestinal nematodes in sheep (in Hungarian). Magyar Állatorvosok Lapja 30:336–343
Vlassoff A, Kettle PR (1980) Benzimidazole resistance in *Haemonchus contortus.* NZ Vet J 28:23–24
Wallnöfer E (1977) Ein Beitrag zur Parasitenbekämpfung bei Schafen in Österreich. Wien. Tierärztl Monatschr 64:129–131
Webb RF, McCully CH (1979) Resistance of *Haemonchus contortus* to oxfendazole. Aust Vet J 55:347–348
Webb RF, McCully CH, Adams BS (1979) The efficiency of oxfendazole against four field populations of benzimidazole resistant *Haemonchus contortus.* Aust Vet J 55:249–250
Wellington AC (1978) Nitroxynil. Anthelmintic activity in cattle following subcutaneous injection. JS Afr Vet Assoc 49:125–126
Werkgroep Wormmiddelen (1973 a) Drugs-anthelmintics (in Dutch). Phenothiazine 98:810–813
Werkgroep Wormmiddelen (1973 b) Drugs-anthelmintics (in Dutch). Befenium en Thenium 98:582–584
Werkgroep Wormmiddelen (1973 c) Drugs-anthelmintics (in Dutch). Methyridine 98:585–588
Wescott RB, Leamaster BR (1982) Efficacy of ivermectin against naturally acquired and experimentelly induced nematode infections in sheep. Am J Vet Res 43:531–533
Wescott RB, Farrell CJ, Gallina AM, Foreyt WJ (1979) Efficacy of albendazole for treatment of naturally acquired nematode infections in Washington cattle. Am J Vet Res 40:369–371
Williams JF, Dade AW, Benne R (1976) Posterior paralysis associated with anthelmintic treatment of sheep. J Am Vet Med Assoc 169:1307–1309
Williams JC, Sheehan D, Fuselier RH (1977 a) Effect of albendazole on gastrointestinal parasites of cattle. Am J Vet Res 38:2037–2038
Williams JC, Knox JW, Sheehan D, Fuselier RH (1977 b) Efficacy of albendazole against inhibited early fourth stage larvae of *Ostertagia ostertagi.* Vet Rec 101:484–486

Williams JC, Sheehan D, Fuselier R (1978) Anthelmintic activity of oxibendazole against gastrointestinal parasites in cattle. Proc Helm Soc Washington 45:129–131
Williams JC, Knox JW, Sheehan D, Fuselier RH (1979a) Further evaluation of the activity of albendazole against inhibited larvae of *Ostertagia ostertagi*. Vet Rec 105:98–100
Williams JC, Knox JW, Sheehan DS, Fuselier RH (1979b) Activity of fenbendazole against inhibited early fourth-stage larvae of *Ostertagia ostertagi*. Am J Vet Res 40:1087–1090
Williams JC, Knox JW, Baumann BA, Snider TG, Hoerner TJ (1981a) Anthelmintic efficacy of albendazole against inhibited larvae of *Ostertagia ostertagi*. Am J Vet Res 42:318–321
Williams JC, Knox JW, Baumann BA, Snider TG, Hoerner TJ (1981b) Further studies on the efficacy of fenbendazole against inhibited larvae of *Ostertagia ostertagi*. Vet Rec 108:228–230
Williams JC, Know JW, Baumann BA, Snider TG, Kimball MG, Hoerner TJ (1981c) Efficacy of ivermectin against inhibited larvae of *Ostertagia ostertagi*. Am J Vet Res 42:2077–2080
Zeakes SJ, Mozier JO, White RG, Hansen MF (1976) Efficacy of coumaphos crumbles and naphtalofos boluses against nematodes of cattle. Am J Vet Res 37:709–710

CHAPTER 7

Chemotherapy of Gastrointestinal Nematodiasis in Equines

M. H. MIRCK

A. Introduction

In modern horse management, infections with nematodes are still an important threat to animal health. A variety of nematodes can be parasitic in the gastrointestinal tract of equids. *Trichostrongylus axei, Draschia megastoma*, and *Habronema* spp. mature in the stomach; *Strongyloides westeri* and *Parascaris equorum* mature in the small intestine; and the strongyles, *Oxyuris equi* and *Probstmayria vivipara* mature in the large intestine. Larval stages of several of these nematodes can be encountered in other parts of the host's body as a result of a possible migratory phase.

B. Strongylidae

The strongyles represent the largest subdivision of nematodes in equids and most of them are cosmopolitan. Many species can be present concurrently in one host. The strongyles are classified in the family Strongylidae, which is divided into the subfamilies Strongylinae (large strongyles) and Cyathostominae (small strongyles). According to LICHTENFELS (1975) the subfamily Strongylinae consists of the genera *Oesophagodontus, Triodontophorus, Strongylus*, and *Craterostomum*. In most literature on equine anthelmintics, however, only *Strongylus* species are considered as large strongyles, while all other members of the family Strongylidae are summarized as small strongyles.

All the Strongylidae have a direct life cycle, involving a period of development in the external environment. After ingestion, larvae of the *Strongylus* species leave the intestinal tract and migrate in the body of the host, following a specific route. *Strongylus vulgaris*, the most harmful of the large stongyles, migrates as fourth-stage larvae in the arterial system and induces arteritis and thrombosis, especially in the anterior mesenteric artery and its main branches. This may lead to functional disorder of the intestine (OGBOURNE and DUNCAN 1977). Larvae of *Strongylus edentatus* reach the liver via the portal system and arrive at the base of the cecum through the hepatorenal ligament (MCCRAW and SLOCOMBE 1974). They deviate easily from this route and can be found in the flanks, lungs, pancreas (MCCRAW and SLOCOMBE 1978), testes (SMITH 1973), and ovaries (MIRCK 1978, unpublished). Little is known about the migratory pathway of *Strongylus equinus*. It is presumed that larvae of *S. equinus* migrate from the liver through the peritoneal cavity to the pancreas (WETZEL 1940).

Of the large strongyles, the incidence of *S. vulgaris* and *S. edentatus* infections is rather high, while *S. equinus* is considered rare (IHLE 1922; WHITLOCK and LEASURE 1970; POYNTER 1970; SLOCOMBE and McCRAW 1973; PECHEUR et al. 1979).

All other members of the subfamily Strongylinae as well as all the Cyathostominae migrate no further than into the mucosa or submucosa of the wall of cecum and colon (SOULSBY 1965; OGBOURNE 1978). Their pathogenic effect consists mainly of injuring the gut wall. As all Strongylidae do, they finally return and mature in the lumen of the large intestine.

I. Epidemiology

In temperate countries the strongyle egg output in horse feces shows a seasonal variation (POYNTER 1954a; DUNCAN 1974; MIRCK 1980). In spring a gradual increase occurs in the egg output of Strongylinae as well as of Cyathostominae. The highest egg output of the large strongyles will be reached by July, while the maximum egg output of the small strongyles may not be attained until the end of the summer.

Because of their long prepatent period, it takes more than half a year for infective larvae of large strongyles to reach maturity, which is mostly in spring of the following year (OGBOURNE 1971). Small strongyles, however, have a rather short prepatent period of about 2 months, which makes possible the development of a second generation within the same year (OGBOURNE 1975; MIRCK 1980). This pattern of development underlies the seasonal variation in egg output.

In autumn a remarkable fall in egg output of the Cyathostominae occurs and at the same time adult, probably senile, worms are expelled (MIRCK 1980). At this time of year a proportionally large number of larvae can be present in the host and most Cyathostominae larvae will be inhibited. During winter, development to maturity will resume gradually and in spring an increasing number of adult strongyles inhabit the large intestine (OGBOURNE 1975; MIRCK 1980).

From strongyle eggs deposited on the land in spring infective larvae will develop and appear on the herbage from July onwards (OGBOURNE 1972). During the grazing season a gradual increase of the pasture larval population occurs (DUNCAN 1974; MIRCK 1980). In temperate countries infective strongyle larvae can overwinter easily, but die out quickly in spring (OGBOURNE 1973; DUNCAN 1974; GRELCK et al. 1977; MIRCK 1980). In June pasture contamination declines to a minimum (DUNCAN 1974; MIRCK 1980).

II. Prevention and Treatment

Because the pathogenicity of all strongyles is mainly determined by their parasitic larval stages, prevention of infection is most important in horse management. For effective parasite control it is necessary to apply the knowledge of parasitic development, epidemiology, and anthelmintics in connection with local management conditions.

The main purpose of prevention must be a diminution of larval intake, which is much easier to achieve in stables than it is at pasture. In most cases hygienic

Table 1. Activity of anthelmintics against gastrointestinal nematodes in equids

	Probstmayria vivipara	*Oxyuris equi* L4	*Oxyuris equi* L5	Small strongyles L4	Small strongyles L5	*Strongylus equinus*	*Strongylus edentatus*	*Strongylus vulgaris*	*Parascaris equorum* L4	*Parascaris equorum* L5	*Strongyloides westeri*	*Habronema* spp.	*Draschia megastoma*	*Trichostrongylus axei*
Phenothiazine (75 mg/kg)	–	–	–	+	+++	+	+	+	–	+	–	–	–	–
Piperazine (200 mg/kg)	–	o	++	–	+++	o	o	+	+++	+++	–	o	–	–
Trichlorfon (40 mg/kg)	–	–	+++	–	–	–	–	–	+++	+++	–	–	–	–
Dichlorvos														
Resin pellet (40 mg/kg)	+++	+++	+++	–	+++	–	o	+++	+++	+++	–	o	o	o
Paste (20 mg/kg)	–	–	–	–	–	–	–	–	++	++	–	–	–	–
Haloxon (60 mg/kg)	+++	+++	+++	–	++	+	++	+++	–	+++	–	o	o	o
Pyrantel (6.6 mg/kg)	+++	+	–	+	+++	+++	+	+++	+++	+++	o	o	o	o
Tiabendazole (50 mg/kg)	+++	+	+++	+++	+++	+++	+++	+++	–	+	+++	–	–	+
Cambendazole (20 mg/kg)	+++	+++	+++	+	+++	+++	+++	+++	–	+++	+++	–	o	+++
Parbendazole (2.5 mg/kg)	–	–	+++	–	+++	–	+++	+++	–	–	o	o	o	o
Mebendazole (8.8 mg/kg)	+++	+++	+++	+	+++	+++	++	+++	–	++	o	o	o	o
Fenbendazole (5 mg/kg)	+++	+	+++	+	+++	+++	+++	+++	–	++	o	o	o	o
Oxfendazole (10 mg/kg)	–	+++	+++	+++	+++	+++	+++	+++	–	+++	o	o	o	+++
Oxibendazole (10 mg/kg)	+++	+++	+++	+	+++	+++	+++	+++	–	+++	+++	o	o	o
Albendazole (5 mg/kg)	–	+++	+++	+	+++	+++	+++	+++	–	+++	–	–	–	–
Tioxidazole (11 mg/kg)	–	+++	+++	–	+++	–	+++	+++	–	+++	o	o	o	o
Febantel (6 mg/kg)	o	+++	+++	–	+++	–	+++	+++	+++	+++	o	o	–	–
Levamisole (10 mg/kg)	o	+	+++	–	+	–	+	+++	+++	+++	–	o	–	o
Ivermectin (0.2 mg/kg)	–	+++	+++	+++	+++	+++	+++	+++	–	+++	+++	–	–	–

+++, 95%–100% efficacy; ++, 80%–100% efficacy; +, 0%–100% efficacy; o, no activity; –, insufficient data

Table 2. Anthelmintics active against gastrointestinal nematodes in equids

Generic name	Trade name(s)	Supplier(s)	Formulation(s)	Dosa (mg/k
Phenothiazine			Powder	75
Piperazine			Powder	200
Trichlorfon	Neguvon Combot	Bayer Haver-Lockhart	97% powder 41% paste	40
Dichlorvos	Equigard Equigel	Shell Shell	19% pellet (PVC) 31% paste	40 20
Haloxon	Equivurm Loxon	Crown Chemical Wellcome	55% paste 77% powder	60
Pyrantel tartrate	Banminth	Pfizer	12.5% powder	6.6
Pyrantel pamoate	Strongid P	Pfizer	43.9% paste	6.6
Tiabendazole	Tibenzole	Merck, Sharpe & Dohme	13.3% susp. 44% paste 75% powder	50
Cambendazole	Equiben	Merck, Sharpe & Dohme	34.1% paste	20
Parbendazole	Helmatac	Smith, Kline & French	9% suspension 30% powder	2.5
Mebendazole	Telmin	Janssen Pharmaceutica	10% granules 20% paste	8.8
Fenbendazole	Panacur	Hoechst	10% suspension 17.8% paste 22% granules	7.5
Oxfendazole	Synantic Systamex	Syntex Wellcome	Different suspensions 6.5% pellets	10
Oxibendazole	Equiminthe	Laboratoires Reading	10% suspension 22.7% paste	10
Albendazole	Valbazen	Smith, Kline & French	Different suspensions 30% paste	5
Febantel	Rintal	Bayer	8.9% paste 10% suspension 10% granules	6
Levamisole	L-Ripercol	Janssen Pharmaceutica	10% solution	10
Ivermectin	Eqvalan	Merck, Sharpe & Dohme	1.87% paste 2% solution	0.2 0.2
Combinations				
Tiabendazole + piperazine	Equizole A	Merck, Sharpe & Dohme	22.2% tiabendazole 66.7% piperazine	Pow
Mebendazole + trichlorfon	Telmin plus	Janssen Pharmaceutica	9% mebendazole 45% trichlorfon	Past
Febantel + trichlorfon	Rintal-Plus	Bayer	7.1% febantel 35.6% trichlorfon	Past

measures alone will not be sufficient and anthelmintics must be used strategically. In spring and early summer, depression of strongyle egg output after anthelmintic treatment lasts not as long as can be observed after treatment during the rest of the year (MIRCK and VAN MEURS 1982). Probably, the development to maturity is much more a continual process during the first 6 months of the year than it is during the second. For successful prevention of pasture contamination, anthelmintics must be administered at monthly intervals, at least during the first half of the grazing season. Later, the intervals can be increased to 8 or even more weeks.

In autumn anthelmintics with special activity against inhibited stages are preferred. However, it is doubtful as to whether anthelmintics which are highly effective against mucosal stages of Cyathostominae can also eliminate inhibited larvae.

Except for the strategic use of anthelmintics, hygienic measures such as the regular disposal of manure also contribute to a reduction of larval contamination of pasture and stable. Pastures grazed by heavily infected horses may still be severely contaminated the following year. These pastures, therefore, should not be grazed by horses before June. Meanwhile they can be safely grazed by ruminants, which is always recommended when pasture contamination threatens to rise too much. Furthermore, mowing also reduces the pasture larval counts.

Because pasture larval contamination increases from July onwards, horses should be moved to clean pasture before the start of this summer increase. If at the same time horses are treated with an anthelmintic, the development of pasture contamination will be largely reduced (EYSKER et al. 1983).

In the case of clinical disease, treatment must be directed at the responsible developmental stages. However, at therapeutic dose levels, most anthelmintics are not sufficiently effective against these larvae. Provided that the safety margin is wide enough, the efficacy can be increased by raising the dose rate. Good results were obtained by administration of elevated dosages once (DRUDGE and LYONS 1970; DUNCAN et al. 1977; DUNCAN and REID 1978), several times a day, or over consecutive days (DRUDGE and LYONS 1970; RENDANO et al. 1979; GEORGI et al. 1980; SLOCOMBE and MCCRAW 1980; DUNCAN et al. 1980; MIRCK 1981). A summary of anthelmintics for horses and their activity is given in Tables 1 and 2.

III. Drug Resistance

In 1961 DRUDGE and ELAM first reported resistance of equine strongyles to phenothiazine. A few years later resistance to tiabendazole was also observed (DRUDGE and LYONS 1965). In both cases only small strongyles were involved. Since 1974 it has been established that side resistance among benzimidazoles does exist (ROUND et al. 1974; DRUDGE et al. 1974b; HOPE and CAMP 1980; KELLY et al. 1981; WEBSTER et al. 1981). However, oxibendazole is still highly effective against strongyles resistant to other benzimidazoles (DRUDGE et al. 1979b; WEBSTER et al. 1981). Benzimidazole-resistant strongyles can also be successfully eliminated by salts of pyrantel and morantel (ROUND et al. 1974; SLOCOMBE and COTE 1977; BARGER and LISLE 1979; HOPE and CAMP 1980; WEBSTER et al. 1981), dichlorvos (SLOCOMBE and COTE 1977), haloxon (WEBSTER et al. 1981), ivermectin

(LYONS et al. 1980b), and mixtures of piperazine and benzimidazoles (SLOCOMBE and COTE 1977; WEBSTER et al. 1981) or piperazine with trichlorfon and phenothiazine (SLOCOMBE and COTE 1977).

Drug resistance has only been demonstrated in small strongyles, particularly in the most prevalent species (DRUDGE et al. 1977, 1979b), but it is most likely that sooner or later other resistant strongyles will appear.

Development of resistance can be prevented or retarded by rotation of anthelmintics between chemical groups. However, when chemically unrelated compounds are used on the same generation, multiple resistance may develop (LE JAMBRE et al. 1977). Therefore, the rotation frequency has to be attuned to the length of the generation interval. Starting from the available epidemiological data, rotation between chemical groups must be recommended at yearly intervals. To prevent the development of resistance it is also important to make sure that anthelmintics are administered in the proper dose.

The existence of resistance must be checked regularly by fecal examination about 2 weeks after treatment. Especially when horses are to be moved to low contaminated or safe pasture after treatment the existence of resistant strains may lead to a next generation with a comparatively much higher degree of resistance (KELLY et al. 1981).

C. Other Important Nematodes

Although strongyles are the most important gastrointestinal nematodes in equines, especially on breeding farms, control must also be directed at *Strongyloides westeri* and *Parascaris equorum*.

Strongyloides westeri infection can provoke diarrhea in foals up to the age of about 6 months. Shortly after birth they become infected by larvae in the mare's milk, which mature in the small intestine within 8–12 days (LYONS et al. 1973), and at the age of 2 weeks large numbers of eggs are expelled with the feces. The way *S. westeri* contributes to the occurrence of diarrhea in foals at the time of the dam's first oestrus is not completely known. When foals lie on their bedding, great numbers of infective larvae can penetrate the skin and within 14 days a new adult population is established (LYONS et al. 1973; MIRCK and FRANKEN 1978). To prevent this rapid accumulation of infection, foals are first treated at the age of about 10 days. In most cases treatment has to be repeated after 2–3 weeks. When mares are treated daily, the lactogenic infection is only prevented during the medication period (LYONS et al. 1977a).

Because the bedding acts as a reservoir of infective larvae, foals must be turned out to pasture as soon as possible. However, in spring attention must be given to the possibility of an overwintered infective strongyle larvae population, which can make a pasture unsuitable for foals.

Parascaris equorum can also give rise to serious problems in young horses. In contrast with *S. westeri*, however, patent ascarid infections are not restricted to foals, but are also found regularly in older horses. Therefore, prevention of infection can only be successful if all the horses on a farm are treated simultaneously at intervals of about 2 months. Stables must be cleaned thoroughly to remove the sticky eggs, which can remain viable for several years. Mowing and alternate grazing can be employed to remove the eggs deposited on the land.

D. Anthelmintics

I. Phenothiazine

At a dose rate of 75 mg/kg body weight, phenothiazine is over 96% effective against adult stages of small strongyles. It has little or no effect on large strongyles, *P. equorum*, and the immature stages of small strongyles (GIBSON 1950; POYNTER 1954b; POYNTER and LLOYD HUGHES 1958). There are individual differences between horses in susceptibility to phenothiazine (MCSHERRY et al. 1966). Therefore, clinical signs of toxicosis may appear at the therapeutic dose level, consisting of anorexia, dullness, muscular weakness, icterus, hemolytic anemia, hemoglobinuria, and sometimes even death (TAYLOR 1942; MCSHERRY et al. 1966; BAIRD et al. 1970).

Modern anthelmintics have pushed aside phenothiazine, but it is still useful in the case of benzimidazole resistance. Although phenothiazine is no longer used frequently in horse management, it is still available in combination with piperazine and trichlorfon.

II. Piperazine

Different salts of piperazine (adipate, citrate, hexahydrate, and phosphate) are used in a water-soluble powder formulation for oral administration. At a dose rate of 200 mg/kg body weight, piperazine base is 90%–100% effective against adult stages of small strongyles and mature as immature stages of *P. equorum*. It removes 80% of adult *O. equi* and about 50% of *S. vulgaris*. It has no effect on *S. edentatus, S. equinus, Habronema* species, and immature stages of *Oxyuris equi* (DOWNING et al. 1955; POYNTER 1955a, b, 1956; GIBSON 1957).

At dose levels of 1,200–1,500 mg/kg only softening of the feces occurs for 24 h (SLOAN et al. 1954; DOWNING et al. 1955).

III. Organophosphates

1. Trichlorfon

For oral administration, trichlorfon is on the market as a 97% water-soluble powder and as a 41% paste. Mixtures with benzimidazoles or piperazine and phenothiazine are also available.

At a dose rate of 40 mg/kg body weight, trichlorfon is 96%–100% effective against mature and immature *P. equorum* and adult *O. equi* (DRUDGE et al. 1975c, 1976; GREVE and PAUL 1976) At dose levels of 60 mg/kg or more it is also highly effective against *S. vulgaris* and small strongyles (GREVE and PAUL 1976).

Although the spectrum is rather small, trichlorfon is frequently used in horse management because of its high efficacy against the larvae of *Gasterophilus* species. At a dose of 40 mg/kg softening of the feces may occur for several days and colic can also develop. At 60 mg/kg moderate to severe colic for 2–6 h is not uncommon (DRUDGE et al. 1976). If administered in the feed trichlorfon is least toxic (DRUDGE et al. 1976), but inappetence may be observed as a result of irritation of the oral mucous membrane.

2. Dichlorvos

Dichlorvos can be orally administered in a 19% resin pellet formulation and as a 31% paste. It is also available as a mixture with benzimidazoles. In resin pellet formulation, 40 mg dichlorvos/kg body weight is 90%–100% effective against adult stages of *S. vulgaris*, small strongyles, *P. equorum, O. equi*, and *P. vivipara*. It is also highly effective against the immature stages of *P. equorum* and *O. equi* (DRUDGE and LYONS 1972; LYONS et al. 1976). The pellet formulation is not effective against *S. edentatus, H. muscae, Draschia megastoma*, and *Trichostrongylus axei* (DRUDGE and LYONS 1972).

In gel formulation, the recommended therapeutic dose of 20 mg/kg body weight is 80%–100% effective against mature and immature *P. equorum* only (BENNETT and BICKFORD 1971; HASS et al. 1973; LYONS et al. 1976). At this dose level, however, it can cause toxic signs such as muscle tremors and incoordination. Later flatulence, frequent passage of soft stools, mild salivation, and lacrimation may occur for several hours (BENNETT and BICKFORD 1971). Side effects of the resin pellet formulation are rare and mostly restricted to self-limited softening of the feces (DRUDGE and LYONS 1972). Some horses reluctantly consume or even refuse the resin pellet formulation, which is a practical disadvantage.

Dosing of mares at any time of pregnancy does not cause ill effects and also has no adverse effects on the foals (JONAS et al. 1972).

Like trichlorfon, dichlorvos is also effective against the larvae of *Gasterophilus* species.

3. Haloxon

Haloxon is available in a powder and a paste formulation for oral administration.

At a dose of 60 mg/kg body weight, haloxon is 99%–100% effective against adult stages of *S. vulgaris, Triodontophorus* spp., *Oesophagodontus robustus, Craterostomum acuticaudatum, P. equorum, O. equi*, and *P. vivipara*. It is also highly effective against fourth-stage larvae of *O. equi*. Removal activity against *S. edentatus* and small strongyles fluctuates and it is only slightly efficacious against *S. equines*. Haloxon is ineffective against *T. axei, H. muscae*, and *D. megastoma* (BOSMAN 1966; NEAVE 1970; COOK 1973; LYONS et al. 1981).

Doses up to 200 mg/kg in the feed caused no ill effects (BOSMAN 1966), but laryngeal paralysis may occur in foals after 2-weekly treatment with haloxon at the recommended dose (ROSE et al. 1981). A dose of 60 mg/kg is safe for pregnant mares (NEAVE 1970).

IV. Tetrahydropyrimidines

Pyrantel and Morantel

Pyrantel and morantel can be administered orally as hydrochloride and tartrate, and pyrantel also as pamoate (syn. embonate) and morantel as fumorate. For horses pyrantel is available as a water-soluble powder (12.5% tartrate) and as a paste (43.9% pamoate).

Independent of salt or method of administration, pyrantel base at a dosage level of 6.6 mg/kg body weight is over 90% effective against adult stages of *S. vulgaris, S. equinus, Triodontophorus* spp., small strongyles, *P. equorum*, and *P. vivipara* (CORNWELL and JONES 1968, 1969; STOYE and ENDE 1969; LYONS et al. 1974, 1975; ENDE and STOYE 1976; BENTLEY et al. 1978). It is also highly effective against immature stages of *P. equorum* and only 62% against immature small strongyles in the gut lumen (CORNWELL and JONES 1968; LYONS et al. 1974). Efficacy against *S. edendatus* and mature and immature stages of *O. equi* is variable (CORNWELL and JONES 1968; LYONS et al. 1974; BENTLEY et al. 1978). *T. axei, Habronema* spp., *D. megastoma*, and *S. westeri* are not susceptible (LYONS et al. 1974, 1975 b).

Morantel shows somewhat greater potency than pyrantel against most worm species in horses (CORNWELL et al. 1973 a, b).

Pyrantel pamoate administered 7 days after experimental *S. vulgaris* infection at a dosage of 52.8 mg base/kg prevented the development of acute arteritis (SLOCOMBE and MCCRAW 1980). Pyrantel hydrochloride at a dose of 40 mg base/kg on the 7th and 8th days after experimental infection in foals was fully effective against migrating larvae of *S. vulgaris*, but a severe toxic reaction developed after the second dose (DRUDGE and LYONS 1969).

The maximum tolerated dose of morantel tartrate given by stomach tube after starvation is about 40 mg base/kg, at which dose level dyspnea, muscular tremors, and incoordination may occur (CORNWELL et al. 1973 b). First signs of toxicosis of pyrantel tartrate are observed at a dose rate of 55 mg base/kg and consist of sweating, dyspnea, and even death (CORNWELL and JONES 1968). Pyrantel pamoate is insoluble in water and even in doses up to 20 times the therapeutic dose no adverse effects occur (SLOCOMBE and SMART 1975).

The reproductive performance of stallions and pregnant mares was not affected by pyrantel (BENTLEY et al. 1978). Morantel is also safe for administration during pregnancy (CORNWELL et al. 1973 b; DOOLE 1970).

V. Imidazothiazoles

Levamisole

Levamisole is available as a drench powder for treatment by stomach tube and as a 10% solution for parenteral administration.

Irrespective of the route of administration a dose of 10 mg/kg body weight is 100% effective against adult stages of *S. vulgaris, P. equorum*, and *O. equi*. Its activity against *S. edentatus*, small strongyles, and immature stages of *T. equi* is limited (LYONS and DRUDGE 1970; CLARKSON and Beg 1971; DRUDGE et al. 1974 a; LYONS et al. 1975 a; DORCHIES et al. 1979). Orally administered at a dose level of 8 mg/kg levamisole is fully effective against 11-day-old migrating larvae of *P. equorum* (LYONS et al. 1976).

Levamisole is ineffective in eliminating migrating fourth- and fifth-stage larvae of *S. vulgaris* (DRUDGE and LYONS 1970). There is no evidence of activity against *T. axei, Habronema* spp. and *P. vivipara* (CLARKSON and BEG 1971; LYONS et al. 1975 a). Oral administration of levamisole at a dose level of 20 mg/kg or more may provoke signs of toxicity within 10 min, such as sweating, lacrimation, nasal discharge, increased respiration, hyperexcitability, and sometimes even death (LYONS and DRUDGE 1970; CLARKSON and BEG 1971). An intramuscular injection may cause a local tissue reaction and at the therapeutic dose level general manifestations of colic can be observed (DORCHIES et al. 1979).

VI. Benzimidazoles

1. Tiabendazole

Tiabendazole is available as a 75% water-soluble powder, a 13.3% suspension, and a 44% paste formulation. It is also on the market as a mixture with piperazine or trichlorfon.

At a dose rate of 50 mg/kg body weight tiabendazole is 90%–100% effective against adult stages of large and small strongyles, *O. equi, P. vivipara,* and *S. westeri.* It is also fully effective against fourth-stage larvae of small strongyles in the gut lumen but efficacy against *P. equorum, T. axei,* and fourth-stage larvae of *O. equi* is insufficient (DRUDGE et al. 1962, 1963; TURK et al. 1962; ENIGK and STOYE 1963; HIEPE et al. 1971). At a dose rate of 100 mg/kg tiabendazole is 100% effective against *P. equorum* (EGERTON et al. 1962).

Two doses of tiabendazole at a level of 440 mg/kg on successive days were fully effective against 12- and 13-day-old larvae of *S. vulgaris* (DRUDGE and LYONS 1969) and 3- and 4-day-old larvae of *S. edentatus* (SLOCOMBE and MCCRAW 1975). At dose levels of 100 mg/kg of more appetite is reduced for at least 24 h (MIRCK 1972–1980, unpublished). At 1,200 mg/kg depression and mild colic may occur for 12 h post-treatment (DRUDGE et al. 1963). Tiabendazole does not influence pregnancy or exhibit other untoward effects on mares or foals (ROUND 1968).

2. Cambendazole

Cambendazole is available as a 34.1% paste formulation. At a dose of 20 mg/kg body weight, cambendazole is 96%–100% effective against adult stages of large and small strongyles, *P. equorum, S. westeri, O. equi, P. vivipara,* and *T. axei.* It is also 100% effective against fourth-stage larvae of *O. equi* and only 77% effective against immature stages of small strongyles in the gut lumen (BELLO et al. 1973; DRUDGE et al. 1975a; CAIRNS and HOLMDEN 1977; COLGLAZIER et al. 1977; LYONS et al. 1977a; SLOCOMBE and COTE 1978). Cambendazole has no effect on *D. megastoma* (DRUDGE et al. 1975a).

At eight times the recommended dose no adverse effects develop (HORTON et al. 1977), but at 600 mg/kg transient depression and fecal softening occur (SCOTT 1977). Cambendazole does not interfere with the reproductive function of stallions (AMMANN et al. 1977).

VII. Benzimidazole Carbamates

1. Parbendazole

Parbendazole is on the market as a 9% suspension and a 30% powder formulation. At a dose level of 2.5 mg/kg body weight, parbendazole is 98%–100% effective against adult stages of *S. vulgaris*, *S. edentatus*, small strongyles, and *O. equi* (LYONS et al. 1980a). At 20 mg/kg it is fully effective against *P. equorum* (LYONS et al. 1980a), but ineffective against 7-day-old larvae of *S. vulgaris* (DRUDGE and LYONS 1970). Parbendazole has no activity against *T. axei*, *Habronema* spp., *D. megastoma*, and *S. westeri* (LYONS et al. 1980a).

Transient diarrhea occurs for 24–48 h after treatment, which may be accompanied by anorexia and listlessness (PUISSET 1974; VERBERNE and MIRCK 1975; LYONS et al. 1980a). No unfavorable effects on the gravidity or on the development of the fetus were observed (VERBERNE and MIRCK 1975).

2. Mebendazole

Mebendazole is on the market as a 10% granule and a 20% paste formulation. A mixture with trichlorfon is also available.

At a dose level of 8.8 mg/kg body weight, mebendazole is 96%–100% effective against adult stages of *S. vulgaris*, *S. equinus*, small strongyles, *P. vivipara*, and mature as well as immature *O. equi*. Some variation in efficacy against *S. edentatus* and *P. equorum* exists, but the mean percentage of effectivity is still over 90% (REINECKE and LE POUX 1972; BENNETT 1973; BRADLEY and RADHAKRISHAN 1973; BENNETT et al. 1974; DRUDGE et al. 1974; MCCURDY et al. 1976; COLGLAZIER et al. 1977; MCCURDY et al. 1977). Only 73% of the fourth-stage larvae of small strongyles in the gut lumen are removed (COLGLAZIER et al. 1977). Larval stages of large and small strongyles outside the gut lumen are not affected (COLGLAZIER et al. 1977). Migrating larvae of *S. vulgaris* were killed by mebendazole at a dose of 120 mg/kg for two consecutive days (KADYROV 1978). At the 8.8 mg/kg-dose level mebendazole is not effective against *T. axei*, *H. muscae*, *D. megastoma*, and *S. westeri* (DRUDGE et al. 1974b). From 50 mg/kg onwards a slight intestinal hyperactivity and fecal softening may occur, with slight diarrhea at 400 mg/kg (MARSBOOM 1973).

3. Fenbendazole

Fenbendazole is available as a 10% suspension, a 17.8% paste, and a 22% granule formulation. At a dose rate of 5 mg/kg body weight, fenbendazole is 97%–100% effective against adult stages of large and small strongyles, *O. equi*, and *P. vivipara* (COLGLAZIER et al. 1977; DRUDGE et al. 1978a). Efficacy against mature *P. equorum* is only 83% (FORSTNER and HASSLINGER 1974). At the same dose level fenbendazole is 78% effective against fourth-stage larvae of small strongyles in the gut lumen (COLGLAZIER et al. 1977), while the efficacy against immature *O. equi* ranged from 43%–100% (DRUDGE et al. 1975b). At 7.5 mg/kg fenbendazole is 92% effective against mature *P. equorum* (DERKMANN and HASSLINGER 1977) and 10 mg/kg removes all mature and immature stages, which also counts for *O. equi* (DRUDGE et al. 1978a).

To be over 80% effective against larval stages of large and small strongyles outside the gut lumen a 60 mg/kg level is necessary (DUNCAN et al. 1977). A dose of 7.5 mg/kg daily for five consecutive days is 94.6% effective against larval stages of small strongyles in the mucosa, 80% effective against migrating larvae of *S.*

vulgaris, and 100% effective against migrating stages of *S. edentatus* (DUNCAN et al. 1980).

At a dose rate of 50 mg/kg fenbendazole is about 90% effective against *S. westeri* (DRUDGE et al. 1981). At 100 mg/kg *S. westeri* is fully eliminated (ENIGK et al. 1974).

Trichostrongylus axei, H. muscae, and *D. megastoma* are barely susceptible at a dose level of 5 mg/kg (COLGLAZIER et al. 1977), but at 30 mg/kg fenbendazole is 98% effective against *H. muscae* (DUNCAN et al. 1977).

At a dose of 100 mg/kg no adverse effects develop. When administered during pregnancy complications are not observed and teratogenic effects were also not registered (BECKER 1975). The reproductive function of stallions is not disturbed by fenbendazole (SQUIRES et al. 1978).

4. Oxfendazole

Oxfendazole is on the market as a 2.3% and 9.1% suspension and as a 6.5% pellet formulation.

At a dose rate of 10 mg/kg body weight, oxfendazole is 99%–100% effective against adult stages of large and small strongyles, *T. axei, P. equorum,* and *O. equi.* Besides, it is fully effective against immature stages of *O. equi* and 97%–100% effective against larvae of small strongyles in the gut lumen as well as in the mucosa (LYONS et al. 1977b; DUNCAN and REID 1978; COLGLAZIER 1979). Efficacy against migrating *S. vulgaris* is incomplete (DUNCAN and REID 1978; LYONS et al. 1977). Oxfendazole is ineffective against *S. westeri, H. muscae,* and *D. megastoma* (LYONS et al. 1977b; COLGLAZIER 1979).

At 100 mg/kg transient liquifying of the feces was observed, although the horse had soft feces before treatment (LYONS et al. 1977b).

5. Oxibendazole

Oxibendazole is available as 3% and 7% pellets, a 10% suspension, and a 22.7% paste formulation. A mixture with dichlorvos in paste formulation is also on the market.

At a dose rate of 10 mg/kg body weight, oxibendazole is 95%–100% effective against adult stages of large and small strongyles, *S. westeri, P. equorum, O. equi,* and *P. vivipara.* It is also highly effective against fourth-stage larvae of small strongyles in the gut lumen (KATES et al. 1975; NAWALINSKI and THEODORIDES 1976, 1977; DRUDGE et al. 1979, 1981; PECHEUR et al. 1980; LYONS et al. 1981a). There is little or no activity against *T. axei, H. muscae, D. megastoma,* and migrating stages of *S. vulgaris* (KATES et al. 1975; NAWALINSKI and THEODORIDES 1976; LYONS et al. 1981a). Oxibendazole is probably safe for horses. Three times the therapeutic dose caused no adverse effects (AGUADO BRESSO 1979).

6. Albendazole

Albendazole is available as a 1.9% and 10% suspension and as a 30% paste formulation. At a dose level of 5 mg/kg body weight, albendazole is 99%–100% effective against adult stages of large and small strongyles, *P. equorum*, and *O. equi*. It is also fully effective against immature *O. equi*, but only 69% against fourth-stage larvae of small strongyles in the gut lumen (COLGLAZIER et al. 1977).

At a dose of 25 mg/kg t.i.d. for 5 days, albendazole was completely effective against migrating larvae of *S. vulgaris*, 1 month after experimental infection (RENDANO et al. 1979). However, at this dose level three out of four foals developed severe diarrhea and one foal died. In naturally infected foals treated the same way, two out of three foals died. At a dosage rate of 50 mg/kg twice a day for 2 days albendazole was effective against fourth-stage larvae of *S. vulgaris* with only minor signs of toxicity (GEORGI et al. 1980).

7. Tioxidazole

At a dose rate of 11 mg/kg body weight, tioxidazole in micronized formulation is 100% effective against adult stages of *S. vulgaris, P. equorum*, and *O. equi*. It is also fully effective against fourth-stage larvae of *O. equi* and over 90% effective against adult *S. edentatus* and small strongyles. When administered in feed it is fully effective against immature *P. equorum*. There is little or no activity against *T. axei, S. westeri, H. muscae, D. megastoma*, and migrating stages of *S. vulgaris*. No adverse effects are observed at the therapeutic dose level (DRUDGE et al. 1980; LYONS et al. 1981).

VIII. Febantel

Febantel is available as an 8.9% paste, a 10% suspension, and a 10% granule formulation. At a dose rate of 6 mg/kg body weight, febantel is 95%–100% effective against adult stages of *S. vulgaris, S. edentatus*, small strongyles, *P. equorum*, and *O. equi*. It is also highly effective against immature stages of *P. equorum* and *O. equi*. Migrating stages of large strongyles are not affected (DRUDGE et al. 1978b, 1979a). To eliminate *T. axei* the dose level has to be increased to at least 20 mg/kg, and in the case of *S. westeri* even ten times the recommended dose is necessary (ENIGK and DEY-HAZRA 1978). Febantel has no effect on *H. muscae* (ENIGK and DEY-HAZRA 1978). Febantel is also available in combination with trichlorfon.

IX. Avermectins

Ivermectin

Ivermectin is available as a 1.87% paste for oral use and as a 2% w/v micellar solution for intramuscular administration.

After parenteral administration at a dose level of 0.2 mg/kg body weight, ivermectin is 96%–100% effective against adult stages of large and small strongyles, *T. axei, S. westeri, P. equorum*, and *O. equi*. It is also highly effective against fourth-stage larvae of *O. equi* and small strongyles in the gut lumen (KLEI and TORBERT 1980; EGERTON et al. 1981; CRAIG and KUNDE 1981; MIRCK and VAN

MEURS 1982). Partial activity exists against mucosal stages of small strongyles and parenteral stages of *S. vulgaris* and *S. edentatus* (KLEI and TORBERT 1980). In experimental infections parenterally administered ivermectin was fully effective against 7-day-old larvae of *S. vulgaris* at the 0.2-mg/kg dose level (SLOCOMBE and McCRAW 1980, 1981). There might be some activity against *Habronema* spp. (KLEI and TORBERT 1980).

Although little information is available yet, about the same anthelmintic acitivity can be achieved after oral administration of ivermectin at the same dose rate (LYONS et al. 1980 b).

Irrespective of the route of administration, no adverse effects occur at the recommended dose level; only a small swelling may appear at the site of the injection (LYONS et al. 1980 b; SLOCOMBE and McCRAW 1981).

Like trichlorfon and dichlorvos, ivermectin is also effective against the larvae of *Gasterophilus* spp.

E. Conclusions

In addition to hygienic measures, anthelmintics play an important part in helminth control in horses. On most farms regular anthelmintic treatments are necessary to keep the degree of infection between acceptable limits. Which anthelmintic has to be chosen depends a great deal on the kind of worms which have to be eliminated but also on their stage of development. However, the anthelmintic of choice must fit into the strategy recommended for the prevention of resistance and the drug formulation must be attuned to local management conditions, success depending only on proper administration.

References

Aguado Bresso J de J (1979) Pruebas con oxibendazole en equinos y su efecto sobre *Parascaris equorum* (Abstract of thesis). Veterinaria Mexico 10:94

Amman RP, Bowen JM, Pickett BW, Berndtson WE, Stasmak RS, Vos JL (1977) Reproductive function in stallions treated with cambendazole. J Am Vet Med Assoc 170:730–732

Baird JD, Hutchins DR, Lephard EE (1970) Phenothiazine poisoning in a thoroughbred horse. Aust Vet J 46:496–499

Barger IA, Lisle KA (1979) Benzimidazole resistance in small strongylids of horses. Aust Vet J 55:594–595

Becker W (1975) Die Anwendung von Panacur® bei trächtigen Tieren. In: Proc 2nd European multi-colloquium of parasitology. Trogir, Yugoslavia, pp 105–106. Izdaje: Drustuo Parazitologija Jugoslavije

Bello TR, Amborski GF, Torbert BJ, Greer GJ (1973) Anthelmintic efficacy of cambendazole against gastrointestinal parasites of the horse. Am J Vet Res 34:771–777

Bennett DG (1973) Efficacy of mebendazole as an anthelmintic in horses. Vet Med Small Animal Clin 68:604–609

Bennett DG, Bickford AA (1971) Efficacy of dichlorvos paste against parasites of horses. Vet Med Small Anim Clin 66:441–444

Bennett DG, Bickford AA, Lund JE (1974) Safety evaluation of mebendazole in horses. Am J Vet Res 35:1003–1004

Bentley OE, Burns SJ, McDonald DR, Drudge JH, Lyons ET, Kruckenberg SM, Vaughn JT (1978) Safety evaluation of pyrantel pamoate administered with trichlorfon as a broad-spectrum anthelmintic in horses. Vet Med Small Animal Clin 73:70–73

Bosman CJ (1966) Haloxon as an anthelmintic for horses. J S Afr Vet Assoc 37:421–424

Bradley RE, Radhakrishnan CV (1973) Critical test evaluation of mebendazole against gastrointestinal parasites of horses and ponies. Am J Vet Pes 34:475–477

Cairns GC, Holmden JH (1977) The anthelmintic efficacy of cambendazole in horses. N Z Vet J 25:35–37

Clarkson MJ, Beg MK (1971) Critical tests of levamisole as an anthelmintic in the horse. Ann Trop Med Parasitol 65:87–91

Colglazier ML (1979) Critical anthelmintic trials in ponies with oxfendazole and caviphos and concomitant studies on the spontaneous elimination of small strongyles. Am J Vet Res 40:384–386

Colglazier ML, Enzie FD, Kates KC (1977) Critical anthelmintic trials in ponies with four benzimidazoles: mebendazole, cambendazole, fenbendazole and albendazole. J Parasitol 63:724–727

Cook TF (1973) The anthelmintic efficacy of haloxon in horses. NZ Vet J 21:82–84

Cornwell RL, Jones RM (1968) Critical tests in the horse with the anthelmintic pyrantel tartrate. Vet Rec 82:483–484

Cornwell RL, Jones RM (1969) Activity of pyrantel against *Parascaris equorum*. Vet Rec 85:196–197

Cornwell RL, Jones RM, Pott JM (1973a) Critical trials of morantel tartrate in equine strongylosis. Vet Rec 93:94–98

Cornwell RL, Jones RM, Pott JM (1973b) Critical trials with morantel tartrate against *Parascaris equorum*. Res Vet Sci 14:134–136

Craig TM, Kunde JM (1981) Controlled evaluation of ivermectin in Shetland ponies. Am J Vet Res 42:1422–1424

Derkmann K, Hasslinger MA (1977) Zur Bekämpfung des Pferdespulwurmes, *Parascaris equorum* (Goeze, 1782) mit Panacur®. Berl Munch Tierarztl Wochenschr 90:95–98

Doole WJ (1970) Morantel tartrate as an anthelmintic for horses. NZ Vet J 18:202

Dorchies P, Franc M, Lahitte JD de (1979) Utilisation du levamisole comme anthelmintique chez le cheval. Rev Med Vet 130:417–418

Downing W, Kingsbury PA, Sloan JEN (1955) Critical tests with piperazine adipate in horses. Vet Rec 67:641–644

Drudge JE, Elam G (1961) Preliminary observations on the resistance of horse strongyles to phenothiazine. J Parasitol 47:38–39

Drudge JH, Lyons ET (1965) Newer developments in helminth control and *Strongylus vulgaris* research. In: Proc 11th Ann Condention Am Assoc Eq Pract, Guelph, Ontario, Canada, pp 381–389

Drudge JH, Lyons ET (1970) The chemotherapy of migrating strongyle larvae. In: Bryans JT, Gerber M (eds) Equine infections diseases. Proc 2nd Int Conf Eq Inf Dis, Paris, pp 310–322, Karger, Basel

Drudge JH, Lyons ET (1972) Critical tests of a resin-pellet formulation of dichlorvos against internal parasites of the horse. Am J Vet Res 33:1365–1375

Drudge JH, Szanto J, Wyant ZN, Elam G (1962) Critical tests on thiabendazole against parasites of the horse. J Parasitol 48 [Suppl]:28

Drudge JH, Szanto J, Wyant ZN, Elam G (1963) Critical tests of thiabendazole as an anthelmintic in the horse. Am J Vet Res 24:1217–1222

Drudge JH, Lyons ET, Taylor EL (1976) Critical tests and safety studies on trichlorfon as an antiparasitic agent in the horse. Am J Vet Res 37:139–144

Drudge JH, Lyons ET, Swerczek TW (1974a) Critical tests and safety studies on a levamisole-piperazine mixture as an anthelmintic in the horse. Am J Vet Res 35:67–72

Drudge JH, Lyons ET, Tolliver SC (1974b) Critical and clinical test evaluations of mebendazole against internal parasites of the horse. Am J Vet Res 35:1409–1412
Drudge JH, Lyons ET, Tolliver SC (1975a) Critical tests of suspension, paste and pellet formulation of cambendazole in the horse. Am J Vet Res 36:435–439
Drudge JH, Lyons ET, Tolliver SC (1975b) Critical tests of the benzimidazole anthelmintic fenbendazole in the horse. Vet Med Small Anim Clin 70:537–540
Drudge JH, Lyons ET, Tolliver SC (1975c) Critical and controlled tests of the antiparasitic activity of liquid and paste formulations of trichlorfon in the horse. Vet Med Small Anim Clin 70:975–978
Drudge JH, Lyons ET, Tolliver SC (1977) Resistance of equine strongyles to thiabendazole: critical tests of two strains. Vet Med Small Anim Clin 72:433–438
Drudge JH, Lyons ET, Tolliver SC (1978a) Critical and controlled tests and clinical trials with suspension and granule formulations of the anthelmintic fenbendazole in the horse. J Eq Med Surg 2:22–26
Drudge JH, Lyons ET, Tolliver SC (1978b) Critical tests of the anthelmintic febantel in the horse: activity of a paste formulation alone or with a trichlorfon paste. Am J Vet Res 39:1419–1421
Drudge JH, Lyons ET, Tolliver SC (1979a) Critical tests of febantel in the horse: antiparasitic activity of a suspension alone or with liquid trichlorfon. J Eq Med Surg 3:135–140
Drudge JH, Lyons ET, Tolliver SC (1979b) Benzimidazole resistance of equine strongyles – critical tests of six compounds against population B. Am J Vet Res 40:590–594
Drudge JH, Lyons ET, Tolliver SC (1980) Critical tests of new benzimidazole anthelmintic tioxidazole in the horse. Am J Vet Res 41:1383–1387
Drudge JH, Lyons ET, Tolliver SC, Kubis JE (1979) Critical tests and clinical trials on oxibendazole in horses with special reference to removal of *Parascaris equorum*. Am J Vet Res 40:758–761
Drudge JH, Lyons ET, Tolliver SC, Kubis JE (1981) Clinical trials with fenbendazole and oxibendazole for *Strongyloides westeri* in foals. Am J Vet Res 42:526–527
Duncan JL (1974) Field studies on the epidemiology of mixed strongyle infection in the horse. Vet Rec 94:337–345
Duncan JL, Reid JFS (1978) An evaluation of the efficacy of oxfendazole against the common nematode parasites of the horse. Vet Rec 103:332–334
Duncan JL, McBeath DG, Best JMJ, Preston NK (1977) The efficacy of fenbendazole in the control of immature strongyle infections in ponies. Eq Vet J 9:146–149
Duncan JL, McBeath DG, Preston NK (1980) Studies on the efficacy of fenbendazole used in a divided dosage regime against strongyle infections in ponies. Eq Vet J 12:78–80
Egerton JR, Brokken ES, Suhayda D, Eary CH, Wooden JW, Kilgore RL (1981) The antiparasitic activity of ivermectin in horses. Vet Parasitol 8:83–88
Egerton JR, Cuckler AC, Ames ER, Bramel RG, Brightenbach GE, Washko FV (1962) Anthelmintic effect of thiabendazole on intestinal nematodes in horses. J Parasitol 48:29
Ende H, Stoye M (1976) Banminth-Paste zur planmäßigen Strongylidenbekämpfung beim Pferd. DTW 83:431–470
Enigk K, Stoye M (1963) Versuche zur Behandlung des Strongylidenbefalls der Pferde mit Thiabendazol. DTW 70:257–261
Enigk K, Dey-Hazra A (1978) Die Wirksamkeit von Rintal auf den Rundwurmbefall des Magen-Darm-Kanals beim Pferd. DTW 85:350–354
Enigk K, Dey-Hazra A, Batke J (1974) Zur klinischen Bedeutung und Behandlung des galaktogen erworbenen *Strongyloides*-Befalls der Fohlen. DTW 81:605–628
Eysker M, Jansen J, Mirck MH, Wemmenhove R (1983) Alternate grazing of horses and sheep as a preventive method for gastro-intestinal helminth infections in the horse. Vet Parasitol 13:273–280
Forstner MJ, Hasslinger MA (1974) Untersuchungen über die Wirkung des Anthelmintikums Fenbendazol an Pferden. Berl Munch Tierarztl Wochenschr 87:325–327

Georgi JR, Rendano VT, King JM, Bianchi DG, Theodorides VJ (1980) Equine verminous arteritis: efficacy and speed of larvicidal activity as influenced by dosage of albendazole. Cornell Vet 70:147–152

Gibson TE (1950) Critical tests of phenothiazine as an anthelmintic for horses. Vet Rec 62:341–342

Gibson TE (1957) Critical tests of piperazine adipate as an equine anthelmintic. B Vet J 113:90–92

Grelck H, Hörchner F, Wöhrl HE (1977) Entwicklungsfähigkeit und Überlebensdauer von Larven der Pferdestrongyliden im Freiland. Prakt Tierarzt 58:265–268

Greve JH, Paul JW (1976) Evaluation of an enteric-coated microencapsulated formulation of trichlorfon in horses. Vet Med Small Anim Clin 71:1737–1742

Hass DK, Albert JR, Pillow BG, Brown LJ (1973) Dichlorvos gel formulation as an equine anthelmintic. Am J Vet Res 34:41–43

Hiepe Th, Siebeke F, Nickel S (1971) Thiabendazol gegen Strongyloidesbefall bei Fohlen. Angew Parasitol 12:65–67

Hope JJ, Kemp GK (1980) Apparent Trichonema resistance to fenbendazole. NZ Vet J 28:80–81

Horton FL, Griffiths OV, McMullan MJ (1977) Field safety evaluation of cambendazole in horses. NZ Vet J 25:69–70

Ihle JET (1922) The adult strongylids (sclerostomes) inhabiting the large intestine of the horse. Report of the commission appointed to enquire into sclerostomiasis in Holland. I Zoological Part, vol I, 118 pp, Algemene Landsdrukkerijs Gravenhage, Netherlands

Jonas D, Hasslinger MA, Wolpert E (1972) Neue Aspekte zur Endoparasitenbekämpfung beim Pferd. Prakt Tierarzt 10:427–430

Kadyrov NT (1978) The treatment of *Delafondia (Strongylus vulgaris)* infection in horses (in Russian). Vestnik Sel'skokhozyaistvennoi Nauki Kazakhstana 11:68–71

Kates KO, Colglazier ML, Enzie FD (1975) Oxibendazole: critical anthelmintic trials in equids. Vet Rec 97:442–444

Kelly JD, Webster JH, Griffin DL, Whitlock HV, Martin JCA, Gunawan M (1981) Resistance to benzimidazole anthelmintics in equine strongyles. I. Frequency, geographical distribution and relationship between occurrence, animal husbandry procedures and anthelmintic usage. Aust Vet J 57:163–171

Klei TR, Torbert BJ (1980) Efficacy of ivermectin (22,23-dihydroavermectin B_1) against gastrointestinal parasites in ponies. Am J Vet Res 41:1747–1750

Le Jambre LF, Southcott WH, Dash KM (1977) Resistance of selected lines of *Ostertagia circumcincta* to thiabendazole, morantel tartrate and levamisole. Int J Parasitol 7:473–479

Lichtenfels JR (1975) Helminths of domestic equids. Proc Helminthol Soc Wash 42[special issue]1–92

Lyons ET, Drudge JH (1970) Critical tests on *dl*-tetramisole against internal parasites of the horse. Am J Vet Res 31:1477–1480

Lyons ET, Drudge JH, Tolliver SC (1973) On the life cycle of *Strongyloides westeri* in the equine. J Parasitol 59:780–787

Lyons ET, Drudge JH, Tolliver SC (1974) Critical tests of three salts of pyrantel against internal parasites of the horse. Am J Vet Res 35:1515–1522

Lyons ET, Drudge JH, Tolliver SC (1975a) Critical tests of levamisole alone or in mixtures with piperazine or thrichlorfon against internal parasites of horses. Proc Helminthol Soc Wash 42:128–135

Lyons ET, Drudge JH, Tolliver SC (1975b) Field tests of three salts of pyrantel against internal parasites of the horse. Am J Vet Res 36:161–166

Lyons ET, Drudge JH, Tolliver SC (1976) Studies on the development and chemotherapy of larvae of *Parascaris equorum* (Nematoda: Ascaridoidea) in experimentally and naturally infected foals. J Parasitol 62:453–459

Lyons ET, Drudge JH, Tolliver SC (1977a) Observations on the development of *Strongyloides westeri* in foals nursing dams treated with cambendazole or thiabendazole. Am J Vet Res 38:889–892

Lyons ET, Drudge JH, Tolliver SC (1977b) Critical tests of oxfendazole against internal parasites of horses. Am J Vet Res 38:2049–2053
Lyons ET, Drudge JH, Tolliver SC (1980a) Antiparasitic activity of parbendazole in critical tests in horses. Am J Vet Res 41:123–124
Lyons ET, Drudge JH, Tolliver SC (1980b) Antiparasitic activity of ivermectin in critical tests in equids. Am J Vet Res 41:2069–2072
Lyons ET, Drudge JH, Tolliver SC (1981a) Oxibendazole: anthelmintic activity in horses. Am J Vet Res 42:685–686
Lyons ET, Drudge JH, Tolliver SC (1981b) Haloxon: critical tests of antiparasitic activity in equids. Am J Vet Res 42:1043–1045
Lyons ET, Drudge JH, Tolliver SC (1981c) Tioxidazole: evaluation of antiparasitic activity of a micronized formulation in horses by the critical test method. Am J Vet Res 42:1048–1049
Marsboom R (1973) Toxicologic studies on mebendazole. Toxicol Appl Pharmacol 24:371–377
McCraw BM, Slocombe JOB (1974) Early development and pathology associated with *Strongylus edentatus*. Can J Comp Med 38:124–138
McCraw BM, Slocombe JOB (1978) *Strongylus edentatus:* development and lesions from ten weeks postinfection to patency. Can J Comp Med 42:340–356
McCurdy HD, Sharp ML, Sweeny WT (1976) Evaluation of mebendazole in paste formulation in the horse. Vet Med Small Anim Clin 71:97–100
McCurdy HD, Sharp ML, Kruchkenberg SM (1977) Critical and clinical trials of mebendazole and trichlorfon in the horse. Vet Med Small Anim Clin 72:245–249
McSherry BJ, Roe CK, Milne FJ (1966) The haematology of phenothiazine poisoning in horses. Can Vet J 7:3–12
Mirck MH (1980) An investigation into the epidemiology of Strongylidae infections in equids in the Netherlands. Thesis, Utrecht, The Netherlands, 117 pp.
Mirck MH (1981) Anthelmintic treatment in the case of cyathostominosis in the horse. Tijdschr Diergeneeskd 106:1281–1283
Mirck MH, Franken P (1978) *Strongyloides westeri* Ihle, 1917 (Nematoda: Strongyloididae) II Parasitological and haematological features of experimental infection. Tijdschr Diergeneeskd 103:355–360
Mirck MH, Meurs GK van (1982) The efficacy of ivermectin against *Strongyloides westeri* in foals. Vet 4:89–91
Mirck MH, Meurs GK van (1982) The influence of albendazole and cambendazole treatment on the faecal egg output of Strongylidae in horses. Tijdschr Diergeneeskd 107:731–736
Nawalinski T, Theodorides VJ (1976) Critical tests with oxibendazole against gastrointestinal parasites of ponies. Am J Vet Res 37:469–471
Nawalinski T, Theodorides VJ (1977) Efficacy of three forms of oxibendazole against gastrointestinal parasites of ponies. Vet Med Small Anim Clin 72:96–101
Neave RMS (1970) Clinical use of haloxon in the horse. Eq Vet J 2:87–90
Ogbourne CP (1971) Observations on the fecundity of strongylid worms of the horse. Parasitology 63:289–298
Ogbourne CP (1972) Observations on the free-living stages of strongylid nematodes of the horse. Parasitology 64:461–477
Ogbourne CP (1975) Survival in herbage plots of infective larvae of strongylid nematodes of the horse. J Helminthol 47:9–16
Ogbourne CP (1975) Epidemiological studies on horses infected with nematodes of the family Trichonematidae (Witenberg, 1925). Int J Parasitol 5:667–672
Ogbourne CP (1978) Pathogenesis of cyathostome *(Trichonema)* infections of the horse. A review. CIH Miscellaneous Publications no. 5, Commonwealth Agricultural Bureau, Farnham Royal, UK, 25 pp
Ogbourne CP, Duncan JL (1977) *Strongylus vulgaris* in the horse: its biology and veterinary importance. CIH Miscellaneous Publications no. 4, Commonwealth Agricultural Bureau, Farnham Royal, UK, 40 pp

Pecheur M, Detry-Pouplard M, Benakhla A (1980) Activité anthelmintique de l'oxibendazole chez les equids. Ann Med Vet 124:609–612
Pecheur M, Detry-Pouplard M, Gerin G, Tinar R (1979) Les helminthes parasites du système digestif de poneys abattus en Belgique. Ann Med Vet 123:103–108
Poynter D (1954a) Seasonal fluctuations in the number of strongyle eggs passed by horses. Vet Rec 66:74–78
Poynter D (1954b) Observations on the relative increase of *Strongylus* species following the administration of phenothiazine to horses. Vet Rec 66:101–105
Poynter D (1955a) Piperazine adipate as an equine anthelmintic. Vet Rec 67:159–163
Poynter D (1955b) The efficacy of piperazine adipate administered in bran mash to horses. Vet Rec 67:625
Poynter D (1956) A comparative assessment of the anthelmintic activity in horses of four piperazine compounds. Vet Rec 68:291–297
Poynter D (1970) Some observations on the nematode parasites of horses. In: Bryans JT, Gerber M (eds) Equine infectious diseases. Proc 2nd Int Conf Eq Inf Dis Paris, Karger, Basel, pp 269–289
Poynter D, Lloyd Hughes D (1958) Phenothiazine and piperazine, an efficient anthelmintic mixture for horses. Vet Rec 70:1183–1188
Puisset B (1974) Essai de traitement de nematodes banales (oxyurose, ascaridose, strongyloses) des equides par le parbendazole. Thesis, Toulouse
Reinecke RK, Le Roux DJ (1972) Anthelmintic activity of mebendazole in equines. J S Afr Vet Med Assoc 43:287–294
Rendano VT, Georgi JR, White KK, Sack WO, King JM, Bianchi DG, Theodorides VJ (1979) Equine verminous arteritis. An arteriographic evaluation of the larvicidal activity of albendazole. Eq Vet J 11:225–231
Rose RJ, Hartley WJ, Baker W (1981) Laryngeal paralysis in arabian foals associated with oral haloxon administration. Eq Vet J 13:171–176
Round MC (1968) Experiences with thiabendazole as an anthelmintic for horses. Br Vet J 124:248–258
Round MC, Simpson DJ, Haselden CS, Glendinning ESA, Baskerville RE (1974) Horse strongyles' tolerance to anthelmintics. Vet Rec 95:517–518
Scott P (1977) A review of some modern equine anthelmintics. NZ Vet J 25:373–378
Sloan JEN, Kingsbury PA, Jolly DW (1954) Preliminary trials with piperazine adipate as a veterinary anthelmintic. J Pharm Pharmacol 6:718–724
Slocombe JOD, Cote JF (1977) Small strongyles of horses with cross resistance to benzimidazole anthelmintics and susceptibility to unrelated compounds. Can Vet J 18:212–217
Slocombe JOD, Cote JF (1978) Evaluation of cambendazole paste against nematodes in horses in a field trial. Can Vet J 19:184–186
Slocombe JOD, McCraw BM (1973) Gastrointestinal nematodes in horses in Ontario. Can Vet J 14:101–105
Slocombe JOD, McCraw BM (1975) Suppression of the pathogenic effects of *Strongylus edentatus* larvae with thiabendazole. Can J Comp Med 39:256–260
Slocombe JOD, McCraw BM (1980) Evaluation of pyrantel pamoate, nitramisole and avermectin B_1a against migrating *Strongylus vulgaris* larvae. Can J Comp Med 44:93–100
Slocombe JOD, McCraw BM (1981) Controlled tests of ivermectin against migrating *Strongylus vulgaris* in ponies. Am J Vet Res 42:1050–1051
Slocombe JOD, Smart J (1975) Evaluation of pyrantel pamoate against strongyles in horses. Can Vet J 16:310–312
Smith JA (1973) The occurrence of larvae of *Strongylus edentatus* in the testicles of stallions. Vet Rec 93:604–606
Soulsby EJL (1965) Textbook of veterinary clinical parasitology, vol I Helminths. Blackwell, Oxford
Stoye M, Ende H (1969) Versuche zur Behandlung des Strongylidenbefalles der Pferde mit Pyranteltartrat. Tierarztl Umsch 24:428–431

Squires EL, Amann RP, Pickett BW, Berndtson WE, Shideler RK, Vos JL (1978) Effect of fenbendazole on reproductive function in stallions. Theriogenol 9:447–455

Taylor EL (1942) A note on phenothiazine poisoning with special reference to reports of its occurrence in horses. Vet Rec 54:95–98

Turk RD, Ueckert BW, Bell RR (1962) Observations on thiabendazole as an equine anthelmintic. J Am Vet Med Assoc 141:240–242

Verberne LRM, Mirck MH (1975) Concerning the toxicity of parbendazole to horses and ponies. Tijdschr Diergeneeskd 100:1143–1153

Webster JH, Baird JD, Gunawan M, Martin ICA, Kelly JD (1981) Resistance to benzimidazole anthelmintics in equine strongyles. II. Evidence of side-resistance and susceptibility of benzimidazole-resistant strongyles to non-benzimidazole compounds. Aust Vet J 57:172–181

Wetzel R (1940) Palisadenwürmer *(Strongylus equinus)* im Pferd. Arch Wiss Prakt Tier 76:81–118

Whitlock JH, Leasure EE (1939) Studies upon *Strongylus vulgaris*. I. The incidence of *Strongylus vulgaris* in midcontinental North America and the reaction of the infected ceca. Am J Hyg 29:83–87

CHAPTER 8

Chemotherapy of Gastrointestinal Nematodiasis in Pigs

F. Rochette

A. Introduction

Sus scrofa, the Eurasian wild pig, was, after the sheep (8,500 B.C.) and dog (8,400 B.C.), the first animal ever domesticated. The earliest archeological source which was found in Cayönü in Turkey and dates back to about 7,000 B.C., tells us that the human race regarded *Sus scrofa* as a domestic animal. In the Oriental as well as the Western world, the pig has become one of man's most important nutritional resources. Despite the fact that there is large range of various sorts of meat, 760 million pigs are consumed annually. Europeans eat 30–40 kg pork per person per year.

The importance of the pig as a nutritional resource is far from surprising: pigs are easy to keep, they are omnivorous, and they reproduce at a ratio of 12–18 piglets/sow per year. Nowadays, the descendants of the Eurasian wild pig are dispersed throughout all continents, except some parts of Asia and Africa because of Jewish or Islamic prohibition rules concerning the eating of impure pig meat. These rules probably originate from archaic behavioral rules, which were very useful in the past in protecting people against parasitic diseases caused by the consumption of raw meat. The "dirty pig" which, even in the dirtiest circumstances, can exist on offal and excrements, indeed transmitted helminthiases such as trichinosis and tapeworms to humans.

The almost complete elimination of these zoonoses in Western Europe (Bourée et al. 1979) is a classic example of the establishment of preventive measures. On the other hand the prevalence of gastrointestinal parasites, which are harmful for the pig itself, remains high.

During the past 10–20 years, tremendous changes in methods of pig production have involved totally new techniques of housing, system control, and large-scale capital investment, not only in the West, but even in developing countries.

Through intensive breeding methods and economic measures, the fattening period has been shortened considerably and fertility has been improved. Simultaneously with this increase in production, a number of risk factors have emerged, such as the increasing susceptibility to stress and parasitosis, which can undermine productiveness. The economic pressures on the pig industry are such that production efficiency is of critical importance, so that no losses due to parasitosis can be afforded.

The diagnosis of gastrointestinal nematodiasis is simple, the biology of the parasites is well known, and many very active anthelmintics are available today. So it is possible, without prohibitive costs, to eliminate completely, or at least reduce markedly, most gastrointestinal helminthiases by the adoption of strenuous management, sanitary techniques, and deworming programs.

B. Pig Nematodes

Parasitosis is continuously prevalent throughout the modern pig industry (THIENPONT et al. 1969; BATTE 1974, 1977; PATTISON et al. 1980; AUGST 1981), and five gastrointestinal nematodes are especially economically important. In breeding animals incidence is highest for *Oesophagostomum* and *Hyostrongylus* and low for *Ascaris, Trichuris,* and *Strongyloides.* In weaners and fattening pigs *Ascaris* and *Trichuris* are most commonly diagnosed. *Strongyloides* infection may cause severe problems in suckling piglets.

Various Spiruroidea species parasitize the stomach of the pig, mostly in tropical and subtropical regions.

Table 1. Gastrointestinal nematodes in pigs

Localization	Worm species
Stomach	*Hyostrongylus rubidus* *Gnathostoma hispidum* *Physocephalus sexalatus* *Simondsia paradoxa* *Gongylonema pulchrum*
Small intestine	*Globocephalus urosubulatus* *Strongyloides ransomi* *Ascaris suum* *Trichinella spiralis*
Large intestine	*Oesophagostomum spp.* *Trichuris suis*

I. *Ascaris suum*

Ascaris suum or the large roundworm is one of the commonest and most pathogenic nematodes of pigs. It is the largest of the worms occurring in the small intestine. Incidence is highest in piglets and fattening pigs and declines with age. Less than 25% of sows are infected and the number of worms per adult animal is low, averaging only single figures. Partial age immunity appears to begin to operate at about 4–5 months.

The main effect of adult worms in the gut is mechanical and only in severe infection may subacute catarrhal enteritis associated with digestive disturbances occur. The worms may wander into the stomach or migrate into the bile duct causing stenosis of the biliary system (GEORGI 1980). A large number sometimes cause perforation of the intestine or become twisted into a bundle and cause intestinal obstruction. The larval stages migrating through the liver and lungs are more pathogenic than the adults. When the larvae reach the liver for the first time the site of arrest is sensitized and primary lesions, initially denoted by a hemorrhagic focus, occur. A mass or permanent reinfection gives rise to focal lesions in the gut, peritoneal invasions, and the characteristic "milk spots." ERIKSEN et al (1981) suggested that the finding of white spots on the liver at slaughter is an indication of a recent massive infection. The main damage caused by the larvae occurs in the lungs, leading to pneumonia and bacterial and viral superinfections (ANDERSEN 1977).

Clinically, ascariasis with identifiable symptoms is seen in young pigs between 2 and 5 months of age. The older pigs are free from infections or asymptomatic carriers of low-grade infections. In severe infections pulmonary signs of "thumps" pneumonia and coughing are seen. Heavy infections may be associated with some diarrhea and with potbelly and unthriftiness. Large numbers of ascarids seriously retard growth and prolong the fattening period (SUPPERER 1973; PACIEJEWSKI 1980). Pig livers may be condemned as unfit for human consumption because of the presence of "milk spots." TIELEN et al. (1976) reported diversity in the incidence of white spots: 20%–73% in Scandinavia, 65.5% in the Netherlands, and even 90% in Poland. The percentage of condemned livers is well below the incidence figures; only 1.5% in Sweden and 9.2% in the Netherlands of pig livers are totally condemned for human consumption. WERTENBROEK (1981) recorded a difference in growth of 40 g daily between baconers without white spots and those with totally involved livers.

II. *Strongyloides ransomi*

The females of the small intestinal threadworm *S. ransomi* are found in the anterior part of the small intestine of pigs, where they lay embryonated eggs. *Strongyloides* has a worldwide distribution and is most important in warmer, humid areas. Poor hygienic conditions such as dirty pens and damp bedding with unventilated houses are ideal for the development of these worms.

The infective larvae invade the host via the skin and reach the bloodstream. They migrate through the lungs and arrive in the duodenum, where they become adult. In pregnant sows the infectious larvae reach the subcutaneous tissue. They remain there in a resting phase until just a few hours before parturition, when they migrate into the mammary glands. The major part of the larvae will reach the piglets via the colostrum and will become adults after a shortened prepatent period of 2–3 days. As soon as from the 4th day after parturition on, the piglets produce worm eggs which, in turn, will lead to massive percutaneous infections. Sows can also be infected (STEWART et al. 1976). Even transplacental infection has been proved (ENIGK et al. 1974b). The various modes of infection, which can take place in the same litter of pigs, and the extremely short prepatent period of strongyloidosis make it difficult to control (ENIGK and DEY-HAZRA 1971). Infected piglets should be treated on the 3rd day after birth and then periodically every 8–10 days because the sow infects her piglets with infective larvae via the milk until 6 weeks after birth (SUPPERER 1972; ENIGK 1978).

Pathogenicity is associated with the adult worms in the intestine and with the migrating larvae in the skin and lungs. During the phase of skin penetration there may be erythema and pustular eruption. In the lungs hemorrhages, edema, and pneumonia may occur. The infection with adult worms is highly pathogenic in the small intestine. In acute infections, in the intestines there is a catarrhal reaction, a general congestion, edema and local hemorrhage with dehydration, loss of cations, and diarrhea. Death may occur early after infection. Mortality may approach 75% or more.

An even greater economic loss results from stunting, anemia, and unthriftiness (MONCOL and BATTE 1967). The piglets remain stunted for a long period after the acute signs have subsided, and for practical purposes in fattening pigs the effects of strongyloidosis may be accepted as permanent (DUNN 1969).

III. *Hyostrongylus rubidus*

In Western countries the red stomach worm is reported to occur in 40%–85% of sows and boars (TINAR 1975; AUGST 1981; PATTISON et al. 1980). The highest incidence of infection is in adult pigs which are at pasture and particularly in those in small paddocks, but the worm also occurs in housed animals. Most of these sows have very few worms, but about 20% harbor 1,000–1,500 worms in the stomach (STOCKDALE 1974). Both larvae and adult worms cause pathological changes in the stomach. The parasitic phase is somewhat similar to that of *Ostertagia* in cattle, with invasion of the gastric glands.

An infection with *Hyostrongylus* is usually a chronic, wasting disease with occasional acute outbreaks. The adult worms produce chronic catarrhal gastritis leading to the formation of a diphtheritic membrane and gastric ulceration (BASKERVILLE and ROSS 1970). A marked thickening of the mucous membrane and abundance of slimy tenacious mucus cover the infected parts. The gastric secretion is disturbed and losses of plasma proteins in the intestines are increased (DEY-HAZRA 1972). Clinically the affected pigs show unthriftiness, loss of weight, and sometimes diarrhea. The main features are anemia and inappetence with occasionally dark coloration of the feces. Mostly progressive loss in condition, without any other signs of illness, is characteristic . In severe cases, acute gastric hemorhage occurs with death or perforation of the stomach wall. High mortality rates have been noted in young pigs as well as in breeding sows (BOCH and SUPPERER 1977).

IV. *Oesophagostomum dentatum, O. quadrispinulatum*

The nodular worm *Oesophagostomum* is the most important nematode of the large intestine in pigs. It is cosmopolitan in distribution and has a high incidence of 60%–90% in sows. Even in piglets and in fattening pigs an incidence of 10% –60% is noted (AUGST 1981). Though infection is chiefly confined to pigs at pasture or paddocks for exercise, it may even occur in pigs under continuous housing (PATTISON et al. 1980). Infection may occur very early in life. *Oesophagostomum* larvae have been recovered from piglets 3 days old and less (DUNN 1979).

The *Oesophagostomum* larvae provoke nodular reaction by invasion through the intestinal mucosa. The fourth-stage larvae may remain in the nodules for periods exceeding 2 months. The typical lesion is of a circumscribed nodule about 4–5 mm in diameter which may be raised or flattened, with or without a central depression (TAFFS 1966).

Clinical signs are usually seen in young pigs, older animals being better able to resist the effect of infection. Heavy infections may be responsible for occasional diarrhea or constipation, diminished weight gain, emaciation, and disturbance of the reproductive cycle in sows. Even sterility and significantly lower litter performance are observed in young sows with normal growth and without clinical signs (SCHOOP et al. 1967; PATTISON et al. 1980).

V. *Trichuris suis*

The whipworm *Trichuris suis* is a nematode found in the cecum, colon, and rectum of pigs throughout the world. Infections with adult worms are commonly found in fattening pigs (2%–39%) and somewhat less in piglets and sows in western Europe (AUGST 1981) and 34%–77% in the United States (BATTE 1974, 1977). Outbreaks of clinical trichuriasis are rare and mainly confined to pigs kept outside or under extensive conditions. A slight infection develops subclinically. Severe natural infections exhibit watery, bloody, profuse diarrhea during 17–21 days postinfection. Clinical manifestations include anemia, anorexia, dysentery, pronounced weight loss, and death. Differential diagnosis is essential as the signs of trichuriasis mimic those of swine dysentery and other diseases (BATTE 1980). Pig trichuriasis can be a disease of economic importance to the pig industry particularly in fattening pigs (8–36 weeks of age) (BEER 1973).

VI. Spiruroidea

Of the five species of Spiruroidea parasitizing the stomach of the pig, one is from the family Gnathostomidae, i.e., *Gnathostoma hispidum*, and four are from the family Spuridae, i.e., *Ascarops strongylina, Physocephalus sexalatus, Simondsia paradoxa,* and *Gongylonema pulchrum*.

1. *Gnathostoma* ist found in eastern Europe and in Asia (Thailand). Pigs are infected by crustacean intermediate hosts or by ingestion of paratenic hosts like frogs, lizards, and fish. The adult worms are found deeply embedded in the gastric mucosa, where they may produce marked ulcerations.
2. The other spiruroids are found in the stomach. They need intermediate hosts such as beetles to complete their life cycle. A large number of spirurid worms causes inflammation of the mucosa, diffuse catarrhal gastritis, and sometimes the formation of pseudomembranes with ulceration covered with yellowish mucus (SOULSBY 1965). A spirurid infection should be differentiated from hyostrongylosis. Clinical signs such as loss of appetite, excessive thirst, and frequent eating of soil are attributable to the gastric inflammation.

VII. *Trichinella spiralis*

Trichinella spiralis parasitizes the small intestine of man and numerous other mammals such as rodents, bears, and pigs. It has been reported as a cause of zoonosis in almost every country of the world. Tropical areas, the Orient, Australia, and west European countries have a very low incidence; arctic regions, Eastern and Middle European countries (Poland, USSR, Rumania), and North American have a high incidence.

The chemoprophylaxis of trichinosis in swine is, as Campbell and Cuckler (1966) stated, primarily of academic interest, since there are more direct methods of interrupting the transmission of this infection. But nowadays anthelmintics are available, giving a high degree of protection against the enteral, migrating, and even encysted phase of *Trichinella* (Thienpont et al. 1978; Bogan 1980).

C. Pen Hygiene and Pasture Management

Modern industrial pig farms have led to enormous concentrations of pigs in a limited space, in warm and sometimes moist pigpens. Unintentionally, the pig farmer has created an ideal environment for the development of worms and their infectious eggs and larvae. In those modern industrial pig farms with intensive breeding and a high throughput, infection and reinfection with gastrointestinal worms remain a continuous problem. Theoretically it should be easy to obtain worm-free pig farms. The diagnosis is simple (Thienpont et al. 1979), the biology of the parasites is fairly well known, and there are many very active anthelmintics available. Despite all this, parasitism is continuously prevalent throughout the pig industry, and most herds are parasitized by several worm species. Multiple infections with two, three, or even four species of worm are still common (Thienpont et al. 1969; Pattison et al. 1980; Batte 1974). In a comparative survey (De Deken et al. 1982) of the endoparasites of pigs in Belgium from 1969 to 1980 it became clear that there had been a spectacular reduction in the general incidence. Certain technical factors such as the "all in – all out system," the frequency of anthelmintic treatment of the sows, cleanliness of the sties, and availability of straw to the piglets and pastures to the sows had a statistically significant influence on the incidence. Levels of parasitism appear to be influenced by the housing system and a number of management practices. Any action which increases the separation of the host from fecal material must limit the chances of infection or reinfection. Conversely, significant worm burdens may be expected when fecal material is allowed to accumulate and remains accessible to pigs, such as on pasture or in deep litter (Pattison et al. 1980). So a run is only meaningful if, apart from the value of exercise, it provides a substantial saving in food. Wallows are sources of infection and can be avoided by regularly rotating paddocks or by ringing the sows. If no paddock is available, a concrete run, which is easy to clean, is the best solution (Enigk 1978).

For each pen separate footwear and working materials (wheelbarrow, shovel, pitchfork) should be made available. If possible the pens must be mucked out regularly. Drinking and feeding installations must be kept as clean as possible. The pens should be disinfected especially when new animals are brought in . A blowtorch and boiling water are practically the only means of killing worm eggs and larvae. Before the sow is brought into the farrowing pen, she must be thoroughly washed and scrubbed. The sow is indeed the most important source of infection for the piglets. Infectious worm eggs or larvae stick to the claws, skin, and udders and the suckling piglets easily become infected.

New animals are first dewormed and placed in quarantine for at least a week.

D. Herd Deworming

Individual treatment of pigs with anthelmintics such as deworming a sow 1–2 weeks before farrowing, or deworming new animals in quarantine has limited and temporary benefits for the treated animals only. It has little or no effect on the degree of infection of the entire stock. The mean EPG (eggs per gram) measure of the farm remains almost constant because the newly treated animals reinfect themselves in the environment contaminated with worm eggs. In addition, the animals that remain untreated continue to infect the environment. Such a constant reinfection of the entire stock can, for the greater part, be avoided by periodically treating all the animals simultaneously with a several-day treatment program (De Keyser 1980; Rogiers 1974; Thomas 1981). This total herd deworming is achieved at tactical intervals, with the aim of obtaining and keeping the whole farm worm free and thus preventing the production of further worm populations. If there is no guarantee that new arrivals at the fattening farm are worm free they should be dewormed with an appropiate anthelmintic.

The veterinary surgeon working out a deworming schedule for a particular farm with the purpose of obtaining worm free animals must take into consideration: the housing system; the type of farm (open or closed, all in – all out, fattening and breeding or mixed farm); and the hygienic situation of the farm including the run. With regular coprological examinations, including differentiation of *Oesophagostomum* and *Hyostrongylus* larvae, and by recognizing the clinical symptoms, the veterinary surgeon can evaluate the infection and determine the appropriate anthelmintic and frequency of the deworming. The time of worming depends to a large extent on the prepatent period of the worm species found (Table 2). When various worm species must be dealt with, the shortest prepatent period should be considered.

If all the animals are wormed again as soon as the larvae have reached the adult stage, new production of millions of worm eggs can be avoided. After a certain period even the worm eggs already present before the worming program will lose their viability. The stock become almost egg as well as worm free if there are optimal hygienic conditions and if the systematic treatment of stock is regularly repeated. If this schedule is followed long enough and the stock become not only free of worms but also free of infective larvae and eggs, the treatments can be spread out. It is then strongly advised to make regular fecal examinations, especially for stock at pasture; the hygienic conditions must always be optimal.

Table 2. Treatment frequency based upon the prepatent period of the worm species

Worm species	Prepatent period	Treatment frequency
Strongyloides ransomi	2–10 days (Enigk 1978; Theodorides 1980)	Every 8–10 days
Ascaris suum	60–70 days (Supperer 1973; Theodorides 1980) 40–49 days in piglets (Euzeby 1963; Dunn 1969)	Every 2 months
Hyostrongylus rubidus	17–26 days (Plonait 1980)	Every 3–4 weeks
Oesophagostomum spp.	50–55 days (Soulsby 1965)	Every 2 months
Trichuris suis	41–47 days (Beer 1973)	Every 2 months

Table 3. Anthelmintics active against gastrointestinal nematodes in pigs

Chemical class	Generic name	Trade name(s)	Supplier(s)	Formulation	Dosage regime
1. Amines	Piperazine	Various	Various	Powder (soluble)	250–300 mg/kg
2. Organo-phosphates	Trichlorfon (metrifonate)	Neguvon	Bayer	Powder	50 mg/kg (for 2 days)
	Dichlorvos	Atgard, Tenac	Shell	Polyvinyl chloride, pellets, premix	30–40 mg/kg
	Haloxon	Eustidil, Galloxon 77% Cavoxon, Loxon	Wellcome/Cooper	Powder, premix 8%	30–50 mg/kg
3. Tetrahydro-pyrimidines	Pyrantel	Banminth	Pfizer	Soluble powder, 12.5% granules	12.5 mg/kg
4. Imidazothia-zoles	Levamisole	L-Narpenol, L-Tramisol Nemicide/Pig Wormer Concurat, Citarin Anthelsol Levasole Tramisol, Ripercol	Janssen Pharmaceutica ICI Bayer Rhone Poulenc Pitman-Moore American Cyanamid	5 % parenteral solution/ 7.5% parenteral solution/ 1.8% aqueous solution, 10 %granules, 1.5% aqueous solution, soluble powder	5–8 mg/kg
5. Benzimidazoles	Tiabendazole	Thibenzole	MSD	Powder 75%, permix paste 14.3%	50 mg/kg 100 mg/kg *Strongyloides*
	Cambendazole	Camdan, Neminil Porcam 5%	MSD	Granules	20–40 mg/kg
6. Benzimidazole carbamates	Parbendazole	Helmatac 30	SKF	Premix 30%, powder 10%	30 mg/kg
	Mebendazole	Mebenvet	Janssen Pharmaceutica	Powder 5%/50%	30 ppm for 5–10 days
	Fenbendazole	Panacur, Axilur	Hoechst	Powder 4%	5 mg/kg
	Oxfendazole	Synanthic, Systamex	Syntex/Wellcome		4.5 mg/kg
	Oxibendazole	Loditac, AM 313, Bovinol	SKF/Labo Thersa	Premix 5%/30% Powder 5%, granules 4.5 g/100 g, suspension 5%	15 mg/kg 100 ppm for 6 days 15 ppm for 50 days
	Flubendazole	Flubenol	Janssen Pharmaceutica	Powder 5%/50%	5 mg/kg 30 ppm for 5–10 days
7. Probenzimida-zoles	Febantel	Rintal	Bayer	Granules 10%, premix 0.6%	5 mg/kg 15–30 ppm for 6 days
	Thiophanate	Nemafax 14	May & Baker	Premix	5–12 mg/kg for14 day
8. Avermectino	Ivermectin	Ivomec	MSD	1% solution	200 μg/kg

E. Anthelmintics (Tables 3 and 4)

The first anthelmintics were used to relieve physical distress of pigs diagnosed to be parasitized by large numbers of *Ascaris*. Sodium fluoride, cadmiums, and hygromycin B had already been adapted for treatment of whole herds. Their spectrum and safety margin was too narrow. The newer anthelmintics used for treating pigs are mostly spin-offs from the ruminant dewormers, with the exception of piperazine. This old compound is specifically active against the ascarid class of worms.

I. Piperazines

Simple salts of piperazine (adipate, citrate, phosphate, sulfate, tartrate, hydrochloride), used to maintain the stability of the piperazine base, are among the oldest drugs still used in pigs. Except for the phosphates and adipates they can be given either in the feed or the drinking water. Various dose rates, mostly from 250 to 300 mg/kg, have been prescribed to control adult *Ascaris* and *Oesophagostomum* (see Table 4). Piperazines are useful for mass treatment of herds when directed against adult ascarids and nodular worms. Piperazine salts have a wide margin of safety, as they are virtually nontoxic at the recommended therapeutic dose levels . No serious form of intoxication has been reported with doses which are four to ten times the therapeutic ones. Intestinal irritation and vomiting may occur when an excessive dose has been taken (SOULSBY 1965).

II. Organophosphates

1. Trichlorfon

The organophosphate trichlorfon (metrifonate) given in the feed at a dosage of 50 mg/kg for two consecutive days is effective against adult *Ascaris suum, Trichuris suiss* and *Ascarops strongylina.* It has an effect against *Strongyloides, Hyostrongylus* and *Trichinella* but not against *Oesophagostomum* (CHANG and WESCOTT 1970; MAUCK and MICKWITZ 1965). The cholinesterase inhibitor trichlorfon may cause transient side effects such as diarrhea and muscular tremors at therapeutic doses (MAUCK and MICKWITZ 1965). Atropine can be used as antidote.

2. Dichlorvos

The insecticide dichlorvos has been subjected to extensive formulation development as an anthelmintic for pigs. Since the pure substance is too toxic as an anthelmintic, it has been formulated in an extruded polyvinylchloride resin pellet under varying concentrations and particle size for administration as a feed dressing. A coated version was designed for use in premix feedstuffs and as a formulation for incorporation into pelleted feedstuffs. The active ingredient dichlorvos is released slowly as the pellets pass through the pig gastrointestinal tract. The rate of drug release is designed to provide maximum anthelmintic activity and safety. At 30–40 mg/kg dichlorvos is an effective broad-spectrum anthelmintic in pigs;

Table 4. Activity of anthelmintics against some adult gastrointestinal nematodes in pigs (see

Anthelmintic at the recommended dose	*Ascaris suum*	*Strongyloides ransomi*	*Hystrongylus rubidus*	*Oesophagostomum* spp.	*Trichuris suis*
Piperazine, 250–300 mg/kg	++	0	(+)	+	0
Trichlorfon, 50 mg/kg for 2 days	++	++	+	+	++
Dichlorvos, 30–40 mg/kg	+++	+	++	+++	++
Haloxon, 30–50 mg/kg	+++		+	+++	+
Pyrantel, 12.5–25 mg/kg	+++	+	++	++	0
Levamisole, 5–8 mg/kg	+++	+++	++	++	++
Tiabendazole, 50–100 mg/kg 100–500 ppm in feed	+	++	++	++	0
Cambendazole, 20–40 mg/kg	++	+++	+++	+++	+
Parbendazole, 30 mg/kg	+++	+++	++	+++	+
Mebendazole, 30 ppm for 5–10 days	+++	++	++	+++	+++
Fenbendazole, 5 mg/kg	++	+	+++	+++	+
or 5–20 ppm for 6–10 days	+++	+++	N.D.	+++	+++
Oxfendazole, 4.5 mg/kg	+++	+	+++	+++	+
Oxibendazole, 5–15 mg/kg or 100 ppm for 6 days	+++	++	N.D.	++ – +++	+
Flubendazole, 5 mg/kg or 30 ppm for 5–10 days	+++	+++	++	+++	+++
Febantel, 5 mg/kg or 15–30 ppm for 6 days	+++	+	+++	++	++

+++, 95%–100%; ++, 80%–100%; +, 0%–100%; 0, 0%; ( ), insufficient data; ND, no data

it is active against roundworms, whipworms, and strongyles (see Table 4). It is effective for the control of mature ascarids and their fourth-stage larvae (BATTE et al. 1965) and for the adult, but not immature, stomach worm *Hyostrongylus rubidus (*TAFFS et al. 1973; STEWART et al. 1975).

Dichlorvos has a good effect against adult *Oesophagostomum* but does not affect the larvae in the subcutaneous nodules (SCHOOP et al. 1967). JACOBS et al. 1971, reported 42% and 61% efficacy against 2-week-old *Oesophagostomum* larvae. *O. quadrispinulatum* appeared to be more susceptible to dichlorvos therapy than *O. dentatum*. Efficacy against *Strongyloides* is variable to high (MARTI et al. 1978; EUZEBY and COTTEREAU 1969; PFEIFFER 1969; DINGELDEIN et al. 1973). At 35–40 mg/kg it is effective against *T. suis* (MARTI et al. 1978). Dichlorvos has no ovicidal effect but can reduce the infective larvae slightly (JACOBS 1968).

The dichlorvos-medicated feed is eaten without hesitation by all pigs and no side effects are observed. Even severe overdoses (11.52 g dichlorvos/sow for 1–2 text for details)

References
SEYFARTH (1960), JUNGMANN and SPLISTESER (1961), BOCH and MATZKE (1958), MANUEL and JOVES (1980)
ENIGK (1966), CHANG and WESCOTT (1970)
EUZEBY and COTTEREAU (1969), ROE et al. (1970), TAFFS et al. (1973), FORSTNER and MATZKE (1969), BATTE et al. (1965), JACOBS et al. (1971), HASS (1975), BEER et al. (1971–1973), MARTI et al. (1978)
CZIPRI (1970), WHITE et al. (1972)
ENIGK et al. (1971), ARAKAWA et al. (1971), HASSLINGER (1974), STEWART et al. (1972), WESCOTT and WALKER (1970)
OAKLEY (1974, 1977), JACOBS et al. (1977), ENIGK and DEY-HAZRA (1973), FERGUSON and WHITE (1975), PROBERT et al. (1973), MARTI et al. (1978), WARD and MCINTOSH (1978), JOHNSON et al. (1972), KUTZER (1978), LINDQUIST et al. (1971)
TAFFS (1968a, b), ENIGK and DEY-HAZRA (1971), DAVIDSON and TAFFS (1965), LELAND and COMBS (1965) THOMAS and SMITH (1968)
ENIGK et al. (1971), PROBERT et al. (1973), BARTH (1980), EGERTON et al. (1970), TAFFS (1971), SIBALIC et al. (1975), POUPLARD (1976)
THEODORIDES et al. (1968), PECHEUR et al. (1971), TAFFS (1970), CHANG and WESCOTT (1969), BATTE and MONCOL (1968)
VAN DEN BOSSCHE et al. (1982), NITZ (1974), ENIGK et al. (1976), ROGIERS (1974)
DÜWEL (1980), ENIGK et al. (1974a), KIRSCH and DÜWEL (1975), STEWART et al. (1981a), VAN DEN BOSSCHE et al. (1982)
CORWIN et al. (1979), KINGSBURY et al. (1981), FURMAGA et al. (1980)
STOYE and BÜRGER (1981), GRISI and LIMA (1981), VANDAELE and CHATON-SCHAFFNER (1980)
DE KEYSER (1980, THIENPONT and VANPARIJS (1980), KUTZER (1978), THIENPONT et al. (1982)
CONNAN (1978), BANKOV (1979), ČORBA (1981), ENIGK and DEY HAZRA (1978), KUTZER (1981)

weeks) are well tolerated (JACOBS 1968). A dose of 80–120 times the therapeutic dose is lethal. The product cannot be used together with other organophosphates (insecticides). The resin pellets are not digested and appear in the feces. These residual pellets are toxic to other animal species, especially birds. The antidote is atropine sulfate.

3. Haloxon

Haloxon, well documented as an anthelmintic for sheep, cattle, and horses (see Chap. 6, this volume), can be used as a wettable powder or premix for pigs. At 30–50 mg/kg it has a high efficacy against *A. suum* and both immature and mature *Oesophagostomum*. Efficacy against *H. rubidus* and *T. suis* is moderate and variable (CZIPRI 1970; WHITE et al. 1972). At a higher dosage (75 mg/kg) it was 74% effective against *H. rubidus* (CZIPRI 1970).

Although the anthelmintic has been widely used without untoward effects, sometimes a delayed neurotoxicity has been observed. Typically, posterior paralysis was seen about 3 weeks after worming with a dose up to 50% above the recommended dose (STUBBINGS et al. 1976).

III. Tetrahydropyrimidines

1. Pyrantel

Pyrantel, available as a 12.5% water-soluble powder or incorporated in the pig feed, given at 12.5 mg/kg is active against *Ascaris, Oesophagostomum*, and *Hyostrongylus* (Table 4). In severe infection the dose has to be doubled (25 mg/kg). It is not active against *Trichuris*. According to WESCOTT and WALKER (1970), pyrantel at 22 mg/kg is 96%–100% active against adult *Ascaris*. At 60.6 mg/kg it has an efficacy against the immature worms in the intestines and against the migrating larvae (ARAKAWA and CONWAY 1969). Continuous treatment with 100 ppm in the feed reduces lung and liver lesions and the number of larvae in the lungs due to *Ascaris*.

ENIGK et al. (1971) reported 84%, 96%, and 96% reduction of *Hyostrongylus* 5, 12–14, and 24 days postinoculation respectively, after a treatment of artificially infected piglets with a dose of 40 mg/kg. At the recommended dosage pyrantel is not toxic and does not provoke side effects. The oral LD_{50} in pigs is 72.3 mg/kg.

2. Morantel/Oxantel

Morantel, a close analogue of pyrantel, is several times more active against *A. suum*. At 5 mg/kg it is 100% effective against adult and immature *Ascaris*. At a dose of 7.5–12 mg/kg it is 70%–80% effective against *Oesophagostomum* and 75%–90% against *Hyostrongylus* (RAYNAUD 1972). According to CONWAY and RAYNAUD (1978) morantel at 30 ppm in the feed can be used in preventing *Ascaris* migration.

Oxantel at 4–5 mg/kg is highly effective against *Trichuris* (ROBINSON 1979). It has no effect on the other pig nematodes. The combination of 4 mg/kg oxantel and 12.5 mg/kg morantel is active against *Ascaris, Oesophagostomum, Hyostrongylus*, and *Trichuris* (JONES and CORNWELL 1974).

IV. Imidazothiazoles

Tetramisole, Levamisole

The racemic mixture tetramisole, whose anthelmintic activity has been shown to be predominantly due to its levo isomer, is soluble in water. Various formulations to be administered parenterally, or admixed in the feed or water, are available (Table 3). Single doses of 5–8 mg/kg levamisole are effective against adult and immature gastrointestinal nematodes (Table 4). OAKLEY (1974) reported anthelmintic efficacy of 100%, 100%, 92%, and 64% after s.c. treatment at 7.5 mg/kg against adult *A. suum* and 35- to 37-day-old, 11- to 13-day-old, and 5- to 7-day-old infections respectively. Administered in the feed or in drinking water at 8 mg/kg it was 100% effective against natural infections with ascarids (FERGUSON and WHITE 1975; JOHNSON et al. 1972).

ENIGK (1973) reports that levamisole at 5 mg/kg s.c. gave a 97% clearance of 10-day infections of *Strongyloides ransomi* in 8-week-old piglets. After dosing sows at 7 mg/kg twice daily for the first 10 days after parturition, larvae were no longer excreted in the milk after the 1st day. PROBERT et al. (1973) evaluated s.c. injections of 7.5 mg/kg as 93% effective against adult *H. rubidus*, 36% effective against 10- to 11-day-old larvae, and 60% effective against 7- to 8-day-old larvae. High efficacy (93%–96%) was obtained against adult *Oesophagostomum* and against 30- to 32-day-old (97%), 10- to 12-day-old (92%), and 4- to 6-day-old (65%) infections at 7.5 mg/kg s.c. (OAKLEY 1977). At 8 mg/kg in-water and in-feed clearances of 86% and 91% were recorded against the adult nodular worm (JOHNSON et al. 1972).

Tetramisole has only a low activity against *Trichuris*. The parenteral formulation of levamisole showed a high degree of anthelmintic activity (91%–100%) against *Trichuris* (FERGUSON and WHITE 1975; JACOBS et al. 1977). The in-feed administration was less active (JACOBS et al. 1977). Based on egg counts KUTZER (1978) reported high efficacy against *Globocephalus urosubulatus* in wild boars.

At therapeutic dose levels levamisole injected (5 mg/kg) and levamisole given in the feed or drinking water (8 mg/kg) are safe for use in pigs. Minute local reactions are detectable at the injection site following injection. Pigs tolerate up to five times the therapeutic dose of 7.5 mg/kg levamisole by s.c. injection. Adverse findings were not observed at three times the recommended dosage given in the drinking water or at five times the recommended dosage given in the feed. Sometimes vomiting occurred but it was of a transient nature (OAKLEY 1974a, c; OAKLEY et al. 1978).

V. Benzimidazoles

1. Tiabendazole

Two formulations of tiabendazole, i.e., a 14.3% paste and a 75% powder, are currently used as anthelmintics in pigs. One single dose of 50–100 mg/kg has high efficacy against *Hyostrongylus*, *Oesophagostomum*, and *Strongyloides*, but is not effective against *Ascaris* or *Trichuris* (Table 4). It is combined with piperazine to broaden the spectrum to include ascarids (TAFFS 1968).

Patent *Strongyloides* infections in piglets and sows are cured with 22–100 mg/kg (ENIGK and FLUCKE 1962; ENIGK and DEY-HAZRA 1971; MONCOL and BATTE 1967). Complete removal was not always achieved and reinfections were quickly established. At 100 mg/kg it was effective against *Strongyloides* infections and cured diarrhea during the 1st week after birth (BRAUNE and FREITAG 1970; SCHÄFER and PFEIFFER 1973). A treatment on the 8th day and a second treatment when the animals are 4 weeks old are effective against intestinal *Strongyloides*. Sows treated a few days before farrowing expelled the total intestinal worm burden, but tiabendazole was ineffective against the larvae which were later passed in the colostrum (PFEIFFER and SUPPERER 1969). TAFFS (1968a, b) reported 57% efficacy against 5-day-old larvae, 81% efficacy against 16-day-old larvae, and 96% efficacy against adult *Hyostrongylus* at 66 mg/kg. At 50 mg/kg tiabendazole was 100% effective against adult *Oesophagostomum* but it had no effect on 5-day-old larvae.

Pigs fed a diet containing 0.1% tiabendazole and exposed to larvae of *T. spiralis* developed either no infection or an infection of negligible severity. The majority of the larvae in the muscles of the treated pigs were killed by the medication (CAMPBELL and CUCKLER 1962). Tiabendazole is ovicidal 24 h after dosing (TAFFS 1968a, b). Low-level medication (5–10 mg/kg for 10–20 days) was 100% effective against strongylids (MOSER 1975) and 0.01% tiabendazole in the feed as a long-term treatment was active against *Strongyloides* (LELAND et al. 1968). Tiabendazole is well tolerated in pigs even in pregnant sows.

2. Cambendazole

Cambendazole, a derivative tiabendazole, is several times more potent than tiabendazole. It is available for pigs in granules to medicate the feed. At 20–40 mg/kg it is highly effective against *Ascaris, Strongyloides, Hyostrongylus,* and *Oesophagostomum* (Table 4). Cambendazole at 20 mg/kg eliminates the adult and most of the immature larvae of *A. suum* (POUPLARD 1976; ENIGK 1978). At dietary concentrations of 0.03% fed prophylactically 4 days before until 8 days after artificial infection with *Ascaris* eggs, it was effective in controlling a severe infection (EGERTON et al. 1970).

One single dose of 7.5 mg/kg is more than 99% effective in reducing *Strongyloides* worms recovered from the intestines (EGERTON et al. 1970). It has a better effect on the immature stages than tiabendazole (ENIGK and DEY-HAZRA 1971). A 10-day-treatment of sows with 2.5 mg/kg (5 days before and 5 days after farrowing) reduced infection by 99%–92% in 8- to 21-day-old piglets so that treatment of the piglets normally was no longer required (BARTH 1980). Cambendazole is highly effective at 20–40 mg/kg against adult and immature *Oesophagostomum* and *Hyostrongylus* (TAFFS 1971; ENIGK et al. 1971; POUPLARD 1976). It has an ovicidal effect of *Hyostrongylus* eggs (TAFFS 1971). Cambendazole is well tolerated in pigs. Pregnant sows must not be treated during the first 5 weeks of pregnancy.

VI. Benzimidazole Carbamates

1. Parbendazole

From the benzimidazole parbendazole two formulations are available in pigs, i.e., a premix 30% and a powder 10%. At the common therapeutic dose of 30 mg/kg, it is highly effective against *Ascaris, Strongyloides*, and *Oesophagostomum*. Efficacy against *Hyostrongylus* is somewhat lower and variable against *Trichuris* (Table 4). PECHEUR et al. (1971) reported 94% efficacy against adult and 47% against 14-day-old *Hyostrongylus* at 30 mg/kg.

An ovicidal effect on the eggs of *Oesophagostomum* and *Hyostrongylus*, or an influence of parbendazole on subsequent larval development in fecal culture, was noted by TAFFS (1970). Parbendazole has been shown to be a safe anthelmintic in pigs. Even single doses of 500–1,000 mg/kg showed no side effects during a 14-day observation period (THEODORIDES et al. 1968).

2. Mebendazole

Mebendazole is available as a 5% or 50% powder to medicate the feed. It has about the same parasitological properties as flubendazole. When given at 30 ppm in the feed for 5–10 days it is active against *Ascaris, Strongyloides, Oesophagostomum, Hyostrongylus*, and *Trichuris*. Evan at 4–8 ppm in the feed for 5 days, or 1.25 mg/kg at one intake, it is 100% active against *Ascaris* (VAN DEN BOSSCHE et al. 1982). It has an effect on the migrating larvae in the lungs (ROGIERS 1974). The pig is slightly sensitive to mebendazole: upon overdosage or inadequate mixing of the feed a transient softening of the feces or sometimes diarrhea is observed.

3. Fenbendazole

To deworm pigs fenbendazole can be given as a 4% powder or as a drench suspension at a single dose of 5 mg/kg. To improve the anthelmintic activity, especially against *Trichuris* and *Strongyloides*, the total therapeutic dose of 5 mg/kg should be divided over several days. It can be mixed in the feed at 5–20 ppm for 5–10 days.

One to three doses of 3–6 mg/kg are highly effective against adult *Ascaris, Oesophagostomum*, and *Hyostrongylus* and are moderately active against *Trichuris* and *Strongyloides* (MARTI et al. 1978; DÜWEL 1980; STEWART et al. 1981 a, b). A patent infection with *Ascaris* is cured with 3–6 mg/kg. At 8 mg/kg fenbendazole has a larvicidal effect on the migrating larvae (TIEFENBACH 1976). The effect on *Strongyloides* is 28%–99% when 40–70 mg/kg are given. A divided dose of six times 5 ppm gave 100% efficacy (ENIGK et al. 1974 b, 1977). Administration of 3–6 mg/kg fenbendazole is 73%–78% active against 5-day-old larvae and 96% effective against 16-day-old larvae of *Hyostrongylus* (KIRSCH and DÜWEL 1975). ENIGK et al. (1974 b) reported 80%, 69%, and 94% efficacy with a dose of 3 mg/kg against 6, 12, and 24-day-old larvae. For *Oesophagostomum* 56%–73% efficacy was recorded for 5-day-old larvae, 44% efficacy for 16-day-old larvae (KIRSCH and DÜWEL 1975), and at 6 mg/kg 61%–100% efficacy is seen for 8- to 30-day-old larvae (ENIGK et al. 1974 b). From 65%–97% of adult *Trichuris* are eliminated with 15–30 mg/kg and up to 100% are eliminated with six times 15 ppm in the feed. (ENIGK et al. 1977). Fenbendazole is well tolerated by pigs. No clinical signs are observed (KIRSCH and DÜWEL 1975).

4. Oxfendazole

Oxfendazole can be used in pigs although no specific formulations are available. At 4.5 mg/kg it is effective in removing the common nematodes of pigs. This was particularly obvious against *A. suum, Oesophagostomum*, and *Hyostrongylus* (Table 4). The effect against *Trichuris* was variable, with fluctuations in efficacy unrelated to the progressive increase in dose (CORWIN et al. 1979). At 7.5 mg/kg it was 80% effective against *Strongyloides* (FURMAGA et al. 1980). High larvicidal activity was observed against *Hyostrongylus* and *Oesophagostomum* 2-, 10-, and 20-day-old (KINGSBURY et al. 1981).

5. Oxibendazole

Various formulations of oxibendazole (Table 3) can be used in pigs. It is given at three dose levels: 15 mg/kg as a single dose, medicated feed at a concentration of 100 ppm for 6 days, and medicated feed at a concentration of 15 ppm for 50 days.

Efficacy against *Ascaris* and *Oesophagostomum* is 100% for the three treatment schedules. Efficacies for the three dosage regimens against *Trichuris* were 75%, 100%, and 80% respectively (GRISI and LIMA 1981). Oxibendazole at a dose of 15 mg/kg was 93% effective against *Strongyloides* (STOYE and BURGER 1981).

6. Flubendazole

The parafluor analogue of mebendazole, flubendazole, is available as a 5% or a 50% powder. It can be given in a single dose of 5 mg/kg or at 30 ppm in the feed for 5–10 days. It differs from mebendazole by its better tolerance in the pig.

At both dosage regimens flubendazole is highly active against *Ascaris, Strongyloides, Oesophagostomum*, and *Trichuris. Hyostrongylus* seems to be less sensitive (92%) but the clinical data reveal high activity (Table 4). A treatment of 30 ppm flubendazole for 10 days kills the migrating larvae of *A. suum* and the immatures of *T. suis* (THIENPONT et al. 1978, 1982). Administration of 32–125 ppm flubendazole for 14 days is 100% active against *Trichinella*, even against the encysted phase (BOGAN 1980; THIENPONT and VANPARIJS 1980). Flubendazole is also an effective anthelmintic against the most important wild boar nematodes (*Globocephalus, Trichuris*) at 100–150 ppm for 10 days (KUTZER 1978). Flubendazole is well tolerated by all animals. Piglets and fattening pigs received up to 20 and 40 times the therapeutic dose for 5 days with no side effects (DE KEYSER 1980). No harmful effects were provoked by flubendazole in gravid sows or in their piglets after administration of a therapeutic dose from the 8th to 50th day of gestation.

7. Albendazole

Albendazole is not available in a special formulation for pigs. Only preliminary data indicate that doses of 5–10 mg/kg are effective against *Ascaris, Oesophagostomum*, and *Trichuris* (THEODORIDES et al. 1976).

VII. Probenzimidazoles

1. Febantel

Febantel, a new guanidine derivative, is formulated in granules or premix as an anthelmintic for pigs. A single dose of 5 mg/kg or long-term treatment of 6 days with 15–30 ppm in the feed is highly active against *Ascaris, Hyostrongylus*, and *Oesophagostomum*.

Results against *Strongyloides* and *Trichuris* at these dosage regimens are moderate and variable (Table 4). At 5–10 mg/kg febantel removes all adult and immature *Ascaris* in the intestines and up to 69% of the larvae in the lungs (BANKOV 1979; ENIGK and DEY-HAZRA 1978). ENIGK (1978) found 76% efficacy against adult *Strongyloides* at 40 mg/kg. At both therapeutic dosage regimens febantel is highly active against adult *Oesophagostomum* and *Hyostrongylus*. It has larvicidal activity against 7-, 14-, and 21-day-old larvae (CORBA 1981; CONNAN 1978; ENIGK and DEY-HAZRA 1978; BANKOV 1979). At 15–20 mg/kg moderate to high efficacy is obtained against *Trichuris*. A long-term treatment of 60 ppm in the feed for 5 days or 30 mg/kg are required for 100% efficacy (Corba 1981; Connan 1978; Enigk and Dey-Hazra 1978). Febantel at 60 ppm/kg feed given for 5 days is active against *Ascaris* and *Globocephalus* but not against *Trichuris* in boars (Kutzer 1981).

At therapeutic doses the probenzimidazole febantel is well tolerated in pigs. No side effects of any kind have been observed at dose rates of up to 800 mg/kg. Only after 1,600 mg/kg did slight transient reduction in appetite occur (Enigk and Dey-Hazra 1978). Sows treated during the critical days of gestation (12th–14th day) with five times the therapeutic dose gave birth to healty piglets (Sachs and Will 1979).

2. Thiophanate

The probenzimidazole thiophanate is, at 50 mg/kg, highly active against *Oesophagostomum, Hyostrongylus*, and *Trichuris*. It is not active against *A. suum* and *S. ransomi* (Baines et al. 1976). Given as a 14-day low-level in-feed anthelmintic to gips (4–12 mg/kg) it is active against strongylids and *Trichuris* and has some effects against *Ascaris* (Baines et al. 1979).

VIII. Avermectins

Ivermectin

Avermectins are macrocyclic lactones produced by the actinomycete *Streptomyces avermitilis*. Several of the natural components have nematocidal and insecticidal (against e.g., the pig louse and the mange mite) properties. The B_1 fraction, one of the most potent components, can be given orally or parenterally at 200–500 μg/kg as an anthelmintic. At this dosage it is highly active against *Ascaris* and *Strongyloides* and moderately active against adult and immature *Oesophagostomum* and *Hyostrongylus*. Ivermectin B_1 has no effect on *Trichuris*. Clinical signs of toxicosis were not seen (Barth et al. 1980; Stewart et al. 1981 b).

Acknowledgments. I thank H. Van Hove, R. Jacobs, and C. Maes for their assistance in the preparation of this manuscript. I gratefully acknowledge J. Boersema, R. Marsboom, M. Rogiers, L. Desplenter, and D. Thienpont for a number of fruitful discussions and their criticism.

References

Andersen S (1977) Der Einfluß einer Askarideninfektion auf die Wachstumintensität des Ferkels. Tierarztl Prax 5:329–338

Arakawa A, Conway DP (1969) Hemagglutination tests for antibiotics to *Ascaris suum* in pigs treated with pyrantel hydrochloride. Am J Vet Res 30:1613–1699

Arakawa A, Conway DP, De Goosh C (1971) Therapeutic efficacy of Pyrantel tartrate against *Ascaris* and *Oesophagostomum* in swine. Vet Med Small Anim Clin 66:108–109

Augst M (1981) Wirtschaftliche Bedeutung der Magen-Darm-Nematoden bei Zucht- und Mastschweinen – Prophylaxe und Therapie unter besonderer Berücksichtigung des neuen Anthelminthikums Flubendazol. Eine Literaturauswertung. Thesis, Hannover

Bakker J (1984) Long term effect of a deworming program with flubendazole and levamisole upon the percentage of condemned livers in slaughter pigs. (D) Tijdschr Diergeneeskd 109:815–819

Baines DM, Dalton SE, Eichler DA (1976) Experimental and field studies with thiophanate in pigs. Vet Rec 99:119–122

Baines DM, Evans P, Lake P, Frape DL (1979) Field studies with thiophanate given as a 14-day low level in-feed anthelmintic to pigs. Vet Rec 105:81–82

Bankov D (1979) Clinical trials and field trials with febantel, a new nematocide substance II. The efficacy of febantel against *Ascaris suum, Oesophagostomum dentatum* and *Trichuris suis*. Vet Med Rev 1:74

Barth D (1980) Zur chemoprophylaxe der galaktogenen Strongyloidesinfektion beim Schwein mit Cambendazol. Prakt Tierarzt 2:119–120

Barth D, Sutherland IH, Roncalli RA, Leaning WHD (1980) The efficacy of ivermectin as an antiparasitic agent in the pig. In: Nielsen NC, Høgh P, Bille N (eds) Porceedings 1980 congress, IPVS, Copenhagen, June 30–July 3 1980, p 275. Available from: The Royal Veterinary and Agricultural University, Bülwosvej 13, DK-1870, Copenhagen V, Denmark

Baskerville A, Ross JG (1970) Observations on experimental and field infections of pigs with *Hyostrongylus rubidus*. Br Vet J 126:538–542

Batte EG (1974) Advances in swine parasitology 1973. Proceedings 22nd Pfizer research conference, Chicago 1974, pp 119–135. Available from: North Carolina State University, Raleigh, North Carolina

Batte EG (1977) A review and update of swine parasite control JAVMA 170:343–344

Batte EG (1980) Differential diagnosis and control of trichuriasis, 2nd international symposium veterinary laboratory diagnosticians, Lucerne/Switzerland. Available from North Carolina State University, Raleigh, North Carolina

Batte EG, Moncol DJ (1968) Evaluation of parbendazole, a new broad spectrum anthelmintic for swine and sheep. Vet Med Small Anim Clin 63:984–985

Batte EG, Moncol DJ, Todd AC (1965) Critical evaluation of an anthelmintic for swine. Vet Med 50:539–545

Beer RJS (1973) Studies on the biology of the life-cycle of *Trichuris suis* Schrank 1788. Parasitology 67:253–262

Beer RJS, Taffs LF, Jacobs DE, Lean IJ, Curran MK (1971) Evaluation of Dichlorvos (V_3 formulation) against larval and adult *Trichuris suis* and observations on experimental infection in growing pigs. Vet Rec 88:436–441

Beer RJS, Lean IJ, Jacobs DE, Curran MK (1973) Clinical trichuriasis produced experimentally in growing pigs. Part II Anthelmintic efficacy of Dichlorvos. Vet Rec 93:195–197

Boch J, Matzke P (1958) Vorkommen, Schadwirkung und Bekämpfung parasitischer Würmer bei Schweinen. Berl Munch Tierarztl Wochenschr 71:168–172

Boch J, Supperer R (1977) Parasitosen der Schweine. In: Parey P (ed) Veterinärmedizinische Parasitologie. Parey, Berlin, pp 295–328

Bogan JA (1980 Veterinary drug. Flubendazole. Drugs of today 16:306–310

Bourée P, Bouvier JB, Passerou J, Galanaud P, Dormont J (1979) Outbreak of trichinosis near Paris. Br Med J 1:1047–1049

Braune S, Freitag H (1970) Erfahrungen mit Thibenzole-Paste bei der Bekämpfung des Ferkeldurchfalls in der ersten Lebenswoche. Umschau 7:356–359

Campell WC, Cuckler AC (1962) Thiabendazole treatment of the invasive phase of experimental trichinosis in swine. Ann Trop Med Pharmacol 56:500–505

Campbell WC, Cuckler AC (1966) Further studies on the effect of thiabendazole on trichinosis in swine, with notes on the biology of the infection. J Parasitol 52:260–279

Chang J, Wescott RB (1969) Anthelmintic activity of parbendazole in swine. Am J Vet Res 30:77–79

Chang J, Wescott RB (1970) An evaluation of trichlorfon as an anthelmintic for swine. Am J Vet Res 31:2197–2200

Connan RM (1978) Trial of febantel against *Hyostrongylus rubidus, Oesophagostomum* spp. and *Trichuris suis* in pigs. Vet Med Rev 2:145–149

Conway D, Arakawa A (1968) Prophylactic efficacy of pyrantel against *Ascaris suum* in swine. Cornell Vet 59:605–610

Conway DP, Raynaund JP (1978) Ascariasis in pigs and new chemoprophylactic agents. In: Miroslav Herak, Marijan Sviben (eds) 5th International Pig Veterinary Society congress, Zagreb, Yugoslavia, June 13–15 1978, KA51. Available from: Zrinski-Čakovec, Zagreb, Yugoslavia

Čorba J (1981) The efficacy of febantel (Rintal) against gastrointestinal and lungnematodes of pigs. Vet Med Rev 1:10–14

Corwin RM, Kennedy JA, Pratt SE (1979) Dose titration of oxfendazole against common nematodes of swine. Am J Vet Res 40:297–298

Czipri DA (1970) The efficiency of haloxon against *Ascaris, Hyostrongylus* and *Oesophagostomum* in pigs. Vet Rec 86:306–309

Davidson JB, Taffs LF (1965) Gastro-intestinal parasites in pigs. Vet Rec 77:403

De Deken R, Sierens G, Hubrechts A, Jochems M, Bechter M (1982) A comparative survey of the endoparasites of swine in Belgium and their treatment. Vl. Diergeneesk Tijdschr 51:35–47

De Keyser H (1980) Einzel- und Bestandsentwurmung bei Schweinen mit Flubendazol. Tierarztl Prax 8:163–170

Dey-Hazra A (1972) Eiweiß- und Blutverlust bei Rundwurminfektionen des Schweines. Proceedings 2nd International Pig Veterinary Society Congr, Hannover 1972, p 45. Available from: Institute for Parasitology, Tierärztliche Hochschule Hannover, West Germany

Dingeldein W, Sperling H, Manz D (1973) Untersuchungen zur Anwendung und anthelmintischen Wirkung von Atgard C unter Praxisbedingungen. Tierarztl Umschau 28:352–355

Dunn AM (1969) Veterinary helminthology. Heinemann, London

Düwel D (1980) Panacur, Axilur. Summary and evaluation of the worldwide published investigations. Hoechst Aktiengesellschaft-Ressort Veterinärmedizin, Frankfurt am Main

Egerton JR, DiNetta J, Neu DC, Walther RJ, Campbell WC (1970) The efficacy of cambendazole against *Ascaris suum* and *Strongyloides ransomi* in swine. Res Vet Sci 11:590–592

Enigk K (1966) Auftreten und Bekämpfung des Helminthenbefalles beim Schwein. DTW 73:613–616

Enigk K (1978) Die biologischen Grundlagen zur Behandlung und Vorbeuge des Helminthenbefalles beim Schwein. DTW 85:77–81

Enigk K, Dey-Hazra A (1971) Zur Therapie des Strongyloidesbefalles beim Schwein. DTW 78:419–422

Enigk K, Dey-Hazra A (1973) Die Wirkung von Levamisole auf den Strongyloides-Befall des Schweines. Tierarztl Umsch 28:76–80

Enigk K, Dey-Hazra A (1978) The treatment of helminth infestations in pigs with Rintal. Vet Med Rev 2:134–144

Enigk K, Flucke W (1962) Zur Therapie des *Strongyloides*-Befalls beim Schwein. DTW 69:519–522

Enigk K, Dey-Hazra A, Gerlach G (1971) Zur Therapie des *Hyostrongylus*-Befalles beim Schwein. DTW 78:569–572

Enigk K, Dey-Hazra A, Batke J (1974a) Zur Wirkung von Fenbendazol auf den Nematodenbefall des Magen-Darmkanals beim Schwein. DTW 81:177–200

Enigk K, Weingartner F, Hazem AS, Schmelzle HM, Stoye M (1974b) Zur pränatalen Strongyloides-Infektion des Schweines. Tierarztl Umsch 29:265–268

Enigk K, Dey-Hazra A, Batke J (1976) Zur Wirksamkeit von Mebendazole auf den Helminthenbefall des Schweines. Tierarztl Umsch 31:360–362

Enigk K, Batke J, Dey-Hazra A, Düwel D, Tiefenbach B (1977) Weitere Erfahrungen mit Fenbendazol bei der Bekämpfung des Magen-Darm-Nematodenbefalls beim Schwein. Tierarztl Umsch 8:414–420

Eriksen L, Andersen S, Nielsen K, Nielsen J, Pedersen A (1981) White spots in the liver of swine. New understanding of a current problem through experimental infection with *Ascaris suum* eggs. Dansk Veterinaertidsskrift 64:488–492

Euzéby J (1963) Les maladies vermineuses des animaux domestiques et leurs incidences sur la pathologie humaine. I Maladies dues aux némathelminthes. Fascicule deuxième. Vigot Frères, Paris

Euzéby J, Cottereau Ph (1969) Activité anthelminthique du phosphate de 2–2 dichlorovinyl-dimethyl (Dichlorvos) sur les nématodes parasites du tractus gastro-intestinal du porc. Revue Med Vet 120:121–129

Ferguson DL, White RG (1975) Anthelmintic activity of levamisole against *Ascaris, Trichuris* and *Metastrongylus* in swine. J Anim Sci 40:838–843

Forstner MJ, Matzke P (1969) Untersuchungen über Wurmwirksamkeit und Mastbeeinflussung von Atgard V auf Schweine. DTW 76:283–287

Furmaga S, Gundlach JL, Sadzikowski A, Uchacz S (1980) The usefulness of Systamex in the control of intestinal helminthiases in pigs (Pol). Med Vet 36:473–476

Georgi JR (1980) Parasitology for veterinarians, 3rd edn. Saunders, Philadelphia, pp 389–396

Grisi L, Lima MM (1981) Efficacy of oxibendazole against gastrointestinal parasites of swine. Proceedings 9th international conference of the World Association for the Advancement of Veterinary Parasitology, Budapest 13–17 July 1981, p 213. Available from: Dept Animal Biology, University Federal Rural do Rio de Janeiro, Brazil

Hass DK (1975) Anthelmintic efficacy of Dichlorvos against *Hyostrongylus rubidus* and *Oesophagostomum dentatum* in swine at timed intervals after exposure to infective larvae. Vet Med Small Anim Clin 70:187–190

Hasslinger MA (1974) Experimentelle Untersuchungen zur Bekämpfung präadulter Magen- und Knötchenwurmstadien beim Schwein mit Thiabendazol und Pyranteltartrat. DTW 81:379–382

Jacobs DE (1968) Experiences with a broad-spectrum anthelmintic, dichlorvos in the adult pig. Vet Rec 83:160–164

Jacobs DE, Curran MK, Taffs LF (1971) The efficacy of Dichlorvos (V_3 formulation) against larval and adult *Oesophagostomum* spp. in the pig. Res Vet Sci 12:189–191

Jacobs DE, Lean IJ, Oakley GA (1977) Levamisole: efficacy against *Trichuris suis*. Vet Rec 100:49

Johnson WP, Eggert RG, Poeschel GP, Wang GT (1972) Levamisole as an anthelmintic for swine. JAVMA 16:1221–1225

Jones RM, Cornwell RL (1974) Activity of oxantel against *Trichuris suis*. Proceedings 3rd International Congress of Parasitology, München 1974, vol III, pp 1435–1436. Facta Publication, Egermann, Vienna

Jungmann R, Splisteser H (1961) Ein Beitrag zur Bekämpfung der Magen-Darm-Parasiten des Schweines mit Piperazinchlorhydrat unter den Bedingungen des Feldversuches. Mh Vet Med 16:685–689

Kingsburry, Rowlands T, Reid JFS (1981) Anthelmintic activity of oxfendazole in pigs. Vet Rec 108:10–11

Kirsch R, Düwel D (1975) Laboratory investigations on pigs with the new anthelmintic fenbendazole. Res Vet Sci 19:327–329

Kutzer E (1978) Die Behandlung der Metastrongylose in Wildschweingehegen. Tierarztl Prax 6:325–334

Kutzer E (1981) The anthelmintic action of febantel (Rintal) in wild boars (*Sus scrofa*). Vet Med Rev 1:34–41

Leland SE, Combs GE (1965) Test of anthelmintic activity against the migratory stages of *Strongyloides ransomi* in pigs. Am J Vet Res 26:932–938

Leland SE, Combs GE, Wallace LJ (1968) Anthelmintic activity of thiabendazole and trichlorfon against migrating and adult *Strongyloides ransomi* in suckling and weaning pigs. Am J Vet Res 29:797–806

Lindquist WD, Leland SE, Ridley RK (1971) Field experiments on levamisole against certain helminths in pigs, with emphasis on test of activity against lungworms. Am. J. Vet. Res. 32:1301–1304

Manuel FM, Joves ER (1980) Efficacy of some anthelmintic preparations against gastrointestinal parasites in swine. Philippine J Vet Med 19:67–80

Marti OG, Stewart TB, Hale OM (1978) Comparative efficacy of fenbendazole, dichlorvos and levamisole HCl against gastrointestinal nematodes of pigs. J Parasitol 64: 1028–1031

Mauck C, Mickwitz G (1965) Neguvon treatment of mange and helminth infections in weaned pigs. DTW 72:521–525

Moncol DJ, Batte EG (1967) Porcine strongyloidosis treatment and control. JAVMA 151:1177–1180

Moser, S (1975) Zur Wirksamkeit von Thiabendazole beim Schwein nach fraktionierter Verabreichung über mehrere Tage. Tierarztl Umsch 30:24–26

Nitz KJ (1974) Die Anthelmintische Wirkung von Mebendazol als Medizinalfutter bei Schweinen. Tierarztl Umsch 29:495–496

Oakley GA (1974a) The anthelmintic efficacy of parenterally administered levamisole against common nematode parasites in the pig. 3rd international congress (International Pig Veterinary Society), Lyon, June 12–14 (1974). Available from L'imprimerie, ESPIC-Toulouse, France

Oakley GA (1974b) Activity of levamisole hydrochloride administered subcutaneously against *A. suum* infections in pigs. Vet Rec 95:190–192

Oakley GA (1974c) The anthelmintic activity of levamisole administered subcutaneously to pigs at 7.5 mg/kg. Br Vet J 130:XXXVI

Oakley GA (1977) Efficacy of levamisole hydrochloride administered subcutaneously against *Oesophagostomum dentatum* infection in pigs. Vet. Rec. 100:310–312

Oakley GA, Froyd G, Cooper RG (1978) The safety of levamisole administered by subcutaneous injection. Proceedings 5th International Pig Veterinary Society congress, KB 41 (1978). Available from: ICI, Pharmaceutical Division, Alderly Park, Macclesfield, Cheshire, UK

Paciejewski S (1980) Economic loss due to experimental larval ascariasis (Pol). Med Welt 36:463–466

Pattison HD, Thomas RJ, Smith WC (1980) A survey of gastrointestinal parasitism in pigs. Vet Rec 107:415–418

Pecheur M, Dewaele A, Brasinne M, Pandey VS (1971) Action du parbendazole vis-à-vis de *Hyostrongylus rubidus* chez des porcs infestés experimentalement. Ann Med Vet 115:175–180

Pfeiffer A (1969) Prophylaxe und Therapie beim Helminthenbefall im Schweinebestand. DTW 76:488–491

Pfeiffer H, Supperer R (1969) Über die Bekämpfung der Strongyloidose der Saugferkel mit Thiabendazol. Wien Tierarztl Monatschr 56:116–120

Plonait H (1980) Parasitäre Erkrankungen. In: Schulze W, Bickhardt, Bollwahn W, Mickwitz GV, Plonait H (eds) Klinik der Schweinekrankheiten. Schaper, Hannover, pp 164–173

Pouplard L (1976) Les anthelminthiques en médecine vétérinaire. I Les Nématodes. Ann Med Vet 120:515–529

Probert AJ, Smith BDS, Herbert IV (1973) The efficacy of orally and subcutaneously administered levamisole against mature and immature stages of *Hyostrongylus rubidus*, the stomach worm of pigs. Vet Rec 93:302–306

Raynaud JP (1972) Controle de l'efficacité des anthelminthiques chez le porc cas particulier du morantel tartrate. Proceedings 2nd International Pig Veterinary Society congr, Hannover 1972, p 133

Robinson M (1979) Efficacy of oxantel tartrate against *Trichuris suis* in swine. Vet Parasitol 5:223–235

Roe CK, Stockdale PHG, Wilson MR (1970) The efficacy of dichlorvos against *Oesophagostomum* spp. in swine. Can Vet J 11:72–73

Rogiers M (1974) The anthelmintic action of mebendazole in pig-breeding. Proc 3rd International Pig Veterinary Society Congr Lyon 1974, p 11, 1–12. Available from: L'imprimerie, ESPIC-Toulouse, France

Sachs, H, Will R (1979) Febantel – ein neues Breitbandanthelminthikum. Thesis XXI world veterinary congress 2 Moscow (III), p 12

Schäfer H, Pfeiffer A (1973) Zur Therapie der Strongyloideserkrankung der Saugferkel mit Thiabendazol. DTW 80:145–172

Schoop G, Lamina J, Bohnhardt H (1967) Untersuchungen über die Anwendungsmöglichkeiten von Dichlorvos bei *Oesophagostomum*-Befall des Schweines. DTW 74:81–87

Seyfarth D (1960) Beitrag zur Bekämpfung des Askaridenbefalles beim Schwein mit „Piavetrin" Bernburg. Mh Vet Med 15:404–408

Sibalic S, Cvetkovic LJ, Thomanovic B, Lepojev O (1975) Studies on the effect of Cambendazole on *Ascaris suum* migrating larvae in artificially infected piglets. Proceedings 2nd European multicolloquy parasitol, Trogir, Yugoslavia 1975, pp 439–443

Soulsby EJL (1965) Textbook of veterinary clinical parasitology. Blackwell, Oxford

Stewart TB, Johnson JC, Hale OM (1972) Effects of pyrantel HCI and dietary protein on growing pigs infected in different sequences with *Strongyloides ransomi, Ascaris suum* and *Oesophagostomum* spp. J Anim Sci 35:561–568

Stewart TB, Hale OM, Marti OG (1975) Efficacy of two Dichlorvos formulations against larval and adult *Hyostrongylus rubidus* in swine. Am J Vet Res. 36:771–772

Stewart TB, Stone WM, Marti G (1976) *Strongyloides ransomi:* prenatal and transmammary infection of pigs of sequential litters from dams exposed to weanlings. Am J Vet Res 37:541–544

Stewart TB, Marti OG, Hale OM (1981 a) Efficacy of fenbendazole against five genera of swine parasites. Am J Vet Res 42:1160–1162

Stewart TB, Marti OG, Hale OM (1981 b) Efficacy of ivermectin against five genera of swine nematodes and the hog louse *Haemotopinus suis*. Am J Vet Res 42:1425–1428

Stockdale HG (1974) The pathogenesis of *Hyostrongylus rubidus* in growing pigs. Br Vet J 130:366–373

Stoye M, Bürger HJ (1981) Anthelmintic activity of oxibendazole against *Strongyloides ransomi.* Proceedings 9th International Conference World Association for Advancement of Veterinary Parasitology, Budapest 1981, p 212. Available from: Institute of Parasitology, Hannover, School of Veterinary medicine, Bünteweg 17, D-3000 Hannover 71, Federal Republic of Germany

Stubbings DP, Gilbert FR, Giles N, Holmes RG, Jackson G, Nicholson TB (1976) An organophosphorous worming compound and paraplegia in pigs. Vet Rec 76 99:127–128

Supperer R (1972) Parasitenbekämpfung beim Schwein. Schweiz Arch Tierheilkd 114:591–600

Supperer R (1973) Parasitosen im Intensivbetrieb: Schwein. Tierarztl Prax 1:33–42

Taffs LF (1966) Helminths in the pig. Vet Rec 79:671–693

Taffs LF (1968 a) Oral thiabendazole. Effect on immature and adult *Hyostrongylus rubidus* in experimentally-infected pigs. Vet Rec 83:119–121

Taffs LF (1968 b) An evaluation of the efficiency of thiabendazole. Vet Rec 83:219–221

Taffs LF (1970) Anthelmintic activity of parbendazole in swine naturally infected with lungworms and gastro-intestinal nematodes. Res Vet Sci 11:515–522

Taffs LF (1971) The effect of oral cambendazole against *Hyostrongylus rubidus* and *Oesophagostomum* spp. in experimentally infected pigs. Vet. Rec. 89:165–168

Taffs LF, Lean IJ, Jacobs DE, Curran MK (1973) Efficacy of four dichlorvos formulations against adult *Hyostrongylus rubidus* and *Oesophagostomum* spp. in pigs. Br Vet J 129:XXI–XXVI

Theodorides VJ (1980) Antiparasitic drugs in: Georgi JR (ed) Parasitology for veterinarians, 3rd edn Saunders, Philadelphia, pp 397–448

Theodorides VJ, Laderman N, Pagano JF (1968) Parbendazole in treatment of intestinal nematodes of swine. Vet Med Small Anim Clin 63:370–371

Theodorides VJ, Gyurik RJ, Kingsbury WD, Parish RC (1976) Anthelmintic activity of albendazole against liver flukes, tapeworms, lung and gastrointestinal roundworms. Experientia 32:702–703

Thienpont D, Vanparijs O (1980) Prophylactic and curative action of flubendazole against experimental trichinellosis in pigs. Proc 5th Int Conf on trichinellosis. Noordwijk aan Zee, The Netherlands Sept 1–5, 1980, pp 343–346

Thienpont D, Sierens G, Vanparijs O, Lauwers H, Hermans L (1969) Remarks about the research into and the control of worm infections in piggeries (D). Tijdschr Diergeneeskd 94:1667–1678
Thienpont D, Vanparijs O, Niemegeers C, Marsboom R (1978) Biological and pharmacological properties of flubendazole. Arzneimittelforsch 28:605–612
Thienpont D, Rochette F, Vanparijs OFJ (1979) Diagnosis of helminthiasis through coprological examination. Janssen Res Found Beerse, Belgium, pp 91–106
Thienpont D, Vanparijs O, Hermans L, Roose P De (1982) Treatment of *Trichuris suis* infections in pigs with flubendazole. Vet Rec 110:517–520
Thomas RJ (1981) The ecological basis of parasite control: nematodes. Proceedings 9th International Conference World Association for the Advancement of Veterinary Parasitology, Budapest 1981, pp 18–19. Available from: Dr Thomas, School of Agriculture, University of Newcastle upon Tyne, Newcastle upon Tyne, UK
Thomas RJ, Smith WC (1968) Anthelmintic treatment of sows with thiabendazole. Vet Rec 83:489–491
Tiefenbach B (1976) Panacur-Weltweite klinische Prüfung eines neuen Breitband-Anthelminthikums. Die Blauen Heften 55:204–218
Tielen MJM, Truyen WT, Remmen JWA (1967) The incidence of diseases of the lung and liver in slaughtered pigs as a criterion in the detection of herds in which the disease is a recurrent problem (D). Tijdschr Diergeneeskd 101:962–971
Tinar R (1975) Fréquence de *Hyostrongylus rubidus* chez le porc en Belgique. Ann Med Vet 119:337–341
Vandaele WM, Chaton-Schaffner M (1980) Oxibendazole – an ideal anthelmintic for pigs. In: Nielsen NC, Høgh P, Bille N (eds) Proceedings 6th International Pig Veterinary Society Congress, Kopenhagen 1980, 272. Available from: The Royal Veterinary and Agricultural Society, Bülowsvej 12, DK-1870, Copenhagen V, Denmark
Vanden Bossche H, Rochette F, Hörig C (1982) Mebendazole and related compounds. Adv Pharmacol Chemother 19:67–128
Ward CJ, McIntosh DAD (1978) A review of the anthelmintic efficacy of levamisole in pigs. Proc 5th IPVS Congr KB 42 (1978)
Wertenbroek ACJM (1981) Field studies on the incidence of damage to the liver caused by migrating *Ascaris* larvae in baconers and its treatment. Tijdschr Diergeneeskd 106:662–670
Wescott RB, Walker JH (1970) Efficacy of pyrantel tartrate as an anthelmintic in swine. Am J Vet Res 31:567–569
White RG, Danielson DM, Ferguson DR, Hibbs CM (1972) Loxon feed additive as an anthelmintic in swine. J Anim Sci 35:196

CHAPTER 9

Chemotherapy of Gastrointestinal Nematodiasis in Carnivores

F. ROCHETTE

A. Introduction

No animal species has, in the course of human civilization, better deserved the denomination "pet animal" than the descendants of the wolf and the wild Nubian cat. Dogs, and to a lesser extent cats, are not only one of the earliest domesticated animal species; they are the animals that have been by far the most intensively modulated by the domesticating process, into hundreds of breeds and races, to meet all kinds of human needs. The dog became a companion, a watchdog, a hunter, a tracker dog, a guide dog, and in the first place – as did cats – a pet; in some countries it still serves as meat for human consumption. There are about 70 million dogs and cats in the United States. During the 1960s the population of dogs increased by more than 40% whereas the human population increased by only about 10% (FAULKNER 1975). The ratios of cat/man and dog/man vary between 1:26.5 for West Germany and 1:6.2 for the United States (BECK 1975). This increase in the number of pets relates to the population growth and the rising standard of living. One of the most important aspects of pet ownership is that dogs and cats are responsible for more than 65 zoonoses, e.g., rabies, ringworm, echinococcosis, ancylostomiasis, and visceral larva migrans (FELDMAN and CARDING 1973; WOODRUFF 1975).

In 1952 BEAVER identified *Toxocara canis* larvae in a liver biopsy and proposed the term visceral larva migrans. The infective larvae of *Ancylostoma braziliense* produce in man "creeping eruption", a dermatitis accompanied by intense itching. The other hookworm species may cause comparable lesions but the symptoms are less severe and more transient (WOOD and PANKAVICH 1961). There have also been several reports of human intestinal infection with an adult *Toxocara cati* worm from cats (WISEMAN and LOVEL 1969; VON REYN et al. 1978).

B. Gastrointestinal Nematodes of Dogs and Cats

The three main types of nematodes found in dogs and cats are ascarids, hookworms, and whipworms. The incidence of other nematodes is low (Table 1).

The prevalence and the ubiquity of the parasites are well documented (LAMINA 1970; ECKERT 1972; VANPARIJS and THIENPONT 1973; JACOBS et al. 1977; REP 1980). The prevalence and distribution of the common helminths vary widely. Mostly the dog or cat is infected with one species, but 12%–16% of animals have a polyinfestation with two to four different worm species (VANPARIJS and THIENPONT 1973; GERIN et al. 1980).

Table 1. Gastrointestinal nematodes of dogs and cats

Common name	Dog	Cat
Stomach		
Stomach worms	*Physaloptera spp.* *Gnathostoma spinigerum*	*Capillaria putorii* *Spirura ritypleuritis* *Ollulanus tricuspis* *Physaloptera spp.* *Gnathostoma spinigerum*
Small intestine		
Ascarids	*Toxocara canis* *Toxascaris leonina*	*Toxocara cati* *Toxascaris leonina*
Hookworms	*Ancylostoma caninum* *Ancylostoma braziliense* *Uncinaria stenocephala*	*Ancylostoma caninum* *Ancylostoma braziliense* *Ancylostoma tubaeforme* *Uncinaria stenocephala*
Trichina worm	*Trichinella spiralis*	*Trichinella spiralis*
Threadworm	*Strongyloides stercoralis*	*Strongyloides stercoralis*
Hairworm		*Capillaria putorii*
Large intestine		
Whipworm	*Trichuris vulpis*	

I. Ascarids

Toxocara canis has been reported from nearly all parts of the world. The infection rate in pups approaches 100% in some kennels. In western Europe 10%–25% of adult dogs are infected with *Toxocara* and *Toxascaris* (GLICKMAN et al. 1979; CONNAN 1979). In a humid and warmer climate, the infection rate is usually higher and reaches 80%. There have been no signs of a reduction in incidence during recent years. The extensive investigation that was undertaken in Great Britain has only shown that show dogs and pets are less infected (±7%) than street dogs, breeding dogs, and kennel dogs (13%–14%) (JACOBS et al. 1977).

These worm species are very fertile. A female worm of *Toxocara* can shed 200,000 eggs daily. One gram of feces from a heavily infected pup may contain 10,000 eggs. It has been estimated that in the United States dogs burden the environment with 3,500 tons of feces daily (DJERASSI et al. 1973), containing millions of worm eggs. Examinations of soil in gardens, parks, and exercise paddocks in different countries have demonstrated worm eggs of *Toxocara* to be present (DUBIN et al. 1975; JACOBS et al. 1977).

The life cycle of *T. canis* is rather complex (SPRENT 1958). After oral infection with embryonated eggs second-stage larvae may remain in the tissues of the adult animals for years, especially in bitches. These larvae in the bitch infect the puppies before and/or after (e.g., colostrum) they are born. Unfortunately, current drugs are insufficient at normal therapeutic doses to kill all the larvae, although the benzimidazole carbamates mebendazole, fenbendazole, and oxfendazole have some effect on *Toxocara* larvae. Only strategic and periodic deworming and rigorous hygiene can reduce the number of adult worms. In severe infections hemorrhagic zones in the lungs may be lethal in heavily prenatally infected pups within a few days after birth. Pot belly, some diarrhea, and retarded growth are the common symptoms in dogs infected with adult worms.

The ascarid *Toxascaris leonina* occurs in both dogs and cats. In European countries it is less common in cats (0.2%, NICHOL et al. 1981; 0.9%, ECKERT 1972) than in dogs (5.1%, ECKERT 1972; 7.2%, VANPARIJS and THIENPONT 1973). Since prenatal infections with *T. leonina* do not occur control measures are much easier than those appropriate to *Toxocara canis*. However, paratenic hosts, e.g., rodents, may bear a large number of infective larvae and as such infect dogs. This will affect control measures. *Toxocara cati* is endemic in all countries. Surveys in domesticated cats revealed that in London 11.5% were infected; kittens had the highest incidence (22%–69%) (NICHOL et al. 1981). In stray cats 65% were infected with ascarids and 39% with hookworms (VANPARIJS and THIENPONT 1973). The general signs are usually confined to pot belly, diarrhea, rough coat, and retarded growth.

II. Hookworms

The geographical distribution of the three common species of canine hookworms depends upon climatic conditions. *Ancylostoma caninum* and *A. braziliense* are found most frequently in subtropical and tropical climates. *U. stenocephala* is more common in temperate regions. In the Netherlands 2.6% of the dogs surveyed had hookworm infections, 3.3% in Belgium, 6.1% in England, and 21% in Poland (REP 1979). Probably more than 50% of kenneled greyhounds or foxhounds under 2 years of age are infected with *Uncinaria*, but the prevalence declines in older animals (HOVELL and WESTON 1970; JACOBS and PROLE 1976). It is rather rare in companion animals.

Hookworms are hematophagic [0.12 ml blood/worm per day (CLARK et al. 1961)]. They may cause considerable mortality and morbidity but *Uncinaria* is only very slightly pathogenic. Puppies infected with *Ancylostoma* have a high death rate. The chief sign is anemia and in chronic infections there is emaciation, poor appetite, pica, a rough coat, and darkish diarrhea. There may be abortion and the pups have a poorer chance of survival (DUNN 1969).

III. Whipworms

Dogs are not infrequently infected with *Trichuris* (11.9%, ECKERT 1972) but usually the number is low. *Trichuris* is more a parasite of kenneled dogs than of companion dogs. *Trichuris* is also a bloodsucker. In young dogs the whipworm may cause periodic, sometimes even severe, blood-tinged diarrhea. The whipworm problem relates particularly to kennels, where hygienic conditions are usually insufficient. Emaciation, diarrhea, and anemia are the major problems.

C. Prevention and Treatment

There are good reasons for protecting pet animals and humans from these parasites with hygienic measures and anthelmintics. The first objective is to obtain a clinical cure. All worm species are more or less harmful to dogs or cats and may even be fatal in puppies. Most important of all, certain gastrointestinal nematodes carried by pets do present a hazard to human health (e.g., visceral larval migrans, creeping eruption).

An effective control program for gastrointestinal nematodes should include sanitation, control of paratenic hosts, good nutrition and husbandry, isolation of new animals until checked or dewormed, decontamination of the environment, and periodic deworming of all animals (ROUDEBUSH 1980). Even with vigorous hygienic measures such as cleaning the kennel each day, destroying or burning the feces, cleaning baskets and drinking bowls, and keeping the kennel as dry as possible, one can reduce the infective ova in the environment. Stringent hygiene precautions alone have proved insufficient to overcome worm infections in dogs and cats, especially in kennels (THIENPONT et al. 1968; JACOBS et al. 1977). Supportive and prophylactic therapy must be considered, apart from the administration of anthelmintics. This includes: increasing the resistance of the host and specific symptomatic therapies, e.g., iron and vitamins (PRESSCOT 1978).

The use of anthelmintics (see Table 2) for the control of nematodes is limited by many factors, such as formulation, toxicity, and drug resistance, as reviewed by GIBSON (1980). The ideal anthelmintic for dogs or cats should be a routine dewormer with the largest spectrum and the lowest toxicity. Important in the choice for a routine dewormer is that it should be 100% active against *Toxocara canis*. The drug must be very safe, especially for young puppies and kit-

Table 2. Measures to free dogs and cats of nematodes and to maintain them in this state (THIENPONT, personal communication)

1. *For individually kept animals*
   Examination on arrival, followed by periodic microscopic fecal examination
   Treatment of infected animals with an effective anthelmintic
2. *The newly bought pup or kitten*
   Not allowing children to contact puppies and kittens, unless after quarantine and a treatment that guarantees a 100% efficacy against *Toxocara*
   Subsequently, treatment every 3 months if the animals were infected
3. *Bitches and their litter*
   Besides the periodic treatment, additional treatment 10 days before and 10 days after whelping
   Treatment of the pups twice: once at an age of approximately 1–3 weeks and a second time at 6 weeks, in an infected kennel a couple of days before weaning
4. *Kennel dogs or cats*
   Stringent hygienic measures: removal and destruction of the feces daily; clean baskets, drinking bowls, etc.
   Deworming of *all* animals periodically
   No sand runs
   Maintenance of the kennel as dry as possible
   Periodic disinfection of boxes, walls, and runs by steaming

tens, and for debilitated and pregnant animals. It should be easy to administer. Most anthelmintics have little or no effect on the migratory stages of the ascarids. So repeated strategic dosing is necessary to bring the infection of *T. canis* and *T. cati* under control.

D. Older and Superseded Anthelmintics

According to GIBSON (1977), anthelmintic discoveries have passed through four stages: the era of uncritical empiricism, the era of critical empiricism, the era of critical testing, and finally the era of anthelmintic screening.

In the first period, anthelmintic efficacy was mainly based on the fact that worms were passed following their administration. The anthelmintics were mostly of vegetable origin. For example, the oil of *Anacardium* (i.e., cashew nut oil) has an effect on ancylostomiasis in dogs. In the early 1900s arsenic compounds, powdered rhizomes of male ferns, minced pumpkin seeds, the sap of fig trees (*leche de higuera*; the active agent seems to be, a proteolytic enzyme, ficin), alkaloids, and calomel became the dewormers for dogs and cats. The efficacy was rather low, but the capsules and tablets were often so bulky and unwieldy that administration was a skilled job. Fasting was often imperative prior to treatment (JACOBS 1977). In the era of critical empiricism, more and more substances such as tetrachlorethylene, hexylresorcinol, and chenopodium oil were used in human medicine and replaced the older remedies. In the early years of the twentieth century, the accurate testing of anthelmintics began with the critical test devised by HALL and FOSTER (1918).

The first anthelmintics with a narrow spectrum such as phenothiazine, *N*-butylchloride, methylbenzene and dichlorophene combinations, piperazine, diethylcarbamazine, phthallofyne, and dithiazanine were developed from 1940 to 1957. Most of these substances, reviewed by DE CARNERI et al. (1973), not only had a narrow spectrum but their efficacy was rather low and/or their toxicity high. Nevertheless, some of them are still being used, e.g., in the United States. They are still present in the latest edition of ARONSON et al. (1978). *The Complete Desk Reference of Veterinary Pharmaceuticals and Biologicals 78/79*.

I. Piperazine

Various piperazine salts (adipate, citrate, phosphate, dihydrochloride, hexahydrate) in various formulations (tablet, syrup, solution, paste, powder) have been used over the past 30 years for treating ascarid infections in carnivores. The therapeutic dose for treating infections with adult ascarids is 100–250 mg/kg. Against immature forms a dose of 200 mg/kg has proved to be most effective. Piperazine is 80%–100% effective against adult worms in the intestine (ENGLISH and SPRENT 1965; FORSTNER 1974; ROUDEBUSH 1980). A second dose should be given after 10 days. In heavily infected animals a third dose should be given after another 10-day rest period. The treatment suffers from its bulk and insufficient effect against the immature intestinal stages of *Toxocara* during the prepatent development phase (KINGSBURY et al. 1977). Piperazine has a moderate effect on *Uncinaria* but not against *Ancylostoma* (BRANDER and PUGH 1971; ROUDEBUSH 1980).

Although piperazine is a drug with a high degree of safety, an occasional animal may show nausea, vomiting, or muscular tremors. To avoid these side effects 100 mg/kg may be given for two consecutive days instead of 200 mg/kg at once.

II. Diethylcarbamazine

Diethylcarbamazine (DEC), a piperazine derivative, is given orally at 50–100 mg/kg or three times at 20 mg/kg for treatment of ascarid infection in dogs and cats (ROUDEBUSH 1980). Combined with styrylpyridinium (3 mg DEC/kg combined with 5 mg styrylpyridinium/kg) it is effective for the control of hookworms, large roundworms, and heartworm disease. It is relatively non-toxic, though it may produce vomiting in fasted animals (PRESCOTT 1978).

III. Methylbenzene

Methylbenzene is active against ascarids. At 200 mg/kg it is moderately active against hookworms and has very limited activity against whipworms. It has a mild purgative effect. Fasting – 12 h prior to treatment and 4 h after treatment – is required. Combined with dichlorophene a partial removal of cestodes is seen. Overdosage may result in transitory incoordination, vomiting, and central nervous system side effects.

IV. Dithiazanine

The cyanine dye, dithiazanine iodide, is still used at 22 mg/kg per day for 3–5 days against ascarids, for 7 days against hookworm and whipworm, and for 10–12 days against *Strongyloides*. Some activity was noted against *Physaloptera rara* (SHUMARD and HENDRIX 1962). Vomiting, severe diarrhea, and anorexia may occur.

V. Disophenol

The nitrophenol disophenol is an injectable drug effective against hookworms. At 7.5–10 mg/kg s.c. it is indicated for treatment against adult *A. caninum, A. braziliense, U. stenocephala,* and *A. tubaeforme,* but not against other nematodes (WOOD and PANKAVICH 1961; BALBO and PANICHI 1972). To determine the accurate dosage each animal should be weighed. The margin of safety for the recommended single s.c. dose of 7.5 mg/kg is three- to fourfold. Doses of 34 mg/kg and above are fatal. At therapeutic doses it is safe for young puppies and pregnant females. Cumulative toxicosis may occur when it is administered repeatedly. Death due to disophenol toxicosis occurs because of circulatory collapse, acidosis, and hyperthermia (LEGENDRE 1973; PENUMARTHY et al. 1975). The parenteral solution of disophenol is not indicated, the side effects being too severe. Treatment must not be repeated within 21 days or given with other anthelmintics (ROUDEBUSH 1980).

VI. Thenium

Thenium closylate is a derivative of the bephenium series and is a quarternary ammonium compound. It is effective against *A. caninum* and *U. stenocephala*. Its efficacy against ascarids is insufficient (20%–50%) so that thenium closylate has been combined with piperazine. Both anthelmintics act synergetically to improve the effectiveness of each drug against ascarids and hookworms (BROWN 1962). Since thenium is insoluble and has a direct action on the adult parasite in situ, a simplified dosage range is based on gut volume rather than on the body weight of the animal. The treatment should be repeated after 2 or 3 weeks. At therapeutic doses, emesis, diarrhea, salivation, or depression may be observed. Contraindications are: dogs weighing less than 2.5 kg, suckling pups, or recently weaned puppies. A high fat content in the bitch's milk facilitates absorption of thenium in unweaned pups with the risk of systemic toxicosis. The product cannot be used in felines.

VII. Metyridine

Metyridine, which is more efficacious when administered subcutaneously, is effective on *Trichuris vulpis*, and orally only partially active on *Toxocara canis* and *A. caninum*. The therapeutic dose of 150–200 mg/kg causes excessive salivation, vomiting, diarrhea, and ataxia (COLGLAZIER et al. 1966). The subcutaneous injection of a large dose is painful, but i.m. injections are not (GIRALDO et al. 1979). The most marked local effect is edema at the site of injection, followed by necrosis.

VIII. Nitrodan

Continuous feeding for 8 weeks (about 32 mg/kg per day) of 100 ppm nitrodan (nidanthel) provides an efficient means of reducing infections of *T. canis, A. caninum,* and *U. stenocephala* in dogs. Removal of both hookworm species was not complete (18%–89%). Better results were obtained with 230 ppm fed for 14 weeks against hookworms (94%). Nitrodan is not active against *Toxascaris leonina* (MCGUIRE et al. 1966). Nitrodan has no side effects or contraindications and there is no evidence of toxicity.

E. Organophosphates

The organophosphates, e.g., vincofos (HASS and COLLINS 1974) and uredofos (ROBERSON and ARBA 1976), have toxic potential for man and animals. Only a few anthelmintics of this type have stood the test of time. The organic phosphate trichlorfon (metrifonate) is used more against ectoparasites than as an anthelmintic.

Dichlorvos

The formulation of dichlorvos consists of nondigestible, bead-shaped resin pellets. The active ingredient dichlorvos is released slowly as the pellets pass through the dog's gastrointestinal tract. The rate of drug release is designed to provide maximum anthelmintic activity and toxicological safety. For dogs the pellets are prepared in gelatin capsules for oral administration or in packets for mixing with canned dog feed or ground meat. Moisture is necessary to obtain adhesion of the pellets to the feed (ROBERSON et al. 1977). The available dog formulations are contraindicated for cats. Only the special small tablets may be used in cats and puppies after weighing each animal prior to dosing. In dogs, dichlorvos is effective at 27–33 mg/kg against ascarids, hookworms, and whipworms. In some dogs the efficacy against *Trichuris vulpis* may be erratic and the animal should be treated again 14 days later (OLSEN et al. 1977). There is little or no activity against the migrating larval forms of the roundworm or hookworm. *Physaloptera* responds to dichlorvos treatment (GREVE 1980).

The acute oral LD_{50} for drug-grade, unformulated dichlorvos in dogs falls in the range of 28–45 mg/kg body weight. The acute oral LD_{50} in the young adult dog for formulated dichlorvos ranges from 387 to 1,262 mg/kg. The drug is safe for pregnant bitches.

Side effects or symptoms of acute intoxication resulting from overdosage are: salivation, myosis, vomiting, watery diarrhea, muscle tremors, general muscular weakness progressing toward paralysis, low blood pressure, and lowered respiratory rate with dyspnea. At therapeutic doses signs of emesis within 30–90 min after dosing may appear, especially in cats and puppies. In clinical trials mild emesis was reported in 3% of cats and in 8% of weaned puppies. It is advisable in high-risk patients to split the normal dosage and to give it at 8–24 h intervals. Atropine is the animal antidote. Atropine and pyridine-2-aldoxine methiodide (2-PAM) are the human antidotes (ARONSON et al. 1978).

Dichlorvos is a cholinesterase inhibitor and there are too many contraindications for use of this anthelmintic as a routine dewormer. It may not be administered in conjunction with cholinesterase-inhibiting drugs, pesticides, other anthelmintics, muscle relaxants, tranquillizers, or modified live vaccines. Animals showing signs of constipation or mechanical blockade of the intestinal tract must not be treated. The drug must not to be administered to dogs with impaired liver function or circulatory failure or to dogs recently exposed to or showing signs of infectious disease. Dogs with active dirofilariasis must not be treated. Whippets and greyhounds are too sensitive to organic phosphate (TODENHÖFER 1970).

Some practical warnings are necessary. The product should be stored in the refrigerator. Pellet contact with the skin is to be avoided. Packet contents should be used shortly after opening and unused drugs should not be stored. The resin pellets pass undigested through the dog and appear in the feces. These residual pellets are toxic for birds.

F. Tetrahydropyrimidines

Pyrantel, Morantel

From the pyrantel base, various salts (hydrochloride, tartrate, and pamoate) have been studied in dogs and cats. The anthelmintic activity has been found to be directly proportional to the amount of free base present. The pamoate (=embonate) form is the most insoluble of the present pyrantel anthelmintics and is likely to be the least toxic.

In *dogs* a single oral dose of 15 mg/kg eliminates ascarids and hookworms. There appeared to be little activity against *Trichuris,* nor was there any indication of anticestodal activity (HOWES and LYNCH 1967).

Pyrantel pamoate is well tolerated, with no signs of vomiting, salivation, or diarrhea. It is safe for young puppies, pregnant or lactating bitches, or debilitated dogs.

The drug concentration of pyrantel embonate in the paste for *cats* is 5.33 times higher than that for dogs. The dosage of 20–30 mg/kg body weight is active against ascarids and hookworms. Some cats spit out the paste when it is injected in the mouth, or refuse to eat when the paste is mixed in their food. Due to a possible underdosing it is advisable to treat cats again 14 days after the first treatment against ascarids (SCUPIN et al. 1978).

Although a higher potency was recorded for the other tetrahydropyrimidine *morantel* pamoate in mice and sheep, there appeared to be little difference in potency in dogs (CORNWELL and JONES 1970).

Pyrantel combined with oxantel is effective against *Trichuris.*

G. Imidazothiazoles

Tetramisole, Levamisole

The activity of the imidazothiazole *dl,*tetramisole was first reported by THIENPONT et al. (1966). Most of the anthelmintic activities of this racemate reside in its levorotatory isomer levamisole, which is twice as potent as tetramisole (JANSSEN 1976).

In comparison with its extensive application in swine, cattle, sheep, and humans, the use of levamisole in dogs has been limited. Only a few specific dog or cat formulations based on levamisole have been developed (Table 3). Levamisole is highly effective against the common nematode species of dogs and cats: ascarids and hookworms, but not against whipworms and tapeworms. It has a marked inhibitory effect on the development of infective stages of the eggs as well as on the infective and migrating larvae of *A. caninum* (BANERJEE and PRAKASH 1971; LÄMMLER et al. 1970).

At a therapeutic dose of 5–10 mg/kg levamisole is well tolerated. The potential side effects of levamisole are apparently similar to those of tetramisole. Adverse reactions are: nausea, muscular tremors, vomiting, salivation, lassitude, and, occasionally, ataxia. Side effects appear to be a greater hazard following injection of the drug. They subside within 3 h without supportive treatment. In their safety studies ALFORD and BURKHART (1975) stated that levamisole should not pose an unusual or unexpected safety hazard if given orally at the rate of 11 mg/kg for 6–10 days as a microfilaricide. Contraindications for a levamisole treatment are: chronic hepatic or renal disease and concurrent use of organophosphates or carbamates. Parenteral treatment of breeds of dogs particularly sensitive to drugs, such as boxers and very small and toy dogs, is not recommended. To avoid vomiting (5% of cases) it is better to treat the animals in the morning after fasting.

Levamisole has been used as an anthelmintic in other carnivores such as the lion, tiger, panther, leopard, and puma (GASS 1971; KAGERUKA and VAN PUYENBROECK 1967; THIENPONT et al. 1967).

H. Nitroscanate

Nitroscanate is one of the few anthelmintics available for treatment of either nematodes or cestodes in dogs and cats. At 100 mg/kg (or 50 mg/kg when micronized nitroscanate is used) it is efficacious against *Toxocara canis, Toxascaris leonina, U. stenocephala,* and *A. caninum.* Although reduction of *Trichuris vulpis* infection is achieved with the drug, efficacy is erratic (BORAY et al. 1974; RICHARDS and SOMERVILLE 1980). At therapeutic dosage delayed vomiting after 4–24 h occurred in 10% of the dogs treated, which normally does not interfere with anthelmintic efficacy (RIGBY 1978). Slight transient incoordination and a tranquilizing effect is occasionally observed in dogs in poor condition or suffering from chronic nutritional deficiency (BORAY et al. 1974). Nitroscanate can only be used for cats if accurately weighed.

J. Benzimidazoles

While benzimidazoles have been used extensively for cattle and sheep, only a few have so far been developed for cats and dogs.

I. Tiabendazole

Tiabendazole was one of the first real broad-spectrum anthelmintics that were discovered by screening helminths of laboratory animals. The various formulations (bolus, powder, paste, suspension) available for large domestic animals can be used in dogs. A dose of 50–60 mg/kg given once daily, 3 days monthly, is active against ascarids and hookworms (ROUDEBUSH 1980). This dosage and higher ones provoke vomiting several hours after treatment. The prophylactic control of the common intestinal nematodes of dogs with tiabendazole-medicated feed has been studied by YAKSTIS et al. 1968. Mixed into commercial dog food at 0.025% and fed three times daily to young dogs almost completely prevents infections with *Toxocara canis, A. braziliense, A. caninum, S. stercoralis,* and *Trichuris vulpis.* CONGDON and AMES (1973) eliminated prepatent *Toxocara canis* infections acquired in utero with a dosage schedule of 150 mg/kg per day tiabendazole paste given from the 5th to the 20th or 25th day postpartum.

II. Mebendazole

The benzimidazole carbamate mebendazole appears to have the broadest spectrum of activity of all anthelmintics, with activity against larval and adult stages of both nematodes and cestodes. Because of its wide safety margin, mebendazole may be given in standard doses of 100-mg tablets or powder (therapeutic dose ± 22 mg/kg). High anthelmintic efficacy in dogs and cats has been shown against

Table 3. Anthelmintics active against gastrointestinal nematodes in dogs and cats

Anthelmintic	Tradename (s)	Supplier (s)	Formulation	Dosage regime	Indications
Piperazine salts	Various, e.g., Pipertab, Piperazine	Various, Burns Biotec, etc.	Various tablets, capsules, pastes, solutions, syrups	1 × 100–250 mg/kg (2nd dose after 10 days) 100–150 mg/kg (2 days)	Ascarids
Diethyl-carbamazine (DEC)	Various, e.g., Caricide, Dirocide	Various: American Cyanamid, Squibb, etc.	Tablets, syrup, powder	1 × 50–100 mg/kg 3 × 20 mg/kg	Ascarids
Methylbenzene + dichlorophene	Methacide, Vermiplex, etc.	Beecham Pitman-Moore	Gelatine capsules, capsules	200 mg/kg	Ascarids, hookworms (+ cestodes)
Dithiazanine iodide	Diazan	Lilly/ Pitman-Moore	10, 50, 100, 200-mg coated tablets; powder	22 mg/kg once daily 3–5 days 22 mg/kg once daily 7 days 22 mg/kg once daily 10–12 days	Ascarids hookworms, whip-worms, threadworms
Disophenol	DNP	American Cyanamid	4.5% and 9% solution	7.5–10 mg/kg	Hookworms
Thenium closylate	Canopar	Burroughs Wellcome	500-mg tablets	1 × 500 mg → > 5 kg 2 × 250 mg → 2.5 → 5 kg	Hookworms
+ piperazine	Ancaris	Burroughs Wellcome	216 mg thenium + 260 mg piperazine phosphate per tablet	2 × 1 tablet → 1–2 kg 2 × 2 tablets > 2 kg	Hookworms, ascarids
Nitrodan (nidanthel)	Everfree	Cooper	Granules Premix	230 ppm in diet – 8 weeks 0.016%–0.1% in feed	Ascarids, hookworms Ascarids, hookworms

Table 3. (continued)

Anthelmintic	Tradename (s)	Supplier (s)	Formulation	Dosage regime	Indications
Dichlorvos	Task	Squibb	Tablets for cats and puppies	5–11 mg/kg	Ascarids, hookworms
	Tenac		Bead-shaped resin pellets in capsules	27–33 mg/kg	Ascarids, hookworms, whipworms
	Canogard	Shell	Capsules	30–35 mg/kg	Ascarids, hookworms, whipworms
Pyrantel pamoate	Banminth, Dogminth, Catminth, Strongid, Nemex	Pfizer	Paste, suspension	15 mg/kg (dog) 20–30 mg/kg (cat)	Ascarids, hookworms
Pyrantel + oxantel	Canex plus	Pfizer	100-mg tablets		Ascarids, hookworms, whipworms
Levamisole	Nemisol 0.7% Némicanisol 0.7%	Specia France R. Bellon	Injectable solution	5 mg/kg	Ascarids, hookworms
Nitroscanate	Lopatol	Ciba-Geigy	1-g tablets 500 mg and 100 mg tablets	100 mg/kg Micronized 50 mg/kg	Ascarids, hookworms
Mebendazole	Telmin KH	Janssen Pharmaceutica	100-mg tablets	½ tablet bid. for 2 days < 2 kg 1 tablet bid. for 2 days > 2 kg	Ascarids
				½ tablet bid. for 3–5 days < 2 kg 1 tablet bid. for 3–5 days > 2 kg	Ascarids, hookworms, whipworms
	Telmintic	Pitman-Moore	Powder 4%	22 mg/kg for 3 days	
Fenbendazole	Panacur	Hoechst	Granules	100 mg/kg once 20 mg/kg for 5 days	Ascarids, hookworms, whipworms

ascarids (2-day treatment) and hookworms and whipworms (3- to 5-day treatment) (Table 3). The stomach worm *Physaloptera* is sensitive to mebendazole (McCurdy and Guerrero 1977).

At therapeutic dose levels mebendazole is a very safe drug. Only very few side effects, such as vomiting and soft unformed stools, have been reported in clinical investigations. These symptoms may be attributed to the worm diseases rather than to mebendazole because the placebo-treated dogs had the same symptoms. It is not embryotoxic or teratogenic in dogs when administered in a single dose of 20 mg/kg each day beginning on the 1st day of pregnancy and continuing for 56 days (Marsboom 1973). It is safe for use in heartworm-infected dogs (Guerrero 1973). Mebendazole is safe for felines. In cats no signs of toxicosis were detected after treatment with high dosages ($LD_{50} > 640$ mg/kg). Mebendazole can be mixed in meat or meatballs for wild carnivores such as the cheetah, puma, panther, bear, and leopard, either during a shorter period at high dosage (15 mg/kg for two consecutive days) or during a longer period at low dosage (3 mg/kg in the feed for ten consecutive days (Dollinger 1973).

III. Fenbendazole

The benzimidazole carbamate fenbendazole is very effective agains the important gastrointestinal nematodes in dogs and cats at 100 mg/kg once or 20 mg/kg for 5 days. Multiple dosing, especially at the higher doses, is more effective than single dosing (Burke and Robertson 1978). Worm elimination extends over several days depending on the parasite species. Dry formulations such as granules or powder give better anthelmintic effects than liquid formulations. However, these differences in efficacy disappear if the suspension is mixed with the feed (Düwel 1980). Fenbendazole has activity against the somatic larvae of *Toxocara*. After treatment with 50 mg/kg each day during gestation of pregnant bitches, helminth-free whelps were born (Düwel and Strasser 1978; Dubey 1979).

Fenbendazole is a very safe drug. Dogs treated with fenbendazole show no signs of toxicosis during or after the treatment period with any dosage level or single or multiple treatments. The following maximum doses of fenbendazole were tolerated by dogs: 1 × 500 mg/kg orally and 30 × 250 mg/kg orally (Baeder et al. 1974). Tasteless fenbendazole given one to three times at 10 mg/kg is taken up readily by wild carnivores such as the lion, tiger, puma, wildcat, lynx, leopard, panther, jaguar, cheetah, and fox. Overdoses which inevitably occur from time to time during voluntary ingestion of the drug can be regarded as harmless and present no risk of adverse side effects (Düwel 1980).

IV. Albendazole

For albendazole only preliminary data are available. Administration of 50 mg/kg albendazole for 3 days was fully active against *T. canis* and *A. caninum* (Theodorides et al. 1976).

K. Avermectins

Avermectins are a family of new anthelmintic agents produced by fermentation of a new species of *Streptomyces (S. avermitilis)*. The natural products and synthetic derivatives are extremely active nematocides with additional biological activity against arthropods and histotrophic stages of certain insects. Most published studies have used ivermectin (avermectin B_{1a} and B_{1b}).

They are extremely potent, being active against a wide variety of parasites at dosages of only a fraction of a milligram per kilogram of body weight (Burg et al. 1979; Egerton et al. 1979). In *dogs* they have been found to be highly efficacious against the hookworm *A. caninum* at doses as low as 5–15 µg/kg (Blair and Campbell 1978). Their major use in dogs will probably be as a preventive and microfilaricidal treatment for heartworm (*Dirofilaria immitis*). To date insufficient data are available on toxicity.

L. Ticarbodine

Ticarbodine given in a single oral dose of 50–100 mg/kg has a high degree of efficacy against ascarids, hookworms, and even tapeworms. Little effect against *Trichuris vulpis* was observed (Slonka et al. 1972). At therapeutic dose levels transitory side effects of delayed vomiting and relaxed nictating membranes occur in some dogs. At 100 mg/kg 1% vomited between 30 min and 2 h, 22.6% between 2 and 6 h, and 7.6% between 6 and 24 h after treatment. Vomiting did not interfere with anthelmintic efficacy or general well-being and was usually very mild and of the "projectile" type (Boisvenue et al. 1972).

M. Tioxidazole

In preliminary experiments in dogs, tioxidazole at a single dose of 200 mg/kg was active against *Toxascaris leonina*. Daily doses of 100 mg/kg for 3 days or 50 mg/kg for 5 days were also effective against hookworms and *Trichuris* (Panitz et al. 1978).

N. Conclusions

Many valuable anthelmintics have now been made available. The use of anthelmintics with a limited spectrum makes sense when a specific infection is diagnosed. Otherwise, it is more practical and effective to deworm dogs and cats with a safe easily administered broad-spectrum anthelmintic.

References

Akusawa M, Deguchi N (1975) Anthelmintic effect of mebendazole against *Trichuris vulpis* in dogs. Jpn J Parasitol 24:357–361

Alford BT, Burkhart RL (1975) Safety studies of levamisole in dogs. Proceedings of the heartworm symposium 1974, Bonner Springs, Kansas 66012 USA, VM Publishing, Bonner Springs, pp 82–84

Arenas TLK (1971) Tetramisole in dogs and cats (Es). Gac Vet 33:75–76

Aronson CE, Powers TE, Scheidy SF (1978) The complete desk reference of veterinary pharmaceuticals & biologicals 78/79. Harwal, Pennsylvania

Austin WC, Courtney W, Danielewicz JC, Morgan DH, Conover LH, Howes HL, Lynch JR (1966) Pyrantel tartrate, a new anthelmintic effective against infections of domestic animals. Nature 212:1273–1274

Baeder C, Bähr H, Christ O, Düwel D, Kellner HM, Kirsch R, Loewe H (1974) Fenbendazole: a new, highly effective anthelmintic. Experientia 30:753–754

Balbo T, Panichi M (1972) A study on ancylostomiasis in cats: spread of hookworms among the cats in Turin and comparative treatment of natural and experimental infections. Nuova Vet 48:156–187

Banerjee D, Prakash O (1971) Inhibition of development of *Ancylostoma caninum* with tetramisole. Trans Soc Trop Med Hyg 65:526

Batte EG, Moncol DJ, McLamb RD (1966) Critical evaluation of an anthelmintic for dogs. Small Anim Clin 61:567–570

Beaver PC, Snyder CH, Carrera GM (1952) Chronic eosinophilia due to visceral larva migrans. Pediatrics 9:7–19

Beck AM (1975) The public health implications of urban dogs. Am J Public Health 65:1315–1317

Blair LS, Campbell WC (1978) Efficacy of avermectins against *Ancylostoma caninum* in dogs, J Helminthol 52:305–307

Boisvenue RJ, Hendrix JC, Potter HD (1972) Efficacy of single oral doses of ticarbodine against nematodes and cestodes of dogs. Am J Vet Res 33:709–712

Boray JC, Von Orelli M, Sarasin G (1974) Cantrodifene, a broad spectrum anthelmintic for dogs. Third international congress of parasitology. Proc 3 Sect E5. München, 25–31 Aug 1974. World Federation of Parasitologists. Available from: Egermann Druckereigesellschaft mbH & Co KG, 1170 Wien, Hernalser Hauptstrasse 196

Brander GC, Pugh DM (1971) Veterinary applied pharmacology and therapeutics, 2nd edn. Balliere Tindall, London

Brown CCD (1962) Thenium and piperazine combined in the treatment of hookworm and roundworm infestation in the dog. Vet Rec 74:787–791

Burg RW, Miller BM, Baker EE, Birnbaum J, Currie SA, Hartman R, Kong Y-L, Monaghan RL, Olson G, Putter I, Tunac JB, Wallack H, Stapley EO, Oiwa R, Omura S (1979) Avermectins, new family of potent anthelmintic agents: producing organism and fermentations. Antimicrob Agents Chemother 15:361–367

Burke TM, Roberson EL (1978) Critical studies of fenbendazole suspension (10%) against naturally occurring helminth infections in dogs. Am J Vet Res 39:1799–1801

Cabaleyro OR (1972) Anquilostomiasis (Su tratamiento con tetramizole). Gac Vet 34:24–27

Clarck CH, Kling JM, Woodley CH, Sharp N (1961) A quantitative measurement of the blood loss caused by ancylostomiasis in dogs. Am J Vet Res 22:370–373

Colglazier ML, Enzie FD, Burtner RH (1966) The systemic action of methyridine against helminths, especially whipworm, in dogs. Proc Helminthol Soc (Wash) 33:40–41

Congdon LL, Ames ER (1973) Thiabendazole for control of *Toxocara canis* in the dog. Am J Vet Res 34:417–418

Connan RM (1979) The use of anthelmintics in dogs and cats. In: Yoxall AT, Hird JFR (eds) Pharmacological basis of small animal medicine 1979, pp 189–197

Cornwell RL, Jones RM (1970) A critical test of morantel pamoate against *Ancylostoma caninum* in dogs. Res Vet Sci 11:485–486

De Carneri I, Vita G (1973) In: Cavier R and Hawking F (eds) Chemotherapy of Helminthiasis. Pergamon Press, Oxford

Djerassi C, Israel A, Jöchle W (1973) Planned parenthood for pets? Bull Atomic Sci (January 1973) 10–19

Dingeldein W, Manz D (1970) Zur Behandlung des Spul-, Haken- und Peitschenwurmbefalls des Hundes mit Dichlorvos. Prakt Tierarzt 51:275–278

Dollinger P (1973) Zur Wirksamkeit des anthelmintikums Mebendazol bei Zootieren. Verhandlungsbericht des XV. Internationalen Symposiums über die Erkrankungen der Zootiere. Kolmarden 1973. Available from: Dr Peter Dollinger, Institut für Parasitologie der Universität Zürich, Winterthurer Strasse 260, CH-8057 Zürich

Dubey JP (1979) Effect of fenbendazole on *Toxocara canis* larvae in tissues of infected dogs. Am J Vet Res 40:698–699
Dubin S, Segall S, Martindale J (1975) Contamination of soil in two city parks with canine nematode ova including *Toxocara canis*. A preliminary study. Am J Public Health 65:1242–1245
Duclós MSV, Ayllón CRM (1973) Ensayos para el tratamiento y control de la ancylostomiasis canina. Rev Inst Zoonosis Invest Pecuar II 1,2:53–71
Dunn AM (1969) Veterinary helminthology. Heinemann, London
Düwel D (1980) Panacur, Axilur. Information brochure of Hoechst Aktiengesellschaft. Available from: Dr D Düwel, Ressort Veterinärmedizin, Hoechst Aktiengesellschaft, Postfach 800 320, 6230 Frankfurt 80
Düwel D, Strasser H (1978) Versuche zur Geburt helminthen – freier Hundewelpen durch Fenbendazol-Behandlung. DTW 85:239–241
Eckert J (1972) Parasitosen von Hund und Katze. Kleintier Prax 17:97–124
Egerton JR, Ostlind DA, Blair LS, Eary CH, Suhayda D, Cifelli RF, Campbell WC (1979) Avermectins, new family of potent anthelmintic agents: efficacy of the B_{1a} component. Antimicrob Agents Chemother 15:372–378
English PB, Sprent JFA (1965) Aust Vet J 41:50
Faulkner LC (1975) Dimensions of the pet population problem. JAVMA 166:477–478
Feldman BM, Carding TH (1973) Free-roaming urban pets. Health Serv Rep 88:956–962
Forstner (1974) Parasitenbekämpfung beim Hund. Berl Munch Tierarztl Wochenschr 87:228–231
Gass H (1971) Citarin in der Kleintierpraxis und bei Zootieren. Vet Med Nach 1:70–73
Gerin T, Pecheur M, Gianfreda H (1980) Fréquence des parasites intestinaux chez les carnivores domestiques. Ann Med Vet 124:133–136
Gibson TE (1977) Perspectives in the control of parasitic disease in animals in Europe. 3rd Symp Assoc Vet Industry, London, October 10–11 1977, pp 13–19
Gibson TE (1980) Factors influencing the application of anthelmintics in practice. Vet Parasitol 6:241–254
Giraldo C, Pancaldi P, Valle VC, Guziano E (1979) Methyridine therapy for dogs with whipworms (*Trichuris vulpis*). Ann Facolta Med Vet Torino 26:398–405
Glickman LT, Schautz PM, Cypess RH (1979) Canine and human toxocariasis: review of transmission, pathogenesis and clinical disease. JAVMA 175:1265–1269
Greve JM (1980) Vomiting roundworms (correspondence). Canine Pract 7:64
Grevel V, Eckert J (1973) Untersuchungen über Mebendazol ein neues Breitspektrumanthelminthikum für die Kleintierpraxis. Schweiz Arch Tierheilkd 115:559–578
Guerrero J (1978) Telmintic (mebendazole) powder: a new broad spectrum anthelmintic for canine use. Pract Vet 49:15–17
Guerrero J, Pancari G, Michael B (1981) Comparative anthelmintic efficacy of two schedules of mebendazole treatment in dogs. Am J Vet Res 42:425–427
Güralp N, Tinar R (1978) The anthelmintic action of fenbendazole against nematodes in cats and dogs (in Turkish). Ankara Univ Vet Fak Derg 25:440–447
Hall MC, Foster WD (1918) Efficacy of some anthelmintics. J Agric Res 12:397
Hass DK, Collins JA (1974) Evolution of an anthelmintic: vincofos. Am J Vet Res 35:103–106
Hovell GJR, Weston R (1970) Cramp in greyhounds. Correspondence in members' Information Supplement. Vet Rec 87:193
Howes HL, Lynch (1967) Anthelmintic studies with Pyrantel I. Therapeutic and prophylactic efficacy against the enteral stages of various helminths in mice and dogs. J Parasitol 53:1085–1091
Jacobs DE (1977) Recent developments in the chemical control of helminths in dogs and cats. 3rd symposium of the association of veterinarians in industry, London, England. October 10–11 1977, pp 45–52. Available from: Tunstall Laboratory, Shell Research Ltd, Sittingbourne, Kent, UK
Jacobs DE, Prole JHB (1976) Helminth infections of British dogs: prevalence in racing greyhounds. Vet Parasitol 1:377–387

Jacobs DE, Pegg EJ, Stevenson P (1977) Helminths of British dogs: *Toxocara canis* – a veterinary perspective. J Small Anim Pract 18:79–92
Janssen PAJ (1976) The levamisole story. Prog Drug Res 20:347
Kageruka P, Van Puyenbroeck B (1967) Contribution a la connaissance de l'activité anthelmintique du tetramisole chez les carnivores sauvages. Acta Zool Patholog Antverpiensa 44:101–117
Kingsbury PA, Rees TA, Piercy DWT (1977) Haloxon as an anthelmintic for dogs and cats. Vet Rec 101:477–479
Lamina J (1970) Das biologische Verhalten von *Toxocara*-Arten bei spezifischen und nicht spezifischen Wirten im Hinblick auf Infektionen des Menschen. Kleintier Prax 14:107
Lämmler G, Srivastava VK, Zahner H (1970) The efficacy of various anthelmintics against the parasitic larval stages of *Ancylostoma caninum* in *Mastomys natalensis*. Br Vet J 126:427–439
Legendre AM (1973) Disophenol toxicosis in a dog. JAVMA 163:149–150
Linquist WD (1975) Drug evaluation of pyrantel pamoate against *Ancylostoma, Toxocara* and *Toxascaris* in eleven dogs. Am J Vet Res 36:1387–1389
London CE, Roberson EL, McCall JW, Guerrero J, Pancari G, Michael B, Newcomb K (1981) Anthelmintic activity of mebendazole against induced and naturally occurring helminth infections in cats. Am J Vet Res 42:1263–1265
Marsboom R (1973) Toxicological studies on mebendazole. Toxicol Appl Pharmacol 24:371–377
McCurdy HD, Guerrero J (1977) Controlled critical anthelmintic evaluation of mebendazole powder in the dog. Vet Med Small Anim Clin 72:1731–1733
McGuire WC, O'Neill CO, Brody G (1966) Anthelmintic activity of 3-methyl-5-[(*p*-nitrophenyl)azo]rhodanine. J Parasitol 52:528–537
Nichol S, Ball SJ, Snow KR (1981) Prevalence of intestinal parasites in domestic cats from the London area. Vet Rec 109:252–253
Noujaim AA, Gaafar SM, Christian JE (1968) Efficacy of tetramisole on nematode infections of dogs. Vet Med 63:986
Olsen JL, Rollins LD, Rosenberg MC, Gundlach CE (1977) Efficacy of dichlorvos administered orally in single and repeated doses for removal of canine whipworms. JAVMA 171:542–544
Panitz E, Daniels PJL, Loebenberg D, Nafissi VMM, Waitz JA (1978) Anthelmintic activity of tioxidazole (Sch 21480) against gastrointestinal roundworms. Specialia 733
Penumarthy L, Oehme FW, Menhusen MJ (1975) Investigations of therapeutic measures for disophenol toxicosis in dogs. Am J Vet Res 36:1259–1262
Prescott CW (1978) Veterinary therapeutics-anthelmintics. Refresher course in the therapeutic jungle, August 14–18. Proc No 39, vol 2, pp 666–682
Puccini V, LO Muzio F (1972) Experimental study on the subcutaneous injection of tetramisole in the dog in the treatment of infection with intestinal nematodes. (It). Acta Med Vet 18:155–165
Rep BH (1979) *Uncinaria stenocephala* infections in dogs in the Netherlands (in Dutch). Tijdschr Diergeneeskd 104:475–478
Rep BH (1980) Ascarid infections in dogs in the Netherlands (in Dutch). Tijdschr Diergeneeskd 105:282–289
Richards RJ, Somerville JM (1980) Field trials with nitroscanate against cestodes and nematodes in dogs. Vet Rec 106:332–335
Rigby JP (1978) Vomiting after anthelmintic. Vet Res 104:248
Roberson EL, Arba LA (1976) Uredofos: anthelmintic activity against nematodes and cestodes in dogs with naturally occurring infections. Am J Vet Res 37:1480–1482
Roberson EL, Burke TM (1982) Evaluation of granulated fenbendazole as a treatment for helminth infections in dogs. JAVMA 80:53–55
Roberson EL, Anderson WI, Hass KD (1977) Anthelmintic drug evaluation: dichlorvos-medicated dry dog feed. Am J Vet Res 38:597–600
Roudebush P (1980) A practical guide to the chemotherapy of small animal intestinal parasites. Canine Pract 7:67–80

Scupin E, Brandes B, Niessen C, Scupin E (1976) Praxiserfahrungen über die Anwendung von Pyrantel-Pamoat in Pastenform bei Katzen und die Wirksamkeit gegen natürliche Ascarideninvasionen. Kleintier Prax 21:222–226

Sharp ML, Sepesi JP, Collins JA (1973) A comparative critical assay on canine anthelmintics. Vet Med Small Anim Clin 68:131–132

Shumard RF, Hendrix JC (1962) Dithiazanine iodide as an anthelmintic for dogs. Vet Med 57:153–157

Slonka GF, Leland SE, Anderson NV (1972) Critical and clinical evaluation of ticarbodine as a canine anthelmintic. Am J Vet Res 33:1075–1078

Sprent JFA (1958) Observations on the development of *Toxocara canis* (Werner 1782) in the dog. Parasitology 48:184

Theodorides VJ, Gyurik RJ, Kingsburry WD, Parish RC (1976) Anthelmintic activity of albendazole against liver flukes, tapeworms, lung and gastrointestinal roundworms. Experientia 32:702–703

Thienpont D, Vanparijs OFJ, Raeymaekers AHM, Vandenberk J, Demoen PJA, Allewijn FTN, Marsboom RPH, Niemegeers CJE, Schellekens KHL, Janssen PAJ (1966) Tetramisole (R 8299) a new, potent broad spectrum anthelmintic. Nature 209:1084

Thienpont D, Mortelmans J, Vercruyse J, Kageruka P, Van Brabant R, Van Puyenbroeck B (1967) Anthelmintic activity of tetramisole in zoo animals. Verhandlungsbericht des IX Int Symp über die Erkrankungen der Zootiere, Prag. Available from: Dr D Thienpont, Janssen Pharmaceutica, Turnhoutseweg 30, Beerse 2340, Belgium

Thienpont D, Vanparijs O, Spruyt J, Marsboom R (1968) The anthelmintic activity of tetramisole in the dog. Vet Rec 83:369–372

Todenhöfer H (1970) Die Anwendung von Tenac (Dichlorvos) als Breitspektrum-Anthelminthikum beim Hund. Kleintier Prax 15:63–66

Vanden Bossche H, Rochette F, Hörig C (1982) Mebendazole and related compounds. Adv Pharmacol Chemother 19:67–128

Vanparijs OFJ, Thienpont DC (1973) Canine and feline helminth and protozoan infections in Belgium. J Parasitol 59:327–330

Von Reyn F, Roberts TM, Owen R (1978) Infection of an infant with an adult *Toxocara cati*. J Pediatr 93:247–249

Weissenburg H (1968) Citarin (Tetramisole) als Anthelminthikum beim Hund. Berl Munch Tierarztl Wochenschr 81:69–71

Wiseman RA, Lovel TW (1969) Human infection with adult *Toxocara cati*. Br Med J 3:454–455

Wood IB, Pankavich JA (1961) The parenteral therapy of ancylostomiasis in dogs. Cyanamid Int Vet Bull 3(1):1–10

Woodruff AW (1975) *Toxocara canis* and other nematodes transmitted from dogs to man. Br Vet J 131:627–632

Yakstis JJ, Egerton JR, Campbell WC, Cuckler AC (1967) Use of thiabendazole medicated feed for prophylaxis of four common roundworm infections in dogs. J Parasitol 54:359–367

CHAPTER 10

Chemotherapy of Gastrointestinal Nematodiasis in Birds

J. H. Boersema

A. Introduction

Poultry keeping has gone through an enormous development in the past years. It has now become one of the most intensive of all branches of livestock farming. With changes in breeding, important changes in the parasitic fauna have occurred simultaneously. Nowadays nematodes, once very common in poultry, have disappeared almost entirely on farms using modern methods of poulty management. However, many domestic birds are still kept in the old-fashioned way, and there is a high chance that they will be infected with nematodes.

B. Nematodes in Domestic Birds

Apart from a few more or less seldomly seen or locally important nematodes, the following genera can be found in domestic birds:

I. Ascaridia

Ascaridia is one of the most common nematodes in various domestic birds. Worms of this species are considered not very harmful as they live free in the lumen of the small intestine without damaging the wall. However, they grow, move, and produce eggs. So they demand energy, which only can be withdrawn form the food destined for their host. Occasionally they cause obstructions or perforations of the intestine. The larvae can spend a part of their developing cycle in the mucosa. This may lead to enteritis in the 2nd week of infection, considered as the most pathogenic time of the infection. During the tissue phase the larvae are less suspectible to anthelmintics.

Several *Ascaridia* species have been found in domestic birds. In chickens *Ascaridia galli* is the most common and is also found in other Galliformes. In turkeys *A. dissimilis* is the dominant species and *A. columbae* can be found in pigeons.

II. Heterakis

Heterakis gallinarium is one of the commonest nematodes living in the cecum. It is considered nonpathogenic, but is important because it can act as a vector of *Histomonas meleagrides*. *Heterakis isolonche,* the predominant species in pheasants, can be pathogenic by causing nodular proliferations in the cecum.

III. Capillaria

Many species have been described in domestic birds. They are, however, not very host-specific and many species are probably identical. They can be found in domestic birds in various sites in the digestive tract. *Capillaria contorta* lives in the esophagus and crop, *C. obsignata* in the small intestine, and *C. anatis* in the cecum. The life cycle can be direct or indirect; in the latter, earthworms are the intermediate host. The adult parasites burrow in the mucosa of the intestinal tract, causing hemorrhagic inflammation. They are among the most pathogenic and most difficult to treat nematodes in domestic birds.

IV. Amidostonum

The most common species is *Amidostonum anseris,* which lives in the gizzard (bird's second stomach for grinding food) of geese. It causes severe inflammation with hemorrhages of the gizzard wall. The horny layer is often fully destroyed. Mortality in young geese can be very high. Adult geese are less susceptible.

C. General Remarks

The choice of anthelmintics that can be used in domestic birds is limited. Many anthelmintics which are very succesful in other animals have never been tested in domestic birds. Of the anthelmintics that can be used, many have a narrow spectrum, sometimes being only effective against one species. Next the method of administration can limit our choice. For administration in the drinking water, only compounds which are soluble can be used. So an important group of anthelmintics, the benzimidazoles, is excluded. Administration by way of the food can also have limitations. Many anthelmintics have only been tested on their efficacy after a single dose. Because many farmers use automatic feeders and bulk feed tanks, it is often only possible to mix the anthelmintic in the total feed for 1 week or more. Only a few anthelmintics, mainly mebendazole and fenbendazole, have been tested for their efficacy after administration in the food during several days. The kind of food can also be a limiting factor. It is very difficult to get a homogeneous mixture of an anthelmintic in food consisting of cereals, as for instance pigeon food. This needs special equipment and can certainly not be done by hand.

D. The Anthelmintics

The most important findings about the activity of anthelmintics against gastrointestinal nematodes in domestic birds are summarized here (results are presented in Table 1–6).

Table 1. Efficacy of the anthelmintics against gastrointestinal nematodes in chickens

Classification[a]	Anthelmintics	Dosage	*Ascaridia*		*Capillaria*		*Heterakis*	
			Adults	Developing larvae	Adults	Developing larvae	Adults	Developing larvae
I.	Phenothiazine	1,000 mg/kg p.o.	–	–	–	–	++	+
II.	Piperazine	250 mg/kg p.o.	+++	+	–	–	–	–
		5,000 ppm[b]	+++	–	–	–	–	–
		3,000 ppm[c]	++	–	–	–	–	–
III.	Metyridine	200 mg/kg s.c.	+	–	+++	+++	–	–
		3,000 ppm[b]	+	–	+++	+++	–	–
IV.1.	Coumafos	40 ppm/10 days[c]	+++	–	+++	–	+++	–
2.	Haloxon	50–100 mg/kg p.o.	–	–	++	–	–	–
VI.1.	Tiabendazole	1,000 mg/kg p.o.	+	–	+	–	+	–
		500 ppm/3 days[c]	+++	++	–	–	–	–
3.	Cambendazole	10 mg/kg p.o.	+++	–	–	–	–	–
		30 mg/kg p.o.	+++	+++	–	–	–	–
		50 mg/kg p.o.	+++	+++	+++	–	+++	–
		70 mg/kg p.o.	+++	+++	+++	+++	+++	–
4.	Mebendazole	10 mg/kg/3 days	+++	+++	–	–	–	–
		20 mg/kg/3 days	+++	+++	+++	+++	–	–
		60 ppm/3 days[c]	+++	+++	+++	+++	–	–
5.	Fenbendazole	5 mg/kg p.o.	–	–	–	–	+++	–
		15 mg/kg p.o.	–	–	+++	+++	+++	–
		8 mg/kg 3 days	+++	+++	–	–	+++	–
		60 ppm/3 days	+++	+++	+++	+++	–	–
		30 ppm/6 days	+++	+++	+++	+++	–	–
VII.	Pyrantel	15 mg/kg p.o.	+++	+	–	–	–	–
		100 mg/kg p.o.	+++	+++	–	–	+	–
		120 mg/kg p.o.	+++	+++	+++	–	+	–
VIII.	Levamisole	20 mg/kg p.o.	+++	+++	–	–	–	–
		40 mg/kg p.o.	+++	+++	+++	+++	–	–
X.	Ivermectin	0.1 mg/kg p.o.	–	+++	+++	–	–	–

Classification of efficacy: +++, 95%–100%; ++, 80%–100%; +, 0%–100%; –, not effective or insufficient data

[a] Numbers correspond to those in text
[b] In the drinking water
[c] In the food

Table 2. Efficacy of the anthelmintics against gastrointestinal nematodes in pheasants

Classification	Anthelmintics	Dosage	*Ascaridia*		*Capillaria*		*Heterakis*	
			Adults	Developing larvae	Adults	Developing larvae	Adults	Developing larvae
VI.4.	Mebendazole	60 ppm/6 days[a]	+++	–	+++	–	+++	–
5.	Fenbendazole	60 ppm/6 days[a]	–	–	+++	–	+++	–
IX.1.	Febantel	10 mg/kg p.o.	+++	+++	–	–	+++	+++

Classification of efficacy: +++, 95%–100%; –, not effective or insufficient data

[a] In the food

Table 3. Efficacy of the anthelmintics against gastrointestinal nematodes in turkeys

Classification	Anthelmintics	Dosage	*Ascaridia*		*Capillaria*		*Heterakis*	
			Adults	Developing larvae	Adults	Developing larvae	Adults	Dev opir larv
II.	Piperazine	4,000 ppm/6 h[a]	+++	–	–	–	–	–
		4,000 ppm/2 days[b]	+++	–	–	–	–	–
III.	Metyridine	200 mg/kg s.c.	–	–	+++	–	–	–
VI.2.	Parbendazole	30 mg/kg	–	–	–	–	+++	–
		500 ppm/1 day[b]	+++	+	+	–	+++	–
		1,000 ppm/1 day[b]	+++	+	++	–	+++	–
VII.1.	Levamisole	30 mg/kg p.o.	+++	+++	++	–	+++	–
		300 ppm/1 day[a]	+++	+++	+	–	+++	–

Classification of efficacy: +++, 95%–100%; ++, 80%–100%; +, 0%–100%; –, not effective insufficient data

[a] In the drinking water

[b] In the food

Table 4. Efficacy of the anthelmintics against gastrointestinal nematodes in geese

Classification	Anthelmintics	Dosage	*Amidostomum*	
			Adults	Developing larvae
IV.3.	Trichlorphon	75 mg/kg p.o.	+++	++
V.1.	Disophenol	10 mg/kg s.c.	+++	–
VI.4.	Mebendazole	10 mg/kg/3 days p.o.	+++	–
		60 ppm/6 days[a]		
5.	Fenbendazole	5 mg/kg p.o.	+++	–
		60 ppm/6 days[a]	+++	–
VII.	Pyrantel	50 mg/kg p.o.	+++	+++
VIII.	Levamisole	15 mg/kg p.o.	+++	+++

Classification of efficacy: +++, 95%–100%; ++, 80%–100%; –, not effictive or insufficient data

[a] In the food

Table 5. Efficacy of the anthelmintics against gastrointestinal nematodes in pigeons

Classification	Anthelmintics	Dosage	*Ascaridia*		*Capillaria*	
			Adults	Developing larvae	Adults	Developing larvae
III.	Metyridine	200 mg/kg s.c., p.o.	–	–	+++	–
IV.2.	Haloxon	50 mg/kg p.o.	–	–	+++	–
VI.1.	Tiabendazole	5,000 ppm/10 days[a]	+++	–	–	–
5.	Fenbendazole	7.5 mg/kg p.o.	+++	–	–	–
		100 ppm/3 days[b]	+++	+++	+++	+++
VIII.1.	Levamisole	20–40 mg/kg p.o.	+++	–	+++	–

Classification of efficacy: +++, 95%–100%; –, not effective or insufficient data
[a] In the food
[b] See contraindication on p. 514–515

Table 6. Anthelmintics effective against gastrointestinal nematodes in domestic birds

Classification	Generic name	Supplier	Trade names	Formulations
I.	Phenothiazine	Various	Various	Powder
II.	Piperazine	Various	Various	Powder, tablets
III.	Metyridine	ICI	Mintic, Promintic	Solution, injectable solution
IV.1.	Coumafos	Bayer, Chemagro	Baymix, Co-Ral	Crumbles
2.	Haloxon	Cooper	Halox, Loxon, Verloxon	Suspension
3.	Trichlorphon	Bayer	Neguvon	Powder
V.1.	Disophenol	Cyanamid	Ancylol	Injectable solution
VI.1.	Tiabendazole	MSD	Thibenzole	Powder
2.	Parbendazole	Smith Kline	Helmatac	Powder
3.	Cambendazole	MSD		
4.	Mebendazole	Janssen Pharmaceutica	Mebenvet	Powder
5.	Fenbendazole	Hoechst	Panacur, Axilur	Powder
VII.1.	Pyrantel	Pfizer	Banminth	Powder
VIII.1.	Levamisole	Janssen Pharmaceutica	L-Ripercol, L-Spartakon	Injectable solution tablets
IX.1.	Febantel	Bayer	Rintal	Suspension
X.1.	Ivermectin	MSD		

I. Phenothiazine

Chickens

Phenothiazine can be given at a dose of 1,000 mg/kg for efficient control of adult *H. gallinarum*. Efficacy against developing stages is low (ENIGK and DEY-HAZRA 1968, 1971). There is hardly any effect against *Ascaridia* and *Capillaria*.

II. Piperazine

a) Chickens

Piperazine citrate given at a single dose of 250 mg/kg was very effective against adult *A. galli*. Its efficacy against developing stages is low (ENIGK and DEY-HAZRA 1971). Piperazine citrate given in the drinking water at a concentration of 0.5% for 1 day was also highly effective (COLGLAZIER et al. 1960). Piperazine adipate administered in the food at a concentration of 0.3% for 1 day had a moderate effect (HORTON-SMITH and LONG 1956).

b) Turkeys

Piperazine hexahydrate given in the drinking water at a concentration of 0.4% for 6 h was very effective against *A. dissimilis* (EDGAR et al. 1957). Piperazine citrate given at a level of 0.4% in the food for 2 days was very effective against adult *Ascaridia* (KATES et al. 1969).

III. Metyridine

a) Chickens

Metyridine administered at a dose of 200 mg/kg subcutaneously was fully effective against adults and developing stages of *C. obsignata* (HENDRIKS 1962; THIENPONT and MORTELMANS 1962; THIENPONT et al. 1963; FRIEDHOFF 1963; GANGADHARA RAO 1976). A high efficacy can be reached with a dose of 150 mg/kg given subcutaneously (BROOME 1963; NORTON and JOYNER 1965). Given orally at a dose of 200–225 mg/kg a high efficacy was also found (HENDRIKS 1963; NORTON and JOYNER 1965; KIENE and GREUEL 1969). For mass treatment metyridine can be given in the drinking water at a concentration of 0.30%–0.35%. High efficacy with this method was found by HENDRIKS (1963), BROOME (1963), and FRIEDHOFF (1963).

Metyridine has only a very limited effect against other nematodes. Only adults of *A. galli* are affected to some extent (THIENPONT et al. 1963; BRUYNOOGHE et al. 1968). The drug has to be given strictly subcutaneously, because an intramuscular injection can cause myositis, myodegeneration, and necroses (THIENPONT et al. 1963).

Toxic effects of metyridine can be seen with the therapeutic dose. After a subcutaneous dose of 200 mg/kg, dullness and cyanosis of the comb and wattles were seen (HENDRIKS 1962; THIENPONT and MORTELMANS 1962). Paralysis and even death was seen after a dose of 400 mg/kg (THIENPONT et al. 1963). In laying hens a drop in the number of eggs laid of 3%–10% for 1 week after a subcutaneous dose of 200 mg/kg was seen (THIENPONT et al. 1963). Metyridine given in the drinking water can depress the water uptake considerably (BROOME 1963; GRATTAN 1963), which may cause production losses.

b) Turkeys

A dose of 200 mg/kg given subcutaneously was, based on egg counts and clinical findings, very effective against *C. obsignata*. No toxic effects were seen (WEISMAN and DISON 1973).

c) Geese

A dose of 133 mg/kg given subcutaneously was, based on egg counts, fully effective against *C. anatis* (FRIEDHOFF 1963). According to ENIGK et al. (1975b) metyridine is too toxic to use in geese.

d) Pigeons

Metyridine at a dose of 100–200 mg/kg given subcutaneously or orally was very effective against *C. obsignata* (FIEVEZ et al. 1963; WEHR et al. 1967; THIENPONT and MORTELMANS 1962; STAM 1963). Given in the drinking water at a dose of 200 mg/kg the efficacy was low (GEERAERTS 1964). At the therapeutic dose of 200 mg/kg given subcutaneously toxic symptoms like vomiting and ataxia were seen. One to two hours after administration these symptoms disappeared. A dose of 300 mg/kg can be fatal (THIENPONT and MORTELMANS 1962).

IV. Organic Phosphorus Compounds

1. Coumafos

Chickens

Coumafos given at a concentration of 40 ppm in the food for 10 days was very effective against *Ascaridia* and *Capillaria*. Efficacy against *Heterakis* was moderate (ELEAZER 1969).

2. Haloxon

a) Chickens

The results of haloxon against *Capillaria* are conflicting. Doses of 50–100 mg/kg gave a high to moderate efficacy only against adult *Capillaria* (CLARKE 1962; HENDRIKS 1964; NORTON and JOYNER 1965; BEECH 1967; KIENE and GREUEL 1969). No toxic effects were seen up to a dose of 100 mg/kg. A dose of 200 mg/kg caused dullness and diminished appetite (HENDRIKS 1964).

b) Pigeons

Haloxon at a dose of 50 mg/kg given orally was fully effective against adult *C. obsignata*. At this dose vomiting occurred accasionally (LÜTHGEN and BERNAU 1967).

3. Trichlorphon

Geese

Trichlorphon given orally at a dose of 75 mg/kg was very effective against adult *Amidostomum anseris*. Efficacy against developing stages was moderate (Enigk and Dey-Hazra 1967).

V. Nitrophenols

Disophenol

Geese

Disophenol at a dose of 10 mg/kg given subcutaneously was very effective against adult *A. anseris*. Its efficacy against developing stages was low (Enigk and Dey-Hazra 1967).

VI. Benzimidazoles

1. Tiabendazole

a) Chickens

Tiabendazole at a single dose of 1,000 mg/kg has only a minor effect against the common nematodes in chickens (Long and Wakelin 1964; Hendriks 1965; Norton and Joyner 1965; Enigk and Dey-Hazra 1968). Given at a concentration of 0.05% in the feed daily for three consecutive days, it was fully effective against adult *Ascaridia galli*. The effect against the larval stages was moderate, however. At a concentration of 0.1% given daily for 8 days in the feed it had no effect against adult *C. obsignata* (Long and Wakelin 1964).

b) Pigeons

Tiabendazole given at a concentration of 0.5% in a mash food daily for 10 days was fully effective against *A. columbae* in naturally infected pigeons (Wehr and Colglazier 1968).

2. Parbendazole

Turkeys

Parbendazole at a dose of 30 mg/kg given by gelatine capsule was very effective against adult *H. gallinarum*. There was hardly any effect against adults and developing stages of *A. dissimilis* and adult *C. obsignata*. Given in the food at a concentration of 0.05% for 1 day it was fully effective against adult *A. dissimilis* and adult *H. gallinarum*. The effect against developing stages of *A. dissimilis* and adult *C. obsignata* was low. A concentration of 0.1% in the food for 1 day had a moderate effect against *C. obsignata* (Kates et al. 1969).

3. Cambendazole

a) Chickens

Cambendazole at a dose of 10 mg/kg was very effective against adult *A.galli.* A dose of 30 mg/kg was necessary to obtain a high efficacy against developing stages of this nematode. At doses of 50 mg/kg it was very effective against adult *H.gallinarum* and adult *C.obsignata*; at 70 mg/kg it had a high efficacy against developing larvae of *C. obsignata* (ENIGK and DEY-HAZRA 1971).

b) Geese

Cambendazole at a dose of 60 mg/kg was very effective against adults and developing stages of *Amidostomum anseris* (ENIGK and DEY-HAZRA 1971).

4. Mebendazole

a) Chickens

For effective control of adults and developing stages of *Ascaridia galli* and adult *H.gallinarum* mebendazole can be given at a dose of 10 mg/kg daily for three consecutive days. To obtain a high efficacy against adults and developing stages of *C.obsignata* a dose of 20 mg/kg given in the same way was necessary (ENIGK et al. 1975). A concentration of 60 ppm given in the food for 3 days was very effective against *Ascaridia* and *Capillaria* (ENIGK et al. 1975 a).

b) Pheasants

Mebendazole given in the food at a concentration of 125 ppm for 15 days was very effective against *Capillaria.* A concentration of 60 ppm permanently in the food prevented outbreaks of capillariasis in pheasants. This treatment had no adverse effect upon laying, fertility, and hatching (SCHRICKE et al. 1973). ENIGK and DEY-HAZRA (1975) found, based on egg counts, that a concentration of 60 ppm given in the food for 6 days was enough to obtain a high efficacy against *Ascaridia, Heterakis,* and *Capillaria.*

c) Geese

Mebendazole at a dose of 10 mg/kg given daily on three consecutive days was very effective against *Amidostomum anseris* and *Trichostrongylus tenuis* (ENIGK et al. 1973, 1975b). The same effect can be achieved by mixing 60 ppm in the food for 6 days (ENIGK et al. 1975).

d) Pigeons

Mebendazole at a dose of 5 mg/kg given twice a day on four consecutive days was very effective against *Tetrameres americana* (YOUNG 1981). Due to possible side effects mebendazole is not recommended in pigeons.

5. Fenbendazole

a) Chickens

A single dose of 5 mg/kg fenbendazole was very effective against adult *H. gallinarum*. A dose of 15 mg/kg, however, is necessary to obtain a high efficacy against adults and developing stages of *C. obsignata*. A high efficacy against adults and developing stages of *Ascaridia galli* was found at a dose of 8 mg/kg given on three consecutive days. High efficacy against *Ascaridia* and *Capillaria* in naturally infected chickens was found after giving a concentration of 60 ppm in the food for three consecutive days or 30 ppm for 6 days (Enigk et al. 1975a).

b) Pheasants

A concentration of 60 ppm fenbendazole daily for days was very effective against *Heterakis* and *Capillaria* in naturally infected pheasants and other game birds (Enigk and Dey-Hazra 1976). Administered at a concentration of 200 ppm in the food of quails for 30 days it had no effect on laying, fertility, embryo mortality, and hatching (Sambeth 1980).

c) Geese

Fenbendazole at a dose of 5 mg/kg was very effective against *Amidostomum anseris*. The same effect was found when fenbendazole was given at a concentration of 60 ppm in the food for six consecutive days (Enigk et al. 1975b).

d) Pigeons

A single dose of 7.5 mg/kg was, based on egg counts fully effective against *A. columbae* in naturally infected pigeons. For the same effect against *C. obignata* a dose of 20 mg/kg was necessary (Kirsch et al. 1978). High efficacy against developing stages of *C. obsignata* was found by Vindevogel et al. (1978) after a dose of 27.5 mg/kg daily for 3 days.

Given in a special pelleted food at a concentration of 100 ppm for three consecutive days it was very effective against *Ascaridia* (Kirsch et al. 1978). The treatment with the pelleted food, however, had conflicting results in the treatment of *Capillaria*. The reason for this was the poor intake of this kind of food in some pigeon flocks (Kirsch et al. 1978; Vindevogel et al. 1978). When fenbendazole was mixed in a normal pigeon food at a concentration of 100 ppm (4 ml 2.5% suspension/kg food) and given for three consecutive days, it was very effective against adults and developing stages of *Ascaridia* and *Capillaria* (Vindevogel et al. 1978; Kirsch and Degenhardt 1979). It is very difficult, however, to get a homogeneous mixture of a suspension and a food consisting of cereals. So it is conceivable that overdosing may occur in some animals. Because a dose of 200 mg/kg can cause toxic symptoms such as vomiting (Kirsch et al. 1978) and higher doses can cause hepatitis, nephritis, and necrosis of the crop wall (Lüthgen 1979), this method of administration is not without danger. More important is that treatment at the therapeutic dose during the molt brings about serious damage to the molting feathers (Kirsch et al. 1978; Lüthgen 1979). This damage consists of defects in the featers and has also been seen in young pigeons still fed by their parents. In these animals even necrosis of the tip of the feathers was seen. For this reason fenbendazole can only be used during the winter months.

VII. Tetrahydropyrimidines

Pyrantel

a) Chickens

Pyrantel tartrate at a dose of 30 mg/kg was very effective against adult *Ascaridia galli,* but the effect against developing stages was moderate (ENIGK et al. 1975a). OKON (1975) found a high efficacy against adult *A. galli* even at a dose of 15 mg/kg. At this dose, however, the efficacy against developing stages was low. A dose of 125 mg/kg was necessary to obtain a high efficacy against developing stages (OKON 1976). Pyrantel tartrate up to a dose of 100 mg/kg only had a low efficacy against *H. gallinarum* (ENIGK and DEY-HAZRA 1968). To achieve a high efficacy against *C. obsignata* a dose of 120 mg/kg has to be given (KIENE and GREUEL 1969; ENIGK and DEY-HAZRA 1971, 1975a). Up to a dose of 500 mg/kg no toxic symptoms were seen (KIENE and GREUEL 1969).

b) Geese

Pyrantel tartrate given at a dose of 50 mg/kg was very effective against adults and developing stages of *Amidostomum anseris* (ENIGK and DEY-HAZRA 1967, 1971; ENIGK et al. 1975b). A dose of 250 mg/kg had no toxic effects.

VIII. Imidazothiazoles

Levamisole

a) Chickens

Levamisole diluted with water, the quantity of which was not mentioned, given by esophageal tube at a dose of 25 mg/kg was very effective against adults and developing stages of *Ascaridia galli.* The effect against adult *C. obsignata* was moderate. There was no effect against developing stages of *C. obsignata* (CLARKSON and BEG 1970). ENIGK et al. (1975a) found a high efficacy against adults and developing stages of *A. galli* after an oral dose of 20 mg/kg. For a high efficacy against adults and developing stages of *C. obstignata* a dose of 40 mg/kg was necessary. Up to a dose of 16 mg/kg the efficacy against *H. gallinarum* was low. A dose of 18 mg/kg administered in the drinking water for 1 day was sufficient for a high efficacy against adult *A. galli* (PANKAVICH et al. 1973; CRUTHERS et al. 1975).

With a dose of 36 mg/kg a high efficacy against *H. gallinarum* was found by PANKAVICH et al. (1973). However, 48 mg/kg was necessary for a high efficacy against *C. obsignata.* In these trials the total amount of levamisole was mixed in one-half to one-third of the amount of water previously consumed daily. At a concentration of 0.07% (48 mg/kg) water consumption was a little delayed but the total amount was consumed within 14 h. Intoxications were not observed at this dose. Given subcutaneously at a dose of 30 mg/kg it was found to be very effective against adults and developing stages of *C. obsignata* (GANGADHARA RAO 1976).

b) Turkeys

Levamisole given at a dose of 30 mg/kg by gelatin capsule was very effective against adults and developing stages of *A. dissimilis* and adult *H. gallinarum*. The effect against adult *C. obsignata* was moderate. When given in the food for 1 day at a concentration of 0.1% the food intake was decreased and only a high efficacy against adult *A. dissimilis* was found (KATES et al. 1969). Administered for 1 day in the drinking water at a concentration of 0.03% it was very effective against adults and developing stages of *A. dissimilis* and adult *H. gallinarum*. Efficacy against adult *C. obsignata* was low (COLGLAZIER 1975).

c) Geese

A high efficacy of levamisole at a dose of 25 mg/kg given orally to naturally infected geese against *Amidostomum anseris* was found by FROYD (1970). ENIGK et al. (1975 b) found a high efficacy at the even lower dose of 15 mg/kg against adults and developing stages of *A. anseris* in artificially infected geese. The efficacy of 25 mg/kg against *Heterakis* and *Capillaria* is low (FROYD 1970).

d) Pigeons

Tetramisole administered orally at a dose of 40 mg/kg/bird (equivalent to about 20 mg/kg levamisole) had, based on egg counts, only a moderate effect against *Capillaria* in naturally infected pigeons (SCUPIN and LINKERMANN 1970).

GHENNE (1967) found a high efficacy of tetramisole, based on egg counts, at a dose of 50 mg/kg/animal (equivalent to about 25 mg/kg levamisole) given orally against *A. columbae*. However, 3 out of 11 treated pigeons kept shedding eggs in their feces. Efficacy against *Capillaria* at this dose was low. Given in the drinking water at a concentration of 0.06% for 2–3 days also gave a low efficacy against *Capillaria* (GHENNE 1967).

In contrast to this finding a high efficacy against *Ascaridia* and *Capillaria* was reported of a single oral dose of 20 mg levamisole/bird (±40 mg/kg) (REPORT JANSSEN 1974). Levamisole given orally at a dose of 40 mg/kg can cause regurgitation (ROBINSON and RICHTER 1977). The same dose administered intramuscularly can cause death (BUYS and VAN DER MADE 1977).

IX. Probenzimidazoles

Febantel

Pheasants

Febantel at a dose of 10 mg/kg was very effective against adults and developing stages of *Ascaridia galli* and *H. gallinarum*. No toxic symptoms were seen up to a dose of 500 mg/kg (BANKOV 1978).

X. Avermectins

Ivermectin

Chickens

In naturally infected chickens ivermectin was effective against adult *C. obsignata* and developing stages of *A. galli* at doses of 0.05 and 0.1 mg/kg. It was not effective against *H. gallinarum* but higher doses were not tested (EGERTON et al. 1979).

References

Bankov D (1978) Clinical and field trials with fenbantel, a new antinematode agent. III. Efficacy of fenbantel against *Ascaridia galli, Heterakis gallinarum, Syngamus trachea* and *Raillietina* spp. in birds. Proceedings of the fourth international congress of parasitology, Warsaw, Sect. 30

Beech JA (1967) Field trials with haloxon against *Capillaria* in laying fowls. Vet Rec 80:195–197

Broome AWJ (1963) The anthelmintic activity of methyridine (2(*b*-methoxyethyl)pyridine) against *Capillaria obsignata* in chickens. Vet Rec 75:1326–1328

Bruynooghe D, Thienpont D, Parijs OFJ Van (1968) Use of tetramisole as an anthelmintic in poultry. Vet Rec 82:701–706

Buys SB, Made HN Van der (1977) The toxicity of levamisole as a parenteral treatment for birds. Tijdskrif S Afrikaanse Vet Vereniging 48:284

Clarke ML (1962) *Capillariasis* in poultry. Vet Rec 74:1431–1432

Clarkson MJ, Beg MK (1970) The anthelmintic activity of L-tetramisole against *Ascaridia galli* and *Capillaria obsignata* in the fowl. Vet Rec 86:652–654

Colglazier ML (1975) Anthelmintic activity of levamisole given in the drinking water to turkeys. Proc Helminthol Soc Wash 42:60–61

Colglazier ML, Foster AO, Enzie FD, Thompson DE (1960) The anthelmintic action of phenothiazine and piperazine against *Heterakis gallinae* and *Ascardia galli* in chickens. J Parasitol 46:267–270

Cruthers LR, Al-Khateeb GH, Hansen MF (1975) Efficacy of levamisole (Tramisol) in drinking water against some nematodes of chickens. Proc Oklahama Acad Sci 55:119–121

Edgar SA, Davis DC, Frazier JA (1957) Efficacy of some piperazine compounds in the elimination of helminths from experimentally and naturally infected poultry. Poult Sci 36:495–510

Egerton JR, Ostlind DA, Blair LS, Eary CH, Suhayda D, Cifelli S, Riek RF, Campbell WC (1979) Avermectins, new family of potent anthelmintic agents: efficacy of the BIa component. Antimicrob Agents Chemother 15:372–378

Eleazer TH (1969) Coumaphos a new anthelmintic for control of *Capillaria obsignata, Heterakis gallinarum* and *Ascaridia galli* in chickens. Avian Dis 13:228–230

Enigk K, Dey-Hazra (1967) Zur Behandlung des *Amidostomum*- Befalles der Gans. DTW 74:524–530

Enigk K, Dey-Hazra A (1968) Zur Therapie des Heterakisbefalles beim Huhn. Tierarztl Umsch 23:584–587

Enigk K, Dey-Hazra A (1971) Zur Behandlung der häufigsten Nematodeninfektionen des Hausgeflügels. DTW 78:178–180

Enigk K, Dey-Hazra A (1975) Zur Behandlung des Wurmbefalles bei Fasan, Rebhuhn und Birkhuhn. Wild Huhn 78:236–239

Enigk K, Dey-Hazra A (1976) Die Behandlung des Helminthenbefalles wildlebender Säugetiere und Vögel mit Fenbendazole. Kleintier Prax 21:133–144

Enigk K, Dey-Hazra A, Batke J (1973) Zur Wirksamkeit von Mebendazole bei Helminthosen von Huhn und Gans. Avian Pathol 2:67–74

Enigk K, Dey-Hazra A, Batke J (1975a) Die Behandlung des Ascaridia-, Heterakis- und Capillaria-Befalles des Hausgeflügels. Tierarztl Umsch 30:324–329

Enigk K, Dey-Hazra A, Batke J (1975b) Zur Epizootologie und Behandlung des Helminthenbefalles der Gans. Acta Parasitol Polon 23:367–372
Fievez L, Granville A, Ghyselings R (1963) Traitement de la capillariose du pigeon par le methyridine (Promintic I.C.I.). Am Med Vet 107:479–482
Friedhoff K (1963) Therapie des Capillariabefalles beim Geflügel. Berl Munch Tierarztl Wochenschr 76:151–155
Froyd G (1970) Levamisole in geese. Vet Rec 86:788–789
Gangadhara Rao YVB (1976) Experimental chemotherapy on *Capillaria obsignata* in chickens. Ind Vet J 53:776–777
Geeraerts J (1964) Treatment of capillariosis in pigeons and chickens with Mintic (in Dutch). Vlaams Diergeneeskd Tijdschr 33:103–105
Ghenne P (1967) Traitement de la capillariose et de l'ascaridiose du pigeon voyageur par le tetramisole. Ann Med Vet 11:291–302
Grattan DAP (1963) Anthelmintic activity of methyridine in chickens. Vet Rec 75:1433
Hendriks J (1962) The use of promintic as anthelmintic against infections of *Capillaria obsignata* Madsen, 1945 in chickens. Tijdschr Diergeneeskd 87:314–322
Hendriks J (1963) Methyridine in the drinking water against *Capillaria obsignata* Madsen 1945 in experimentally infected chickens. Tijdschr Diergeneeskd 88:418–424
Hendriks J (1964) The anthelmintic activity of haloxon against *Capillaria obsignata* Madsen 1945 in experimentally infected chickens. Tijdschr Diergeneeskd 89:1218–1224
Hendriks J (1965) The effects of oral administration of thiabendazole upon *Capillaria obsignata* Madsen, 1945 in experimentally infected chickens. Tijdschr Diergeneeskd 90:1062–1066
Horton-Smith C, Long PL (1956) The anthelmintic effect of three piperazine derivatives on *Ascaridia galli* (Schrank 1788). Poult Sci 35:606–614
Kates KC, Colglazier ML, Enzie TD (1969) Comparative efficacy of levotetramisole, parbendazole, and piperazine citrate against some common helminths of turkeys. Trans Am Microsc Soc 88:142–148
Kiene B, Greuel E (1969) Die Wirkung verschiedener Anthelmintika auf *Capillaria obsignata* nach experimenteller Infektion beim Huhn. Berl Munch Tierarztl Wochenschr 82:432–436
Kirsch R, Degenhardt H (1979) Zur Wirksamkeit von Fenbendazol auf unreife und reife Stadien von *Capillaria obsignata* und *Ascaridia columbae* bei Tauben im controlled test. Tierarztl Umsch 34:767–771
Kirsch R, Petri K, Degenhardt H (1978) Zur Behandlung des Ascaridia- und Capillaria-Befalles bei Tauben mit Fenbendazole. Kleintier Prax 23:291–298
Long PL, Wakelin D (1964) The effects of thiabendazole upon experimental infestations of *Ascaridia galli* and *Capillaria obsignata* in chickens. Br Poult Sci 5:187–192
Lüthgen W (1979) Untersuchungen über die Wirksamkeit von Fenbendazol auf den Rundwurmbefall der Tauben (*Columba livia* dom.). Tierarztl Umsch 34:104–112
Lüthgen W, Bernau U (1967) Versuche zur Bekämpfung der Capillariasis der Tauben mit Haloxon. Kleintier Prax 12:17–21
Norton CC, Joyner LP (1965) Experimental chemotherapy of infection with *Capillaria obsignata*. J Comp Pathol 75:137–145
Okon ED (1975) Anthelmintic activity of pyrantel tartrate against *Ascaridia galli* in fowls. Res Vet Sci 18:331–332
Okon ED (1976) Effect of pyrantel tartrate on the third-stage larvae of *Ascaridia galli*. Res Vet Sci 21:104
Pankavich JA, Poeschel GP, Shor AL, Gallo A (1973) Evaluation of levamisole against experimental infections of *Ascaridia, Heterakis,* and *Capillaria* spp. in chickens. Am J Vet Res 34:501–505
Report Janssen (1974) The activity of levamisole (R 12564) against nematodes in pigeons. Janssen Res Found, Beerse, Belgium
Robinson PT, Richter AG (1977) A preliminary report on the toxicity and efficacy of levamisole phosphate in zoo birds. J Zoo Anim Med 8:23–26
Sambeth W (1980) Verträglichkeit von Fenbendazole im Hinblick auf die Fruchtbarkeit von Wachteln. Berl Munch Tierarztl Wochenschr 93:274–275

Schricke E, Goupille F, Heude B (1973) Efficacité d'un nouvel anthelmintique, le Mebendazole sur la Syngamose et les Capillariose du faisan. Rec Med Vet 149:1327–1337
Scupin E, Linkermann H (1970) Die Taubencapillariasis im Raume Göttingen. Behandlungsmöglichkeiten mit Tetramisole. Kleintier Prax 15:174–177
Stam JWE (1963) Capillariasis in pigeons (in Dutch). Tijdschr Diergeneeskd 88:879–882
Thienpont D, Mortelmans J (1962) Methyridine in the control of intestinal capillariasis in birds. Vet Rec 74:850–852
Thienpont D, Bruynooghe D, Mortelmans J (1963) Mass treatment of *Capillaria*- and *Ascaridia*-infected poultry with methyridine. Vet Rec 75:1019–1024
Vindevogel H, Duchatel JP, Fievez L (1978) Traitement de la capillariose du pigeon par le fenbendazole. Ann Med Vet 122:109–115
Wehr EE, Colglazier ML (1968) Thiabendazole as an anthelmintic against *Ascaridia columbae* in pigeon. Proc Helminthol Soc Wash 35:117–118
Wehr EE, Colglazier ML, Burtner RH, Wiest LM (1967) Methyridine an effective anthelmintic for intestinal threadworm, *Capillaria obsignata* in pigeons. Avian Dis II:322–326
Weisman J, Dison MS (1973) *Capillaria obsignata* (Madsen 1945) in turkeys in Israel. Vet Rec 93:205–206
Young RA (1981) Mebendazole treatment of stomach-wall worm in the racing pigeon. Vet Med Small Anim clin 76:426–427

CHAPTER 11

Chemotherapy of Intestinal Trematodiasis in Mammals and Birds

M. M. H. SEWELL

A. Introduction

Trematode parasites occur in the intestinal tract of most types of domesticated livestock and also in wild animals, including those in zoological collections. However, with the main exception of paramphistomes in ruminants, they tend to occur in relatively small numbers and even then in only a small proportion of those hosts of major veterinary importance. They occur with greater frequency in birds and rodents and in some cases these hosts form reservoirs of infection for man or his domestic animals. This happens mainly because trematodes tend to have little host specificity as adults and are therefore often reported in unusual hosts, usually in small numbers.

In general the intestinal trematodes are of low pathogenicity as compared with intestinal nematodes or hepatic trematodes, such as *Fasciola*. This tends to limit their impact on productivity and their significance as agents of disease, except where they are involved in zoonotic infections. In addition some of them are restricted in their geographical range.

Accordingly the need to develop chemotherapeutic agents against these parasites has been less apparent and most studies have been restricted to observations as to the effects of known fasciolocides, cesticides or in some cases nematocides against the intestinal trematodes. Even then, the preponderance of this work has been concerned with paramphistomes in domestic ruminants and in most cases activity against other intestinal trematodes has to be inferred. Nevertheless, in contrast to the situation 20 years ago, there are now several drugs with known and reliable activity against these parasites and it would appear likely that some of the more recently introduced products will be found to possess such activity.

B. Intestinal Trematodes of Mammals

I. Ruminants

1. Paramphistomiasis

Adult paramphistomes occur commonly in the rumen and reticulum of domestic and wild ruminants in most parts of the world, while their immature forms are found in the duodenum and abomasum. The adults are small conical flukes up to about 15 mm in length and 5 mm in maximum diameter, these dimensions varying with both age and species. They have a small oral sucker at the narrower, anterior end and a much larger posterior sucker or acetabulum.

Table 1. Paramphistomes of domestic ruminants

Species	Range
Calicophoron calicophorum	Russia, eastern Asia, Africa, Australia
Carmyerius gregarius	East Africa, Egypt
Ceylonocotyle scolioceolium	India, eastern Asia, Africa
Cotylophoron cotylophorum	India, eastern Asia, Africa, Australia, Americas
Fishoederius elongatus	India, Southeast Asia, Japan
Gastrothylax crumenifer	Russia, India
Gigantocotyle explanatum	India
Homolagaster paloniae	Southern and eastern Asia
Johnsonitrema magnum	India
Liorchis scotiae	Russia, Europe
Olveria indica	India
Paramphistomum cervi	Africa, Asia, North America, Europe
P. daubneyi	Eastern and southern Europe
P. gotoi	Eastern Europe, Asia, Egypt, Brazil
P. gracile	Asia, Brazil
P. hibernae	Brazil, Europe
P. ichikawai	Asia, Australia, Brazil, Europe
P. microbothrium	Africa, Europe, western Asia, Russia
Strephanopharynx compacta	Africa
Zygocotyle lunata	Americas, Africa

Several other species of limited range have been described, mainly in the genus *Paramphistomum*

Paramphistomes occur in ruminants throughout the world but, from the research interest which has been shown in them, it would appear that they are considered to be a more significant problem in Russia, Eastern Europe, the Indian subcontinent and to a lesser extent Africa than they are elsewhere.

Each species is very limited in its range of intermediate hosts and their distribution is accordingly restricted to that associated with the particular snails involved. The major species of paramphistomes and their geographical range are shown in Table 1. *Gigantocotyle explanatum,* a common paramphistome in cattle in the Indian subcontinent, is exceptional in that its characteristic site in the mammalian host is in the bile ducts rather than in the intestinal tract.

The life cycles of these species are all similar. The cercariae released from the snails encyst as metacercariae on herbage and, after they have been ingested by the final host, the juvenile flukes excyst in the duodenum and jejunum. They remain in these sites for about 8 weeks, browsing on the epithelium, with the youngest flukes deeply embedded in the mucosa. Thereafter they migrate anteriorly, passing through the abomasum to reach the forestomach. The adults then remain attached to the wall of the rumen and reticulum, usually concentrated about the rumenoreticular junction.

The most severe pathology associated with paramphistomes occurs following massive infections of sheep and calves (BIDA and SCHILLHORN VAN VEEN 1977; ERBOLATOV 1975; NIKITIN 1978; CHHABRA et al. 1978; HORAK 1971). In these cases the immature stages denude the epithelial lining with consequent severe losses of fluid, protein and even red cells (HORAK 1971). This may result in profuse diarrhoea, dehydration, emaciation, hypoproteinaemia, oedema, and anaemia. In severe outbreaks a large proportion of the flock or herd may succumb to the infection and die (HORAK 1971; NIKITIN 1978).

Until about 1960 there were no reliable drugs available against paramphistomes. OLSEN (1949) had reported successful treatment using a mixed suspension of hexachlorethane and bentonite but later authors had less success with this mixture. Control measures were therefore perforce based entirely on epidemiological considerations. Since then several drugs have been shown to be effective against these parasites, notable among these being resorantel, bithionol, niclosamide, and oxyclozanide.

Drugs which appear to be effective but have been studied less intensively include brotianide (KARRASCH et al. 1975; CORBA et al. 1976b; CORBA et al. 1979) and perhaps clioxanide (CHHABRA and BALI 1976). On the other hand, niclosamide has received considerable attention (BORAY 1969; NATH 1970; ZHARIKOV et al. 1970; SCHILLHORN VAN VEEN and BIDA 1975; CHHABRA and BALI 1976; CHHABRA et al. 1978) but with rather variable results.

Other drugs studied in recent years, which are active against paramphistomes but probably less so than those mentioned above, include difluorotetrachlorethane (GUILHON et al. 1971; ERBOLATOV 1977), fenbendazole (CORBA et al. 1979), hexachlorethane (RUZIEV 1972), hexachloroparaxylene (ZHARIKOV et al. 1970; KHAIDAROV 1972; MEREMINSKII and GLUZMAN 1975; PETKOV et al. 1975; TRIFONOV 1979), levamisole (GEORGIEV and GRUEV 1979), niclofolan (BORAY 1969; KHAIDAROV 1972; SCHILLHORN VAN VEEN and BIDA 1975; CHHABRA and BALI 1976; CHHABRA et al. 1978), oxinide (KHAIDAROV 1972; RUZIEV 1972), tetramisole (STOIMENOV et al. 1976), and trichlorophon (MEREMINSKII and GLUZMAN 1966). The inclusion of fenbendazole in this list is of some interest as it may suggest that others of the commonly available wide-spectrum benzimidazoles, notably the fasciolicidal drug albendazole, might be of value, at least in the emergency treatment of acute paramphistomiasis.

A major difficulty in comparing the results of the various authors lies in the different criteria they have adopted in assessing the efficacy of the treatment. The most reliable procedure is to carry out comparative postmortem counts of the numbers of adult and immature paramphistomes in adequate numbers of treated and control animals, as has been done by such authors as BOSMAN et al. (1961) for hexachlorophene, CORBA et al. (1979) for oxyclozanide, brotianide, and fenbendazole, VASIL'EV et al. (1970) and PAVLOV and GEORGIEV (1976) for bithionol, and CHOWANIEC et al. (1976) for resorantel.

Somewhat less satisfactory is the commonly used procedure of relying on faecal egg counts to give some indication of the initial infection followed by treatment of all the animals and postmortem examination to show what proportion have been completely freed of infection. Still other authors have relied on faecal egg counts before and after treatment, a doubtful procedure since such studies can only demonstrate the effect of the drugs on the mature forms and several drugs have been shown to cause a temporary cessation of egg production, including oxyclozanide (ROMANIUK 1971), hexachloroparaxylene and niclosamide (ZHARIKOV et al. 1970). Other authors have been merely concerned with clinical recovery, which may follow only partial loss of immature paramphistomes from the small intestine.

Russian and other East European authors consistently make use of the concepts of extensefficacy (EE) and intensefficacy (IE). These terms refer respectively to the percentage of animals completely freed of infection and the percentage reduction in burden. The parameters may be assessed either from autopsy findings or from coprological results.

An overall assessment of the findings from all these studies suggests that the drugs of choice in paramphistomiasis at present are resorantel (65 mg/kg), bithionol (70 mg/kg) or bithionol sulphoxide (40 mg/kg). Niclosamide at 75 mg/kg is also effective against the immature stages, while oxyclozanide (15 mg/kg) usually has a useful clinical effect.

2. Eurytremiasis

Eurytrema pancreaticum, E. coelomaticum and *E. dajii* are usually located in the pancreatic duct of domestic ruminants but may be found in the duodenum. They are relatively wide, dorsoventrally flattened dicrocoeliid trematodes up to 16 mm long by about 8 mm broad, with a distinct posteriorly sited brown patch, resulting from the eggs in the uterus. They occur widely throughout the Far East and in Brazil, causing inflammation and fibrosis of the pancreatic duct. Heavy infections result in the loss of condition.

As is typical of the family, their life cycle involves both a molluscan intermediate host and an arthropod transport host, these being a land snail and a grasshopper respectively. They are therefore well adapted to survive in relatively arid areas.

There are relatively few accounts of studies on the chemotherapy of this condition and these have mostly been unsuccessful, using such drugs as bithionol sulphoxide, tiabendazole (NOSAKA et al. 1970), hexachloroparaxylene, hexachlorethane, and chlorophos (KUKHARENKO 1973). There is, however, a recent report that nitroxynil is effective against *E. coelomaticum* in cattle at 20–30 mg/kg per day for 3 days (KONO et al. 1981).

3. Hasstilesiasis

Hasstilesia ochotona and *H. ovis* are small brachylemid trematodes about 1 mm long, which used to be included in the genus *Skrjabinotrema* and are found in the small intestine of sheep in Russia (GVOZDEV and SUBOLEVA 1973). There are no records of treatment directed against this parasite, which appears to be of minimal pathogenicity.

II. Equines

Paramphistomiasis

Gastrodiscus aegypticus is the most commonly encountered paramphistome of horses, donkeys and mules, with some reports of pathogenic infections in Africa (AZZIE 1975; BRACEGIRDLE 1973). Its morphology is not that of a typical amphistome as it has a circular, dorsoventrally flattened body (10–15 × 8–9 mm), with a small posterior sucker on the ventral surface and an anterior cone-shaped projection on the dorsal surface, about 4 mm long, which carries the oral orifice and sucker. Its site in the host is also unusual for this family as it occurs mainly in the small intestine. A similar but smaller (2–5 × 5–10 mm) parasite *Pseudodiscus collinsi* occurs in the large intestine of equines in India (GUPTA and WALIA 1970).

Several of the drugs used for the treatment of paramphistomes in cattle have also been shown to be effective against *G. aegypticus* in horses, including resorantel and oxyclozanide (ROBERTS et al. 1976) bithionol (GRABER 1969), and hexachlorophene and dichlorvos (AZZIE 1975; TAGER-KAGAN 1979).

III. Pigs

1. Fasciolopiasis

Fasciolopsis buski occurs in the small intestine of man and pigs in China, India, and Southeast Asia and may cause a severe enteritis with local ulcerative lesions and diarrhoea (HAQUE and SIDDIQI 1978). Pigs form the only significant animal reservoir (MANNING and RATANARAT 1970). There may be oedema and ascites as a result of hypoalbuminaemia. In man the condition is painful. *F. buski* is a large thick-set fluke up to 75 × 20 mm in size. The small oral sucker and the much larger ventral sucker are close together at the narrover anterior end. The life cycle involves aquatic snails and cercariae which encyst on vegetation – *Trapa natansl* the water chestnut being notorious as a source of human infection. There appear to be no reports of treatment of this condition with modern anthelmintics in pigs but niclosamide at up to 160 mg/kg (SUNTHARASAMAI et al. 1974), piperazine followed by bephenium with a purgative (CHANDRA et al. 1974) or 1.5–4.0 g dichlorophen (MUTTALIB 1978; IDRIS et al. 1980) have been used successfully in man. Drugs recommended in earlier studies include hexylresorcinol, tetrachloroethylene (BROWN et al. 1959) and carbon tetrachloride given by a stomach tube at 0.3 ml/kg.

2. Paramphistomiasis

Gastrodiscus aegypticus occurs in pigs as well as in equines (Sect. II.1) and a similar species *Gastrodiscoides hominis* (syn. *Gastrodiscus hominis*) occurs in both man and pigs (HAQUE and SIDDIQI 1978).

There appear to be no references to the treatment of these parasites in pigs but those drugs of value against *G. aegypticus* in horses might be expected to be effective.

Stichorchis giganteus has been repeatedly found in the caecum of pigs in Brazil (COSTA and FREITAS 1970).

3. Echinostomiasis

The echinostomes are a family of trematodes which mainly occur in birds. They tend to be elongated flukes and may be up to about 20 × 2 mm in size but are usually much smaller than this. Their ventral sucker is very much larger than their oral sucker but their most characteristic feature is a collar, which carries large spines. Echinostomes use various water snails as their intermediate hosts and have cercariae which encyst in snails. The following species have been reported from pigs:

1. *Artyfechinostomum malayanum* (syn. *Paryphostomum sufrartyfex*), which may cause clinical disease in adult pigs and even fatalities in young pigs in India (BHATTACHARYA et al. 1972) and Thailand (DISSAMARN et al. 1966).
2. *Echinochasmus perfoliatus*, which may give rise to fatal infections (SOSIPATROV 1962), but is more commonly reported from dogs.
3. *Echinostoma malayanum*, which also occurs in man in India and eastern Asia (HAQUE and SIDDIQI 1978).
4. *Echinostoma revolutum*, which is normally found in birds but has been reported from pigs in Brazil (KOHN et al. 1972 b).
5. *Stephanoprora deniticulata*, a widespread parasite of birds, has been reported from pigs in Brazil (KOHN et al. 1972 a).
6. *Euparyphium suinum* in Rumania (CIUREA 1921).

Most reports of echinostomes in pigs are incidental postmortem findings and treatment has not been recorded. *A. malayanum* or *E. perfoliatus* infections would probably merit treatment but suitable drugs would need to be chosen by analogy with other conditions. Resorantel, niclosamide, oxyclozanide, or bithionol would appear to be the indicated choices.

4. Other Trematodiases

Other trematodes reported to cause natural infections in pigs include the following:

1. *Brachylaema suis*, a small fluke up to 8×2 mm which has been reported from pigs in several parts of the world including Tunisia (BALOZET 1936), Cuba (JURASEK et al. 1971) and Russia (FATALIEV 1974). In Italy COLELLA (1972) considered that heavy infection with this parasite had caused fatalities in 3- to 4-month-old pigs. Other species in this genus are parasites of birds or rodents.

2. *Metagonimus yokogawai*, a heterophyid which occurs in man and dogs (Sect. IV.1) in eastern Europe and Asia.

There are no records of treatment used specifically against these parasites in pigs.

IV. Dogs

The relatively weak host specificity of adult trematodes has led to a large number of species, mainly heterophyids but with some echistomes and holostomes, which normally occur in birds, seals or rodents, being reported from dogs as shown in Table 2.

Very few of these species can be regarded as primarily parasites of dogs and most of them are only likely to occur in individuals which are prone to eating fish

Table 2. Intestinal trematodes recorded from dogs, cats, and other domesticated carnivores

Family	Species	Hosts	Locality
Clinostomidae	*Clinostomum falsatum*	Cat	Zimbabwe
Diplostomatidae	*Alaria alata*[a]	Dog	Europe, North America, Australia
	Pharyngostomoides sp.	Dog	India
	Pharyngostomum cordatum	Cat	India, Japan, Taiwan
Echinostomatidae	*Artyfechinostomum malayanum*	Dog, cat	India
	A. munchii	Dog	India
	Echinochasmus perfoliatus[b]	Dog, cat	Asia, Europe
	Echinoparyphium sp.	Cat	Korea
	Echinostoma hortense	Dog	Japan
	Isthmiophora melis	Dog, cat, mink	India, Europe, North America
Heterophydae (Holostomes)	*Adleriella minutissima*	Dog, cat	Middle East
	Apophallus donicum	Cat	Belgium
	Ascocotyle sp.	Dog	Brazil
	Cephalophallus obscurus	Mink	North America
	Centrocestus armatus	Dog, cat	Asia
	Cryptocotyle lingua[c]	Dog, silver, fox, mink	Europe
	Galactosomum lacteum	Cat	India
	G. fregatae	Dog	Sri Lanka
	Haplorchis pumilio[d]	Dog	Sri Lanka, Malaysia
	Heterophyes heterophyes	Dog, cat	Asia
	H. pleomorphis	Dog, cat	Uganda
	Heterophyopsis expectans	Dog, cat	Southeast Asia, Africa
	Metagonimus yokogawai	Cat	Russia, Korea
	Phagicolla italica[e]	Dog	Turkey
	P. longa	Cat	Greece
	Pricetrema sp.	Dog	Japan
	Pygidiopsis sp.	Dog	Malaysia
	Stellantchasmus falcatus	Cat	Thailand
	Stictodora sawakinensis	Dog	Sri Lanka, Malaysia
Leoithodendriidae	*Prosthodendrium glandulosum*	Dog	Sri Lanka
Nanophyetidae	*Nanophyetus salmincolla*	Dog	Northwest America, East Russia
Opisthorchiidae	*Phocitrema* sp.	Dog	Japan

[a] Several other species described in dogs in North America
[b] Several other species reported from dogs in India
[c] Two other species described from dogs and mink in Europe and Egypt
[d] Two other species described from dogs and cats in India and Thailand
[e] Two other species described from dogs in Brazil

or rodents. They are rarely pathogenic in the dog and are usually only recorded postmortem, so that treatment is not feasible. However, some of these parasites, including *Heterophyes heterophyes, Nanophyetus salmincola, Metagonimus yokogawi* and, less commonly, *Alaria* spp. and *Echinostoma malayanum* are also parasites of man.

1. Heterophyidiasis

Heterophyids are small or very small distomes not more than 2 mm long or broad and frequently much smaller. Many species have been found in dogs, especially in the Far East, but they are very rarely pathogenic, though *H. heterophyes* may cause diarrhoea in man. The life cycle involves a snail and either a fish or an amphibian second intermediate host. The condition is unlikely to merit treatment.

2. Echinostomiasis

A brief description of the echinostomes has been given above (Sect. III.3). *Echinochasmus perfoliatus*, which is found commonly in dogs in India (SAHAI and SRIRASTAVA 1970) and to a lesser extent in Europe, is a typical small echinostome up to 4 × 1 mm in size. It uses fish as its second intermediate host.

These parasites may cause severe enteritis and therefore merit treatment but there are few reports of studies on the effect of modern anthelmintics against them. However, niclosamide (KREMNER 1970) and brotianide (LEGER and NOTTEGHEM 1975) have been reported to be effective against experimental infections with echinostomes in mice and pigeons respectively. Tetramisole given orally at 10 mg/kg has also been shown to be effective against *Echinochasmus* in dogs (SWIETLIKOWSKI and WROCINSKI 1969), while flubendazole was effective when given as five daily doses to mice experimentally infected with *Echinostoma caproni* (NOTTEGHEM et al. 1979). Older remedies include carbon tetrachloride or male fern extract.

3. Nanophyetiasis

Nanophyetus salmincolla is a very small trematode, about 1 mm long or less, which occurs in man, dogs and wild carnivores in northwest America and eastern Russia. It uses salmonid fish as its second intermediate host. Heavy infections may cause severe or even fatal haemorrhagic enteritis (MISHAKOV 1971; KISTNER et al. 1979) and this parasite is associated with the ricketsial diseases "salmon poisoning" in dogs and "elokomin fluke fever" in man.

There appear to be no reports of the use of modern anthelmintics against this parasite in animals, although hexachloroparaxylol has been used in man. Carbon tetrachloride, extract of male fern and tetrachloroethylene have also been used against these flukes but none of these anthelmintics will have any effect against the intercurrent rickettsial infections.

4. Alariasis

Alaria alata is a relatively commonly encountered holostome in dogs in Europe, North America, and Australia. It is up to 6 mm long, with a short, cylindrical posterior part and a long flattened anterior part carrying two anterolateral tentacle-like processes. The life cycyle involves a water snail and, by analogy with other members of the genus, probably involves a mesocercarial stage in a frog. Metacercariae may then develop in a small rodent as a paratenic host. Several other species of this genus have been described in dogs in North America. There has also been a report of a fatal human infection with the mesocercariae from frogs in Canada (FERNANDES et al. 1976). Otherwise this infection causes only a catarrhal enteritis in the final host and there appear to be no reports of treatment.

V. Other Carnivores

As cats and Mustelidae would probably act as hosts for all the intestinal trematode parasites of dogs and vise versa, many of these parasites are shared (Table 2). Species which appear to have only been reported from cats include:

1. *Pharyngostomum cordatum*, which uses frogs and toads as a second intermediate host and snakes as a paratenic host. This species has been recorded in several parts of Asia (KIFUNE et al. 1967; DUBEY 1970; KONDO et al. 1974).
2. *Stellantchasmus falcatus*, reported as a natural infection in cats in Thailand (KLIKS and TANTACHAMRUN 1974).

Euparyphium melis, which also occurs in hedgehogs, has been reported to cause a severe enteritis in mink.

VI. Elephants

Protofasciola robusta is a common parasite of elephants and may give rise to fatalities (WINDSOR and SCOTT 1976). It has been successfully treated with two doses of 3 mg/kg rafoxanide.

Several species of paramphistomes have also been recovered from elephants, including *Pseudodiscus collinsi*, *Pfenderius papillatus*, and *Hawkesius hawkesi* in India (BHALERAO 1933).

C. Intestinal Trematodes of Birds

There are many species of trematodes which are infective for birds and most of these occur in the intestine. They are particularly common in anserine birds and in sea birds and include a number which may also infect dogs and cats (Sects. B.IV, B.V). They include many plagyorchids which use insect larvae as their second intermediate hosts, echinostomes which use snails or other molluscs and heterophyids which use fish. A number of the more common species in domestic poultry are given in Table 3.

There are relatively few reports in the literature of the treatment of naturally occurring trematode infections of birds and in most cases such treatment has been with oral carbon tetrachloride, as was recommended by SPREHN (1930) and in standard texts (SOULSBY 1968). However, such treatment is not without risk even at the recommended dose of 0.5 mg/kg in liquid paraffin and KREMNER (1970) advised the use of niclosamide at the high dose rate of 1.2 g/kg against *Echinoparyphium paraulum* in racing pigeons.

Table 3. Major intestinal trematode parasites of domestic birds

Family	Species	Hosts
Brachylaemidae	*Brachylaema commutatus*	Galliformes, pigeons
Echinostomatidae	*Echinoparyphium recurvatum* *E. paraulum*	Galliformes, anserines, pigeons, ducks
	Hypodarum conoideum	Galliformes, anserines, pigeons
Microphallidae	*Levinseniella pellucida*	Ducks
Notocotyllidae	*Notocotylus attenuatus*[a]	Galliformes, anserines
	Catatropis verrucosa	Galliformes, anserines
Paramphistomidae	*Zygocotyle lunata*	Galliformes, anserines
Plagiorchidae	*Plagiorchis anatinus*[b]	Ducks
Prosthogonimidae	*Prosthogonimus pellucidus*[c]	Galliformes, ducks
	Schistogonimus rarus	Ducks
Strigeidae	*Apatemon gracilis*	Pigeons, ducks
	Cotylurus cornutus	Pigeons, ducks
	Parastrigea robusta	Ducks

[a] Several other species in fowl and ducks
[b] Several other species in ducks
[c] Several other species in the cloaca, *Bursa fabricii* and oviducts of fowl and anserines

D. Chemotherapeutic Agents

The two main groups of drugs used in the treatment of intestinal trematodiasis are the halogenated hydrocarbons and various modified salicylanides and phenols. The latter group includes all the most effective of the more recently introduced drugs for use against paramphistomes. Most attention has been paid to drugs which were already known to be effective fasciolicides.

I. Halogenated Hydrocarbons

1. Carbon Tetrachloride

This was the first effective drug used against trematode infections, being introduced as a fasciolicide. It is much less effective against paramphistomes although its use in sheep at a relatively high oral dose rate of 7 ml/animal was recommended by BAWA (1939), while KUPPUSWAMY (1948) advocated its use at a smaller oral dose rate of 1–3 ml in sheep or 3–6 ml in cattle, following oral pretreatment with 5–10 ml 10% copper sulphate solution. These recommendations were based solely on clinical observations and other authors have discounted the value of oral carbon tetrachloride in paramphistomiasis (GUSEV 1954; AHLUWALIA and SINGH 1975), although the latter authors did recommend the intramuscular administration of carbon tetrachloride in liquid paraffin (1 : 3 v/v), with sheep receiving 4 ml and cattle 8 ml of the mixture at the same time as oral hexachlorethane or hexachlorophene (AHLUWALIA et al. 1976). Again, their findings were based on clinical improvement and faecal egg counts.

However, since carbon tetrachloride has been shown by many authors to be potentially toxic in both cattle and sheep (GIBSON 1975) and is also of doubtful efficacy it cannot now be routinely recommended for use in these hosts. It may however still be of value in the treatment of these or other hosts, including birds, where other drugs are too expensive or have not been shown to be safe or efficacious.

2. Hexachlorethane

This drug has been extensively used as a fasciolicide in cattle as it is usually less toxic in this host than carbon tetrachloride (HARROW 1959). Its use, as a suspension mixed with bentonite, against paramphistomes was recommended by OLSEN (1949) but this was based on his observations in only two animals, one cow and one ewe, with only the latter result being confirmed at necropsy, when 17% of 168 paramphistomes were still apparently alive. The value of hexachlorethane was later discounted by both ORLOVA (1953) and GUSEV (1954), although on clinical grounds DEUSOV (1955) considered it to be effective at 300–500 mg/kg.

The use of hexachlorethane against paramphistomes would now appear to have been superseded by more effective modern drugs.

3. Tetrachloroethylene

A classical remedy for hookworm infection in dogs, this drug has been used for the treatment of *Fasciolopsis buski* infection in man, with a 77% cure rate but considerable side effects (SUNTHARASAMAI et al. 1974). It might therefore be expected to be effective against this parasite in pigs.

4. Hexachloroparaxylol

This is an efficient fasciolocidal drug but, although it has been shown to reduce the burden of paramphistomes in cattle by 97% (KHAIDAROV 1972) and sheep by 75% (TRIFONOV 1979), it failed to remove completely the burden from any of the cattle or from 97% of the sheep.

5. Hexachlorophene

Having been used for some time as a fasciolicide, hexachlorophene [Bis(2-hydroxy-3,5,6-trichlorophenyl)methane] was shown to be active against *Paramphistomum* sp. at a dose rate of 10 mg/kg in both cattle and sheep by BOSMAN et al. (1961). Nine sheep and 13 cattle which had been excreting paramphistome eggs before treatment were free of infection at autopsy 18–90 h after treatment. These results have generally been confirmed by later authors, although complete removal of the flukes in all animals has not always been achieved (HORAK 1962; CHHABRA and BALI 1976; DUTTA and CHAKRABORT 1971). However, HORAK (1962) also showed that two doses of 10 mg/kg given 7 days apart removed 99.6% of the paramphistomes.

Toxicity has been observed in both cattle and sheep, usually at dose rates of 40 mg/kg or more but sometimes following therapeutic doses (OSINGA 1960; PUGH and CROWLEY 1966).

6. Difluorotetrachloroethane

Commercially available Freon 112, administered orally or more safely by intraruminal injection, has been used as a fasciolicidal drug by several authors. However, it was found to have relatively little efficacy (< 1%) in critical and controlled tests against *Paramphistomum microbothrium* in experimentally infected sheep by HORAK (1962). On the other hand, the isomer Freon BU (1,chloro-2,2,2-trichlorodifluorethane) was shown to be effective at 300 mg/kg against this parasite and also against *Cytolophoron cotylophorum, Gastrothylax crumenifer* and *Fischoederius elongatus* by HORAK (1964), NATH (1970), and GUILHON et al. (1971). ERBOLATOV (1977) also found that Freon 112 given as a mixture in equal parts of vaseline removed all the paramphistomes from five out of seven treated cattle. GUILHON et al. (1971) showed that these isomers were not toxic below 900 mg/kg but animals which inhale orally administered Freon may be rendered unconscious at well below this dose rate (MATEVOSYAN and KRYUKOV 1961).

II. Salicylanilides and Substituted Phenols

Most of the drugs in this group are primarily used in veterinary medicine for the treatment of fascioliasis in cattle and sheep. Among them are the most efficacious drugs available against intestinal trematodes, while several of them have activity against *Haemonchus contortus* and tapeworms. They are potent uncouplers of oxidative phosphorylation (WILLIAMSON and METCALF 1967), their differential toxicity being probably due to their pharmacokinetic behaviour and, in particular, the extent to which they are absorbed, metabolised and bound to plasma protein (PRICHARD 1978). Toxic effects of these compounds include vomiting, salivation, apathy, and diarrhoea.

1. Bithionol

The first report concerned with the efficacy of bithionol [2,2^1-thiobis-(4,5 dichlorophenol)] against paramphistomes was that of GUILHON and GRABER (1962), who found that all the paramphistomes were removed from five of six animals given a dose of 20 mg/kg and from all those given higher doses. Many other authors have since reported on trials using this drug (usually at 70 mg/kg) or its sulphoxide (sulphene) (40 mg/kg) and have usually found it to be very efficacious, although there is considerable variation in the proportion of animals completely freed from the infection and bithionol per se is perhaps somewhat less effective in sheep than in cattle (ERBOLATOV 1975). There is also some evidence of varying efficacy against different species, as when NIKITIN et al. (1969) showed that a dose rate of 70 mg/kg of bithionol would remove all *Liorchis scotiae* from 69% of treated cattle, whereas the entire burden of *Gatrothylax crumenifer* was only removed from 20% of the treated animals. Bithionol has also been shown to be effective against *Paramphistomum microbothrium* in South Africa (HORAK 1965), Bulgaria (PAVLOV and GEORGIEV 1976), and Nigeria (SCHILLHORN VAN VEEN and BIDA 1975) and against *Calicophoron calicophorum* in Russia (KHAIDAROV 1972). Bithionol has also been used when incorporated in mixtures with hexachlorophene (TEUSCHER and BERGER 1965) or dichlorophenol (POPOV et al. 1966; MEREMINSKII et al. 1969). These authors both considered that the mixtures were more efficacious than the single drugs.

GRABER (1969) showed that bithionol was of value in the treatment of *Gastrodiscus aegypticus* infection in horses. However, both NOSAKA et al. (1970) and

KUKHARENKO (1973) found bithionol and bithionol sulphoxide to be ineffective in the treatment of *Eurytrema* infections in cattle and sheep respectively.

There are few reports on the use of this drug in carnivores but it has been used against cestode infections in dogs (REDZHEPOV et al. 1971) at a dose rate of 200 mg/kg.

2. Brotianide

Brotianide [2-acetoxy-3-bromo-5-chloro-*N*(4'bromphenyl)-thiobenzamide] was shown to have good activity against paramphistomes in cattle at a dose of 15 mg/kg by KARRASCH et al. (1975) in Madagascar and by CORBA et al. (1976b) in Czechoslovakia. There are no reports of its activity against other intestinal trematodes apart from that by LEGER and NOTTEGHEM (1975), who found that brotianide was 100% effective against *Echinostoma caproni* at 75 mg/kg in mice, a dose rate which exceeds the LD_{50} for rabbits and would cause toxic signs in dogs.

3. Clioxanide

CHHABRA and BALI (1976) reported that clioxanide (2-acetoxy-4'-chloro-3,5-diidosalicylanilide) cured amphistomiasis in nine of ten cattle and buffalo, as assessed by faecal egg counts. The dose rate they used (50–110 ml) is probably well below the LD_{50} of 420 mg/kg (PEARSON et al. 1970).

4. Dichlorophenol

POPOV et al. (1966) found that a mixture of bithionol and dichlorophenol (Trematol) removed all paramphistomes from both cattle and sheep. Later MEREMINSKII et al. (1969) claimed that 80 mg/kg of a similar mixture of 96%–97% bithionol with 3%–4% 2,4-dichlorophenol (Tremanol) was 94%–100% effective against mixed infections of *Liorchis scotiae* and *Paramphistomum ichikawai* in cattle. Dichlorophenol has also recently been shown to be effective against *Fasciolopsis buski* in man (MUTTALIB 1978; IDRIS et al. 1980).

5. Niclofolan

Several authors have described studies on the paramphistomicidal effect of niclofolan (2,2'-dihydroxy-3,3'-dinitro-5,5'-dichlorodiphenyl), which has also been called menichlopholan.

The dose rate used is in the range 4–6 mg/kg as toxic effects may be seen with doses of only 9 mg/kg (FLUCKE et al. 1969) but the results against paramphistomes have been rather equivocal. Thus niclofolan cured only six out of ten cattle treated by CHHABRA and BALI (1976) and was considered to give a more variable result in sheep than either niclosamide (BORAY 1969) or bithionol (SCHILLHORN VAN VEEN and BIDA 1975). In *Calicophoron calicophorum* infection in cattle KHAIDOROV (1972) reported that 4 mg/kg niclofolan removed 95% of the paramphistomes but completely cured none of the animals.

Niclofolan has also been used in man to treat infection with *Metagonimus yokogawai*, but in other hosts it appears only to have been used against intestinal trematodes in a study on the treatment of sea birds, where it was effective when administered in gelatine capsules at a dose rate of 3 mg/kg, together with niclosamide at 250 mg/kg (BORST et al. 1974).

6. Niclosamide

Niclosamide (2′,5-dichloro-4′-nitrosalicylanilide) is a somewhat unusual member of this group of drugs in that it has little activity against *Fasciola* but considerable activity against tapeworms. The usual dose rate is 75 mg/kg liveweight. Reports of its efficacy against paramphistomes are somewhat variable, being good when the criteria are those of clinical recovery and faecal egg counts (NATH 1970; SCHILLHORN VAN VEEN and BIDA 1975). This is because the drug is much more effective in killing immature than mature paramphistomes (HORAK 1962, 1964; BORAY 1969) but results in a temporary depression of egg production by the latter (ZHARIKOV et al. 1970). Niclosamide has also been shown to have some effect against *Fasciolopsis buski* in man (SUNTHARASAMAI et al. 1974) and at much higher dose rates (250–1,200 mg/kg) against intestinal trematodes in pigeons (KREMNER 1970) and sea birds (BORST et al. 1974).

7. Nitroxynil

Although nitroxynil (4-cyano-2-iodo-6-nitrophenol) is a widely used and effective fasciolicidal drug there have been few studies on its use against intestinal trematodes. GUPTA and MALIK (1979) found it to be ineffective against immature paramphistomes in sheep. However, KONO et al. (1981) have reported that three doses of 20–30 mg/kg nitroxynil eliminated *Eurytrema coelomaticum* from two heavily infected cattle, although a third died during treatment.

8. Oxyclozanide

Oxyclozanide (3,3′-5,5′-6-pentachloro-2,2′-dihydroxysalicylamide) has been extensively used against paramphistomes and most authors have found it to be effective in reducing the numbers of parasites present in the hosts but not in removing all the parasites (KHAIDAROV 1972; CORBA et al. 1976a; CHOWANIEC et al. 1976; GEORGIEV and GRUEV 1979). Where complete success has been claimed this has usually been on the basis of faecal egg counts – e.g. CHRISTOPHER (1974), CHHABRA and BALI (1976) – but ROMANIUK (1971) has shown that at 30 ml/kg the commercial formulation of this drug is ovistatic for at least 1 week. GEORGIEV and GRUEV (1979) found that the commercially available mixtures of oxyclozanide and levamisole tended to be more efficacious than either compound singly.

The only other successful reported use of oxyclozanide against intestinal trematodes is its use against *Gastrodiscus aegypticus* in horses in Zimbabwe (ROBERTS et al. 1976).

9. Rafoxanide

Although it has some activity against mature paramphistomes (PRICHARD 1978) and is a readily available fasciolicidal drug, rafoxanide [3,5-diiodo-3′-chloro-4′(*p*-

chlorophenoxy)salicyanilide] appears to have been little used against intestinal trematodes. It was, however, used successfully against *Protofasciola robusta* in elephants in a zoo park in England (WINDSOR and SCOTT 1976) (see Sect. B.VI).

10. Resorantel

Resorantel (2,6-dihydroxybenzoic acid-4′-bromanilide) is the most consistently successful drug used in the treatment of paramphistomiasis of cattle and sheep and has been mostly used against these parasites, although it is also active against adult cestodes. It is effective against both the immature and mature forms in goats (LÄMMLER et al. 1969), sheep and cattle (OGUZ 1971). In several trials its efficacy against the adult forms in the rumen has equalled or approached 100% (GAENSSLER 1974; SAHAI and PRASAH 1975) and is usually better than that achieved by other paramphistomicidal drugs, including oxyclozanide (CHOWANIEC et al. 1976) and bithionol, but possibly excluding bithionol sulphoxide (GEORGIEV et al. 1977). Its use is usually free from side effects but a reduction in milk yield has been reported (GEORGIEV et al. 1977). Resorantel has also been used successfully for the treatment of horses infected with *Gastrodiscus aegypticus* (ROBERTS et al. 1976).

III. Other Chemotherapeutic Agents

Although the action of many other drugs on intestinal trematodes has been studied, few of them have been found to be effective. In particular most of the benzimidazoles appear to have little effect on paramphistomes, a possible exception being fenbendazole (*S*-phenylthiobenzimidazole-2-methyl carbamate) at 7.5 mg/kg daily for 6 days, which reduced burdens of immature *Liorchis scotiae* by 87% (CORBA et al. 1979, 1981). Flubendazole [methyl 5-(4-fluorobenzoyl) 1-*H*-benzimididazole 2-yl carbamate], a fluorinated derivative of mebendazole, has been shown to be active against *Echinostoma caproni* in experimental infections in mice (NOTTEGHEM et al. 1979) and against *Heterophyes heterophyes* in man in doses of 0.5–1.0 g/day (COMBESCOT and DUONG 1980). It is perhaps surprising that there appear to be no reports as to the activity of the fasciolicidal drug albendazole (5-proprylthio-benzimidazole-2-methyl carbamate) against intestinal trematodes.

There are also few reports of organophosphates being used successfully against intestinal trematodes, although dichlorvos has been shown to be effective against *Gastrodiscus aegypticus* in horses (AZZIE 1975; TAGER-KAGAN 1979). Trichlorphon[(*O*-*o*-dimethyl)-2,2,2-trichloro-1-hydroxymethyl phosphonate], a commonly used nematocide, may give a clinical improvement (NATH 1970) in sheep infected with paramphistomes but is only effective in cattle at toxic dose rates (MERMINSKII and GLUZMAN 1966).

Levamisole [(−)-(*S*)-2,3,5,6-tetrahydrohydrochloride 6-phenyl-imidazo(2,1-b)thiazole] or the equivalent racemic mixture, tetramisole, appears to have little effect against paramphistomes in cattle or sheep on its own (GEORGIEV and GRUEV 1979), although it may enhance the action of oxyclozanide (see Sect. III.7) and praziquantel (YOKOGAWA et al. 1980). Tetramisole was, however, shown to be very effective at a dose rate of 10 mg/kg liveweight when given to dogs infected with *Echinochasmus* sp. (SWIETLIKOWSKI and WROCINSKI 1969).

Finally, praziquantel [2-cyclohexylcarbonyl-1,2,4,6,7,11,b-hexahydro *2H*-pyrazino(2,1-a)isoquindine-4-one], a recently introduced cestocidal drug which has been shown to be effective against cestodes and schistosomes (GÖNNERT and ANDREWS 1977), is now proving to be active against other trematodes including *Clonorchis sinensis* in rats (HA 1980) and man (RIM et al. 1981), *Paragonismus* sp. in dogs (YOKOGAWA et al. 1980) and the intestinal trematode *Metagonimus yokogawai* (20 mg praziquantel/kg) in man (RIM et al. 1978). The intestinal flukes *Heterophyes* sp. have been successfully eliminated from man with 10 mg/kg praziquantel daily for 3 days (98% egg reduction, 88% cure rate) and the same can be expected for *Fasciolopsis buski* and other intestinal flukes. *Isthmiophora melis* has been eliminated from rats and ferrets with single doses of 1 × 50 and 1 × 100 mg/kg (ANDREWS et al. 1983). Since praziquantel is now widely available for use as a cestocide in dogs and cats and is of low toxicity with few side effects or contraindications, it may well prove to be of great value in many other intestinal trematode infections.

References

Ahluwalia JS, Singh AN (1975) Treatment of amphistomiasis in sheep. Curr Sci 44:907–908

Ahluwalia JS, Sinha BK, Singh AN (1976) Efficacy of carbon tetrachloride with hexachlorophene in an outbreak of amphistomiasis among cattle in Bihar. Indian Vet J 53:723–724

Andrews P, Thomas H, Pohlke R, Seubert J (1983) Praziquantel. Med Res Rev 3:147–200

Azzie MAJ (1975) Pathological infection of thoroughbred horses with *Gastrodiscus aegypticus*. J S Afr Vet Assoc 46:77–78

Balozet L (1936) Sur un *Brachylaemus* de l'intestin du porc. Bull Acad Vet France 9:93–99

Bawa HS (1939) Intestinal paramphistomiasis of sheep in Sind (a preliminary report). Indian J Vet Sci 9:425–429

Bhalerao GD (1933) The trematode parasites of the Indian elephant, *Elephas indicus*. Indian J Vet Sci 3:103–115

Bhattacharyya HM, Das SK, Sinha PH, Biswas SN, Bose PK (1972) Mortality in pigs due to *Paryphostomum sufrartyfex* (Lane 1915) Bhalerea 1931. Indian Vet J 49:976–978

Bida SA, Schillhorn van Veen T (1977) Enteric paramphistomiasis in Yankasa sheep. Trop Anim Health Prod 9:21–23

Boray JC (1969) The anthelmintic efficiency of niclosamide and menichlopholon in the treatment of intestinal paramphistomiasis in sheep. Aust Vet J 45:133–134

Borst GHA, Duiven P, Van Soeren JH, Swennen C (1974) Anthelmintic treatment in sea birds. Tijdschr Diergeneeskd 99:122–126

Bosman CJ, Thorold DW, Purchase HS (1961) Investigation into and development of hexachlorophene as an anthelmintic. J S Afr Vet Med Assoc 32:227–233

Bracegirdle JR (1973) A case of *Gastrodiscus aegypticus* infection in a horse in Ethiopia. Vet Rec 93:561–562

Brown HW, Chin-Sung Chan, Chang-Ti Chen, Ke-Hong Lin, Chao-Rang Chang, Lintang Lee, Chin-chuan Hsu, Lien-pin Chow, Hsien-chen Hsieh (1959) The treatment of *Fasciolopsis buski* infection with dithiazanine iodide, 1-bromo-naphthol-(2), ascaridol, piperazine and tetrachlorethylene. J Formosan Med Assoc 58:792–798

Chandra SS, Siddhu CMS, Pandey SN, Nath P (1974) A case of *Fasciolopsis buski* infestation in Uttar Pradesh. Armed Forces Med J India 30:290–293

Chhabra RC, Bali HS (1976) Efficacy of some drugs against amphistomes in cattle and buffaloes under field condition in the Punjab. J Res Punjab Agric Univ 13:226–231

Chhabra RC, Gill BS, Dutt SC (1978) Paramphistomiasis of sheep and goats in the Punjab State and its treatment. Indian J Parasitol 2:43–45

Chowaniec W, Ziomoko I, Paciejewski S (1976) The efficacy of Terenol-Hoechst and Zanil-ICI in the control of *Paramphistomum* sp. in cattle. Medycyna Wet 32:739–741
Christopher J (1974) Zanil (oxyclozanid) in the treatment of amphistomiasis in sheep. Indian J Anim Res 8:79–80
Ciurea I (1921) Sur un nouvel echinostome de l'intestine du porc. CR Soc Biol 84:1010–1013
Colella G (1972) Observation on an outbreak of *Brachylaema suis* Balozet 1936 on a pig farm in the province of Matera. Acta Med Vet 18:145–154
Combescot C, Duong TH (1980) Action of fluoromebendazole (flubendazole) against intestinal helminthiasis. Med Malad Infect 10:735–738
Corba J, Pacenovsky J, Krupicer I, Breza M, Popvic S, Reisz T (1976a) The efficacy of oxyclozanide in cattle naturally infected by *Liorchis scotiae*. Vet Med (Praha) 21:461–465
Corba J, Pacenovsky J, Krupicer I (1976b) Study on the efficacy of brotianide (Dirian®). II. The efficacy of brotianide in cattle naturally infected with *Paramphistomum* spp. Vet Med Rev 2:181–189
Corba J, Legeny J, Krupicer I, Pacenovsky J, Stoffa P (1979) Efficacy of some anthelmintics in paramphistomatidiasis (liorchosis) of cattle. Helminthologia 16:217–229
Corba J, Stoffa P, Legeny J, Krupicer I, Lietava P (1981) Efficacy of fenbendazole (Panacur) on the most important trematodes and cestodes in ruminants. Veterinarstvi 31:118–121
Costa HM, Freitas MG (1970) Lista de helmintos dos animais domésticos du Brazil. Arq Esc Vet 22:33–94
Deusov NL (1955) Paramphistomiasis in calves. Veterinariya 32:(4)36–37
Dissamarn R, Aranyakanda P, Srivoranath P, Chai-Anan P, Thirapat K, Chitrakurn P (1966) The life history of *Paryphostomum sufrartyfex* (Lane 1915) Bhalerao 1931. J Thai Vet Med Assoc 17:11–16
Dubey JP (1970) *Pharyngostomum cordatum* from the domestic cat (*Felis catus*) in India. J Parasitol 56:194–195
Dutta B, Chakrabort AK (1971) Clinical trial with "Distodin" (Pfizer) against mixed infection of fascioliasis and amphistomiasis. Orissa Vet J 6:15–16
Erbolatov KM (1975) Acute course of paramphistomiasis in cattle and sheep (in Russian). Veterinariya 5:78–79
Erbolatov KM (1977) Efficacy of bithionol and Freon 112 in the treatment of paramphistomiasis of sheep (in Russian). Veterinariya 1:72–73
Fataliev GG (1974) The occurrence of the trematode *Brachylaemus suis* Balozet 1936 in wild pigs in Azerbaidzhan. Mater nauch Konf vses obshch G'elmin 26:323–324
Fernandes BJ, Cooper JD, Cullen JB, Freenaw RS, Ritchie AC, Scott AA, Stuart PE (1976) Systemic infection with *Alaria americana* (Trematoda). Can Med Assoc J 115:1111–1114
Flucke W, Wirtz S, Feltkamp H (1969) Niclofolan (Bayer 9015) – activity against liver fluke, tissue levels and elimination. SCI Monograph No 33:12–24
Gaenssler JG (1974) Further trials of the efficacy of Terenol in cattle and goats in South Africa. Blue book for the veterinary profession. no 24. pp 94–98. Hoechst, Frankfurt
Georgiev B, Gruev A (1979) Effectiveness of levamisole and oxyclozanide against paramphistomiasis in sheep and cattle. Vet Med Nauki 16:45–51
Georgiev B, Denev I, Vasilev I (1977) Efficacy of some chemotherapeutic agents against *Paramphistomum microbothrium* infections in ruminants. Vet Sbir Sof 75:22–25
Gibson TE (1975) Veterinary anthelmintic medication, 3rd edn tech comm no 33. Comm Inst Helm, St. Albans
Gönnert R, Andrews P (1977) Praziquantel, a new broad spectrum antischistosomal agent. Z Parasitenkd 52:129–150
Graber M (1969) Etude en Afrique Central du pouvoir anthelminthique due 2-2'-thiobis (4,6-dichlorophénol) ou Bitin ou bithionol ou Actamer sur divers parasites des animaux domestiques. Possibilités d'emploi. Republic du Tchad Fort Lamy. Laboratoire de Farcha, Region de Recherches Vétèrinaires et Zootechniques d'Afrique Centrale

Guilhon J, Graber M (1962) Action de bithionol sur les amphistomes et sur *Fasciola gigantica*. Bull Acad Vét Fr 35:275–278

Guilhon J, Graber M, Barnabe R (1971) Activité du tétrachlorodifluoroéthane sur divers trematodes et sa toxicite à l'égard des ovins. Bull Acad Vet Fr 44:79–86

Gupta RP, Malik PD (1979) Anthelmintic activity of Trodax in sheep. Ind Vét J 56:834–838

Gupta N, Walia S (1970) *Pseudodiscus collinsi* (Cobbold 1875) Stiles and Goldberger, 1910, an amphistome parasite of equines in India. Res Bull Punjab Univ Sci 20:49–55

Gusev NI (1954) Paramphistomiasis in adult cattle. Abstract from a symposium "Anthelmintics for domestic animals". Veterinariya 31(4):25

Gvozdev EV, Suboleva TN (1973) Revision of the subfamily Hasstilesiinae (Trematoda: Brachylaemidae). Problemy obschei i prikladnoi gelmintologii (in Russian). Izdatel'stvo „Nauka", Moscow, pp 41–48

Ha JH (1980) Experimental study on the therapeutic effect of praziquantel (Embay 8440) in rats experimentally infected with *Clonorchis sinensis*. Korea Univ Med J 17:477–495

Haque M, Siddiqi AH (1978) Histopathology of gastro-intestinal trematode parasites of pig and man. Int J Parasitol 2:97–99

Harrow WT (1959) The toxicity of hexachlorethane. Vet Rec 71:111–112

Horak IG (1962) Studies on paramphistomiasis. IV. Modified critical and controlled anthelmintic tests on the conical fluke *Paramphistomum microbothrium*. J S Afr Vet Med Assoc 33:203–208

Horak IG (1964) Studies on paramphistomiasis. VI. The anthelmintic efficacy of Lintex and Freon against *Paramphistomum* spp. in sheep and cattle. J S Afr Vet Med Assoc 35:161–166

Horak IG (1965) The anthelmintic efficacy of bithionol against *Paramphistomum microbothrium, Fasciola* spp. and *Schistosoma matthei*. J S Afr Vet Med Assoc 36:561–566

Horak IG (1971) Paramphistomiasis of domestic ruminants. Adv Parasitol 9:33–72

Idris M, Rahman KM, Muttalib MA, Azad Khan AK (1980) The treatment of fasciolopiasis with niclosamide and dichlorophen. J Trop Med Hyg 83:71–74

Jurasek V, Ovies D, Espaine L (1971) First record of *Brachylaemus suis* Balozet 1936 (Brachylaemidae) in swine in Cuba. Revta cub Cienc Vet 2:57–62

Karrasch SW, Hörchner F, Böhnel H (1975) Zur Wirkung von Dirian gegen *Fasciola gigantica* und Paramphistomiden bei natürlich infizierte Rindern in Madagascar. Berl Munch Tierarztl Wochenschr 88:348–351

Khaidarov U (1972) Testing anthelmintics against *Calicophoron* infections in cattle. Veterinariya 49(4):65–66

Kifune T, Shiraishi S, Takao Y (1967) Discovery of *Pharyngostomum cordatum* (Diesing 1850) in cats from Hyushu, Japan (Trematoda; Strigeoidea; Diplostomatidae). Jpn J Parasitol 16:403–409

Kistner TP, Wyse D, Schmitz JA (1979) Pathogenicity attributed to massive infections of *Nanophyetus salmincola* in a cougar. J Wildl Dis 15:419–420

Kliks M, Tantachamrun T (1974) Heterophyid (Trematoda) parasites of cats in North Thailand, with notes on a human case found at necropsy. Southeast Asian J Trop Med Public Health 5:547–555

Kohn A, Bührnheim U, Costa RMA (1972a) Ocorênce de *Stephanoprora denticulata* (Rudolphi 1902) Odhner 1911 (Trematoda, Echinostomatidae) em porco domestico no Brazil. Atas Soc Biol Rio de Janeiro 15:121–123

Kohn A, Bührnheim U, Costa HMA (1972b) Infestacao natural de *Echinostoma revolutum* (Froelich 1802) (Trematoda, Echinostomatidae) em porco domestico. Atas Soc Biol Rio de Janeiro 16:5–6

Kondo K, Kurimoto H, Oda K, Shimada Y (1974) On *Pharyngostomum cordatum* (Diesing 1850) from cats in Shiga Prefecture, Japan. Jpn J Parasitol 23:8–13

Kono I, Sakamoto T, Yasuda N, Yakamoto Y, Nakagawa H (1981) Pathological findings in the pancreas of cattle infected with *Eurytrema coelomaticum* after anthelmintic treatment, with special reference to globule leucocytes. Bull Fac Agric, Kagoshima Univ No 31:101–106

Kremner E (1970) A contribution towards the chemotherapy of echinostomiasis with *N*-(2′-chloro-4′-nitrophenyl)-5-chlor-salicylamide (=Yomesan). Vet Med Rev 1:27–33
Kukharenko NS (1973) The major helminths in livestock in the Far East and the struggle against them (in Russian). (Collection of scientific works.) Blagoreshchensk Agricultural Institute, pp 20–22
Kuppuswamy PB (1948) "Pitto" and "Gillar" in sheep and goats. Indian Frmg 9:73–74
Lämmler G, Sahai BN, Herzog H (1969) Anthelmintic efficacy of 2,6-dihydroxybenzoic acid-4′-bromanilide (HOE 296V) against mature and immature *Paramphistomum microbothrium* in goats. Acta Vet Acad Sci Hung 19:447–451
Léger N, Notteghem MJ (1975) Étude de l'activité douvicide d'un nouveau composé: le brotianide, sur *Echinostoma caproni* Richard 1964. Annl Pharm Fr 33:273–277
Manning GS, Ratanarat C (1970) *Fasciolopsis buski* (Lankester 1857) in Thailand. Am J Trop Med Hyg 19:613–619
Matevosyan EM, Kryukova KA (1961) Large scale trials of Freon 112 and carbon tetrachloride in liquid paraffin against fascioliasis in cattle (in Russian). Sb nauchno-tekh Inf vses Inst gel'mint KI Skryabina (7/8) 34–42
Mereminskii AI, Gluzman IYa (1966) Testing of chlorophos against chronic paramphistomiasis of cattle (in Russian). Veterinariya (Kiev) 6:24–31
Mereminskii AI, Gluzman IYa (1975) The efficacy of Bitifen in mixed infections of cattle (in Russian). In: Parasitological problems. Materialy VIII nauchnoi Konferentsii parazitologov UkSSR. Chast'2. Kiev, USSR. Naukova Dumka (1975), pp 27–29
Mereminskii AI, Artemenko YuG, Gluzman IYa (1969) Tremanol treatment of paramphistome infection in cattle. Veterinariya 41:(12)40–41
Mishakov NE (1971) Pathological changes in the internal organs of animals infected with *Nanophyetus*. Biol Med Issled. Dal'nem Vost 66–68
Muttalib MA (1978) Dichlorophen in the treatment of *Fasciolopsis buski*. Bangladesh Med J 7:45–48
Nath D (1970) Observations on the effect of some anthelmintics against mature amphistomes in experimentally infected sheep. Indian J Sci Ind 4:53–56
Nikitin VF (1978) The course of active enzootic paramphistomiasis in calves in the lower Volga region (in Russian). Byull vses Inst Gel'min KI Skryabina 22:40–44
Nikitin VF, Lipkin GL, Proshin YuG, Chernov VI (1969) Bithionol tested against *Gastrothylax* and *Liorchis* sp. in cattle (in Russian). Byull vses Inst Gel'min KI Skryabina 3:71–73
Nosaka D, Ashizawa H, Nagata Y (1970) Pathological studies on bovine eurytremiasis. IV. Anthelmintic experiments and pathological findings in cows infected with *Eurytrema* species. Bull Fac Agric Miyazaki Univ 2:286–298
Notteghem MJ, Leger N, Cavier R (1979) Étude de l'activité douvicide du Flubendazole sur *Echinostoma caproni*. Ann Pharm Fr 37:153–156
Oguz T (1971) Treatment trials with Terenol (4-bromo-2,6-dihydroxybenzanilide) against *Paramphistomum* in sheep and cattle. Vet Fac Derg Ankara Univ 18:209–213
Olsen OW (1949) Action of a hexachlorethane-bentonite suspension on the rumen fluke *Paramphistomum*. Vet Med 44:108–109
Orlova KV (1953) *Paramphistomum cervi* infection of young cattle (in Russian). Veterinariya 30(4):20–22
Osinga A (1960) Toepassing van hexachlorofeen (G-11) bij distomatose van runderen en schapen. Tijdschr Diergeneeskd 85:529–533
Pavlov P, Georgiev B (1976) Zur Wirksamkeit von Coriban und Disto-5-Cogla bei der Fasciolose und Paramphistomose der Hauswiederkäuern. Dtsch Tierarztl Wochenschr 83:482
Pearson LG, Whitlock HV, De Goosh CP, Farrington KJ, Jones RC, Haigh JA (1970) Clioxanide, a new anthelmintic against *Fasciola hepatica* and *Haemonchus contortus* in sheep. Aust Vet J 46:480–484
Petkov A, Mes'ov Ya, Rusev I (1975) Hexachloroparaxylene in group treatment of sheep against mixed trematode infections. Vet Sbir Sof 73:25–26
Popov A, Bankov D, Denev I, Georgiev B, Bratanov V, Monov M (1966) Experimental treatment of paramphistomiasis (in Russian). Vet Med Nauki 3:813–888

Prichard RK (1978) Sheep anthelmintic in the epidemiology and control of gastro-intestinal parasites of sheep in Australia. In: Donald AD, Southcott WH, Dineen JK (eds) Division of animal health. CSIRO, Australia, pp 75–107
Pugh DM, Crowley J (1966) Some observations on the toxicity of hexachlorophane for sheep. Vet Rec 78:86–91
Redzhepov A, Stepanov DF, Agapovich Zha, Patishaguliev B (1971) Treatment of cestodiasis in dogs. Veterinariya 48(3):75–76
Rim HJ, Chu DS, Leo JS, Joo KH, Won CY (1978) Anthelmintic effects of various drugs against metagonimiasis. Korean J Parasitol 16:117–122
Rim HJ, Lyu KS, Lee JS, Joo KH (1981) Clinical evaluation of the therapeutic efficacy of praziquantel (Embay 8440) against *Clonorchis sinensis* infection in man. Ann Trop Med Parasitol 75:27–33
Roberts HM, Adams WJE, Danks BC (1976) *Gastrodiscus aegypticus*: a therapeutic trial. Rhodesian Vet J 6:73–76
Romaniuk K (1971) Experimental use of Zanil ICI in the treatment of chronic paramphistomiasis in cattle (in Polish). Medycyna Wet 27:240–241
Ruziev ShM (1972) Test of several anthelmintics against *Gastrothylax* infections in cattle (in Russian). Trudy uzbek nauch Issled 20:129–131
Sahai BN, Prasah KD (1975) Anthelmintic efficacy of Terenol against immature and mature *Cotylophoron cotylophorum* in goats. Riv Parasitol 36:171–176
Sahai BN, Srivastava HD (1970) Studies on *Echinochasmus perfoliatus* (Hutz 1908) Dietz 1909: incidence in dogs and development of the miracidium. J Helminthol 44:315–320
Schillhorn van Veen T, Bida SA (1975) Acute paramphistomiasis in sheep in Zaria, vol 1. In: Proc 20th world vet cong, Thessaloniki, pp 517–519
Sosipatrov GV (1962) *Echinochasmus* infection of pigs. Veterinariya 39(2):30–32
Soulsby EJL (1968) Helminths, arthropods and protozoa of domesticated animals. Bailliere, London
Sprehn C (1930) Wichtige Endoparasiten des deutschen Hausgeflügels. Berl Munch Tierarztl Wochenschr 46:765–774
Stoimenov K, Gruev A, Simov P (1976) Anthelmintic treatment of paramphistomatid infections. Vet Sbir, Sof 74:41–43
Suntharasamai P, Bunnag D, Tesavantij S, Harinasatu T, Migasena S, Vutikes S, Chindanond D (1974) Comparative clinical trials of niclosamide and tetrachorethylene in the treatment of *Fasciolopsis buski* infection. Southeast Asian J Trop Med Public Health 5:556–559
Swietlikowski M, Wrocinski M (1969) Nilverm as an anthelmintic in dogs. Medycyna Wet 25:84–85
Tager-Kagan P (1979) Utilisation du dichlorvos dans les parasitoses gastro-intestinales du cheval au Niger. Rev Elev Med Vet Pays Trop 32:181–183
Teuscher E, Berger J (1965) Observations on the anthelmintic activity of combinations of hexachlorophene and bithionol against *Fasciola gigantica* and paramphistomes in cattle. Bull epiz Dis Afr 13:45–54
Trifonov T (1979) The clinical symptoms of mixed trematode infection in sheep. Vet Sbirk Sof 77:28–29
Vasil'ev AA, Velichko IV, Gluzman IYa, Mereminskii AI, Nikitin VF, Ovenchkin NA (1970) Efficacy of bithionol in acute paramphistomiasis infection of cattle (in Russian). Byull vses Inst Gel'min KI Skryabin 4:23–25
Williamson RL, Metcalf RL (1967) Salicylanilides: a new group of active uncouplers of oxidative phosphorylation. Science 158:1694–1695
Windsor RS, Scott WA (1976) Fascioliasis and salmonellosis in African elephants in captivity. Br Vet J 132:313–317
Yokogawa M, Niimura M, Hata H, Kobayashi M, Tokita K, Tazaki T (1980) Efficacy of praziquantel against *Clonorchis* and *Paragonismus* infections in rats and dogs. Jpn J Parasitol 29:515–522
Zharikov IS, Orlovskii VI, Kaminskii II (1970) Hexochloroparaxylol and phenasal tested in chronic paramphistomiasis of cattle (in Russian). Nauch Trudy nauchno-issled vet Inst Minsk 8:74–77

CHAPTER 12

Chemotherapy of Intestinal Trematodiasis in Man

J. H. CROSS

A. Introduction

Human intestinal trematodiases are associated with eating habit and are usually localized to areas where there is water, snail vectors, and reservoir hosts. Most of the parasitoses are in Asia but foci of infections occur in other population groups throughout the world.

Although a significantly large number of species of trematodes may inhabit the intestinal tracts of man (HEALY 1970) few are considered serious pathogens. Symptoms are usually vague in most of the infections, but when a large number of worms are involved the symptoms can be severe. In some infections the pathology may be associated with the eggs rather than with adult parasites.

Treatment usually involves the oral administration of an anthelmintic and in some cases followed by a purgative. Unfortunately, the development of new anthelmintics in the treatment of intestinal trematodiasis has not advanced as dramatically as treatment for other trematode infection such as blood, liver, and lung flukes. In many instances the anthelmintics used today are the same ones used one-half century or more ago and while these preparations are effective, many cause side effects. However, promising results are now being reported on the use of praziquantel in most trematode infections.

The intestinal trematodes to be discussed in this chapter are members of the families Fasciolidae, Heterophyidae, and Echinostomatidae, and to a lesser extent Gastrodiscidae, Lecithodendriidae, Microphallidae, Plagiorchiidae, and Isoparochiidae.

B. Fasciolopsiasis

I. Introduction

Fasciolopsis buski, Fasciola hepatica, and *Fasciola gigantica* are three species of the family Fasciolidae that infect humans, but only *F. buski* inhabits the intestinal tract.

The distribution of *F. buski* is limited to scattered locations throughout Asia. STOLL (1947) estimated 10 million human infections with most in Chinese on the China mainland. Other endemic areas are Taiwan, Thailand, Vietnam, Laos, Bangladesh, and India; there is a recent report from Indonesia (HADIDJAJA 1982). Reports of infections have been made from other Asian countries but it is not known whether the infections were imported or acquired locally. Reported cases outside of Asia are believed to be of persons who acquired the infection in Asia (CROSS 1969; MALEK 1980).

II. Morphology

Fasciolopsis buski is the largest trematode to infect man and is commonly referred to as the "giant intestinal fluke." The worm is thick and fleshy measuring 20–75 mm in length, 8–20 mm in width, and 1–3 mm in thickness. It lacks a cephalic cone which is present in other fasciolids, has a spinose tegument, and the oral sucker is at the anterior end with the ventral sucker or acetabulum located immediately behind. The two intestinal ceca are unbranched and the paired markedly branched testes nearly occupy the posterior half of the worm. The ovary is centrally located and the coiled uterus is located in the anterior half. The vitellaria are in the lateral fields.

III. Life Cycle

The parasite is found in the small intestine of the definitive host usually in the duodenum or jejunum. The eggs are oval, operculated, and unembryonated when passed and measure 130–154 by 78–98 μm. After reaching fresh water the miracidium develops within the egg in 3–7 weeks, depending upon the temperature. The ciliated miracidium emerges from the egg through the opened operculum and swims in the water in search for a suitable planorbid snail host. The miracidium penetrates the soft tissue of the snail (*Segmentina* and *Hippeutis*), reaches the lymph spaces, and forms into a sporocyst. A mother redia develops within the sporocyst and in turn daughter rediae. Cercariae emerge from the daughter rediae, escape from the snail, and swim free in the water in search of a smooth, more or less hard surface, such as aquatic plants, upon which to encyst and form a metacercaria. It takes 25–29 days from the time the miracidium enters the snail until formation of the metacercaria. The metacercaria is ingested by man, pig, or other susceptible host when uncooked water plants are eaten. The organism excysts in the small intestine, attaches to the mucosa, and develops into an egg-producing adult in 3 months. The adult may live for 6 or more months.

IV. Pathology

In Thailand, it has been shown that in less than massive numbers, *F. buski* is not directly responsible for clinical disease (PLAUT et al. 1969); however, with heavy worm loads, there are often serious disease manifestations. The large sucker of the worm attaches to the mucosa and may cause bleeding, inflammation, or ulceration and may provoke excessive mucus secretion. Intestinal obstruction can occur with a large number of worms. Abdominal distention, hunger pains, increased appetite, and diarrhea are symptoms associated with infection. The stools may be foul smelling, greenish-yellow in color and with undigested food. Absorption of parasite secretions and excretions may lead to toxemia and allergic manifestation, generalized edema, ascites, nausea, vomiting, and possible cachexia. Leukocystosis due to eosinophilia and neutrophilic leukopenia may also develop. Death can occur in untreated infections as a result of toxemia and anasarca.

V. Diagnosis

Although the symptoms may be suggestive of *F. buski* infection in endemic areas, the confirmed diagnosis is made by the detection of characteristic eggs or adult worms in the feces (CROSS 1975). Worms may also be present in the vomitus. The eggs, which are numerous in the stools (21,000–28,000 day per fluke produced, STOLL et al. 1927), are indistinguishable from those of *F. hepatica* and *Echinostoma* sp. Immunological methods for diagnosis are of no value and unnecessary since the eggs are easily found.

VI. Treatment

A number of anthelmintics have been used to eliminate *F. buski* from the intestinal tract. BARLOW (1925) listed oil of chenopodium, oil of terebinthinae, beta-naphthol, thymol, carbon tetrachloride, and native drugs such as powdered betel nut. Betel nut mixed with black prunes and licorice taken once a day for 3–5 days is still recommended by traditionalists in China today. McCOY and CHU (1937) evaluated hexylresorcenol and the drug continues to be used in a single dose of 1 g for adults and lower dosages (400–900 mg) for children. BROWN et al. (1959) treated Taiwanese with dithiazanine iodine, 1-bromo-naphthol-(2), piperazine citrate, piperazine malate, ascaridol, and tetrachloroethylene and found that dithiazanine iodide had some effect in light infections, 1-bromo-naphthol-(2) cured one of five infections, the piperazine preparations were ineffective, and ascaridol cured five of eight infections. Tetrachloroethylene was the most effective, curing seven of nine infections. All drugs, however, caused side effects. In a later study on Taiwan, HSIEH et al. (1963) reported a cure rate of 62% with stilbazium iodide. SHAH et al. (1966) in India found tetrachloroethylene effective but nausea and vomiting were constant and one patient passed as many as 750 worms. In another trial, SHAH et al. (1973) tested tetrachloroethylene, anthephane, iodothymol granules, Yomesan (niclosamide), bephenium hydrochloride, and metronidazole in Indian children in doses prescribed for hookworm, but none were effective except metronidazole, where the cure rate was 60%. Niclosamide and tetrachloroethylene were tested in Thailand; in doses of 43–160 mg/kg body weight niclosamide caused a 41% reduction in eggs while tetrachloroethylene at dosages of 0.08–0.14 ml/kg body weight induced an egg reduction of 97% (SUNTHARASAMAI et al. 1974). Dichlorophen was tested in children by IDRIS et al. (1980) and the first treatment reduced the egg count by 83% and the repeat treatment completely eradicated the infections. Tetrachloroethylene, in dosages of 0.12 ml/kg (maximum 5 ml), although causing side effects of headache, abdominal pain, and dizziness, is the drug of choice; and some physicians recommend a saline purge 2 h after treatment to enhance expulsion of the worms. Recently praziquantel was reported effective and the authors recommended a single dose of 15 mg/kg body weight for treatment of the parasitosis (BUNNAG et al. 1983). Care must also be taken in treating all cases with toxemia associated with the infection.

VII. Socioeconomic, Ecological, and Cultural Aspects

Fasciolopsiasis remains endemic in Asia because of contamination of water by human and pig feces containing eggs. Massive numbers of eggs are produced each day to ensure perpetuation of the life cycle and once in the water the miracidium will develop in a few weeks if the water temperature remains at 27°–30 °C. The miracidium must find specific planorbid snail intermediate hosts (*Segmentina, Hippeutis,* and *Gyraulus* spp.) and factors such as temperature and water vegetation influence survival of the snails. Temperature affects larval development within the snail and cercarial shedding often begins in the spring, decreases in the summer and autumn, and ceases in winter. The cercariae encysts on any hard surface, not only plants. In the laboratory, the metacercariae will form on the snail, vegetation, and even the aquarium glass. The metacercariae, however, must remain in a wet or moist environment to survive.

Vegetation is important in the epidemiology of the disease in both man and pigs. If aquatic plants are not eaten raw, *F. buski* infection does not result. It is only in population groups that have the custom of eating freshwater plants uncooked that infection persists. Water caltrop (*Trapa notans, T. bicornis*), water chestnut, (*Eliorcharis tuberosa*), water bamboo (*Zizania aquatica*), water hyacinth (*Eichornia crassipes*), water morning glory (*Ipomea aquatica*), water cress (*Neptunia oleracea*), and lotus (*Nymphaea lotus*) are plants commonly involved in various endemic areas. Infection occurs when the husk or outer portion of the water plant with metacercariae is peeled with the teeth. Kung-shin tsai (*Ipomea reptans*) is a water plant eaten cooked by Chinese but fed uncooked to their pigs. The leaves and stems of this and other plants are main sources of pig infection. Pig is the major reservoir host but there are areas where man is infected and pigs are not and, conversely, areas where pigs are infected and humans not infected. It was once said that where pigs are infected man will not be infected. This is no longer valid since many areas are known where both are infected. Infection is solely dependent upon eating habits. In some areas humans do not eat water plants but feed them to pigs or the water plants are cooked prior to eating. In some endemic areas pigs may not be present because of religious practices. Unboiled water is also suspected as a source of infection since the metacercariae may become detached from the plants.

Changing of pig-raising practices has influenzed the prevalence of *F. buski*. In a once highly endemic area of Taiwan infection has disappeared from both pig and man. At one time pigs were fed the leaves and stems of water caltrop and kung-shin tsai from nearby ponds. Feces from the pigs and intestinal contents from the pigs at the time of slaughter were permitted to drain into the ponds, thus maintaining the life cycle of the parasite. The practice of feeding water plants to pigs has stopped since the farmers have found that the pigs will grow larger and faster with commercial food preparations. The feces still drain into the ponds to fertilize the water plants and to feed the fish, but the feces no longer contain *F. buski* eggs.

In other parts of Asia infection continue to occur and in most endemic areas the infection rates are higher in children or young people who collect water caltrop and eat it on the way to school or on their return home. In some areas there is no difference in prevalence rates by sex but in Thailand, MANNING and RATANART (1970) found infection rates higher in females. The highest prevalence rates throughout most areas are among those who live closest to infected ponds. Prevalence rates are highly variable for various endemic countries. In China rates of 1%–85% have been reported, 24%–61% in Taiwan, 13%–70% in Thailand, 9%–39% in Bangladesh, and 7%–60% in India (CROSS 1975).

Fasciolopsiasis is not considered a very serious parasitic disease, the distribution is limited, and there is little symptomatology unless infections are heavy. Consequently, very few studies have been carried out on the parasite during the past few decades. Treatment with old established preparations seems to suffice, but some of these may produce side effects. Further studies will most likely show praziquantel to be the drug of choice, however.

C. Heterophyidiasis

I. Introduction

The heterophyids are small ovoidal trematodes found in the small intestines of birds and mammals worldwide. Reports of human infections have been extensive and some workers consider all heterophyid species as potential human parasites. In Asia alone 19 different species have been reported from humans at least once but the two most important species, and more commonly reported, are *Heterophyes heterophyes* and *Metagonimus yokogawai*. All species, however, are acquired by the definitive host through eating of raw or partially cooked freshwater fish.

Heterophyes heterophyes is reported from Asia (Japan, Korea, China, Taiwan, the Philippines), Mediterranean countries (Egypt, Israel, Greece, Turkey, Maroc-co, Spain), and parts of Africa (Nigeria, Senegal). The prevalence rates are usually low except in some Asian countries. In areas endemic for *Clonorchis* and *Opisthorchis* species, it is difficult to differentiate the eggs of these opisthorchids from the heterophyids.

Metagonimus yokogawai has been reported from the Philippines, China, Taiwan, Japan, Korea, Russia, and Siberia. European reports, however, are questionable since they may be of a related heterophyid. The highest prevalence rates are in Japan and Korea.

Other heterophyids reported in humans, most in Asians, are: *H. hatsuradai, M. minutus, Centrocestus formosanus, C. kurokawai, Pygidiopsis summa, Haplorchis taihokui, H. microrchis, H. yokogawai, H. vanissimus, H. taichui, Procercovum calderoni, Diorchitrema formossanum, D. amplicalcale, Stellantchasmus falcatus, S. pseudocirratus, S. formosanus,* and *Stichtodora fuscata.*

II. Morphology

Adult *Heterophyes heterophyes* are very small, measuring 1–2 by 0.3–0.4 mm. They are elongated, oval, or pyriform in shape with a broadly rounded posterior end and an attenuated anterior end. The body surface is spinose. The oral sucker is anterior and the ventral sucker is located in the middle third of the anterior part of the body. The genital sucker has rows of tiny spines and is posterior and contiguous with the ventral sucker. The digestive tract divides at the midbody and extends to the posterior end. Two oval testes lie in the posterior fifth of the body and the rounded ovary is midline in the anterior portion of the posterior third of the body. The vitelline glands consist of about 15 polygonal follicles.

Metagonimus yokogawai is similar to *H. heterophyes* and measures 1.0–2.5 by 0.4–0.8 mm. The ventral sucker is to the right of the midline and the genital sucker is inconspicuous since the outer rim is fused to the ventral sucker. The tegumentary spines are more prominent at the anterior end around the oral sucker.

The other heterophyid species reported from man are small and ovoid to piriform in shape. There are slight variations in morphology but the location and relationship of ventral sucker to the genital sucker is an important diagnostic feature.

III. Life Cycle

Adult heterophyids reside in the small intestines and are found in the lumen attached to the mucosa or between the villi reaching into the crypts of Lieberkühn. The eggs contain a fully developed miracidia when passed in the feces. The eggs must reach water containing the snail intermediate hosts: prosobranch or operculate snails of the families Pleuroceridae, Thiaridae = Melaniidae, Potamididae = Cerithiidae, and Hydrobiidae (MALEK 1980). Snails ingest the eggs and the miracidiae hatch within the snail and develop into sporocysts followed by one or two radial generations. Cercariae are produced, escape from the snail, and swim freely in the water in search of a suitable fish second intermediate host. The cercariae encyst and form into metacercariae under the scales of the fins, tail, and gills or in the muscle, depending on the heterophyid species and host species. Many species of fishes serve as second intermediate host for the parasites and some heterophyids use frogs rather than fishes. Infection in birds and mammals is acquired by eating raw or inadequately cooked second intermediate hosts. The metacercariae excyst in the intestinal tract and develop into adults in 1 or 2 weeks; the adults may live for a few months to 1 year.

IV. Pathology

Adult heterophyids in the mucosa of the jejunum or upper ileum may cause mild inflammation and necrosis. Abdominal tenderness, colicky pain, and mucus diarrhea are usual symptoms with heavy infection. Most cases, however, are asymptomatic. AFRICA and his co-workers (1935a, 1935b, 1937) in the Philippines reported severe effects of heterophyidiasis in which the eggs filtered through the intestinal wall and were carried to the heart and central nervous system by the lymphatics or venules. These ectopic foci caused lesions in the viscera, cardiac valves, myocardium, brain, and spinal cord. Adult *H. heterophyes* were also reported responsible for neurological disorders in two patients (DESCHIENS et al. 1958). In the Philippines cases of ectopic heterophyiasis may have involved several heterophyid species.

V. Diagnosis

Heterophydiasis is diagnosed by the detection of eggs in the feces. The operculated eggs are small (26–33 by 14–20 μm) ovoidal and yellowish to brown in color with slight thickening at the opercular fitting. The eggs of this group are difficult to speciate and must also be differentiated from opisthorchid eggs. Species identification can be made of the adult worms recovered from intestinal scrapings at autopsy or from the feces following anthelmintic therapy.

VI. Treatment

Oil of chenopodium, oleoresin of aspidium, carbon tetrachloride, tetrachloroethylene, bephenium hydroxynaphthoate, hexylresorcinol, and niclosamide have been used in the treatment of *H. heterophyes* and *M. yokogawai*. KHALIL et al. (1964) treated cases of *H. heterophyes* with niclosomide (2 g/day for three alternate days) and obtained an 80% cure rate. In Korea, RIM (1972) obtained an egg reduction of 96% in treating *M. yokogawai* with niclosamide in dosages of 1.5–2.0 g followed 2 h later by an additional dose of 1.0–2.0 g. Radical cure was obtained in children using a dosage of 100–125 mg/kg body weight. AHN et al. (1978) recommended niclosamide for metagonimiasis in dosages of 2 g/day for three successive days. In a comparative study in Korea, RIM et al. (1978) evaluated bithionol, niclosamide, niclofolan, and praziquantel and all were found to be highly effective against metagonimiasis in a single or two daily doses. Praziquantel, however, was considered the most effective when given in two doses in one day of 20 mg/kg body weight. The drug was well tolerated without side effects and was recommended for mass treatment against metagonimiasis. In Japan, YOKOGAWA and his co-workers (1965, 1973) used kamela in a single dose of 5, 7, and 10 g followed by a sodium sulfate purgative and obtained a reduction in eggs in most patients and complete cures in others. Three heterophyid species were recovered from some of the patients: *H. heterophyes*, *M. yokogawai*, and *Pygidiopsis summa*. One woman given 7.5 g kamela passed 55,310 *M. yokogawai* worms following treatment and the woman was without clinical or subjective symptoms.

The drug of choice will probably by praziquantel when it becomes available for general use, but in the meantime older preparations such as tetrachloroethylene, 0.12 ml/kg body weight for a maximum of 5 ml, or niclosamide 2 g/day for 2 to 3 days are recommended for *H. heterophyes* and *M. yokogawai* as well as some of the lesser known heterophyid infections.

VII. Socioeconomic, Ecological, and Cultural Aspects

Heterophydiasis is a zoonotic disease, the heterophyids being parasites of fish-eating animals. Natural hosts for the group consist of a number of bird and mammal species whose diet consists of freshwater, brackish water, or sometimes marine fish. Humans acquire infections from eating raw or incompletely cooked fish. *H. heterophyes* in endemic areas of Egypt is acquired from the brackish water mullet, *Mugil cephalis*, and *Tilapia nilotica* which are eaten raw, pickled, or salted. Fishermen and boatmen are usually infected since they lack cooking facilities and eat their catch raw. Sanitation facilities are also lacking and the people usually defecate into the water, depositing heterophyid eggs. The important snail host of *H. heterophyes* in Egypt is *Pirenella conica.*

In Korea, the silver carp, *Carassius carassius,* and the sweetfish, *Plecoglossus altivelis,* are major sources of *Metagonimus yokogawai. P. altivelis* has the highest rates of metacercarial infection in the summer months and from June to September the people prefer to eat the fish uncooked. After September, eating raw fish is no longer favored and they are eaten either dried or cooked (KIM et al. 1979). Prevalence rates for *M. yokogawai* for certain localities vary from 0.5% to 29%, higher rates are seen in males than females, and the highest rates are in the middle age group. The major snail vectors in Korea are *Semisulcospira libertina* and *S. coreana.*

The metacercariae of *M. yokogawai* have been found in the Japanese fishes *Salangichthys microdon, Tribolodon hakonensis,* and *P. altivelis.* The latter seems to be the most important host and is called Ayu. Mountain stream sports fishermen often become infected by eating it freshly caught. *H. heterophyes* and *P. summa* metacercariae are found in *Mugil cephalus,* which is also eaten raw. The snail host of *Metagonimus yokogawai* in Japan is *S. libertina* and that of *H. heterophyes* is *Cerithidea cingulata.* Prevalence rates of human infection with *M. yokogawai* in Japan vary from 20% to 78%; rates for *H. heterophyes* are reputed to be 8% to 9% in endemic areas.

In Thailand, where the eating of freshwater fish is common practice, heterophyid infections are also reported in humans; *Haplorchis pumilio, H. yokogawai, Haplorchis* sp. (VAJRASTHIRA 1975), and *H. taichui* (MANNING et al. 1971) have been reported on a number of occasions and most recently *Stellantchasmus falcatus* was reported in three persons in northern Thailand (TANTACHAMRUA and KLIKS 1978). The prevalence rates in other parts of Asia for heterophyids is not well documented. In stool surveys on Taiwan and the Philippines the rates were less than 1% for Taiwan and approximately 1% for the Philippines (CROSS 1975). In the Philippines, only certain population groups, such as the Ilocanos, relish the eating of raw fish and this group is commonly infected with heterophyids. As long as Asians and others continue to eat raw or inadequately cooked freshwater fish, heterophyid infections will continue.

D. Echinostomatidiasis

I. Introduction

Echinostomids are primarily intestinal parasites of birds and some mammals that on rare occasions become parasites of man. There are about a dozen species reported from humans and although infections with certain members of the group have been reported from various locations throughout the world, most human infections have been reported in Asians. *Echinostoma ilocanum* and *E. lindoense* are the most often reported, and to a lesser extent *E. revolutum, E. malayanum, E. metis, E. recurvatum, E. cinetorchis, E. macrochis, Echinochasmus perfoliatus, Hypoderaeum conideum, Paryphostomum surfrartyfex,* and *Himasthla muehlensi.*

II. Morphology

The echinostomids are relatively small elongated flukes with a large ventral sucker and with one or two rows of large spines surrounding the oral sucker. The number and arrangement of the circumoral spines are helpful in species identification. The anterior tegument is provided with smaller spines. The genital pore is anterior to the ventral sucker, the two testes are round and centrally situated in the posterior part of the body, and the ovary is anterior to the testes. The uterus occupies the space between the gonads and the ventral sucker and the vitillaria are lateral. The adults measure 2–6 mm in length by 1–1.5 mm in width and both ends are attenuated.

III. Life Cycle

The adult flukes are located in the jejunum and the eggs are unembryonated when passed in the feces. The miracidium develops within the egg and hatches in 14 days or more. It emerges from the operculated egg and swims in the water in search of the first snail intermediate host. The miracidium penetrates a pulmonate or operculate snail and passes through a sporocyst and one or two redial stages before producing cercariae. The cercariae swim in the water and eventually encyst in the same or another snail species, clams, fishes, or tadpoles, all of which can serve as second intermediate hosts. Humans and other definitive hosts acquire infection by eating the second intermediate host usually uncooked.

IV. Pathology

Most echinostomid infections in man are without symptoms unless the worm load is extensive. Inflammatory lesions may develop at the site of attachment in the jejunum and there may be abdominal pain and diarrhea. In the Philippines, where *E. ilocanum* infections are common, clinical disease is not usually seen. Similarly, in areas of Indonesia endemic for *E. lindoensis* and in areas in Thailand highly endemic for *Hypoderaeum conoideum* little morbidity has been directly attributed to infections.

V. Diagnosis

Echinostomatidiasis can be diagnosed by finding eggs in the feces, but species identification is not possible unless the adult flukes are recovered following anthelminthic therapy. The eggs of the different species vary in size, i.e., *E. ilocanum,* 83–116 by 53–82 μm; *E. lindoensis,* 97–107 by 65–73 μm; *E. revolutum,* 90–126 by 59–71 μm; and *H. conoideum,* 137 by 75 μm. The eggs are thin shelled, oval, operculated, and unembryonated when passed in the feces.

VI. Treatment

Drugs similar to those used for the treatment of fasciolopsiasis are effective in the treatment of echinostomiasis: tetrachloroethylene, carbon tetrachloride, oil of chenopodium, hexylresorcinol, and male fern extract. Filamon oil, santonin, and kamala are also reportedly effective (Malek 1980). Mebendazole while treating cases of intestinal capillariasis was also found effective against concomitant *E. ilocanum* infections in the Philippines. In Korea, bithionol with a cathartic was recently reported effective in the treatment of *E. cinetorchis* (Seo et al. 1980).

VII. Socioeconomic, Ecological, and Cultural Aspects

Echinostomid infections although widespread in nature are rare in man except in a few areas of Asia where population groups eat molluscan, amphibian, and fish second intermediate hosts uncooked. In Northern Luzon in the Philippines, *E. ilocanum* eggs were found in the feces of over 10% of persons examined (Cross et al. 1970). The infections are usually acquired by eating a large rice field pulmonate snail, *Pila luzonica*. Sanitary facilities are not well developed in some of the endemic areas and the water irrigating the rice fields is easily contaminated with human and animal feces. The first intermediate host, a small freshwater planorbid, *Gyraulus prashadi*, abounds in the water as does *P. luzonica*. The Ilocanos of Luzon collect the snails from the water in the rainy season and from the soil in the dry season and usually eat them uncooked. Infections are not long lasting but reinfection is common. Rats are considered reservoir hosts.

Echinostoma lindoensis, once very common in the Lindu Lake region of central Sulawesi, has nearly disappeared from the area. The major first intermediate host was *Anisus sarasinorum*, and the clam *Corbicula lindoensis* was the second intermediate host. The clam was the primary source of human infection along the shores of Lake Lindu since it was a substantial part of the diet of the people. In 1950 the fish *Tilapia mossambica* was introduced into the lake; it thrived and became the most common fish in the lake and a major part of the population. At the same time, the molluscan population began to decline because of competition for food and predation by the fish on the molluscan larval stages (Carney et al. 1980). It is very unusual to find eggs of *E. lindoensis* in humans in the area today while in 1956 the prevalence of infection in three villages ranged from 42% to 85%.

In northern Thailand the prevalence of echinostomid infection was approximately 50% among the people in five villages. Most of the infections were due to *H. conoideum* but *E. malayanum* and *E. revolutum* were also found. A first intermediate host in the area is *Indoplanorbis exustus* and the second *I. exustus, Lymnea rubiginosa, G. convexiusculus*, and tadpoles, which are all eaten uncooked (Sornmani 1969).

In Japan, freshwater fish are the source of infection for *E. perfoliatus* and *E. hortense*. In one study of four patients with *E. hortense*, three had eaten raw loaches, *Misgurnus anguillicaudatus*, and raw green frogs (Malek 1980).

Echinostomid infections, when they occur in humans, are generally accompanied by a variety of other helminthic infections. Alone, they cause little disease, but when with other parasites they can contribute to the overall morbidity. Echinostomatidiasis is usually self-limiting and treatment may not be necessary. Reinfection in highly endemic areas of Thailand and the Philippines is common, however.

E. Gastrodisciasis

I. Introduction

Only one amphistome of the family Paramphistomatidae, *Gastrodiscoides hominis*, is a parasite of man, with infections reported from parts of India, particularly Assam, Bangladesh, Vietnam, China, the Philippines, and Russia. In a survey conducted in an Indian population in Assam, 41% of those examined were infected. Animal infections have also been reported from Malaysia, Thailand, Burma, Indonesia, and Japan.

II. Morphology

Adult *G. hominis* is pyriform in shape with a large broad discoidal posterior end and a narrow conical anterior end and may measure 5–14 by 5–8 mm in flattened specimens. The conical anterior end measures 2 mm. The mouth is situated in the anterior sucker and the acetabulum is large, occupying the ventral rear of the posterior portion of the body. The tegument is without spines. The digestive tract consists of a pharynx with two pharyngeal pouches and bifurcated ceca which extend to the anterior margin of the ventral sucker. The large, lobate, tandem testes are between the ceca. The ovary is round, in the midline, and posterior to the testes. The vitellariae are in the discoidal region.

III. Life Cycle

Gastrodiscoides hominis eggs are similar to *Fasciolopsis buski* and are unembryonated when passed in the feces. The miracidium develops in about 2 weeks and upon hatching from the egg searches for a snail intermediate host. The complete life cycle has not been established but cercariae are known to encyst on aquatic plants. Man and pig acquire the infection by eating the plants containing metacercariae.

IV. Pathology

If only a few worms are involved the infection causes no pathological condition. In heavy infections, however, inflammation may develop in the mucosa of the colon or cecum at the site of attachment. A mucus diarrhea may also develop. Nearly 1,000 worms have been recovered following treatment of one patient and death has been reported in some patients.

V. Diagnosis

The eggs, unembryonated and operculated, are similar to those of *F. buski*. They are greenish-brown in color and measure 150–170 by 60–70 μm. They are narrower than *F. buski* and may have a thickening of the shell at the abopercular end.

VI. Treatment

Drugs used in the treatment of fasciolopsiasis are effective against *G. hominis*: thymol, hexylresorcinol, carbon tetrachloride, and tetrachloroethylene. The latter is the drug of choice at present, but some of the newer anthelminthics may be more efficacious.

VII. Socioeconomic, Ecological, and Cultural Aspects

Gastrodisciasis occurs in many of the areas of Asia endemic for fasciolopsiasis. The life cycle and mode of transmission of the two parasitoses are similar, but more information must be obtained on the epidemiology of *G. hominis*. Pig and man are the most common definitive hosts, and aquatic plants such as water caltrop are the source of infection. Monkeys, rats, and the Malayan mouse deer are also reported as hosts, but are probably not involved in the transmission of the parasite to man.

F. Lecithodendriidiasis

I. Introduction

There are two lecithodendriids reported as intestinal parasites of man and both are often found in the same person. *Prosthodindrium molenkampi* and *Phaneropsolus bonnei* are small flukes commonly found in bats and other insectivorous vertebrates. Both were first reported from autopsies in Indonesia and later in Thailand.

II. Morphology

Prosthodindrium molenkampi is a small fluke measuring 0.4–0.8 by 0.37–0.58 mm. The body is round and the tegument covered with dark spots and spines. The oral sucker is at the anterior end and the smaller ventral sucker is in the middle of the body. The testes are round and in the anterior half of the body at each side of the ventral sucker. The ovary is located near the right testis adjacent to the ventral sucker. The vitellaria are anterior to the testes. The uterus nearly fills the posterior two-thirds of the body below the acetabulum. The digestive tract consists of a pharynx and bifurcated ceca which extend to the midbody close to the testes.

Phaneropsolus bonnei is ovoid, measuring 0.48–0,78 by 0.22–0.34 mm. The oral sucker is at the anterior end, and the ventral sucker, about the same size, is in the midbody. The ovoid testes, slightly larger than the acetabulum, are in the anterior half of the body. The ovary is smaller than the testes and is dorsal and posterior to the ventral sucker. The vitellaria are symmetrical and anterior to the testes. The uterine coils wind through the posterior part of the body and the digestive tract is bifurcated and short.

III. Life Cycle

The life cycles of *Pr. molenkampi* and *Ph. bonnei* have not been completely elucidated. The first intermediate hosts are probably aquatic pulmonate snails and the metacercariae encysts in aquatic insects. In Thailand, MANNING and LERTPRASERT (1973) suggested *Bithynia ganiomphalus* as the first intermediate host for both trematodes and found insects of the order Odonata (*Crocothemis servilia, Orthetrum sabina, Trithemis pallidinervis, Brachythemis contaminata*) as the second intermediate hosts. It was postulated that man became infected by eating the naiads.

IV. Pathology

Clinical manifestations of lecithodendriidiasis have not been documented. In northern Thailand, however, where both species have been found in humans, it would be difficult to separate symptoms associated with this disease from other helminthiases.

V. Diagnosis

It is quite difficult to differentiate the eggs of the lecithodendriids from those of heterophyids and opisthorchids. The eggs of *Pr. molenkampi* are operculated, dark-brown in color, and measure 24–26 by 8–10 μm. The shell is thick with a knob-like thickening at the posterior end and there is no operculate shoulder. The eggs are unembryonated when passed in the feces. *Ph. bonnei* eggs measure 23–33 by 13–18 μm. The eggs are oval and thin shelled without an aboperculated projection or knob. The operculum and the operculate shoulders are not always evident. They are dark-brown in color and unembryonated when passed.

VI. Treatment

Little information is available on the treatment of lecithodendriidiasis but it is assumed that anthelmintics used for other intestinal trematodiases would be effective. MANNING et al. (1970) reported the recovery of *Ph. bonnei* from three persons treated with hexylresorcinol.

VII. Socioeconomic, Ecological, and Cultural Aspects

Infection of *Pr. molenkampi* and *Ph. bonnei* are associated with the unique eating habits of some Southeast Asian populations. In Thailand, MANNING (1971) reported prevalence ranges of 10%–40% for both species by stool examination and adults of both worms were found in over 50% of autopsies from the same area. Eggs of the parasites were also found in stool specimens from Laos.

Humans acquire the parasites by eating the aquatic stage or naiads of dragonflies. Natural hosts for *Pr. molenkampi* are bats and rats and infections in these hosts are believed to be by eating adult dragonflies. Only the cynomolgus monkey, *Macaca fascicularis*, has been found naturally infected and it is believed that the monkey acquires the parasite by eating adult dragonflies. As many as 150 metacercariae have been recovered from the abdomen of a single dragonfly in Thailand (MANNING 1971).

Since the eggs from these parasites are similar to other trematode eggs, it is likely that they are being missed in routine stool examination. In northeastern Thailand *Opisthorchis viverrini* is highly prevalent and eggs of these intestinal flukes could easily be confused for eggs from the liver fluke. Eggs of *Haplorchis yokogawai* and *Haplorchis taichui* have also been found in the same persons with *O. viverrini, Pr. bonnei*, and *Ph. molenkampi* (Manning et al. 1971). These findings indicate the unique eating habits of some Thai populations.

G. Other Human Intestinal Trematodiasis

As mentioned previously there are probably a great many trematode parasites that occasionally infect humans. It is apparent that most are of no significance since reports of these infections are rare. A few of those that have been reported are members of the families Microphallidae, Plagiorchiidae, and Isoparorchiidae.

The microphallid, *Spelotrema brevicaeca*, has been reported on several occasions in Filipinos and like the heterophyids the tiny eggs (15–16 by 9–19 μm) are suspected of causing lesions in the heart, brain, and spinal cord. The adults are usually found in birds and mammals and transmission is by eating raw crustaceans.

Plagiorchis philippinensis has been found in the Ilocanos of Luzon in the Philippines, who are also infected with *E. ilocanum* and *S. brevicaeca*. *Plagiorchis javanensis* was found at autopsy in an Indonesian who also had an echinostomid infection. *Plagiorchis muris* was recovered from the feces of a Japanese treated for metagonimiasis.

The isoparorchid, *Isoparorchis hypselobagri*, a natural parasite of catfish and eels, has been reported from humans twice. Thymol was used to expel the worm from one patient and because of heavy infections in fish throughout Southeast Asia and Southeast Asians enjoy eating raw fish, human infection may be occurring undetected or the eggs of the parasite may be confused for those of another species.

H. Comment

Intestinal trematode infections in humans are generally not considered serious public health problems and generally do not cause significant clinical disease except in heavy infections. In most endemic areas the population is usually infected with a number of parasites and it is often difficult to determine the real cause of clinical manifestations.

Since the diseases are not usually serious and have limited geographical distributions very little effort has been made to carry out treatment trials with new or developing drugs. Most of the drugs currently in use have been around for a long time. Most are effective and inexpensive, but most cause side effects. Some of the more recently developed drugs, such as praziquantel should be field tested against all of the intestinal trematodiases and if found effective could be made available for mass treatment especially for fasciolopsiasis, heterophyidiasis, and echinostomatidiasis.

The trematodiases will exist as long as indigenous populations continue to eat uncooked aquatic plant and animal life and continue to practice indiscriminate defecation. These customs have been in existence for generations and are difficult to alter.

References

Africa CM, Garcia EY, Leon W de (1935a) Intestinal heterophyidiasis with cardiac involvement: a contribution to the etiology of heart failure. Philipp J Public Health 2:1–19

Africa CM, Leon W de, Garcia EY (1935b) Heterophyidiasis. II. Ova in sclerosed mitral valves with other chronic lesions in the myocardium. J Philipps Is Med Assoc 15:583–592

Africa CM, Leon W de, Garcia EY (1937) Heterophyidiasis. V. Ova in the spinal cord of man. Philipp J Sci 62:393–397

Ahn YK, Chung BS, Soh CT (1978) Niclosamide in treatment of metagonimiasis (in Korean). Korean J Parasitol 16:65–68

Barlow CH (1925) The life cycle of the human intestinal fluke *Fasciolopsis buski* (Lankester). Am J Hyg Monogr Ser 4:99

Brown HW, Cheng CC, Chen CY, Lin KE, Chang CR, Lee LT, Hsu CC, Chow LP, Hsieh HC (1959) The treatment of *Fasciolopsis buski* infections with dithiazanine iodide, 1-bromo-naphthol-(2), ascaridol, piperazine and tetrachlorethylene. J Formosan Med Assoc 58:792–798

Bunnag D, Radomyos P, Harinasuta T (1983) Field trial on the treatment of fasciolopsiasis with praziquantel. SE Asian J Trop Med Public Health 14:216–219

Carney WP, Sudomo M, Purnomo (1980) Echinostomiasis: a disease that disappeared. Trop Geogr Med 32:101–106

Cross JH (1969) Fasciolopsiasis in Southeast Asia and the Far East: a review. In: Proceedings of the fourth southeast Asian seminar on parasitology and tropical medicine: schistosomiasis and other snail transmitted helminthiasis, Manila, 24–27 Feb 1969, pp 177–199. Seameo Central Coordinating Board for Tropical Medicine and Public Health Project, 420/6 Rajvithi Road, Bangkok 4, Thailand

Cross JH (1975) Diagnostic methods in intestinal fluke infections: a review. In: Diagnostic methods for important helminthiasis and amoebiasis in Southeast Asia and the Far East, Tokyo, 5–8 Feb 1974, pp 87–108. Seameo Central Coordinating Board for Tropical Medicine and Public Health Project, 420/6 Rajvithi Road, Bangkok 4, Thailand

Cross JH, Banzon TC, Murrell KD, Watten RH, Dizon JJ (1970) A new epidemic diarrheal disease caused by the nematode *Capillaria philippinensis*. Ind Trop Health 7:124–131

Deschiens R, Collomb H, Demarchi J (1958) Distomatose cerebrale a *Heterophyes heterophyes*. In: 6th international congress tropical medicine and malaria, Lisbon, p 265

Hadidjaja P, Dahri HM, Roesin R, Margono S, Djalins J, Hanafiah M (1982) First autochthonous case of *Fasciolopsis buski* infection in Indonesia. Am J Trop Med Hyg 31:1065

Healy GR (1970) Trematodes transmitted to man by fish, frogs and crustacea. J Wildl Dis 6:255–261

Hsieh HC, Brown HW, Chen ER, Chen CY, Shih CC (1963) Treatment of *Fasciolopsis buski, Ancylostoma duodenale, Ascaris lumbricoides, Trichuris trichiura* and *Enterobius vermicularis* infections with stilbazium iodide. J Formosan Med Ass 58:792–798

Idris M, Rahman KM, Muttalib MA, Khan AKA (1980) The treatment of fasciolopsiasis with niclosamide and dichlorophen. J Trop Med Hyg 83:71–74

Khalil HM, Rifaat MA, Koura M (1964) A further trial of "Yomosan" in *Heterophyes heterophyes* infection. J Trop Med Hyg 67:286–287

Kim DC, Lee OY, Jeong EB, Han EJ (1979) Epidemiological conditions of *Metagonimus yokogawai* infection in Hadong Gun, Gycongsang Nam (in Korea). Korean J Parasitol 17:51–59

Malek EA (1980) Snail-transmitted parasitic diseases, vol II. CRC, Baton Rouge, p 324

Manning GS (1971) Study of novel intestinal parasites in Thailand. In: Report of the first international seminar of the South-East Asia Treaty Organization Medical Research Laboratory, Bangkok, 22–25 Feb 1971, pp 43–46 (no longer available)

Manning GS, Lertprasert P (1973) Studies on the life cycle of *Phaneropsolus bonnei* and *Prosthodendrium molenkampi* in Thailand. Ann Trop Med Parasitol 67:361–365

Manning GS, Ratanarat C (1970) *Fasciolopsis buski* (Lankester, 1857) in Thailand. Am J Trop Med Hyg 19:613–619

Manning GS, Diggs CL, Viyanant V, Lertprasert P, Watanasirmkit K (1970) Preliminary report on *Phaneropsolus bonnie* Lie Kian-Joe, 1951 a newly discovered human intestinal fluke from Notheastern Thailand (In Thai). J Med Assoc Thai 53:173–178

Manning GS, Lertprasert P, Watanasirmkit K, Chamroen C (1971) A description of newly discovered intestinal parasites endemic to Northeastern Thailand. J Med Assoc Thai 54:466–474

McCoy OR, Chu T (1937) *Fasciolopsis buski* infection among children in Shaoshing and treatment with hexylresorcinol. Chin Med J 51:937–944

Plaut AG, Kampanart-Sanyakorn C, Manning GS (1969) A clinical study of *Fasciolopsis buski* infection in Thailand. Trans R Soc Trop Med Hyg 63:470–478

Rim HJ (1972) Chemotherapy of trematode infections excluding schistosomiasis. In: Proceedings of the tenth Seameo tropical medicine seminar. Symposium on chemotherapy in tropical medicine of Southeast Asia and the Far East. Bangkok, 26–30 Oct 1972, Seameo Central Coordinating Board for Tropical Medicine and Public Health Project, 420/6 Rajvithi Road, Bangkok 4, Thailand

Rim HJ, Chu DS, Lee JS (1978) Anthelmintic effects of various drugs against metagonimiasis (in Korean). Korean J Parasitol 16:117–122

Seo BS, Cho SY, Chai JY (1980) Studies on intestinal trematodes in Korea: 1. a human case of *Echinostoma cinetorchis* infection with an epidemiological investigation. Seoul Med J 21:21–29

Shah A, Gadgil RK, Manohar KD (1966) Fasciolopsiasis in Bombay: a preliminary communication. Indian J Med Sci 20:805–811

Shah PM, Udani PM, Manjarumkar PV, Naik PA (1973) *Fasciolopsis buski* infestation in children. Indian Pediatr 10:721–724

Sornmani S (1969) Echinostomiasis in Thailand: a review. In: Proceedings of the fourth southeast asian seminar on parasitology and tropical medicine: schistosomiasis and other snail transmitted helminthiasis, Manila, 24–27 Feb, pp 171–175, Seameo Central Coordinating Board of Tropical Medicine and Public Health Project, 420/6 Rajvithi Road, Bangkok 4, Thailand

Stoll NR (1947) This wormy world. J Parasitol 33:1–18

Stoll NR, Cort WW, Kwei KS (1927) Egg-worm correlations in cases of *Fasciolopsis buski:* with additional data on distribution of this parasite in China. J Parasitol 13:166–172

Suntharasamai P, Bunnag D, Tejavanij S, Harinasuta T, Migasena S, Vutikes S, Chindanond D (1974) Comparative clinical trials of niclosamide and tetrachloroethylene in the treatment of *Fasciolopsis buski* infection. Southeast Asian J Trop Med Public Health 5:556–559

Tantachamruna T, Kliks M (1978) Heterophyid infection in human ileum: report of three cases. Southeast Asian J Trop Med Public Health 9:228–231

Vajrasthira S (1975) A note on microscopic diagnosis of some human intestinal flukes. In: Diagnostic methods for important helminthiasis and amoebiasis in Southeast Asia and the Far East, Tokyo, 5–8 Feb 1974, pp 132–134, Seameo Central Coordinating Broad for Tropical Medicine and Public Health Project, 420/6 Rajvithi Road, Bangkok 4, Thailand

Yokogawa M, Sano M, Itabashi T, Kachi S (1965) Studies on the intestinal flukes II. Epidemiological studies on heterophyid trematodes of man in Chiba Prefecture (in Japanese). Jpn J Parasitol 14:577–585

Yokogawa M, Sano M, Arakik, Kobayashi M, Kihata M (1973) Epidemiological studies on metagonimiasis in Chokai Village, Akita Prefecture. 2. Results of the treatment with various doses of kamala for *Metagonimus* infections (in Japanese). Jpn J Parasitol 22:362–368

CHAPTER 13

Chemotherapy of Tapeworm Infections in Animals

M. D. RICKARD and J. H. ARUNDEL

A. Introduction

Adult and larval stages of tapeworms occur in domesticated animals throughout the world. However, the economic importance of cestode infections is generally less than that of nematodes and trematodes and the development of compounds effective against cestodes has been neglected until relatively recently. The major economic impact of cestode infections derives from the condemnation of infected livestock carcasses or offal for human consumption rather than through the direct effects of adult or larval stages upon the health of animals. Losses due to condemnation are more difficult to quantitate than the more overt disease or production losses occasioned by other parasites. The public health significance of some adult and larval stages of tapeworms of domesticated animals has probably provided the major impetus for development of new cestocidal drugs.

In a series of lectures to medical students in 1872, COBBOLD gave the most important remedies as male fern, kousso, kamala, turpentine, panna, pumpkin seeds, and pomegranate root bark. Powdered areca nut was acknowledged to be of value but as it lost its strength quickly after crushing it was less favoured. In 1963, STANDEN gave extract of male fern as still the most favoured treatment in man, although it was being replaced by mepacrine and dichlorophen, while in veterinary medicine dichlorophen, arecoline, lead arsenate and inorganic and organic tin compounds were used. In recent years there have been major advances in the chemotherapy of cestode infections, extending even to activity against the larval stages. This review concentrates on recent developments, although the more important older compounds still in use are also considered. For information concerning older compounds not mentioned in this review, the reader should consult GIBSON (1975).

The section dealing with the cestodes cannot, within the scope of this review, include an exhaustive description of all facets of each parasite. It is intended only as a summary of important information concerning major diagnostic features, biology, transmission, and significance in the host for readers who are not familiar with this group of organisms. This information is presented in the belief that an understanding of these factors is desirable, often essential, for proper application of chemotherapeutic agents in the treatment and control of parasitic diseases. For more detailed information concerning the parasites the reader should consult more comprehensive works (WARDLE and MCLEOD 1952; YAMAGUTI 1959; ABULADZE 1964; SOULSBY 1965; SMYTH 1969; WARDLE et al. 1974). The list of parasites does not include all genera and species which are, or may be found, in domesticated animals and birds. Only the more common and important tapeworms are dealt with. The system of classification used is mostly according to WARDLE and MCLEOD (1952) in preference to their more recent version (WARDLE et al. 1974).

B. Cestodes of Veterinary Importance

The cestodes or "tapeworms" are members of the class Cestoda within the phylum Platyhelminthes (the flatworms). All adult members of this group are parasitic in the alimentary tracts, or associated ducts, of vertebrates. Their bodies are usually flat, elongate, lack a body cavity or alimentary system, and are usually divided into three major regions; the scolex ("head" or holdfast), the neck, and the body (strobila). The scolex bears organs of attachment such as suckers or bothridia which assist the worms in maintaining their position in the gut. The scolex may also have a protrusible part, the rostellum, which may be armed with one or more rows of hooks. The neck is a short, undifferentiated area behind the scolex, and is an area of very active cell division. It is from this region that the rest of the body originates. The strobila consists of a series of proglottids or segments. Each proglottid is a complete unit in itself and has its own set of male and female reproductive organs. In most tapeworms the proglottids vary in sexual development along the length of the strobila so that they become mature as they move further from the neck and finally the terminal segments are gravid. Tapeworms vary widely in size from a few millimetres to several metres in length.

The outer coating of the tapeworm is the syncytial tegument, which bears numerous small projections called microtriches. These important structures serve like intestinal villi in providing a vast surface area for absorption or excretion into the surrounding fluid; microtubules in each microthrix communicate with the tegumental syncytium. The tegument contains many organelles and vacuoles and has been shown to be a very actively metabolising area. These parasites rely entirely for their nutrition, and probably a significant part of their excretion, upon the activity of the tegument. It therefore becomes a very important organ, affording much more than simply protection from the environment. Because cestodes lack an alimentary system, the function and permeability of the tegument play an important role in determining the activity of chemotherapeutic substances used to kill these parasites.

Underneath the tegument is a loose, sponge-like mass of tissue termed the parenchyma, within which are located the other internal organs of the tapeworm, i.e. osmoregulatory system, nervous system, reproductive system and musculature. Scattered throughout the parenchyma are numbers of free cells, of unknown function, and the calcareous corpuscles. The musculature consists of two major layers, subtegumental muscle and parenchymal muscle. The subtegumental muscle consists of an outer circular layer and an inner longitudinal layer. The parenchymal musculature is peculiar to the cestodes, and divides each segment into an outer cortical and inner medullary area. It consists of an outer layer of longitudinal fibres and an inner layer of transverse fibres. The well-developed musculature of tapeworms makes them highly contractile. In a freshly opened cadaver of a dog infected with one of the large *Taenia* spp., it is often possible to pick the location of the worm in the gut by the manner in which it holds the intestine of the host in a contracted state. Undoubtedly this contractility assists the worms in both maintaining and probably altering their position in the gut. For instance, *Hymenolepis diminuta* worms in rats alter their position in the gut in response to varying conditions in the alimentary tract (READ and KILEJIAN 1969; HOPKINS 1970). Detached gravid proglottids of many of these tapeworms can actively migrate out of the faecal mass and disseminate eggs over a wider area.

The primitive nervous system generally consists of the central ganglia with their commissures in the scolex, and nerve trunks which pass forward to the scolex and backward down the strobila. Ganglia with commissures between them are located in each proglottid. The osmoregulatory system originates in flame cells in the parenchyma with capillaries leading into longitudinal collecting vessels. There are two ascending dorsal vessels and two descending ventral vessels all located in the lateral edges of the medullary parenchyma. The ventral canals are connected by anastomoses in the posterior part of each proglottid, and the ventral and dorsal canals all join together in the scolex. The last segment often contains a bladder into which the dorsal and ventral canals open. When the terminal segment is shed, the canals open to the exterior.

Cestodes are hermaphrodites, and normally protandrous, i.e. the male reproductive system matures before the female system. The male system consists of testes, vasa efferentia, a vas deferens, sometimes a seminal vesicle and a cirrus (sometimes in a cirrus sac), which opens into a lateral (more common) or ventral genital pore. Each testis is a spherical or ovoid mass of cells in which the spermatozoa are formed. In the female reproductive system the bilobed ovary lies in the medullary parenchyma and is linked by a short oviduct to the ootype, where the eggs are formed. The ootype is surrounded by Mehlis' gland. The vitellarium, or yolk gland, is usually a compact body at the rear of the proglottid, but in some cestodes, notably the Diphyllobothriidae, it takes the form of scattered follicles; a vitelline duct leads to the ootype. The vagina leads from the ootype to the common genital atrium and may have a blind pouch, the seminal receptacle. The uterus leads forward from the ootype. Oocytes, which are fertilised by sperm (from other tapeworms, other segments of the same worm or from the same segment) pass into the ootype, where eggs characteristic of the particular tapeworm are formed. These eggs then pass forward into the uterus. In the majority of tapeworms of veterinary importance, the uterus acts as a storage organ and eggs are released only after the terminal "gravid" proglottid has been detached, a process known as apolysis. There are many variations in morphology of the uterus in gravid proglottids, and special structures such as uterine or parenchymal egg capsules and the par-uterine organ may be present. These special characteristics are often useful in the identification and diagnosis of cestode infections. In the Diphyllobothriidae the uterus opens to the ventral surface at a uterine pore, and eggs are shed continuously into the faeces.

Almost all cestodes have at least one intermediate host in their life cycle. The cycles vary widely, as do the larval forms, and these will be discussed when considering the various parasites. Generally the intermediate host ingests the egg, and the mature metacestode which develops in it is ingested by the definitive host when it eats the intermediate host. Intermediate hosts vary from insects, crustacea, amphibians, reptiles, fish, birds, and mammals.

I. Order Pseudophyllidea

Members of this order are found mainly in fish, but also occur in mammals and birds. Only one family, the Diphyllobothriidae, contains parasites of veterinary importance.

Family Diphyllobothriidae

The scolex is unarmed and has dorsal and ventral longitudinal grooves, the bothria, as holdfast organs. Each segment has a ventral uterine pore through which eggs are shed continuously into the digestive tract of the host. They are anapolytic, i.e. terminal segments are not shed serially from the strobila, but when senescent, chains of segments are shed from the end of the parasite. The genital pore opens onto the ventral surface of the segment and the vitelline follicles are scattered throughout the parenchyma. Eggs are operculated and immature when released from the uterus, and eventually develop to contain a ciliated larva, the coracidium, which is characterised by the presence of three pairs of hooks. The parasites have two intermediate hosts, a crustacean and a vertebrate. The coracidium must be ingested by a copepod larva within 12 h of hatching, and within the haemocoel of these organisms a solid-bodied larva, the procercoid, develops within 18 days. The copepod is eaten by a suitable vertebrate and the procercoid bores through the gut and develops into the plerocercoid larva. The plerocercoid is club shaped with a solid, cylindrical, unsegmented body with an invaginated scolex. The final host is infected by ingesting the plerocercoid in the second intermediate host.

a) *Diphyllobothrium latum (Dibothriocephalus latus)*

The taxonomy of the genus *Diphyllobothrium* is confused and many species which have been described are undoubtedly invalid. In fact it has been advocated that specific identification should ideally be based on the study of many factors such as the morphology, biology, physiology, immunology, and biochemistry (VIK 1964). This is especially so with plerocercoid stages, which are devoid of special morphological characteristics. Recently BYLUND and DJUPSUND (1977) distinguished four species of *Diphyllobothrium* on the basis of protein profiles constructed using isoelectric focussing.

Diphyllobothrium latum, the "broad tapeworm" or "fish tapeworm," is a large, weakly muscular worm growing up to 10 m in length depending upon the host species. Its natural host is probably man, but it has been found in many animals including the dog, cat, fox, bear, seal, sea lion, walrus, and domestic pig. A useful experimental host has been the golden hamster (*Mesocricetus auratus*) (GNEZDILOV 1957). It is most common in the far Northern Hemisphere in the USSR, the Baltic Sea countries, the Far East and North America, but also occurs in central and southeastern Europe, Africa, the Middle East, and southern South America. Its distribution is determined by availability of the intermediate hosts and the temperature requirements of the free-living stages. With increased mobility of people the parasite is now recorded from many countries in which it is undoubtedly not endemic.

The parasite has a spatulate scolex, and the uterus in each segment has a rosette-like appearance with four to eight loops on each side. The eggs are ovoid and operculate with rounded ends and are approximately 65 × 45 μm in size. They must pass into water for development of the coracidium within the egg, which takes approximately 2 weeks. The first intermediate hosts are crustacea of the genera *Diaptomus* (HUMES 1950) or *Cyclops*. The intermediate hosts have special habitat requirements such as fresh or slightly brackish water (maximum salt concentration 0.2%–0.4%) with a temperature mostly under 22 °C; relatively shallow lakes and rivers are the best habitat (VON BORNSDORFF 1978). Many kinds of freshwater fish can act as second intermediate hosts such as trout, pike, burbot, perch, and salmon and the plerocercoids develop mainly in the muscles but also in the viscera. Small fish can be eaten by larger fish which then act as transport hosts. Dogs are not as suitable as final hosts as man. The worms are smaller and as few as 1% of eggs produced will develop and hatch. Thus, dogs probably play only a minor role in the dissemination of this parasite (ESSEX and MAGATH 1931; KUHLOW 1953). The parasite can produce a variety of gastrointestinal symptoms in man, but its most serious effect in some instances is a pernicious anaemia-like syndrome caused by massive uptake of vitamin B_{12} by the worm, especially when it is present in the upper part of the intestinal tract. Because the parasite does not develop to the same extent in dogs as in humans it is only rarely harmful. Infection is prevented either by not providing fish or by adequate treatment of the fish to destroy plerocercoids before consumption. SALMINEN (1970) carried out extensive studies on factors affecting survival of plerocercoids and provides a detailed list of treatments required to render them non-infective.

b) Genus *Spirometra*

Members of this genus differ morphologically from *Diphyllobothrium* in that the uterine loops form a spiral rather than a rosette, the eggs have pointed ends (62 × 34 μm) and the male and female genital pores open separately rather than into a common sinus (BEARUP 1953). The life cycle is basically similar but *Cyclops* rather than *Diaptomus* is the preferred first intermediate host (MUELLER 1938) and a wider range of amphibians, reptiles, and mammals (but not fish) serve as second intermediate or transport hosts. The final hosts are a variety of carnivores, especially felines, but not man.

As with *Diphyllobothrium,* the taxonomy of this genus also presents problems. MUELLER (1974) considered that the only member which could be defined firmly was *Spirometra mansonoides* but LEVINE (1978) describes four species of *Spirometra. S. mansonoides* in North and South America uses principally cats as the final host, but also develops in dogs, pigs and other mammals. The plerocercoid is found in a number of vertebrate hosts (except fish) but the water snake *Natrix* is probably the most important natural second host (MUELLER 1974). *S. erinacei* in Australia is common in foxes and cats, and will also infect dogs. Tadpoles are the second intermediate host. However, a wide range of vertebrates can be infected, and infection can pass from animal to animal along the food chain. Feral pigs are commonly infected in Australia (BEARUP 1953) and man can become infected by eating improperly cooked pork. *S. mansoni* in the Far East uses dogs and cats as final hosts and has a similar intermediate host range to *S. erinacei.*

Frogs and snakes seem to be important sources of infection. *S. theileri* in Africa uses canids as final hosts and various antelopes, buffaloes, baboons, warthogs, etc. as second intermediate hosts; amphibians and reptiles seem to play no part in this cycle (OPUNI and MULLER 1974).

The adult tapeworms are of little significance to animal health. The major importance of these parasites results from the lack of specificity of the plerocercoid. This stage is often referred to as a "Sparganum," a name which was given generic status until it was realized that the sparganum was an intermediate stage of Diphyllobothriid tapeworms. Man can become infected by ingestion of any vertebrate harbouring the plerocercoid, by ingesting the copepod containing the procercoid or by local application of infected flesh as a poultice to wounds or to the eye. This latter means of infection has been reported from the Orient. Normally the sparganum remains as a single organism in the fascial planes of the muscle and subcutaneous tissue of the host. However, proliferating forms "*Sparganum proliferum*" have been described, and MUELLER and STRANO (1974) suggested that a virus may be responsible for this aberrant form.

NELSON et al. (1965) postulated that in East Africa man may be a natural intermediate host of *Spirometra theileri* as the dead bodies of Masai are traditionally laid out for the hyenas to eat. If plerocercoids of *S. mansonoides* are injected into the peritoneal cavities of dogs and cats, some remain as plerocercoids in the tissues, whilst others penetrate the gut and develop into adult worms (CORKUM 1973). An interesting feature of infection with the plerocercoid of *S. mansonoides* is the production of a sparganum growth factor (SGF) (MUELLER 1963) which stimulates rapid growth in hypophysectomized rats. This growth-promoting effect does not occur with all species of *Spirometra* (MUELLER 1965, 1970). *S. mansonoides* has been grown in vitro from plerocercoid to gravid adult (BERNTZEN and MUELLER 1972).

II. Order Cyclophyllidea

This group contains most of the tapeworms of veterinary importance. They vary widely in size ranging from a few millimetres to 30 m or more in length. Typically, the scolex has four cup-shaped suckers and a rostellum with or without hooks may be present. The male and female genital pores open close together on the lateral aspect of each segment. The vitellarium is a compact body posterior to the ovary. There is no uterine pore, and the uterus typically functions as a storage organ. Eggs are released only after apolysis of the terminal segment and rupture of the uterus. The eggs contain a fully developed hexacanth embryo, or oncosphere, with three pairs of hooks and surrounded by the embryophore. The embryo and embryophore are equivalent to the pseudophyllidean coracidium, except that in this case the embryophore is not ciliated. The embryophore is in turn surrounded by various other membranes including the true "shell," which is not operculated.

Almost all cyclophyllidean tapeworms have an intermediate host which is infected by ingesting the egg. Two processes are involved in preparing the oncosphere for invasion of the host tissue. Firstly, the outer layers of the egg including the embryophore are broken down to release the oncosphere, and secondly the oncosphere is stimulated ("activated") to become motile and tear its way out of its enclosing oncospheral membrane using its hooks. These two processes may be mediated by independent stimuli. With cyclophyllidean tapeworms other than those belonging to the family Taeniidae, the process of hatching is often initiated by mechanical disruption of the outer coatings by the mouthparts of the invertebrate intermediate hosts, probably aided by digestive secretions. Activation of the oncosphere of these tapeworms is poorly understood, but factors which have been implicated are temperature change, the concentration of inorganic ions and in some cases enzymes such as trypsin and amylase. In the family Taeniidae, although limited hatching and activation can occur in simple solutions with some species, optimum results are achieved in vitro by mimicking the passage of eggs through the mammalian stomach and duodenum, i.e. preincubation in pepsin/hydrochloric acid followed by incubation in various combinations od sodium bicarbonate, trypsin, pancreatin, bile salts, and cholesterol. Under these conditions the embryophore darkens, swells and bursts apart, releasing myriads of tiny embryophoric blocks. These keratinaceous embryophoric blocks (MORSETH 1966) are thought to be held together by some interstitial substance which on exposure to the intestinal secretions becomes hydrophilic, swells and forces the blocks apart (LAWS 1968a). The mechanism of activation is not known.

Once the oncosphere is activated, it penetrates the gut of the host and, on reaching its final site of election, develops into the mature infective stage (for the definitive host) or metacestode. There are several larval forms amongst the Cyclophyllidea.

The *cysticercoid* usually occurs in invertebrate intermediate hosts. It consists of a double-walled bladder, with essentially no cavity, containing the scolex of the future tapeworm in its normal, everted position. There is a small bladder-like tail, the cercomer.

The *cysticercus* and its various modifications are often called the "bladder worms" because of the large amount of fluid they may contain. They are larval stages of parasites in the family Taeniidae all of which have vertebrate intermediate hosts. The cysticercus is a fluid-filled bladder with a single scolex invaginated in an "inside-out" fashion at one end. In the host the cysticercus becomes surrounded by a connective tissue host capsule.

The *Coenurus* is a large type of larval bladder worm with many scoleces in single or multiple groups invaginated over its surface.

The *hydatid* cyst has a germinal layer which buds off internally large numbers of brood capsules. Each brood capsule contains many inverted scoleces, called protoscoleces. Daughter cysts may develop within the parent cyst. The germinal layer is surrounded by the laminated membrane, of parasite origin (HEATH and OSBORN 1976), and this in turn becomes encapsulated in a tough, connective tissue host capsule. Single hydatid cysts can contain several hundred thousand protoscoleces. The brood capsules and protoscoleces are known collectively as "hydatid sand."

The *strobilocercus* is a specialised larva of *Taenia taeniaeformis* and consists of a scolex followed by a solid strobilated region and terminal bladder; the strobilated region does not contain any reproductive organs.

The *tetrathyridium* is found only in the family Mesocestoididae. It has a contractile, threadlike body, and an invaginated scolex with four suckers and without a rostellum.

Many of these larval forms have, in the past, been erroneously accorded generic status, e.g. *Cysticercus ovis, Coenurus serialis*. Strictly speaking this is not correct, i.e. *Cysticercus ovis* is the cysticercus stage of *Taenia ovis*, but the names are in such common usage that they will be used here.

The final or definitive host is infected by ingesting the mature metacestode, which is freed from its surrounding membranes and tissue (excystment) by chewing and digestion. The larva must then evaginate and become active. This process is brought about by the digestive secretions of the host, bile playing an especially important role. It has been suggested that the composition of the host bile may play a role in determining specificity (Smyth 1969). Once the evaginated larva becomes active it attaches to the intestinal wall. All of the larval tissue apart from the scolex and neck are digested away and the worm commences to bud off segments to form the adult strobila.

1. Family Mesocestoididae

This family contains a single genus, *Mesocestoides*, and although classified in the order Cyclophyllidea it has several pseudophyllidian characteristics. The scolex has four prominent suckers, but has neither rostellum nor hooks. The genital atrium opens onto the midventral aspect of each segment but no uterine pore is present. Instead, the eggs are massed in a thick-walled par-uterine organ at the posterior end of each gravid segment. The oncospheres are enclosed in a thin embryonic membrane and the egg measures approximately 24 × 19 µm. Williams et al. (1975) point out that neither freed par-uterine organs nor free eggs float in saturated sugar or zinc sulphate solutions, and diagnosis rests upon identification of the highly motile segments in faeces.

A number of species of *Mesocestoides* have been described, but the taxonomy of the group is rather confused. The two most common species identified in dogs and cats are *M. corti* and *M. lineatus*, although Witenburg (1934) considered that *M. lineatus* was the only species of this parasite in carnivores and that all others were subspecies of this. The parasite is found in Europe, Asia, Africa, and North America. Soulsby (1965) stated that the parasite was not common in Britain, but recently Thompson (1976a) found that 9 of 38 foxes from Scotland and South East England were infected. Williams et al. (1975) suggested that infection with *Mesocestoides* spp. in domesticated carnivores is probably often confused with *Dipylidium caninum*, and that it may be more common than is apparent.

The life cycle of *Mesocestoides* has similarities to the Pseudophyllidea in that two intermediate hosts are required. Oribatid mites can act as first intermediate hosts (Soldatova 1944) (although a role for other arthropods has not been excluded) and in these mites a cysticercoid develops. Many species of vertebrates (amphibians, reptiles, birds, and mammals) can act as second intermediate hosts. These ingest the cysticercoid, which becomes a tetrathyridium. The tetrathyridia are most commonly found in the peritoneal cavity of the intermediate host, but can also invade the liver, pleural cavities, and other organs. They undergo rapid multiplication by asexual longitudinal splitting (SPECHT and VOGE 1965), and appear to be remarkably robust. MUELLER (1972) found that they were still infective after storage for 7.5 months at 4 °C in Medium 199 plus fetal calf serum without any medium changes in the interim period. In laboratory animals the infection can be transferred by the intraperitoneal inoculation of tetrathyridia, and the mouse has been extensively used for experimental work. The carnivore definitive host is infected by ingesting tetrathyridia, which develop into adult worms measuring up to 1.5 m in length. If the wrong host ingests the tetrathyridia they can become encapsulated in the body until eaten by a favourable host. A very unusual feature of this parasite is its ability also to multiply in the intestine of the definitive host (ECKERT et al. 1969; SCHMIDT and TODD 1978); a dose of 2,000 tetrathyridia to a dog yielded 53,410 worms 45 days after infection (SCHMIDT and TODD 1978). Tetrathyridia can also invade and multiply in the body cavities of the definitive host.

Generally speaking the adult tapeworms are less pathogenic, although digestive disorders, disturbances of appetite, diarrhoea, anal pruritis, and even disturbances of the central nervous system (BICIK and LYSEK 1970) may occur. Multiplication in the body cavities can cause serious disease. BARSANTI et al. (1979) describe in detail a severe case of peritonitis in a dog. *Mesocestoides* spp. have been recorded on several occasions from man in Europe, Japan, Africa, and North America (GLEASON and HEALY 1967).

2. Family Taeniidae

Except for the genus *Echinococcus*, these are all large tapeworms, up to 10 m in length and with many hundred segments. The scolex has four suckers and a hemispherical rostellum armed with two rows of hooks. The hooks have a characteristic shape, consisting of a blade, guard, and handle. The genital pores are usually prominent on the lateral aspect of the segment and are irregularly alternate. The uterus is quite characteristic in this family, consisting of a medium longitudinal stem with lateral branches. Eggs are typically spherical to ovoidal with a thick embryophore made up of tiny keratinaceous blocks which give the egg a striated appearance. The eggs of all species are approximately 30–40 μm in diameter and have no differences which can be used for specific diagnosis of infection by faecal examination.

The definitive hosts of these parasites are carnivorous or omnivorous mammals, and the intermediate hosts are herbivores or omnivores. Each segment may contain up to 70,000 eggs (except *E. granulosus*, where there are less than 1,000 eggs/gravid proglottid) and these commence to be released from the uterus when the segment detaches from the strobila. When segments are released individually the anterior branches of the uterus are ruptured and the majority of eggs are discharged into the gut of the host so that the segment in the faeces may contain a few hundred eggs only. When a number of proglottids are shed together in a chain, the uteri in all segments except the most anterior one remain intact and eggs are retained in the segments until they are passed in the faeces. Muscular contractions of the segments assist in releasing the eggs. Eggs released from individual segments shed in the anterior part of the digestive tract can hatch there and be lost to the transmission cycle (COMAN and RICKARD 1975). Adult worms may shed several segments/day (GREGORY 1976).

Taeniid eggs are quite resistant to harsh environmental conditions and can survive for many months with moderate temperatures and available moisture (LAWS 1968 b; COLLI and WILLIAMS 1972; COMAN 1975). Heat and dryness kill taeniid eggs rapidly, but their resistance to common chemical disinfecting agents makes it difficult to sterilise the environment (PEREZ-ESANDI et al. 1974). Following ingestion of the egg by the intermediate host the hatched oncosphere penetrates the intestine and travels via the portal venous system or the mesenteric lymphatics to the site of election. The time taken to develop to the mature metacestode depends upon the species, but in general it is 6–12 weeks for cysticercus stages and much longer, e.g. up to 12 months, for a hydatid cyst to become fertile. The larval forms that occur are the cysticercus, coenurus, strobilocercus and hydatid, and these were described earlier. The larval forms can survive for some time in carcasses in the field or in meat or organs stored in the refrigerator. Freezing or boiling kills all metacestode stages, but the conditions necessary to bring this about may vary, e.g. with a large hydatid cyst in sheep offal it may take 40 min boiling to guarantee death of all protoscoleces (FASTIER 1949) and supercooling may occur when hydatid cysts are frozen so that some protoscoleces may survive (ARUNDEL 1972). The final host is infected by ingesting the mature metacestode.

Diagnosis of infection with these tapeworms in the definitive host depends mostly on identifying the characteristic segments in the faeces. Eggs will float in saturated sugar, sodium nitrate or zinc sulphate solutions, but identification of these will only allow a diagnosis of taeniasis. *E. granulosus* segments are very tiny and the only practical means of diagnosis is by arecoline purging; this is discussed later. Segments of the larger tapeworms have to be distinguished from *Dipylidium caninum, Diplopylidium* spp., *Mesocestoides* spp., and *Joyeuxiella* spp. This is easy because of the characteristic uterus and eggs. However, differentiating the various large *Taenia* spp. from one another is not so simple. The most commonly used criteria are hook sizes (especially the large hooks), the number of uterine branches, appearance of the genital atrium, the relationship of the cirrus to the excretory canals, the presence or absence of a vaginal sphincter and the distribution of the testes. For many of these characteristics to be determined accurately segments must be stained or even histologically sectioned. A detailed consideration of the taxonomy and identification of members of this group is outside the scope of this review, and the reader is referred to ABULADZE (1964), VERSTER (1969), and BEVERIDGE and GREGORY (1976).

The adult tapeworms are of little significance to the definitive host. As with *Mesocestoides* spp. a variety of mild disorders or alterations in appetite have been ascribed to them. Of more significance are the larval stages occurring in both man and domesticated animals. These can be important for two reasons, firstly because of disturbances to the health of the individual, and secondly because of economic losses due to downgrading or rejection of carcass meat and offal. The reader wanting more detailed descriptions of pathogenesis of infection with larval cestodes is referred to SLAIS (1970), SMYTH and HEATH (1970), and ARUNDEL (1972).

Table 1. The most prevalent members of the family Taeniidae in domesticated animals

Adult worm	Definitive host[a]	Intermdiate host(s)[a]	Type of larval stage	Preferred site of larva	Name of larva	Geographical distribution
Taenia hydatigena	Dog	Sheep, goat, pig	Cysticercus	Liver, peritoneal cavity	*Cysticercus tenuicollis*	Cosmopolitan
T. ovis	Dog	Sheep, goat	Cysticercus	Striated muscle	*C. ovis*	Cosmopolitan
T. pisiformis	Dog	Rabbit, hare	Cysticercus	Liver, peritoneal cavity	*C. pisiformis*	Cosmopolitan
T. saginata	Man	Cattle	Cysticercus	Striated muscle	*C. bovis*	Cosmopolitan
T. solium	Man	Pig, man	Cysticercus	Striated muscle, brain	*C. cellulosae*	Cosmopolitan
T. taeniaeformis	Cat	Rat, mouse	Strobilocercus	Liver	*C. fasciolaris*	Cosmopolitan
Multiceps serialis	Dog	Rabbit, hare	Coenurus	Subcutaneous, fascial planes	*Coenurus serialis*	Cosmopolitan
Multiceps multiceps	Dog	Sheep, goat, cattle	Coenurus	Muscle, brain	*C. cerebralis*	Cosmopolitan
Echinococcus granulosus	Dog	Sheep, goat, pig, cattle, horse, man, and other mammals depending upon parasite strain	Hydatid (unilocular)	Liver, lung	Hydatid	Cosmopolitan
E. multilocularis	Dog	Microtine rodents	Hydatid (multilocular)	Liver	Hydatid	Northern hemisphere, mainly holarctic
E. vogeli	Dog	Paca (*Cuniculus paca*)	Hydatid (polycystic)	Liver, lung	Hydatid	Central and South America

[a] Only the major domesticated animal host is given where applicable. Many of these parasites utilise wild carnivores, omnivores or herbivores as hosts

It is impossible to cover all species which have been found in domesticated animals, and worms considered in some texts as species are almost certainly synonymous. The major parasites and their various hosts and larval stages are listed in Table 1.

a) *Taenia hydatigena*

The strobilate stage of this parasite grows up to 2 m in length in the dog. The larval stage, commonly known as the "false hydatid," is called *Cysticercus tenuicollis* because of the long neck of the bladder, and it grows up to the size of a hen's egg. It is commonly found in sheep, goats, pigs, and cattle. Activated oncospheres migrate from the intestine to the liver where the young larvae grow and migrate for 2–4 weeks and may reach a size of 0.5 cm. After this they leave the liver via its serosal surface and complete their development in the peritoneal cavity, usually attached to the mesentery. Most damage is caused by the young migrating cysticerci in the liver. They cause extensive tissue destruction leaving large haemorrhagic tracts in their wake. Massive infection can cause death at this stage, or can trigger off "black disease" due to *Clostridium novyii,* especially in sheep. More commonly the lesions resolve, but residual fibrosis may result in rejection of livers for human consumption. The larva matures in 7–10 weeks and can survive for some years when fully developed.

b) *Taenia ovis*

The strobilate stage of this parasite grows up to 2 m in length in the dog. A very closely related, if not identical, parasite called *T. krabbei* utilises various deer as intermediate hosts in the northern hemisphere. The larvae develop in striated muscle anywhere in the body of sheep and goats. The so-called predilection sites are the heart, diaphragm, and masseter muscles and these organs are often searched during meat inspection after slaughter (SWEATMAN and WILLIAMS 1963). Certainly in heavy infections these organs are almost invariably infected, but in our experience cysticerci in light infections can occur in other parts of the body without infection of the predilection sites. The condition in sheep is known as "sheep measles." *Cysticercus ovis* normally grows to the size of a small pea and is mature 7–8 weeks after infection. However, the parasite leads a very precarious existence in this host and the majority of larvae are destroyed by the host reaction forming a caseous, later calcified, nodule. The rapidity with which lambs destroy larvae is highlighted by the extreme measures, such as blanket corticosteroid treatment, which have to be employed to obtain large numbers of cysticerci for experimental purposes (COMAN and RICKARD 1975). The parasite causes little harm to the animal and its major significance is the loss of meat due to rejection at the abattoir. Such rejection is based purely on aesthetic grounds as the parasite is not harmful to man.

c) *Taenia pisiformis*

The adult tapeworm in the dog grows to about 1.5 m in length. The cysticerci are about the size of a pea, and have a very similar course of infection and pathogenesis in rabbits and hares as does *T. hydatigena* in sheep. It has been used extensively as an experimental model.

d) *Taenia saginata (Taeniarynchus saginatus)*

The strobilate stage in man grows to 10 m in length and is of little pathogenic significance. It is unique amongst the Taeniidae in that it has an unarmed rostellum. The larval stage, *Cysticercus bovis,* causes "beef measles" in cattle. Like *C. ovis, C. bovis* is found in striated muscle and is often described as having similar predilection sites. However, as with *C. ovis* these sites are not a reliable guide in light infections. The larva and the host reaction to it are very much like *C. ovis* in sheep, and are described in detail by SLAIS (1970). It is of little pathogenic significance in cattle, but is obviously of public health significance because of its infectivity for man. In some parts of the world, e.g. East Africa and the Middle East, the parasite is extremely common; this is particularly related to the consumption of beef in an undercooked state. In countries where sanitation is good, the parasite is much less common. However, certain agricultural practices such as feedlot feeding of cattle where feed can be contaminated with human faeces if poor hygiene is observed (MCANINCH 1974; SLONKA et al. 1978) or the use of sewage for irrigation or fertilization of pastures grazed by cattle (GREENBERG and DEAN 1958; RICKARD and ADOLPH 1977; ARUNDEL and ADOLPH 1980) can result in high infection rates. Cattle develop very high levels of immunity to reinfection with *C. bovis* and immunisation has shown some promise in controlling infection in a sewage irrigation situation (RICKARD et al. 1981). SLAIS and MANN (1976) have reported prenatal infection of calves in an area of East Africa with a high endemic rate of infection.

e) *Taenia solium*

The strobilate stage in the small intestine of man grows to 8 m in length and has an armed rostellum. It is of little pathogenic significance itself. The larval stage, *Cysticercus cellulosae,* occurs in pigs, mainly in striated muscle causing "pork measles." However, cysticerci are often found in other organs including the brain. The cysticerci take about 10 weeks to become infective in pigs, and degenerated or calcified cysts are not as frequent as with *C. bovis* and *C. ovis*. There is usually little clinical evidence of infection. The major importance of the parasite is its public health risk because man can become infected with the larval stage of this parasite, thereby serving as both definitive and intermediate host. The source of infection is probably mostly faecal contamination from other infected persons, although self-infection from eggs released into the upper digestive tract or ingested due to poor personal hygiene are possible routes. The cysts locate most commonly in the subcutaneous tissues, muscle and brain, but any organ can be infected. Cysticerci in the brain tend to be on the surface and it is the tissue reaction to degenerating cysts that produces major clinical signs. Where *T. solium* infection is endemic, cysticercosis occurs not uncommonly in dogs. Cerebral cysticercosis in dogs can cause marked behavioural disorders. Cysticerci are killed in pork by adequate freezing or cooking.

f) *Taenia taeniaeformis*

The strobilate stage in cats grows to about 60 cm in length. This parasite has quite a distinct appearance because of its serrated appearance and the absence of a neck. It is of little pathological significance in cats, and the strobilocercus larval stage, *Cysticercus fasciolaris*, is found commonly in mice, rats, and other rodents. It has been used very extensively as a laboratory model.

g) *Taenia serialis (Multiceps serialis)*

This parasite grows to about 80 cm in the small intestine of the dog, and unlike most of the other *Taenia* spp. it is quite common to find large numbers of worms present. This is because the larval stage is a coenurus, *Coenurus serialis*, and each cyst can contain many scoleces. *C. serialis* is found in the subcutaneous and intermuscular connective tissue of rabbits, hares, and other lagomorphs, where it commonly grows to the size of a hen's egg or bigger.

h) *Taenia multiceps (Multiceps multiceps)*

This parasite is very similar to *T. serialis* and there have been suggestions that they are synonymous and that differences in host range may be strain variations. However, VERSTER (1969) considers them distinct species. The larval stage, *Coenurus cerebralis*, occurs most frequently in sheep, goats, and other ruminants, commonly in the central nervous system, and can cause serious neurological disturbances. "Gid" or "sturdy" are common names given to infection with this parasite, but care must be taken to distinguish it from other diseases causing localising signs such as listeriosis, abscesses, and plant poisonings. Coenuri may also occur in other parts of the body such as muscle and internal organs.

i) *Echinococcus granulosus*

This tiny parasite in the small intestine of the dog grows to only 0.5 cm in length and consists typically of three to four segments. The worm lives with its scolex buried deep in the crypts and a heavy infection with this parasite can superficially resemble intestinal villi. It is found in most parts of the world and is being reported in countries previously thought to be free from infection (MATOSSIAN et al. 1977). The hydatid cyst occurs in a wide variety of mammals, but in most circumstances sheep are probably the most important intermediate host for perpetuation of the life cycle. However, in certain localities other animals may be more important. Speciation in *Echinococcus* is a taxonomic headache because there seem to be a number of "strains" of the parasite. These have sometimes been accorded subspecific status, e.g. *E. granulosus granulosus* for the sheep-dog cycle and *E. granulosus equinus* for the horse-dog cycle. Morphological differences are often not apparent but there appear to be very real biological differences, for instance, in infectivity for different hosts (HATCH and SMYTH 1975; THOMPSON 1978), behaviour in in vitro culture (SMYTH and DAVIES 1974a), and in chemical composition and metabolism (LERICHE and SEWELL 1978; MCMANUS and SMYTH 1978; KUMRATILAKE et al. 1979).

Infection of the dog with the adult *E. granulosus* is of no pathological significance. The larval stages in domesticated animals, even in heavy infections, do not usually cause discernible harm. The most common sites of infection are the liver and lungs, but many other organs have been reported as being infected. Where infection is common, there can be considerable economic impact due to wastage of infected organs.

The major importance of this parasite is in its infectivity for man. Cysts containing several litres of fluid can develop and multiple surgery is often required to remove infection completely. Death from anaphylaxis following accidental rupture of a cyst can occur. Undoubtedly the domesticated dog and domesticated herbivores are most important in maintaining infection in man, but sylvatic cycles occur in many parts of the world, e.g. dingoes and wallabies in Australia (COMAN 1972) and deer and coyotes in the United States (BRUNETTI and ROSEN 1970; LIU et al. 1970). Because of the variations in host range amongst "strains" of *E. granulosus*, the importance of the sylvatic cycles in infection of man is difficult to assess. One example of this is the relatively benign nature of infection with the Canadian strain of *E. granulosus* in man (WILSON et al. 1968).

Some laboratory animals, e.g. mice, rabbits, and the Mongolian jird, have been useful as laboratory hosts for secondary echinococcosis induced by the intraperitoneal inoculation of protoscoleces (DE COOMAN and DE RYCKE 1970; HEATH 1970; THOMPSON 1976b). Significant progress has been made in *in vitro* cultivation of both the strobilate (SMYTH and DAVIES 1974b) and cystic (HEATH and LAWRENCE 1976) stages although complete development has not been achieved in either case.

j) *Echinococcus multilocularis*

The strobilate stage of this parasite occurs most commonly in wild carnivores, but also develops in the domesticated dog. The intermediate hosts are microtine rodents. The parasite is holarctic in distribution, but cases have been reported in southern Europe, Turkey and as far south as Iran, the United States and recently in India (MATOSSIAN et al. 1977; AIKAT et al. 1978). This parasite causes multilocular (alveolar) hydatid disease in man. Unlike the unilocular cyst of *E. granulosus* this parasite is infiltrative, without a host-tissue barrier. Infection starts in the liver and the parasite buds off new cysts exogeneously and develops a progressively enlarging necrotic cavity internally. It can metastasise to other organs in the body.

k) *Echinococcus vogeli*

This parasite, initially described by RAUSCH and BERNSTEIN (1972), has recently been shown to infect man (D'ALESSANDRO et al. 1979). The strobilate stage occurs in bush dogs (*Speothus venaticus*) in Central and South America and, at least experimentally, develops in domesticated dogs. The larval stage is different to *E. multilocularis* in that it is polycystic with clusters of quite large cysts in either the liver or lungs, and there is no formation of a necrotic cavity (D'ALESSANDRO et al. 1979). The main intermediate host is believed to be the paca, but it has also been found in the spiny rat.

3. Family Anoplocephalidae

This family contains the common tapeworms of horses and ruminants. They are often large and the proglottids are usually wider than long. The scolex is without hooks or rostellum and has four prominent suckers. Genital pores are lateral and there may be one or two sets of genitalia per segment. The uterus assumes a variety of forms and may persist or be replaced by egg capsules or par-uterine organs. Eggs have three envelopes and the innermost chitinous membrane surrounding the oncosphere may have two projections forming the pyriform apparatus. The intermediate hosts are usually pasture mites of the family Oribatidae or Psocids (bark lice, dust lice, book lice). The larval stage is a cysticercoid.

a) Anoplocephalis of Horses

Anoplocephala perfoliata is the most common tapeworm in horses and is cosmopolitan. It usually attaches in the posterior small intestine or caecum, often clustered around the ileocaecal junction. It is normally about 4 cm in length and about 1.5 cm wide and the body is thick and fleshy. Its shape is that of a long triangle with the scolex at the apex. The suckers have posterior projections called lappets. Eggs are 65–80 µm in size and contain a pyriform apparatus. *A. magna* is less common in most areas but heavy infestations can occur. It is usually found in the small intestine and is a large tapeworm measuring up to 80 cm long and 2.5 cm wide. The suckers have no lappets and the pyriform apparatus in the egg is poorly developed. *Paranoplocephala mamillana* is the least common. It is usually in the anterior intestine and is a smaller worm up to 4 cm long. The eggs are like *A. perfoliata* with a well-developed pyriform apparatus.

Moniezia pallida resembles *M. benedeni* in cattle and has been reported in the small intestine of horses in Africa and Angola. It grows up to 4 m in length.

All species have similar life cycles and a variety of oribatid mites act as intermediate hosts. The cysticercoid develops in 2–4 months and horses are infected by accidental ingestion of mites when feeding. The adult tapeworms are mature 6–10 weeks later. Reports of pathogenicity vary. *A. magna* is generally regarded as the most harmful in heavy infections and can cause catarrhal or haemorrhagic enteritis. *A. perfoliata* may cause ulceration and the formation of fibrous tissue around the ileocaecal junction. This can cause constriction of the orifice and rupture of the bowel has been known to occur. *P. mamillana* is rarely harmful and *M. pallida* is not known to be pathogenic.

The degree of infection is associated with availability of large numbers of mites on the pasture and these are most common in spring and summer. The mites prefer well-established pasture with a thick "mat," and one method of control is to reseed the area.

b) Anoplocephalids of Ruminants

Genera of anoplocephalids found in domesticated ruminants include *Moniezia, Thysanosoma, Helictometra, Avitellina,* and *Stilesia.*

Moniezia expansa and *M. benedeni* are cosmopolitan and the most common of this group in calves and lambs. *M. expansa* tends to be more common in lambs and *M. benedeni* more common in calves, although both readily cross-infect. They grow to 4–6 m in length and 1.5–2.5 cm in width. The segments are broad laterally and narrow anteroposteriorily and have paired genitalia. The eggs measure 65–75 µm with a well-developed pyriform apparatus. The life cycles involve oribatid mites, and up to two dozen species have been experimentally infected although many of these may not act as intermediate hosts in natural transmission. The cysticercoid develops in mites within 8–30 weeks depending upon the temperature (STUNKARD 1937) and adult worms mature in calves and lambs after about 6 weeks. These tapeworms occur chiefly in lambs and calves under 6 months of age. After this time, burdens tend to be shed spontaneously and the animal is then resistant to further infection.

Thysanosoma actinioides, the "fringed tapeworm," occurs in the bile ducts, pancreatic ducts and small intestine of sheep, cattle and goats in North and South America. In North America its distribution is limited to the western States. It is smaller and more delicate than *Moniezia* spp., measuring up to 30 cm long by 8 mm wide, and the posterior margin of each segment has a conspicuous "fringe" of papillae. The eggs lack a pyriform apparatus and become enclosed in numerous par-uterine organs. The life cycle of this parasite is incompletely known but psocids have been experimentally infected (ALLEN 1959).

Helictometra (Thysaniezia) giardi is found in the small intestine of sheep, goats, and cattle and is cosmopolitan. It grows to 200 cm and the egg has no pyriform apparatus. The intermediate hosts are probably oribatid mites. Several species of *Avitellina* occur in the intestine of ruminants in Europe, Asia, and Africa. They are long (3 m) delicate worms and the eggs are contained in a paruterine organ. The intermediate hosts are probably psocids (SOULSBY 1968).

Stilesia hepatica is found in the bile duct of ruminants in Africa and *Stilesia globipunctata* in the small intestine of sheep and goats in Europe, parts of the Middle East and India.

There is considerable debate concerning the pathogenesis of infection with tapeworms in ruminants. Mechanisms by which these tapeworms could harm the host are by competing for nutrients, by excreting toxic metabolites or by their sheer physical bulk causing interference with gut function. They are usually thought by farmers to be important, especially *Moniezia* spp., because of the masses of worms that can be found in calves and lambs. REID and ARMOUR (1978) concluded that these parasites were of little economic importance in Britain. Several eastern European workers have recently published papers implicating *Moniezia* spp., *Helictometra* spp., and *Avitellina* spp. as having a direct effect on productivity in sheep, as well as indirectly predisposing to enterotoxaemia (EFNER 1974; VIBE 1976; RADIONOV and KEMEL'BEKOV 1977) although such effects are difficult to establish experimentally. STAMPA (1967) obtained good weight gain responses in lambs treated with niclosamide, more so in arid areas where other gastrointestinal nematodes were less of a problem. *Stilesia globipunctata* has been incriminated as causing more severe pathology, even death, in sheep and goats (AMJADI 1971), and causes the formation of large nodules at its attachment site in the intestine.

Whatever the pros and cons of pathogenicity of these worms, there is usually considerable demand for their removal by chemotherapy when heavy burdens are present in calves and lambs.

4. Family Davaineidae

These are small- or medium-sized tapeworms with a retractible rostellum armed with numerous hammer-shaped hooks and the suckers also have spines at their margins. The segments contain a single set of reproductive organs and the uterus either persists as a sac or the eggs become surrounded by egg capsules or a paruterine organ. All the members of veterinary importance are in domesticated poultry.

Davainea proglottina in chickens is a tiny tapeworm and usually embedded deep between the villi. Being only 4 mm in length and having four to nine segments it can easily be overlooked during casual inspection at postmortem examination. Eggs are passed out in egg capsules and snails act as the intermediate hosts. Cysticercoids develop in snails in about 3 weeks and adult worms develop in chickens in about 2 weeks. The parasite is cosmopolitan. *Davainea meleagridis,* a somewhat larger parasite consisting of 17–22 segments, has been reported in turkeys from the eastern United States (SOULSBY 1965). *D. proglottina* is the most pathogenic of poultry tapeworms causing necrosis and haemorrhagic inflammation of the upper small intestine. The intestinal wall becomes thickened, and although haemorrhagic enteritis may cause death of the bird, a chronic, debilitating disease is more common. The most critical aspect of infection with this parasite is in diagnosis, where large numbers of worms can be overlooked because of their small size. Because a snail intermediate host is required the parasite is less frequent in intensive rearing systems.

Members of the genus *Raillietina* are larger tapeworms, up to 25 cm long with many segments, and the eggs are released in groups rather than individually. There are three common, cosmopolitan species, *R. cesticillus, R. tetragona,* and *R. echinobothrida. R. echinobothrida* utilises beetles as intermediate host whereas cysticercoids of the other two genera are found in ants. *R. echinobothrida* is the most overt pathogen of the group, causing the formation of nodules visible from the peritoneal surface at their site of attachment to the intestinal wall. Emaciation and diarrhoea can occur. BOTERO and REID (1969) were unable to detect any effect of *R. cesticillus* infection in White Rock male poultry and NADAKAL et al. (1971) had similar results with *R. tetragona* infection in White Rock and Desi birds. However, the latter authors found that White Leghorn and White Leghorn X Desi birds suffered considerable weight loss and differences between the breeds of birds were statistically significant at the 1% level. Breed variation and size of infection must obviously be taken into account in experiments assessing pathogenicity.

Cotugnia digonopora occurs in the small intestine of fowls in Asia. It grows to 10 cm in length and eggs are released in single egg capsules. CHAND (1970) showed that *Monomorium (Holcomyrmet) scabriceps* can act as intermediate host. SOULSBY (1965) states that heavy infection can produce diarrhoea and depression of growth.

5. Family Dilepididae

These are small- to medium-sized worms occurring in birds and mammals. The scolex has an armed rostellum and the suckers are usually unarmed. Genitalia are single or double and the uterus often breaks down to form egg capsules or eggs become surrounded with a par-uterine organ. The larval stage is a cysticercoid.

a) Dilepidids in Domestic Birds

Amoebotaenia sphenoides occurs in the small intestine of the fowl and is cosmopolitan in distribution. It is a tiny worm only 2–3 mm in length, roughly triangular in shape and has 20 or so segments. No egg capsules are formed. Earthworms act as intermediate hosts and cysticercoids develop in them within 2 weeks. Tapeworms mature in the fowl approximately 4 weeks after the cysticercoid is ingested. The parasite is generally not harmful but CHANDRA and SINGH (1972) reported catarrhal and haemorrhagic enteritis in experimentally infected chickens, with two of nine birds dying from the infection.

Choanotaenia infundibulum is much larger than *A. sphenoides,* growing upward of 20 cm in length, and is cosmopolitan. The proglottids are bell shaped and eggs are not encapsulated. The cysticercoid develops in houseflies and beetles in 3–8 weeks and mature worms develop in chickens 3 weeks after infection. This worm is not usually associated with any harmful effects.

Metroliasthes lucida occurs in domesticated poultry but is most common in turkeys in Europe, India, Africa, North and South America, and Australia. It grows to 20 cm in length, and in gravid segments the eggs become enclosed in a par-uterine organ. The cysticercoid develops in grasshoppers in 2–6 weeks depending upon temperature, and the adult worm grows to maturity in about 3 weeks. It is of little pathological significance except in very large numbers.

b) Dilepidids in Domestic Animals

Dipylidium caninum is the most common tapeworm found in the small intestine of dogs and cats throughout the world. It grows to 50 cm in length and has an armed rostellum with four to seven rows of characteristic “rose-thorn” hooks. The gravid segments are “melon-seed” shaped and are often pinkish in colour when passed in the faeces. The genitalia are paired and eggs become encapsulated in groups of 20–30 in egg capsules. Segments in freshly passed faeces are highly motile and readily seen macroscopically. They are readily differentiated from segments of *Taenia* spp., and *Mesocestoides* spp., or from fly maggots by their characteristic shape, double genitalia and identification of the egg capsules. Dried segments can be cut and the eggs or egg capsules gently expressed or they can be rehydrated in water and examined. The cysticercoids develop in fleas commonly parasitising dogs and cats and in the dog louse, *Trichodectes canis*. Fleas become infected at the larval stage and the cysticercoid is mature in about 3 weeks when the flea is adult. The adult worm matures in dogs and cats within 6 weeks. There are many other species of this genus described and for details of these the reader should consult WARDLE and MCLEOD (1952).

Two other genera of this family also occur in cats and dogs. *Joyeuxiella* spp. are found in Europe, Africa, and Asia. They are smaller in size and the egg capsules contain only single eggs. The cysticercoids are found in reptiles, but SOULSBY (1965) points out that these may be acting as transport hosts only. *Diplopylidium* spp. are also smaller worms and the eggs are single in capsules. The many species of this genus are detailed in WARDLE and MCLEOD (1952). Reptiles act as intermediate hosts.

Dilepidid tapeworms in dogs and cats are generally of little pathological significance. Almost all animals become infected and may carry heavy burdens of worms. Most of the vague symptoms attributed to other tapeworms have been described in infections with these parasites. The segments of *D. caninum* are very motile and can escape from the anus of their own volition. The resultant anal pruritis may cause behavioural abnormalities like "scooting" or tail biting. The segments present an aesthetic problem and owners generally request that animals are treated. Children can become infected with *D. caninum* by accidentally swallowing fleas.

6. Family Hymenolepididae

These are small- to medium-sized tapeworms and most genera have a cone-shaped rostellum armed with a single row of hooks. There is a single set of genitalia per segment and seldom more than three testes. The larval stage is a cysticercoid.

a) Genus *Hymenolepis*

Species of *Hymenolepis* occur in birds and mammals.

Hymenolepis (Drepanidotaenia) lanceolata is found worldwide in the small intestine of ducks and geese. It grows to 13 cm in length and 1.8 cm in width, and is probably transmitted by the ingestion of cysticercoids in crustacea such as *Cyclops*. It can be quite harmful in heavy infestations. *H. carioca* and *H. cantaniana* are common in fowls and are transmitted as cysticercoids in dung beetles. They can be found in very large numbers but are relatively harmless.

Hymenolepis diminuta and *H. nana* occur in rats and mice, and are worthy of mention because of their frequent use as laboratory models, and because of the frequent occurrence of *H. nana* in man. *H. diminuta* is up to 60 cm long and the scolex is unarmed. It has a variety of intermediate hosts such as moths, earwigs, fleas, beetles, cockroaches, and millipedes. It has occasionally been recorded in man. *H. nana* is the dwarf tapeworm and grows to 4 cm in length. It is commonly found in man and is unusual amongst the cestodes in that the cysticercoid and adult stages both occur in the same mammalian host. Fleas and beetles can act as intermediate hosts, but direct infection is undoubtedly more common. The rat, mouse or man ingest the eggs and the hatched and activated oncospheres penetrate the intestinal villi, where the cysticercoids develop. The mature cysticercoid emerges into the gut lumen, evaginates, attaches, and develops into the adult worm. Although humans can become infected from rats and mice, direct human to human transmission is probably more important as a source of infection. Another interesting feature is that the host becomes immune to infection with the cysticercoid, and this is a major reason why this parasite has been used frequently for studies on immunity to cestodes.

b) Genus *Fimbriaria*

Fimbriaria fasciolaris is cosmopolitan in the intestine of fowls, ducks, and geese. It is unusual in that it not only possesses a scolex, but also has a folded expansion of the anterior chain of proglottids called a pseudoscolex which assists it to attach to the gut wall. Also, the external segmentation does not correspond with the internal organs. It grows up to 50 cm long and 1 cm wide and the cysticercoids develop in crustacea such as *Cyclops* and *Diaptomus*. It is apparently of little pathological significance.

C. Chemotherapeutic Agents

I. Arecoline

Arecoline is an alkaloid obtained from the dried seeds of the betel nut palm (*Areca catechu*). The seeds of this palm have been chewed for hundreds of years and have useful cestocidal activity. The powdered seed was used as areca BVetC[1] for many years in animal and human medicine, but deterioration quickly takes place once the seed is ground. This, and the variation in alkaloid content between seeds, led to variable results and areca is no longer used. Arecoline itself is rather unstable and is used as the hydrobromide (Fig. 1), acetarsol or carboxy phenylstibonate derivatives as a taeniacide in dogs and cats.

Fig. 1. Arecoline hydrobromide

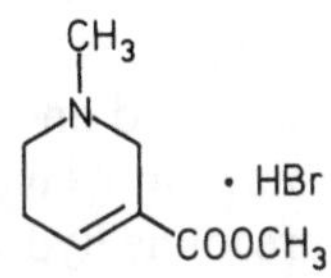

1. Arecoline Hydrobromide

a) Efficacy

This salt (Hydarex, Parke Davis & Co.) is a fine white slightly bitter powder, soluble in water and in alcohol. Solutions should be kept in well-stoppered containers protected from light. The efficacy of arecoline hydrobromide against cestodes of the dog was first reported by LENTZ (1921) and was confirmed in critical work by HALL and SHILLINGER (1923) and ROSS (1924). KORKHAUS (1933) and REINHARDT (1933) also obtained good results in larger numbers of dogs and BATHAM (1946), in more detailed work, reported a high level of efficiency against *Taenia ovis*, *T. hydatigena*, *T. pisiformis*, *T. serialis*, and *Dipylidium caninum*. FORBES (1964a) showed that efficiency was related to purgation and that with a satisfactory purge, 90%–100% of *Taenia*. spp. and 90%–99% of *Echinococcus granulosus* worms were removed from infected dogs.

BATHAM (1946) had noted that some *E. granulosus* persisted in dogs in spite of repeated treatments and FORBES (1964a) reported that four of seven dogs remained infected even though he obtained 99% efficiency. The difficulty of freeing dogs from infection with *E. granulosus* was further examined by GEMMELL (1968), who infected 30 dogs with 50,000 protoscolices each and then treated them every 2nd day using arecoline hydrobromide at 3.5 mg/kg in sugar solution. Examination of the faeces collected 6 h after each treatment showed that 20% of the dogs

1 British Veterinary Codex

were freed of infection after one treatment, 57% were still infected after three treatments and one dog required nine treatments to eliminate the infection. GEMMELL (1968) drew attention to the fact that not only did it require many treatments to eliminate infection in some dogs, but failure to find *E. granulosus* in faeces following two consecutive treatments at 48-h intervals did not imply freedom from infection. TREJOS et al. (1975) did not find *E. granulosus* in the faeces of 9 of 18 dogs treated with arecoline hydrobromide and later found at autopsy to have worms in their intestine. Thus arecoline was effective as a diagnostic agent in only half of the animals. This failure in diagnosis, added to the failure to remove infection completely and so allow continuing contamination, is a limitation of this drug in hydatid control schemes.

Best results are obtained if dogs are dosed when their stomachs are empty and so dogs should not be fed for some hours before dosing. Preliminary treatment should be given to constipated dogs and bones should not be fed for 48 h prior to treatment. Arecoline hydrobromide is bitter and dogs appear to dislike its taste. FERRO (1948) recommended the use of sucrose and FORBES and WHITTEN (1961) investigated various formulations including sugar coating, aqueous solutions with varying concentrations of sucrose some with added saccharine, lozenges with 20% or 60% glycerine or the use of gelatine capsules. The drug was also given as an aqueous solution or as tablets. In tests in 1,500 dogs, it was shown that the action of arecoline was more rapid and more reliable when given in solution and that there was no advantage in using dose rates above 1 mg/kg. The recommended solution was 1.5% arecoline hydrobromide and 15% sucrose and this gave a median purgation time of 30 min with only 19% failing to purge within 2 h. When used in this manner the drug acts for up to 2 h and if the worms are not removed within this time they may reattach.

b) Mode of Action

Arecoline hydrobromide acts by paralysing the worms and by causing purgation which removes the paralysed worms from the intestine. If purgation does not occur then efficiency is less (BATHAM 1946; FORBES 1964a). Efficacy is therefore directly related to purgation and, in various trials, it was found that there was no increase in the proportion of dogs that purged when the dose rate was increased from 1–2 mg/kg to 4 mg/kg (GEMMELL 1958a; FORBES and WHITTEN 1961; JACKSON and ARUNDEL 1971). Under field conditions of mass dosing 75%–80% of dogs will purge, and worms may also be voided in vomit (FORBES 1964a).

FORBES (1961) reported that the use of arecoline hydrobromide enemas using 0.5 mg/kg 45 min after oral dosing with 2 mg/kg increased the purgation rate, but while enemas of arecoline or soap may increase the number of dogs purging they do not aid in the removal of worms (GEMMELL 1968). Injection of arecoline causes purgation but not worm removal (BATHAM 1946) and this is related to the efficiency with which the drug is destroyed by the liver (BELL and BENNETT 1970).

c) Toxicity and Pharmacodynamics

Arecoline has strong parasympathomimetic actions. When given parenterally it causes contractions of most involuntary muscles particularly those of the gastrointestinal tract, uterus and bronchioles and also causes constriction of the pupil, slowing of the heart rate and the production of excessive salivary flow.

When given orally at doses of 1–3.5 mg/kg very few dogs show signs of toxicity other than vomiting and persistent diarrhoea. This latter sign, although not very distressing to the dog, is not welcomed by the owner who has to transport a dog after dosing. With larger doses the incidence of vomiting is increased and convulsions may occur in some dogs. Ross (1924) found that the minimal lethal dose was eight times the therapeutic dose and BATHAM (1946) found a proportion of dogs was severely affected at a dose of 7 mg/kg. Doses as high as 44 mg/kg have been tested in some dogs and while they showed extreme discomfort and some convulsions, there were no deaths (ROBERSON 1977). Whether toxicity occurs and the degree of the toxic reaction depends somewhat on the method of administration. Enteric-coated tablets result in absorption to the portal circulation and thence to the liver, where the drug is rapidly inactivated (BELL and BENNETT 1970), giving minimal toxic reaction. FORBES (1946b) found that toxic reactions such as inhibition of the heart and lungs occurred more commonly if the drug was given as a solution and concluded that these signs are caused by absorption from the mouth and pharynx. When given at five to ten times the normal dose, absorption from the oesophagus, stomach, and small or large intestine did not cause cardiac or pulmonary symptoms. The action of arecoline hydrobromide in causing purgation is a local effect resulting from the cholinergic action on gastrointestinal muscle and glands (FORBES 1971). Arecoline hydrobromide should not be given to pregnant bitches or to pups less than 6 months of age.

Although there is an acceptable safety margin when therapeutic doses of 1–3.5 mg/kg are used, some dogs may collapse and convulsions and unconsciousness may follow. Atropine sulphate, 0.044 mg/kg, is the pharmacological antidote and does not interfere with the effect on the worm (LINK 1965).

d) Use as Diagnostic Agent

Arecoline has now been superseded as a treatment for tapeworms but it remains as a useful tool in control schemes for the diagnosis of cestode infections in dogs. It is not accurate enough for use as a test for individual dogs – see earlier discussion of work by GEMMELL (1968) and TREJOS et al. (1975) – but, if used on a group of dogs on a farm, it gives valuable information as to whether dogs on that farm are infected and if so, that they have been fed improperly. *E. granulosus* is usually found in the duodenum and if a diagnosis is to be made, it is the duodenal purge that should be collected and examined. Some dogs will only pass rectal or colonic material after dosing but unless duodenal faeces are passed, purgation is not satisfactory. Dogs that fail to purge within 45–60 min may do so if allowed to run free or are given walking exercise on a lead. Alternatively they may be given a further half dose.

Arecoline hydrobromide is not recommended for cats as it is believed that the excessive outpouring of mucus that occurs may cause suffocation. BRANDER and PUGH (1971) could find no scientific corroboration for this statement.

2. Arecoline Acetarsol

a) Chemistry

This complex (Cestarsol, May and Baker; Tenoban, Wellcome; Nemural, Winthrop Laboratories) is the arecoline salt of 3-acetamido-4-hydroxyphenyl-arsonic acid. It is a white tasteless odourless powder, soluble in water and alcohol, but is unstable in solution.

b) Efficacy

Early reports by STETTER (1933) and BEYDEMULLER (1934) showed satisfactory results in both cats and dogs while POPESCU and MIRONESCU (1934) established the therapeutic dose rate (5 mg/kg) and reported on its efficacy in dogs. ENZIE et al. (1957) examined the compound in two critical trials in dogs and obtained inconsistent results against *D. caninum* but better results against *Taenia* spp. Two treatments were required to remove all *Taenia* spp. and the drug failed if purgation did not take place. SINGH and RAO (1967) obtained 100% efficiency in two cats and 71% in another cat infected with *T. taeniaeformis*.

The only work on the efficacy of this compound against *E. granulosus* appears to be that of ROSS (1936), who obtained 89% efficiency in one dog. Further work on this compound was not carried out presumably because of the satisfactory results obtained with the less expensive arecoline hydrobromide.

c) Mode of Action

The complex is hydrolysed in the stomach, releasing arecoline, which paralyses the worms and causes purgation.

d) Toxicity

Arecoline acetarsol is generally well tolerated, but is not recommended for puppies less than 3 months of age and cats less than 6 months of age, and should not be used in pregnant animals. Vomiting, excessive salivation, ataxia and increased respiration occasionally occur. It is usually given to dogs after a light meal (ENZIE et al. 1957) and to cats in milk some hours after a meal. Atropine sulphate is the antidote.

3. Arecoline Carboxyphenylstibonate

This derivative (Anthelin) is used at 10 mg/kg for the removal of tapeworms in dogs. It appears to have approximately the same degree of efficiency against *E. granulosus* as arecoline hydrobromide (WHITTEN 1956; MATOFF and KOLEV 1963; BLOOD et al. 1968) and is probably hydrolysed to arecoline. Like all arecoline derivatives it causes purgation which facilitates passage of the paralysed worms. Against mixed infections of *Taenia* spp. and *D. caninum*, 10 mg/kg gave 97% efficiency and cleared 8 of 10 dogs (KARTSONIS and AUSTIN 1950), while ENZIE et al. (1957) cleared 82% of *Taenia* spp. and 66% of *D. caninum* from 18 and 5 dogs respectively. The signs of toxicity include vomiting and depression and may be more severe in dogs in poor condition. It should not be used in pregnant bitches.

II. Dichlorophen

This compound, which is also called diphenthane-70 (Dicestal, May & Baker; Taeniathane, Pitman Moore Inc.), was first introduced into veterinary medicine in 1946. It was an important advance as it gave an alternative to arecoline which, although moderately effective against tapeworms including *E. granulosus*, was unpleasant to use. It has been sold as a single compound effective against cestodes other than *E. granulosus* or as a mixture with toluene (Vermiplex, Pitman Moore Inc.) to increase its spectrum to include roundworms and hookworms. Information on its chemistry, toxicity and mode of action is given in Chap. 4.

Dichlorophen has been shown to have activity against *Taenia* spp. and *D. caninum* in dogs but results have been variable and the drug cannot be relied upon to eliminate infection (Craig and Kleckner 1946; Enzie et al. 1957; Biddis 1950; Frost 1951; Henderson 1951). Many failures in practice are probably due to the destrobilating action of the drug that occurs within the recommended dose rate of 150–300 mg/kg (M. A. Gemmell 1974, personal communication). Combining dichlorophen with toluene increases its spectrum to include nematodes but does not increase the efficiency against cestodes (Blair 1949). Dichlorophen is not active against *E. granulosus* when given as a single dose or twice at 24-h intervals (Whitten 1951; Gemmell 1958 b).

In sheep the compound has limited effect against *Moniezia* spp. (Enzie et al. 1953) while its effect against *Thysanosoma* spp. is variable (Olsen 1953; Allen and Jackson 1953).

III. Di-*n*-Butyl Tin Dilaurate

A number of tin compounds have been tested and found to have some cestocidal activity since the initial work by Guthrie and Harwood (1941). The only one that has been used commercially is dibutyl tin dilaurate and this is still used occasionally in small poultry flocks and in cage birds, although it has been largely superseded by niclosamide.

a) Chemistry

Dibutyl tin dilaurate (Butynorate, Davainex, Tinostat) is a pale yellow, soft crystal or liquid with a melting point of 22°–24 °C. It is practically insoluble in water and methanol, but soluble in ether, benzene, acetone, and carbon tetrachloride.

b) Efficacy

Kerr (1952) found that doses of 150 mg/kg given orally were 100% efficient against *Raillietina* spp. and when the compound was given in the feed at 86 mg/kg and above for varying periods efficiencies of 85% or better were obtained. These results were confirmed by Edgar (1956) and Edgar and Teer (1957), who also showed that it was efficient, but somewhat erratic, against *Choanotaenia* spp. and *Davainea proglottina* whether given as a single oral dose or in medicated feed. Abou (1956) confirmed that this drug was effective against the more pathogenic tapeworm, *D. proglottina*. Doses of 500 mg/kg were needed to remove all worms.

NUGARA and REID (1962) used dibutyl tin dilaurate for the treatment of turkeys infected with *R. georgiensis* and obtained 85% efficiency when turkeys were given 0.07% in the feed for 5 days. The usual dose rate recommended is 100–125 mg/kg given in the feed.

c) Toxicity

When used commercially it had a satisfactory therapeutic ratio. Doses of 1,000 mg/kg caused some diarrhoea (SAWADA 1963) and deaths (KERR 1952). Levels of 0.16% in feed for 5 weeks or 0.01% and 0.02% for 13 weeks did not cause toxic effects (KERR 1952). Other workers (EDGAR 1956; GRABER and GRAS 1962; WILSON et al. 1967; FRY and WILSON 1967) found that a temporary drop in egg production occurred 7–10 days after treatment, that some yolk mottling was seen and that losses could occur if the drug was given to emaciated, heavily parasitised birds.

IV. Niclosamide

Information on the chemistry, pharmacokinetics, toxicity, and mode of action of niclosamide is given in Chap. 4.

a) Efficacy

Niclosamide is used throughout the world to control tapeworms in dogs, cats, sheep, cattle, horses, poultry, and cage birds. It is also highly effective against immature paramphistomes in sheep (HORAK 1964; BORAY 1969). The preparation, Yomesan, which was marketed for use in dogs and cats, has now been withdrawn by the manufacturer and replaced by praziquantel, which is more efficient and includes *E. granulosus* in its spectrum of activity.

Niclosamide is used as the monohydrate although the piperazine salt, which is less hygroscopic than niclosamide itself and therefore more stable, is equally effective (PAGANI and AGOSTI 1969; GEMMELL et al. 1977a). In dogs, doses of 100 mg/kg or greater give high efficiency against *Taenia* spp. (FORBES 1963; GREGOR 1963; GURALP and TIGIN 1966; COX et al. 1966; POOLE et al. 1971). Occasional failures to achieve 100% efficiency have been reported but these infections were removed by a second dose. Few trials where doses less than 100 mg/kg were tested have been reported but GEMMELL et al. (1977a) obtained complete removal of *T. hydatigena* at 32 and 64 mg/kg and of *T. ovis* at 50 mg/kg, while FORBES (1963) failed to remove all *T. hydatigena* with 50 mg/kg. In widespread field usage in New Zealand where regular 6-weekly treatments of 125 mg/kg were given to several thousand dogs, excellent control of *T. hydatigena* and *T. ovis* was obtained (G. A. Thomson 1973, personal communication). Niclosamide is also effective against *T. taeniaeformis* in cats; WESCOTT (1967) obtained 100% efficiency against 3- and 6-week infections with 100 mg/kg while SINGH and RAO (1967) cleared three cats of infection with 400 mg/kg. Repeated doses of 167 mg/kg given every 3 day for four treatments cleared a single dog of *Mesocestoides corti* (SPECKMAN and WEBSTER 1975), but single doses of 160–470 mg/kg gave variable results (TODD et al. 1978).

The results against *Dipylidium caninum* are much more variable. POOLE et al. (1971) obtained 100% efficiency at doses of 110 mg/kg and higher and KURELEC and RIJAVEC (1961) cleared three dogs of infection with 100 mg/kg. However, GURALP and TIGIN (1966) found doses less than 300 mg/kg to be ineffective and SHARP et al. (1973) only obtained 18% efficiency at 157 mg/kg. ROBERSON (1976) failed to clear *D. caninum* from any of 12 dogs dosed at 154–162 mg/kg compared with 12 of 12 dogs cleared with diuredosan and 9 of 11 with bunamidine hydrochloride.

Early reports on the efficacy of niclosamide against *E. granulosus* were conflicting (for references see GEMMELL et al. 1977a) but it is now accepted that, at normal dose rates, it has low efficiency and this is not improved by micronisation (GEMMELL et al. 1977a).

In ruminants excellent results have been obtained against *Moniezia* spp., *Helictometra giardi* and *Avitellina* spp, and it is used throughout the world in those areas where tapeworms are thought to be exerting a pathogenic effect (STAMPA and TERBLANCHE 1961; NUGARA 1963; TEICHERT 1963; ZETTL 1965; HALL 1966; KATIYAR and GARG 1966; PRIETO 1971). The recommended dose rate is 50 mg/kg with a minimum dose of 1 g (STAMPA and TERBLANCHE 1961). Its action against *Thysanosoma actinioides* is less satisfactory, doses of 400–600 mg/kg being required (ALLEN et al. 1967), while its action against *Stilesia hepatica*, another bile-duct-dwelling parasite, is also poor (STAMPA and TERBLANCHE 1961).

The low pathogenicity of tapeworms in the horse is reflected by the sparse literature on therapy in these species, but SAFAEV (1972) obtained efficiencies of 99%–100% against anoplocephalids in horses of all ages when using doses of 200–300 mg/kg. Lower doses were not tried.

Niclosamide is a safe and efficient compound for use in poultry although only limited tests have been reported and work defining the optimal dose rate and the therapeutic spectrum does not appear to have been published. Medication in the feed at doses between 20 and 53 mg/kg has given good results (BOISVENUE and HENDRIX 1965), while doses over 50 mg/kg given as tablets have also been satisfactory (SAWADA 1965a, b; LUNGU et al. 1965). ABRAMS (1976) reported an outbreak of *Choanotaenia infundibulum* in a flock of 90,000 hens which was controlled by two doses of 50 mg/kg 2–3 weeks apart. It was considered that a further dose of 100 mg/kg was necessary to eliminate the infection. In ducklings BANKOV and JUPERLIEV (1965) obtained 100% efficiency against *Hymenolepis* spp. and *Dicranotaenia* spp. using 50, 60, and 80 mg/duck while TERBLANCHE (1966) obtained 100% efficiency against *Raillietina* spp. in pigeons using doses of approximately 200 mg/kg.

b) Toxicity

Niclosamide is a very safe compound. The LD_{50} in rats is not known but they tolerate doses of 5,000 mg/kg (HALL 1966), while 40 times the therapeutic dose in sheep and cattle is non-toxic except for some diarrhoea (PRIETO 1971). Normal usage in sheep and dogs may cause some transient softening of the faeces (FORBES 1963; ZETTL 1965; HALL 1966; ALLEN et al. 1967; GEMMELL et al. 1977a). GEMMELL et al. (1977a) also found that vomiting occurred in up to 34% of dogs depending on dose rate, but this did not appear to interfere with efficiency. This lack of toxicity is probably related to the very poor absorption of niclosamide (HECHT and GLOXHUBER 1960; GREGOR 1963) and because that small fraction that is absorbed is quickly metabolised to 4-aminoniclosamide, which is much less toxic than niclosamide itself (STRUFE and GONNERT 1967). The manufacturers claim that it can be used during pregnancy, lactation, and in animals with liver disorders but it should not be used simultaneously with the organophosphate nematocidal compound, naftalofos, as the combination is toxic. It would be unwise therefore to use it in combination with any organophosphate compound unless there is clear evidence that such a mixture is safe.

V. Bunamidine

Bunamidine (*N,N*-di-*n*-butyl-4-hexyloxy-1-naphthamidine) has the structural formula shown in Fig. 2. It is usually sold as the monohydrochloride but the 3-hydroxy-2-naphthoate, which is less irritant when given orally, has also been tested and is used in ruminants. Another salt, the *p*-toluenesulphonate, is also active but causes severe vomiting. This salt has not been marketed.

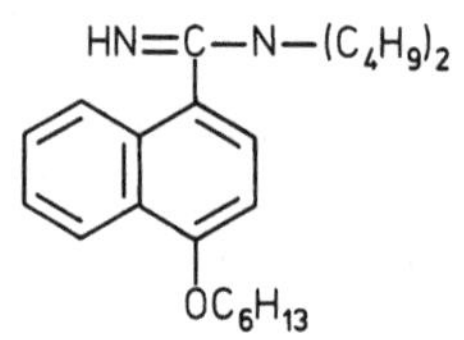

Fig. 2. Bunamidine

1. Bunamidine Hydrochloride

a) Chemistry

Bunamidine hydrochloride (Scolaban, Wellcome) is a white, odourless, crystalline solid, soluble in methanol and hot water. It is available in coated tablets formulated to disintegrate rapidly in the stomach. This is a necessary precaution to prevent transfer of bunamidine hydrochloride, which is irritant, to the eye of the person treating the dog. Care should be taken if the scored tablets are broken.

b) Efficacy

The introduction of bunamidine hydrochloride to replace arecoline was seen as a notable advance in *Echinococcus* therapy. In initial experiments, FORBES (1966) found the compound had good activity against *E. granulosus*. His results were extended by GEMMELL and SHEARER (1968), who also obtained high efficiency against experimental infections of various ages at dose rates between 50 and 200 mg/kg. Increased efficiency was obtained against younger worms if the dose was repeated within 48 h. However, even with the very high level of efficiency obtained in these experiments 10 of 31 dogs retained some degree of infection. This inability to eliminate infection completely from dogs was confirmed by TREJOS et al. (1975) in a controlled trial where 39% of dogs given a single oral dose of 50 mg/kg retained some infection and by BORAY et al. (1979) where five of ten dogs retained a residual burden of 10–900 worms. BANKOV (1977) was also unable to eliminate the infection. Part of the reason for the lack of efficiency obtained by TREJOS et al. (1975) may have been the use of gelatine capsules to hold the drug as this is now known to affect the activity of the drug, probably because the local concentration of the drug in the duodenum may not reach sufficiently high levels to kill the parasites in that region (WILLIAMS and TREJOS 1970). ANDERSEN et al. (1975) obtained considerably better results than other workers. They cleared adult worms from groups of three dogs using 25 and 50 mg/kg as a single dose or two doses of 25 mg/kg 48 h apart, while against immature 36-day-old worms they obtained efficiencies of 98.8%, 85.9%, and 95.8% respectively using the same dose rates. They queried the need to use double doses as suggested by other workers.

HATTON (1965, 1967) reported that 25–50 mg base/kg was highly effective against *Taenia pisiformis*, *T. hydatigena*, and *T. multiceps*, particularly when given to dogs on an empty stomach. Doses of 25 mg/kg or greater completely removed *T. taeniaeformis* from small groups of cats but the efficiency obtained was dependent on the formulation, much better results being obtained with rapidly disintegrating tablets. These results were confirmed by BURROWS and LILLIS (1966) and GURALP and TIGIN (1971) but HROMATKA et al. (1966) obtained poor results against *T. hydatigena*. In large-scale field trials in New Zealand, efficiency against *T. hydatigena* appeared to decrease at doses below 50 mg/kg (G. A. Thomson 1970, personal communication) and this was confirmed in a series of controlled trials by GEMMELL (1972, personal communication), who required three doses of 25 mg/kg 48 h apart or one dose of 50 mg/kg to obtain complete elimination.

There is little published data on the efficacy of bunamidine hydrochloride against *D. caninum* infection. HATTON (1965) cleared 7 of 15 dogs but reported that Kingsbury had eliminated infection from 12 dogs when doses ranging from 7.5 to 25 mg/kg were given in gelatine capsules. Good results were also obtained by HROMATKA et al. (1966), BURROWS and LILLIS (1966) and ROBERSON (1977). The compound has also been shown to be effective against *S. mansonoides* (BURROWS and LILLIS 1966), *M. lineatus* (HROMATKA et al. 1966) and *M. corti* (TODD et al. 1978) in dogs. Bunamidine hydrochloride has been shown to have an ovicidal effect on eggs of *E. granulosus*, *T. pisiformis*, and *T. taeniaeformis*; aqueous solutions in concentrations as low as 0.2 mg/kg for1 h giving highly significant reductions in infectivity of eggs of *T. taeniaeformis* (WILLIAMS et al. 1973). However, eggs of *E. Multilocularis* are not killed (SAKAMOTO et al. 1971) and eggs within the proglottid of *E. granulosus* are not destroyed (THAKUR et al. 1979).

In practice the product is recommended for all common tapeworms of the dog and cat at a dose rate of 25 mg/kg for *Taenia* spp. and *D. caninum* and 50 mg/kg repeated in 48 h for *E. granulosus*. It is suggested that a single dose of 50 mg/kg be used against *Taenia* spp. to ensure elimination of the economically important *T. hydatigena*. It should be given on an empty stomach and the dog should be fed about 3 h later.

c) Mode of Action

Bunamidine acts on the tegument of *Hymenolepis nana*, causing disruption of the outer layers (HART et al. 1977) and this allows digestion of the worm by the proteolytic enzymes in the intestine. The worms are digested in the host. In vitro studies on *H. diminuta* showed that bunamidine hydrochloride caused dose-dependent changes in the tegument and the nephridial epithelium. At maximum drug solubility concentrations the fumarate-reductase system is completely inhibited (CHATFIELD and YEARY 1979). In odd cases, in which the scolex is covered by mucus, the worm is protected and efficacy is reduced (BURROWS and LILLIS 1966).

d) Toxicity and Pharmacodynamics

Experimentally, bunamidine has been shown to have low toxicity other than slight diarrhoea and vomiting. HATTON (1965) reported that in their studies 14% of dogs and 5% of cats vomited, while this symptom was seen in 9% of dogs used by BURROWS and LILLIS (1966). GEMMELL and SHEARER (1968) found that only 1.6% of dogs given a single dose of 50 mg/kg vomited but the proportion rose sharply when doses of 100 and 200 mg/kg were used. While diarrhoea was common it rarely persisted more than 3 h. When repeat doses of 100 and 200 mg/kg were given, some deaths occurred. When the drug was used extensively in mass-dosing programs for hydatid control, reports of deaths increased. Some dogs, which were tied or caged, died within a few hours of dosing, while others appeared normal the morning following dosing, but when released ran up to 50 metres, collapsed and died quickly. The death rate, which was about 1 in 2,000, was about three times higher in country dogs than in city dogs (FASTIER 1972). It is known that there is little difference in absorption rate in dogs that are fed or fasted before dosing and that most of the bunamidine absorbed from the intestine is removed by the liver, little getting into the circulation (VIRJI and LAVERTY 1972). In dogs with hepatic dysfunction higher levels of bunamidine may get into the circulation (BILLS et al. 1970). In excited dogs the high levels of adrenalin may then cause ventricular fibrillation in hearts sensitised by bunamidine to endogenous catecholamines (FASTIER et al. 1973). Under some circumstances bunamidine may cause liver damage (MENRATH et al. 1973). Cases of sudden death are also seen occasionally without evidence of hepatic dysfunction, and it is recommended that excitement and exertion be avoided after treatment (WILLIAMS and KEAHEY 1976). Reduced spermatogenesis was found in dogs but not cats at 4 days and up to 28 days after administration of 50 mg/kg (ROBERSON 1977).

2. Bunamidine Hydroxynaphthoate

a) Chemistry

Bunamidine hydroxynaphthoate (Buban, Wellcome) is a yellow, odourless, crystalline solid, insoluble in water but soluble in 35 parts of alcohol at 20 °C. It is much less irritant to mucous membranes than the hydrochloride and is therefore preferred for use as a drench for ruminants and for administration in the feed for dogs.

b) Efficacy and Toxicity

HATTON (1967) reported that the drug was highly effective against *T. pisiformis* and *T. hydatigena* when given in feed at 25 mg base/kg but was inactive against *T. pisiformis* when given on an empty stomach. This contrasts with results obtained with the hydrochloride which he found to be less effective when given with feed.

Schedules for treating dogs against *E. granulosus* and *T. hydatigena* by continuous low-dose or specific high-dose feeding were investigated by GEMMELL and OUDEMANS (1974, 1975a). Low concentrations could eliminate tapeworms if fed for a sufficient period but higher concentrations fed to give 32 mg base/kg and higher caused feed refusal and vomiting. Two doses of 25 mg base/kg body weight given in the feed 4 days apart are highly effective against *E. granulosus* (SHEARER and GEMMELL 1969).

In sheep and goats doses of 25 mg/kg and 50 mg/kg respectively gave good results against *Moniezia expansa* in naturally infected sheep (CZIPRI et al. 1968; RANATUNGA 1971) and no toxic symptoms were seen at doses up to 200 mg base/kg. Some diarrhoea occurred in sheep given 400 mg base/kg. This compound has also been tested in poultry with natural infections of *Raillietina* spp. and *Amoebotaenia sphenoides* (MCCULLOCH and KASIMBALA 1967). The birds were individually dosed and with this regime 400 mg base/kg was required for high efficiency. A dose of 200 mg base/kg given in the feed had no effect on egg production and no toxic effects were seen in poultry given 400 mg base/kg.

VI. Nitroscanate

a) Chemistry

Nitroscanate (Lopatol, Ciba Geigy Ltd.) has the chemical formula 4-nitro-4′-isothiocyanodiphenyl-ether. Its structural formula is shown in Fig. 3. It is a yellow crystal, insoluble in water but soluble in chloroform (23 g/100 ml) and benzene (16.5 g/100 ml).

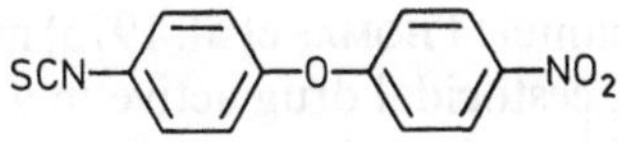

Fig. 3. Nitroscanate

b) Efficacy

Nitroscanate was introduced in 1973 (BORAY et al. 1973) as a broad-spectrum compound effective against roundworms (*Toxocara canis* and *Toxascaris leonina*), hookworms (*Ancylostoma caninum* and *Uncinaria stenocephala*), *Taenia* spp. and *D. caninum* in the dog. Its action against *Trichuris vulpis* was erratic and high doses were necessary to obtain high efficiency against *E. granulosus* and *Spirometra erinacei*. KASSAI et al. (1975), GEMMELL and OUDEMANS (1975b) and SCHANTZ et al. (1976) confirmed that the compound was active against cestodes and that high doses were necessary to achieve acceptable results. GEMMELL et al.

(1977c) found that micronisation (95% of particles less than 5 μm) greatly improved efficiency.

Further work has confirmed that a single dose of 50 mg/kg of the micronised drug has high efficiency against the common nematodes other than *T. vulpis,* and against *Taenia* spp. and *D. caninum.* The compound has given variable results against *E. granulosus* (GEMMELL et al. 1977c; BANKOV 1977; BORAY et al. 1979; GEMMELL et al. 1979a; RICHARDS and SOMERVILLE 1980) and is not recommended against this worm.

BORAY et al. (1979) also obtained high efficiency against *Toxocara cati* and *Ancylostoma tubaeforme* in cats when doses of 25 mg/kg and above were given 24 h apart, and it would presumably also be active against *T. taeniaeformis.*

c) Toxicity

Doses up to 10,000 mg/kg have been given orally to dogs without toxic signs other than vomiting, diarrhoea and inappetance (BORAY et al. 1979). At normal dose rates 10%–20% of dogs may vomit 4–16 h after dosing (BORAY et al. 1979; RICHARDS and SOMERVILLE 1980). Vomiting does not appear to be dose dependent and is less frequent with micronised material (GEMMELL et al. 1977c, 1979a). Recent studies with radioactive nitroscanate have shown that a greater proportion of the drug is absorbed if the stomach of the dog is full at the time of treatment and although efficiency is not impaired, vomiting is more pronounced. If the drug is given on an empty stomach, it passes through the intestines more quickly, low absorption occurs and efficiency is reduced. The present recommendation, to gain maximum efficiency with minimum side effects, is to give the drug to dogs after 12–24 h of fasting followed immediately with a small quantity of feed (J. C. Boray 1981, personal communication).

VII. Praziquantel

Information on the chemistry, pharmacokinetics, toxicity and mode of action of praziquantel is given in Chap. 4.

a) Efficacy

The introduction of praziquantel (THOMAS et al. 1975) made available, for the first time, a safe, highly specific, cestocidal drug active in a single oral, subcutaneous or intramuscular dose against a broad range of tapeworms in dogs, cats, and sheep. It was the first compound to be highly effective against bile duct cestodes.

Many reports quickly appeared confirming the activity of praziquantel against all juvenile and adult *Taenia* spp., *D. caninum, Joyeuxiella pasqualei, D. latum, S. erinacei,* and *M. corti* in dogs or cats (ROMMEL et al. 1976; DEY-HAZRA 1976; GURALP et al. 1976; GEMMELL et al. 1977b; BALDOCK et al. 1977; BYLUND et al. 1977; SAKAMOTO 1977a; THOMAS and GONNERT 1978a). Dose rates of 2.5 mg/kg or less gave complete elimination of *Taenia* spp., *D. caninum* and *M. corti* but higher doses were needed against the pseudophyllidean parasites. Against *D. latum* a single oral dose of 35 mg/kg completely eliminated infection from dogs (SAKAMOTO 1977a) while BYLUND et al. (1977) found 50 mg/kg to be completely effective against the same species in hamsters. SAKAMOTO (1977a) eliminated *S.*

erinacei from cats with two doses of 7.5 mg/kg given on successive days. In practice it is recommended to use a single dose of 5 mg/kg against all species in the dog except *S. erinacei*, where 20 mg/kg is used.

Because of the public health risks of *E. granulosus* and *E. multilocularis* infections, and because of the failure of available compounds to eliminate these parasites from dogs completely, the high activity reported against these species by THOMAS et al. (1975) encouraged many workers to confirm their results (ROMMEL et al. 1976; DEY-HAZRA 1976; GURALP et al. 1976; GEMMELL et al. 1977b; SAKAMOTO 1977a; THOMAS and GONNERT 1977, 1978a; THAKUR et al. 1978; ANDERSEN et al. 1978, 1979; BORAY et al. 1979). A single dose of 5 mg/kg given orally or by injection completely eliminated infection in all trials with the exception of one dog in a group of five infected with *E. multilocularis* which remained infected with two worms, a clearance rate of 99.99% (SAKAMOTO 1977a). In later work GEMMELL et al. (1980) found that the compound was less active when given subcutaneously, a small proportion of dogs retaining some *E. granulosus* when given doses of 5 and 10 mg/kg. BAUDITZ and SACHS (1979) have advised that a 5.68% injectable formulation will be available for subcutaneous or intramuscular use in dogs, but recommended the intramuscular route to ensure high efficacy in *Echinococcus* spp. infections. Micronisation did not improve the efficacy of the drug against *H. nana* in mice (THOMAS and GONNERT 1977). Praziquantel has some ovicidal action against eggs of *E. granulosus* that have been released from the proglottid but not against eggs contained within the proglottid (THAKUR et al. 1979).

In their initial series of papers on praziquantel THOMAS et al. (1975b) reported that it was active against some larval cestodes and later workers (NOVAK 1977; SAKAMOTO 1977b; THOMAS and GONNERT 1978b; HEATH and LAWRENCE 1978) have confirmed the activity against a range of larval forms in mice, rabbits, and sheep. After single or repeated administration, larval stages of *M. corti*, *T. crassiceps*, *H. nana*, *T. taeniaeformis*, *T. pisiformis*, *T. hydatigena*, and *Multiceps multiceps* were killed. THOMAS and GONNERT (1978b) commented that it appeared more active against the older larval stages while HEATH and LAWRENCE (1978), using 50 mg/kg, obtained clearance of *Cysticercus tenuicollis* only in those sheep with less than 100 cysts.

The activity of praziquantel against larval *T. saginata* (*C. bovis*) is of interest as it could provide a method of killing larvae in cattle before slaughter and so reducing the level of infection with *T. saginata* in man. GALLIE and SEWELL (1978) found that it was highly effective against 12-week-old but not 4-week-old cysts but high efficiency has been reported in both natural and experimental infections using dose rates of between 50 and 100 mg/kg (PAWLOWSKI et al. 1978; WALTHER and KOSKE 1979). The cost of such treatment would preclude its routine use. Another important condition caused by a larval cestode for which a chemotherapeutic agent would be of great benefit is hydatid disease due to infection with *Echinococcus* spp. THOMAS and GONNERT (1978b) demonstrated an effect against protoscoleces of *E. multilocularis*. SAKAMOTO (1977b), HEATH and LAWRENCE (1978), and THOMAS and GONNERT (1978b) failed to inhibit the growth of cysts of *E. multilocularis* or *E. granulosus*. As three studies in sheep infected with *E. granulosus* failed to demonstrate an effect of praziquantel (1×50 mg/kg s.c. and 2×100 mg/kg p.o.) on the parasite (ANDREWS et al. 1983), one has to conclude that its use in the treatment of hydatid disease in man is unlikely to succeed.

The activity of praziquantel has not been examined extensively in sheep, probably because of the availability and price advantage of niclosamide, which is highly efficient against the common tapeworm species. However, niclosamide lacks activity against those species (*S. hepatica* and *T. actinioides*) in the bile ducts while praziquantel eliminates them at dose rates of 8–15 mg/kg (BANKOV 1976; DEY-HAZRA 1976) as well as removing *Moniezia* spp. with a single dose of 2.5 mg/kg (THOMAS and GONNERT 1978 a).

Therapeutic trials in chickens, ducks, and geese have shown high activity against the common cestodes of these species (VASSILEV et al. 1977). At 3 mg/kg, 100% efficiency was obtained in chickens infected with *Raillietina cesticillus,* whereas 10 mg/kg was needed to obtain 100% efficiency against *Davainea proglottina* (ANDREWS et al. 1983). These authors also obtained high efficiency against a number of cestode species in ducks and geese.

b) Toxicity

Praziquantel is a very safe compound when given orally or parenterally. The acute oral LD_{50} in mice and rats is more than 2,200 mg/kg and in rabbits is greater than 1,000 mg/kg. Oral toxicity in dogs has not been determined because doses in excess of 200 mg/kg cause vomiting, which removes part or all of the test dose, and it is difficult to introduce sufficient compound parenterally because of formulation difficulties. The only side effect seen when doses up to 40 times those recommended were used was vomiting (BALDOCK and HOPKINS 1977). Dogs tolerated oral treatment with dose rates of 20, 60, and 180 mg/kg/day for over 4 weeks without ill effect. In rabbits, the compound did not cause skin irritation after single and repeated patch tests and there was no evidence of skin absorption (MUERMANN et al. 1976). However, when dissolved in isopropanol or dimethylsulfoxide (DMSO) it is absorbed and has anthelmintic activity (THOMAS and GONNERT 1978 a). The drug had no effect on mucous membranes and there were no embryotoxic or teratogenic effects in pregnant rats or rabbits with daily oral doses of 30, 100, and 300 mg/kg (MUERMANN et al. 1976). The compound is compatible with other anthelmintics and with externally applied insecticides (BALDOCK and HOPKINS 1977) and has no mutagenic effects (MACHEMER and LORKE 1978; BARTSH et al. 1978).

VIII. Benzimidazoles

The introduction of tiabendazole (Merck, Sharpe & Dohme) in 1961 introduced a new era in veterinary anthelmintic medication against nematodes in sheep, cattle, and horses. The benzimidazoles that were developed after tiabendazole had the 5-position blocked to slow down the rate of metabolism and excretion. The nature of the group substituted at the 5-position and the replacement of the thiazole ring by methylcarbamate markedly affects the rate of excretion so that the new compounds persist longer. They can then be given at lower dose rates and because they are in contact with the parasites for longer periods, they tend to have a broader spectrum of activity. For example, tiabendazole, parbendazole, and oxibendazole reach maximum plasma levels in sheep in 4–6 h and are quickly excreted while peak plasma levels of fenbendazole, oxfendazole, and albendazole are reached 15–24 h after dosing and persist for 48–120 h (PRICHARD 1978). The earlier chemicals in this series (tiabendazole, parbendazole, and oxibendazole) were not sufficiently active against cestodes to warrant claims against this group of parasites. Those with activity are discussed in the following section.

1. Cambendazole

Information on the chemistry, pharmacokinetics, toxicity, and mode of action of the benzimidazole derivatives is given in Chap. 4.

a) Efficacy

There are few data on the activity of this compound against cestodes. HORAK et al. (1972) and GIBBS and GUPTA (1972) found that doses between 15 and 30 mg/kg eliminated most of the *Moniezia expansa* scoleces from lambs but was less efficient in calves, while ALLEN (1973) obtained 100% activity against *Thysanosoma* spp. with 100 mg/kg, the only dose used. DRUDGE et al. (1975) reported that *Anoplocephala magna* in the horse was not affected by doses of 10 and 20 mg/kg and GEMMELL et al. (1977d) found little effect against *T. hydatigena* in dogs. CAMPBELL et al. (1975) reported that cambendazole had some activity against the tissue phase of *Taenia crassiceps* in mice. It appears that the cestocidal activity of this drug against *M. expansa* in lambs is a useful adjunct to its nematocidal effect but that it has little use against cestodes in other hosts.

b) Toxicity

Teratogenic effects in rats have been observed (DELATOUR et al. 1975). It is not recommended for use in ewes.

2. Oxfendazole

a) Efficacy

AVERKIN et al. (1975) introduced this compound and described its synthesis, range of activity and preliminary toxicity studies. They claimed greater than 95% activity against a broad range of parasites, including *Moniezia* spp. in sheep, when the recommended dose of 5 mg/kg was used. CHALMERS (1977) and MICHAEL et al. (1979) also reported excellent results against *Moniezia* spp. in lambs, both groups reporting 100% efficiency. In other species the compound has little effect. LYONS et al. (1977) and DUNCAN and REID (1978) stated that oxfendazole was not active against *A. perfoliata* and *A. magna* in the horse, while GEMMELL et al. (1979b) found little effect on *T. hydatigena* or *E. granulosus* in the dog.

b) Toxicity

AVERKIN et al. (1975) reported that oxfendazole has an LD_{50} of greater than 6,400 mg/kg in rats and mouse and 1,600 mg/kg in dogs. Doses of 20 times the therapeutic dose were well tolerated by sheep and repeated dosing of rams from

21 days before the breeding season and of ewes during pregnancy, with three times the recommended dose, had no effect on the ewes, rams or the progeny. Oxfendazole has also been shown to be safe and without teratogenic effect when given to heifers in early pregnancy (Piercy et al. 1979). Oxfendazole and fenbendazole are not compatible with bromsalans in cattle and should not be given within 7 days (Prichard 1978).

3. Fenbendazole

This compound (Panacur, Hoechst) was the first benzimidazole to have high efficiency against hypobiotic larvae of *Ostertagia ostertagi* in cattle and because of the importance of this parasite, the product quickly gained acceptance.

a) Efficacy

Duwell et al. (1975) first showed that fenbendazole had cestocidal activity. They reported that 25 mg/kg was highly efficient against *H. diminuta* in the rat while 10 mg/kg eliminated almost 100% of *Moniezia* spp. in sheep. Other workers quickly confirmed these results in sheep, obtaining good results using single oral doses of 5–15 mg/kg (McBeath et al. 1977; Townsend et al. 1977; Corba et al. 1979; Malan 1980). Preliminary results obtained by Duwell et al. (1975) indicated some activity against *Anoplocephala* spp. in the horse. However, Duncan et al. (1977) found small numbers of *A. perfoliata* in both treated and control horses while Drudge et al. (1978) could not show activity in a series of critical and controlled trials.

Efficacy against tapeworms in the dog, excluding *E. granulosus*, has been reported by Duwell (1978) and Gemmell et al. 1977d) and in cats by Roberson and Burke (1980). High doses appear to be needed, but the recommendation to use this compound at doses of 50 mg/kg on three successive days to give broad-spectrum activity against nematodes of dogs probably results in the expulsion of most cestodes other than *E. granulosus*.

b) Toxicity

Many authors have shown that fenbendazole is a very safe compound. In sheep, single oral doses of 5,000 mg/kg or 30 doses of 45 mg/kg were well tolerated (Baeder et al. 1974) and no teratogenic effects have been detected in rats, sheep, cattle or horses (Delatour et al. 1975; Becker 1975). Doses of 50 mg/kg given daily to pregnant bitches from the 40th day of gestation to 10 days after whelping had no effect on the birth weight or growth of the pups (Duwell and Strasser 1978). In extensive field trials R. E. James (1980, personal communication) treated 23,000 sheep without ill effect and could find no evidence of intolerance when used simultaneously with fasciolocides or insecticides. However, in cattle, Borland et al. (1978) reported an interaction between fenbendazole and bromsalans (Fascol, Ciba Geigy Inc.) that resulted in death within 24–48 h. It is now recommended that fenbendazole should not be given within 7 days of dosing with bromsalans.

4. Albendazole

a) Efficacy

This compound is the most recent benzimidazole to be marketed and has the broadest spectrum of members of this group, having activity against nematodes, cestodes, and trematodes (THEODORIDES et al. 1976a). In sheep SCHALKWYK et al. (1979) obtained 100% activity against *Moniezia* spp. using a single oral dose of 2.5 mg/kg, while THEODORIDES et al. (1976b) also cleared lambs of infection with 10 and 15 mg/kg, the only dose rates they tested. It also has high activity against *T. actinioides* in sheep. Bile duct parasites have proved difficult to eliminate with drugs other the praziquantel but 7.5 mg/kg albendazole removed 98% of *T. actinioides* from experimentally infected sheep (CRAIG and SHEPHERD 1980) and completely eliminated infection from eight of ten naturally infected sheep (BERGSTROM et al. 1979). Albendazole is also highly effective in cattle, 5 mg/kg removing 98%–100% of *Moniezia* spp. (WILLIAMS et al. 1977; CIORDIA et al. 1978). It is also effective against larval *T. saginata* in cattle when given at a dose rate of 50 mg/kg (LLOYD et al. 1978).

Albendazole does not appear to have been tested against cestodes of dogs and cats, except that TODD (1978) completely eliminated *Mesocestoides* from dogs using 100 mg/kg as a single oral dose or 50 mg/kg twice a day for 2 days. Because *M. corti* has the unique capacity to multiply in the definitive host, it is important to obtain 100% efficiency against this species.

b) Toxicity

Single oral doses of 37.5 mg/kg produced no ill effects in sheep and doses of 5 and 15 mg/kg every 10 days for 3 months did not produce clinical symptoms or any histopathological change. Albendazole did not produce teratological effects when ewes were treated 28–32 days after the rams were introduced and there was no effect on sperm production or sperm characters when rams were dosed with 15 mg/kg (JOHNS and PHILLIP 1977).

5. Mebendazole

a) Efficacy

Mebendazole, when introduced in 1972, was reported to have high activity against nematodes and cestodes in man and other mammalian hosts (VANDEN BOSSCHE 1972; VANPARIJS and THIENPONT 1973). The cestocidal activity of benzimidazoles had been known for many years (CAMPBELL 1961), early members of the series had only weak activity but sufficient action was shown by cambendazole for claims to be made against cestodes in sheep (HORAK et al. 1972; ALLEN 1973). Little was known at this time about their effects on larval cestodes and reports that mebendazole was active against secondary cysts of *E. granulosus*, mature and immature cysticerci of *T. pisiformis*, multiplying tetrathyridia of *M. corti* and larval *T. taeniaeformis* (HEATH and CHEVIS 1974; THIENPONT et al. 1974; HEATH et al. 1975) caused considerable interest, particularly with respect to the treatment of hydatid cysts in man. CAMPBELL et al. (1975) examined the effect of a range of benzimidazoles against mice infected with metacestodes of *T. crassiceps* and *E. multilocularis*. In their experiments mebendazole was highly effective against larval *T. crassiceps* when given as a single intraperitoneal injection of 25 mg/kg, while against *E. multilocularis* cysts 75–150 mg/kg given intraperitoneally for 3 days markedly reduced the cyst mass. In contrast 1,000 mg/kg given orally daily for 3 days was only partially effective. PAWLOWSKI et al. (1976a) obtained a marked effect on hydatid disease in pigs fed 25 mg/kg in the feed for 10 days on two occasions, 2 months and 5 months after infection. They found it was less efficient if given intraperitoneally. ECKERT and POHLENZ (1976) demonstrated an effect on larval *E. multilocularis* and KAMMERER and JUDGE (1976) treated mice with long-standing *E. granulosus* infections with 50 mg/kg for 10 days and found a decrease in the number of cysts in treated mice, with many of the cysts ruptured. Some mice died and toxic or anaphylactic reactions could not be excluded from the possible causes of death. HEATH and LAWRENCE (1978) gave 50 mg/kg orally to sheep for 14 days and this retarded the growth of *E. granulosus*. The germinal epithelium of a hydatid cyst must be completely destroyed, as even small surviving portions have the capacity to regrow, so these results could be interpreted as promising only.

REISIN et al. (1977) showed that mebendazole moves across the hydatid cyst wall by passive diffusion and the failure to obtain high concentrations in the cyst is probably due to the lack of absorption of mebendazole from the gastrointestinal tract and the low plasma levels obtained (MACNAIR 1980).

In work on other larval cestodes PAWLOWSKI et al. (1976b) found no effect on larval *T. saginata* in cattle given 40 mg/kg by intraperitoneal injection but HEATH and LAWRENCE (1978) administered 50 mg/kg orally to sheep for 14 days and killed most of the *T. hydatigena* and *T. ovis* larvae. VERSTER et al. (1978) found no activity against *Multiceps multiceps* larvae in sheep, while ECKERT and POHLENZ (1976) and BENNETT et al. (1978) obtained high efficiency against tetrathyridia of *Mesocestoides corti* in mice.

While mebendazole has some activity against larval cestodes, the long course of treatment required and the expense of such treatment precludes its use in animals. Its use against hydatid disease in man is questionable because of toxic side effects and because its low absorption means that even enormous doses give only low levels in plasma (MACNAIR 1980), resulting in poor therapeutic results.

There is less information on its effect on adult tapeworms. GEMMELL et al. (1975) found that a single dose of 20 mg/kg micronised mebendazole eliminated *T. hydatigena* but 160 mg/kg was needed to eliminate *E. granulosus* infection from a group of ten dogs. The compound was not so active when incorporated in the feed (GEMMELL et al. 1978c). BORAY et al. (1979), using two doses of 20 mg/kg 48 h apart, obtained 53.5% efficiency against *E. granulosus* and 50% against *T. hydatigena*. Although mebendazole is used against nematodes in horses and sheep, there appears to be little published information on its efficacy against cestodes in these species. BRADLEY and RADHAKRISHNAN (1973) and DRUDGE et al. (1974) could not demonstrate activity of mebendazole against cestodes of horses but KELLY and BAIN (1975) obtained 96% and 99% activity against *Anoplocephala perfoliata* when horses were given a single oral dose of 15 and 20 mg/kg micronised material. At the usual dose rate of 10 mg/kg only 52% of worms were eliminated. In practice, mebendazole is used in dogs, sheep, and horses at about

10 mg/kg against nematode infections. Repeated treatment is needed in dogs. Its cestocidal effect is secondary to this use.

b) Toxicity

Mebendazole is a very safe compound. The LD_{50} for sheep, cattle, and horses is above 600 mg/kg. Literature from the company states that dogs given 2.5, 10 or 40 mg/kg 6 days a week for 13 weeks remained normal, and on autopsy no drug-induced changes could be found. Further, when given to ewes during pregnancy no effect on the embryo could be detected. It appears to be compatible with other commonly used farm chemicals.

IX. Antibiotics

1. Paromomycin

Paromomycin sulphate is a mixture of sulphates of antimicrobial substances produced by the growth of certain strains of *Streptomyces rimosus* var *paromomycinus*. It is identical to amminosidin sulphate produced by *Streptomyces chrestomyceticus* (SCHILLINGS and SCHAFFNER 1961).

Paromomycin was introduced as an antimicrobial compound active against a range of Gram-positive and Gram-negative bacteria and against some intestinal protozoa, and it was noted incidently that cestodes were passed by patients undergoing therapy (ULIVELLI 1963; SALEM and EL-ALLAF 1969). Its veterinary use was investigated by WAITZ et al. (1966), who found little activity against *Hymenolepsis nana* in mice or *H. diminuta* in rats, but more promising results against *T. taeniaeformis* in the cat when given as a single dose of 250 or 500 mg/kg or as 25 mg/kg twice daily for 5 days. All treated cats had loose stools to moderate diarrhoea. Paromomycin is poorly absorbed from the gastrointestinal tract and most of the dose is passed in the faeces.

2. Axenomycins

Axenomycins are isolated from the fermentation broth of *Streptomyces lisandri*. There are three different fractions A, B, and D, the most active against tapeworms being fraction D (DELLA-BRUNA et al. 1973). These authors showed that 10 mg/kg axenomycin D had high activity against *H. nana* in mice, and *T. pisiformis* and *Diphyllobothrium* spp. in dogs. Preliminary tests using 20 mg/kg of the crude axenomycin complex gave promising results against *Moniezia* spp and *Avitellina centripunctata* in lambs and *Dipylidium caninum* in dogs.

The oral LD_{50} of the D fraction in mice was 100 mg/kg and oral administration of 10 and 20 mg/kg to dogs for 30 days was well tolerated, sporadic vomiting being the only side effect seen.

3. SQ 21,704

The antibiotic SQ 21,704 (E. R. Squibb and Sons) of the streptothricin family is produced from *Streptomyces griseocarneus*, strain S 15-1, and was first used as an antiviral agent. BROWN et al. (1977) reported that it had cestocidal activity against

H. nana in mice, and against cestodes in cats, dogs, and sheep; this was further investigated by GEMMELL et al. (1978 b), SZANTO et al. (1979) and CRUTHERS et al. (1979). These authors found that 25 mg/kg or above given orally as a single dose completely eliminated *T. pisiformis, T. hydatigena,* and *T. taeniaeformis,* while higher doses (37.5–50 mg/kg) were needed against *D. caninum*. In a comparative test CRUTHERS et al. (1979) found that it was more efficient than niclosamide or bunamidine hydrochloride and that administration of the compound mixed in the feed gave good results. GEMMELL et al. (1978 b) using doses as high as 100 mg/kg could not clear all dogs of *E. granulosus* even when the dose was repeated in 2 days. No effect against nematodes was noted in any of the above trials (see also GEMMELL and JOHNSTONE 1981).

No drug-related toxicity was seen in these trials except that GEMMELL et al. (1978b) noted vomiting and diarrhoea in a proportion of dogs given 25, 50, and 100 mg/kg. This did not occur in other trials and it has been suggested that this effect was due to an impurity in the initial batch supplied for that trial (SZANTO et al. 1979).

X. Diuredosan

a) Chemistry

This compound, which is also called uredofos, (Sansalid, Rohm and Haas and Whitmoyer Laboratories) has the chemical formula diethyl-[thio[-*o*-[3-(*p*-tolyl-sulphonyl)-ureido]-phenyl]-carbamoyl]-phosphoramidate. It is a colourless powder with the structural formula shown in Fig. 4.

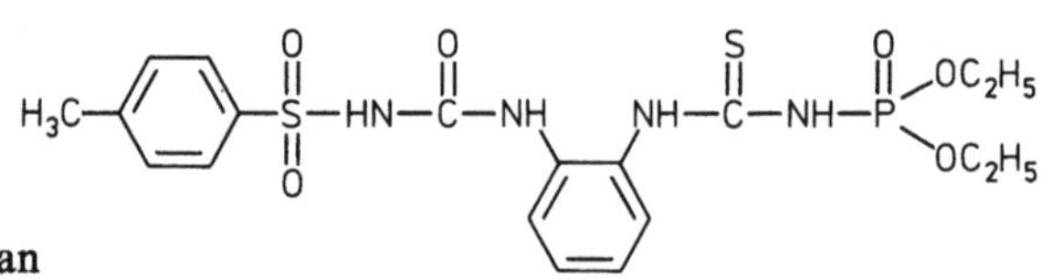

Fig. 4. Diuredosan

b) Efficacy

This compound has been reported to be active against a range of nematodes and cestodes in dogs and cats. At the recommended dose rate of 50 mg/kg, complete clearance of *Taenia* spp. and *D. caninum* (SIEDEL et al. 1975; ROBERSON 1976; ROBERSON and AGER 1976; KLEIN and BRADLEY 1976; GEMMELL et al. 1978 a) and very high efficiency against *M. corti* (TODD et al. 1978) has been reported. No significant effect was attained against *E. granulosus* (GEMMELL et al. 1978 a). SIEDEL et al. (1975), ROBERSON and AGER (1976), TODD and YATES (1976), and KLEIN and BRADLEY (1976) also obtained high efficiency against the common roundworms and hookworms of dogs but not against *Trichuris vulpis*. ROBERSON and AGER (1976) noted that efficiency against whipworms was inversely related to worm burden and only dogs with less than ten worms were cleared. In cats, high efficiency has also been recorded against roundworms and hookworms but only 83% efficiency against tapeworms (ROBERSON 1977).

c) Toxicity

Little has been published on the mode of action, pharmacodynamics or toxicity of this organophosphate. At the recommended dose rate no signs referable to organophosphate toxicity have been noted but up to 30% of dogs may show some diarrhoea and up to 20% may vomit (ROBERSON 1976; ROBERSON and AGER 1976; GEMMELL et al. 1978 a).

XI. Fospirate

a) Chemistry

Fospirate (Torelle, Dow Chemical Co.) has the chemical formula dimethyl 3, 5, 6-trichloro-2-pyridyl phosphate. Its structural formula is shown in Fig. 5.

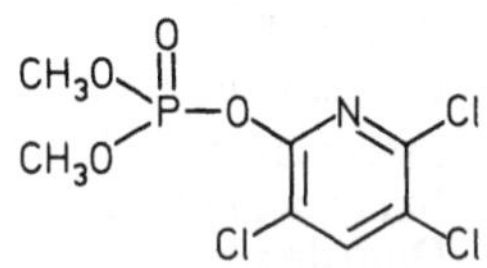

Fig. 5. Fospirate

b) Efficacy

Fospirate was first tested as an insecticide for flea control but has been tested and found to have efficiency against *T. hydatigena* in dogs at 10 mg/kg (GEMMELL and OUDEMANS 1975 c) and against *E. granulosus* when given in divided doses of 40–80 mg/kg (GEMMELL and OUDEMANS 1975 c; SCHANTZ and PREZIOSO 1976). At least three treatments of 40 mg/kg may be required, and vomiting that occurs in some dogs at this dose rate seems to interfere with its efficiency.

XII. Other Compounds

Many compounds other than those discussed in this review have been used commercially, but are not discussed here because there is no new information on them and they have been reviewed by GIBSON (1975). Such compounds as bithionol, mepacrine, copper sulphate with or without added nicotine sulphate and cupric acetoarsenite fall into this category.

Lead arsenate is still used, mainly as an additive to the early benzimidazole compounds that lack cestocidal activity. It is used at a dose rate of 1.0 g/sheep other than lambs, which receive only 0.5 g. As lead arsenate settles quickly it is essential that the amount mixed is used the same day and that the mixture is continuously shaken. Resorantel (Terenol, Hoechst), which is highly effective against paramphistomes in cattle, sheep, and goats, is also effective against cestodes (DUWELL 1970). However, while field trials have given reasonable results (BEHRENS

Table 2. Recommended treatments for cestode infections

DOG		
Taenia spp.	Praziquantel	5 mg/kg
	Niclosamide	100 mg/kg
	Bunamidine HCl	50 mg/kg
	Nitroscanate	50 mg/kg
	Diuredosan	50 mg/kg
Echinococcus granulosus *E. multilocularis*	Praziquantel	5 mg/kg
	Bunamidine HCl	50 mg/kg repeated in 48 h
Spirometra spp. *Diphyllobothrium latum*	Praziquantel	20 mg/kg
	Bunamidine HCl	50 mg/kg
Mesocestoides spp.	Praziquantel	5 mg/kg
	Bunamidine HCl	50 mg/kg
	Diuredosan	50 mg/kg
	Albendazole	100 mg/kg
Dipylidium caninum *Joyeuxiella* spp. *Diplopylidium* spp.	Praziquantel	5 mg/kg
	Bunamidine HCl	50 mg/kg
	Diuredosan	50 mg/kg
CATS		
Taenia taeniaeformis	Praziquantel	5 mg/kg
	Niclosamide	100 mg/kg
	Bunamidine	50 mg/kg
	Diuredosan	50 mg/kg
Dipylidium caninum *Joyeuxiella* spp. *Diplopylidium* spp.	Praziquantel	5 mg/kg
	Bunamidine HCl	50 mg/kg
	Diuredosan	50 mg/kg
SHEEP and CATTLE		
Moniezia spp. *Helictometra giardi* *Avitellina* spp. *Stilesia globipunctata*	Niclosamide	50 mg/kg
	Albendazole	5 mg/kg
	Bunamidine hydroxynaphthoate	50 mg/kg
	Praziquantel	2.5 mg/kg
	Cambendazole	20 mg/kg
	Oxfendazole	5 mg/kg
	Fenbendazole	5 mg/kg
Stilesia hepatica[a] *Thysanosoma actinioides*[a]	Albendazole	7.5 mg/kg
	Bunamidine hydroxynaphthoate	50 mg/kg
	Praziquantel	10 mg/kg
HORSES		
Anoplocephala spp. *Paranoplocephala mamillana* *Moniezia pallida*	Niclosamide	200 mg/kg
	Mebendazole	20 mg/kg
BIRDS		
Fowl and turkey *Raillietina* spp. *Davainea* spp. *Amoebotaenia sphenoides* *Choanotaenia infundibulum* *Cotugnia digonopora* *Metroliasthes lucida* *Hymenolepis* spp. *Fimbriaria fasciolaris*	Niclosamide	50 mg/kg
	di-n-butyl tin dilaurate	125 mg/kg in feed
PIGEON		
Davainea proglottina *Raillietina tetragona* *Cotugnia cuneata*	Niclosamide	200 mg/kg

[a] These tapeworms are found in the bile ducts

and MATSCHULLAT 1970; HUMKE et al. 1970; PFEIFFER 1970), the therapeutic ratio of this compound is small, about threefold the therapeutic dose of 65 mg/kg, and it is unlikely that this compound will be sold for its cestocidal activity.

D. Recommended Treatments for Cestode Infections

The more important and the newer cestocidal compounds have been described in some detail in the preceding section. Table 2 summarises the compounds most efficient against the common cestode infections of various domesticated animals and birds.

References

Abou AH (1956) The use of di-*n*-butyl tin dilaurate for the treatment of chickens experimentally infected with *Davainea proglottina.* J Helminthol 30:121–128

Abrams L (1976) Cestodosis in battery and housed laying hens. J S Afr Vet Assoc 47:171–173

Abuladze KI (1964) Essentials of cestology. In: Skrjabin KI (ed) Vol 4, Taeniata of animals and man and diseases caused by them. Akad Nauk SSR, Moscow (English translation: Israel program for scientific translation 1970)

Aikat BK, Bhusnurmath SR, Cadersa M, Chhuttani PN, Mitra SK (1978) *Echinococcus multilocularis* infection in India: first case report proved at autopsy. Trans R Soc Trop Med Hyg 72:619–621

Allen RW (1959) Preliminary notes on the larval development of the fringed tapeworm of sheep *Thysanosoma actinioides* Diesing, 1834, in psocids (Psocoptera : Corodentia). J Parasitol 45:537–538

Allen RW (1973) Preliminary evaluation of levamisole, parbendazole, and cambendazole as thysanosomicides in sheep. Am J Vet Res 34:61–63

Allen RW, Jackson PK (1953) Evaluation of di-phenthane-70 in removing fringed tapeworms from sheep. Vet Med 48:352–354

Allen RW, Enzie FD, Samson KS (1967) Trials with Yomesan and other selected chemicals against *Thysanosoma actinioides,* the fringed tapeworm of sheep Proc Helminthol Soc Wash 34:195–199

Amjardi AR (1971) Studies on histopathology of *Stilesia globipunctata* infections in Iran. Vet Rec 88:486–488

Andersen FL, Loveless RM, Jensen LA (1975) Efficacy of bunamidine hydrochloride against immature and mature stages of *Echinococcus granulosus.* Am J Vet Res 30:673–675

Andersen FL, Conder GA, Marsland WP (1978) Efficacy of injectable and tablet formulations of praziquantel against mature *Echinococcus granulosus.* Am J Vet Res 39:1861–1862

Andersen FL, Conder GA, Marsland WP (1979) Efficacy of injectable and tablet formulations of praziquantel against immature *Echinococcus granulosus.* Am J Vet Res 40:700–701

Andrews P, Thomas H, Pohlke R, Seubert J (1983) Praziquantel. Med Res Rev 3:147–200

Arundel JH (1972) A review of cysticercoses of sheep and cattle in Australia. Aust Vet J 48:140–155

Arundel JH, Adolph AJ (1980) Preliminary observations on the removal of *Taenia saginata* eggs from sewage using various treatment processes. Aust Vet J 56:492–495

Averkin EA, Beard CC, Dvorak CA, Edwards JA, Fried JH, Kilian JG, Schultz RA, Kistner TP, Drudge JN, Lyons ET, Sharp ML, Corwin RM (1975) Methyl 5(6)-phenyl-sulfinyl-2-benzimidazolecarbamate, a new, potent anthelmintic. J Med Chem 18:1164–1166

Baeder C, Bahr H, Christ O, Duwell D, Kellner HM, Kirsch R, Loewe H, Schultes E, Schutz E, Westen H (1974) Fenbendazole: a new, highly effective anthelmintic. Experientia 30:753–754
Baldock FC, Hopkins TJ (1977) Praziquantel: a new cestocide. Proc 54th Ann Conf Aust Vet Assoc, Perth, pp 127–128
Baldock FC, Flucke WJ, Hopkins TJ (1977) Efficiency of praziquantel, a new cestocide, against *Taenia hydatigena* in the dog. Res Vet Sci 23:237–238
Bankov D (1976) Diagnosis and treatment of *Stilesia* infection in sheep. Vet Med Nauki 13:28–36. From Vet Bull 47:5050 (1977) (abstract)
Bankov D (1977) Comparative assessment of anthelmintics against *Echinococcus granulosus* in dogs. Vet Med Rev 2:145–148
Bankov D (1979) Trials for therapy and chemoprophylaxis of coenurosis in sheep. Vet Med Rev 1:79–80
Bankov D, Juperliev W (1965) Comparative studies of drugs for treatment of cestodes and trematodes of ducklings. Vet Sbirka 3:13. From Vet Med Rev 2:144–145 (1966) (abstract)
Barsanti JA, Jones BD, Bailey WS, Knipling GD (1979) Diagnosis and treatment of peritonitis caused by a larval cestode *Mesocestoides* spp. in a dog. Cornell Vet 69:45–53
Batham EJ (1946) Testing arecoline hydrobromide as an anthelmintic for hydatid worms in dogs. Parasitology 37:185–191
Bauditz R, Sachs H (1979) Droncit injectable: new possibilities of tapeworm control. Vet Med Rev 2:129–133
Bearup AJ (1953) Life history of a spirometrid tapeworm causing sparganosis in feral pigs. Aust Vet J 29:217–224
Becker W (1975) Die Anwendung von Panacur bei trächtigen Tieren. Proc 2nd Eur Multicolloquy Parasitol, Trogir, Yugoslavia
Behrens H, Matschullat G (1970) Behandlungsversuche an Schafen mit dem Bandwurmmittel Terenol., DTW 77:101–104
Bell ME, Bennett EW (1970) Effects of arecoline on dogs: influence of route of administration. Proc Univ Otago Med Sch 48:3–4
Bennet EM, Behm C, Bryant C (1978) Effects of mebendazole and levamisole on tetrathyridia of *Mesocestoides corti* in the mouse. Int J Parasitol 8:463–466
Bergstrom RC, Armstrong DA, Hancock HA (1979) Evaluation of albendazole as a thysanosomicide in sheep. Vet Med Small Anim Clin 74:549–551
Berntzen AK, Mueller JF (1972) In vitro cultivation of *Spirometra* spp. (Cestoda) from the plerocercoid to the gravid adult. J Parasitol 58:750–752
Beveridge I, Gregory GG (1976) The identification of *Taenia* species from Australian carnivores. Aust Vet J 52:369–373
Beydemuller F (1934) Die Spulwurm- und Bandwurmkrankheit der kleinen Haustiere und ihre Bekämpfung mit Nemural und Askaridol „Bayer". Tieraerztl Rundschau 40:43–46
Bičik V, Lýsek H (1970) A contribution to the knowledge of the influence of parasites on the quality of higher nervous activity in experimental animals. Acta Parasitol Pol 18:99–105
Biddis JK (1950) A new taeniacide for dogs. Vet Rec 62:841
Bills GNB, Sharard A, Fastier FN (1970) Possible role of the liver in bunamidine toxicity. Proc Univ Otago Med Sch 48:59–60
Blair HE (1949) Vermiplex: a new anthelmintic for dogs. North Am Vet 30:306–309
Blood BD, Moya V, Lelijveld JL (1968) Evaluation of selected drugs for the treatment of canine echinococcosis. Bull WHO 39:67–72
Boisvenue RJ, Hendrix JC (1965) Prophylactic treatment of experimental *Raillietina cesticillus* infections in chickens with Yomesan. J Parasitol 51:519–522
Boray JC (1969) The anthelmintic efficiency of niclosamide and menichlopholan in the treatment of intestinal paramphistomosis in sheep. Aust Vet J 45:133–134
Boray JC, Orelli M von, Sarasin G (1973) The role of broad spectrum anthelmintics in the control of zoonoses due to helminths of dogs. Proc 6th Symposium World Assoc Adv Vet Parasitol, Vienna

Boray JC, Strong MB, Allison JR, Orelli M von, Sarasin G, Gfeller W (1979) Nitroscanate a new broad spectrum anthelmintic against nematodes and cestodes of dogs and cats. Aust Vet J 55:45–53

Borland R, Sinclair AJ, Allison JF, Embury D, James RE (1978) Toxicity in cattle following exposure to combinations of fenbendazole and bromsalans-type anthelmintics. Proc 55th Ann Conf Aust Vet Assoc, Sydney

Botero H, Reid WM (1969) The effects of the tapeworm *Raillietina cesticillus* upon body weight gains of broilers, poults and on egg production. Poult Sci 48:536–542

Bradley RE, Radhakrishnan CV (1973) Critical test evaluation of mebendazole against gastro-intestinal parasites of horses and ponies. Am J Vet Res 34:475–477

Brander GC, Pugh DM (1971) Veterinary applied pharmacology and therapeutics. Bailliere Tindall, Lond

Brown WE, Szanto J, Meyers E (1977) Taeniacidal activity of streptothricin antibiotic complex S 15-1 (SQ 21, 704). J Antibiot 30:886–889

Brunetti OA, Rosen MN (1970) Prevalence of *Echinococcus granulosus* hydatid in California deer. J Parasitol 56:1138–1140

Burrows RB, Lillis WG (1966) Treatment of canine and feline tapeworm infections with bunamidine hydrochloride. Am J Vet Res 27:1381–1384

Bylund G, Djupsund BM (1977) Protein profiles as an aid to taxonomy in the genus *Diphyllobothrium*. Z Parasitenkd 51:241–247

Bylund G, Bang B, Wikgren K (1977) Tests with a new compound (praziquantel) against *Diphyllobothrium latum*. J Helminthol 51:115–119

Campbell WC (1961) Effect of thiabendazole upon infections of *Trichinella spiralis* in mice, and upon certain other helminthiasis. J Parasitol 47 (Section 2):37

Campbell WC, McCracken RO, Blair LS (1975) Effect of parenterally injected benzimidazole compounds on *Echinococcus multilocularis* and *Taenia crassiceps* metacestodes in laboratory animals. J Parasitol 61:844–852

Chalmers K (1977) The efficacy of oxfendazole against natural infections of nematodes and cestodes in sheep. NZ Vet J 25:266–269

Chand K (1970) Preliminary studies on some common tapeworms of the fowl. Punjab Vet 9:31–35

Chandra R, Singh KS (1972) Histopathological studies on the lesions caused by *Amoebotaenia sphenoides* (Raillet, 1892) in chicks. Indian J Anim Sci 42:45–50

Chatfield RC, Yeary RA (1979) The effects of bunamidine HCl on *Hymenolepis diminuta*. Vet Parasitol 5:177–193

Ciordia H, McCampbell HC, Stuedemann JA (1978) Cestocidal activity of albendazole in calves. Am J Vet Res 39:517–518

Cobbold TS (1872) Worms. Churchill, London

Colli CW, Williams JF (1972) Influence of temperature on the infectivity of eggs of *Echinococcus granulosus* in laboratory rodents. J Parasitol 58:422–426

Coman BJ (1972) A sylvatic cycle for the hydatid tapeworm (*Echinococcus granulosus*) in remote areas of Eastern Victoria. Aust Vet J 48:552–553

Coman BJ (1975) The survival of *Taenia pisiformis* eggs under laboratory conditions and in the field environment. Aust Vet J 51:560–565

Coman BJ, Rickard MD (1975) The location of *Taenia pisiformis, Taenia ovis*, and *Taenia hydatigena* in the gut of the dog and its effect on net environmental contamination with ova. Z Parasitenkd 47:237–248

Corba J, Lietava P, Duwell D, Reisenleiter R (1979) Efficacy of fenbendazole against the most important trematodes and cestodes of ruminants. Br Vet J 135:318–323

Corkum KC (1973) The duality of host function in spirometrid tapeworm infections. Proc Lousiana Acad Sci 36:64–70

Cox DD, Mullee MT, Allen AD (1966) The anthelmintic activity of Yomesan against *Taenia* spp. of dogs and cats. Vet Med Rev 1:49–55

Craig AH Jr, Kleckner AL (1946) Taeniacidal action of di-phenthane-70. North Am Vet 27:26–30

Craig TM, Shepherd E (1980) Efficacy of albendazole and levamisole in sheep against *Thysanosoma actinioides* and *Haemonchus contortus* from the Edwards Plateau, Texas. Am J Vet Res 41:425–426

Cruthers LR, Linkenheimer WH, Maplesden DC (1979) Taeniacidal efficiency of SQ 21704 in dogs by various types of oral administration and in comparison with niclosamide and bunamidine hydrochloride. Am J Vet Res 40:676–678

Czipri DA, Nunns VJ, Shearer GL (1968) Bunamidine hydroxynaphthoate. Activity against *Moniezia expansa* in sheep. Vet Rec 82:505–507

D'Alessandro A, Rausch RL, Cuello C, Aristizabal N (1979) *Echinococcus vogeli* in man, with a review of polycystic hydatid disease in Colombia and neighboring countries. Am J Trop Med Hyg 28:303–317

DeCooman PE, DeRycke PH (1970) Experimental secondary echinococcosis of *Echinococcus granulosus* I. Development in different strains of mice. Z Parasitenkd 34:362–370

Delatour P, Lorgue G, Courtot D (1975) Embryotoxicity of some benzimidazolic anthelmintics. Proc 20th World Vet Congr, Thessaloniki

Della Bruna C, Ricciardi ML, Sanfilippo A (1973) Axenomycins, new cestocidal antibiotics. Antimicrob Agents Chemother 3:708–710

Dey-Hazra A (1976) The efficacy of Droncit (Praziquantel) against tapeworm infections in dog and cat. Vet Med Rev 2:134–141

Drudge JH, Lyons ET, Tolliver SC (1974) Critical and clinical test evaluations of mebendazole against internal parasites of the horse. Am J Vet Res 35:1409–1412

Drudge JH, Lyons ET, Tolliver SC (1975) Critical tests of suspension, paste, and pellet formulations of cambendazole in the horse. Am J Vet Res 36:435–439

Drudge JH, Lyons ET, Tolliver SC (1978) Critical and controlled tests and clinical trials with suspensions and granule formulations of the anthelmintic, fenbendazole, in the horse. J Equine Med Surg 2:22–26

Duncan JL, Reid JFS (1978) An evaluation of oxfendazole against the common nematode parasites of the horse. Vet Rec 103:332–334

Duncan JL, McBeath DG, Best JMJ, Preston NK (1977) The efficacy of fenbendazole in the control of immature strongly infection in ponies. Equine Vet J 9:146–149

Duwell D (1970) Ein neues Zestizid: Terenol – seine Wirkung gegen Bandwürmer von Laboratoriums- und Haustieren. DTW 77:97–101

Duwel D (1978) Die Behandlung des Helminthen-Befalls bei Hunden mit Fenbedazol. Kleintierprax 23:237–242

Duwel D, Strasser H (1978) Versuche zur Geburt helminthenfreier Hundewelpen durch Fenbendazol – Behandlung. DTW 85:239–241

Duwel D, Kirsch R, Reisenleiter R (1975) The efficacy of fenbendazole in the control of trematodes and cestodes. Vet Rec 93:371

Eckert J, Pohlenz J (1976) On the effect of mebendazole on metacestodes of *Mesocestoides corti* and *Echinococcus multilocularis*. Tropenmed Parasitol 27:247–262

Eckert J, Brand T von, Voge M (1969) Asexual multiplication of *Mesocestoides corti* (Cestoda) in the intestine of dogs and skunks. J Parasitol 55:241–249

Edgar SA (1956) The removal of chicken tapeworms by di-*n*-butyl tin dilaurate. Poult Sci 35:64–73

Edgar SA, Teer PA (1957) The efficiency of several compounds in causing elimination of tapeworms from laboratory-infected chickens. Poult Sci 36:329–334

Efner T (1974) (The influence of intestinal tapeworms on weight gains and the composition of carcass halves of wethers.) Medycyna Wet 30:81–83

Enzie FD, Foster AO, Sinclair LR, Colglazier ML (1953) Trials with di-phenthane-70 on the sheep tapeworm, *Moniezia expansa*. J Am Vet Med Assoc 122:29–30

Enzie FD, Foster AO, Colglazier ML (1957) Taeniacides in dogs and cats. North Am Vet 38:119–128

Essex HE, Magath TB (1931) Comparison of the viability of ova of the broad fish tapeworm, *Diphyllobothrium latum*, from man and dogs: its bearing on the spread of infestation with this parasite. Am J Hyg 14:698–704

Fastier LB (1949) The effect of physical agents on scolex viability. Parasitology 39:157–163

Fastier FN (1972) Pharmacological aspects of bunamidine dosing of dogs. NZ Vet J 20:148–151

Fastier FN, Menrath RLE, Sharard A, Ng J (1973) Toxicity of bunamidine I. Cardiovascular effects. NZ Vet J 21:201–204

Forbes LS (1961) Arecoline hydrobromide enemata and their use in dogs to improve purgative efficiency of the drug administered orally. NZ Vet J 9:105–106

Forbes LS (1963) The efficiency of *N*-(2′-chlor-4′-nitrophenyl)-5-chlor-salicylamid against *Taenia hydatigena* and *Echinococcus granulosus* infections in dogs. Vet Rec 75:321–324

Forbes LS (1964a) The use of arecoline hydrobromide in the treatment of Taeniid infections in dogs. Ann Trop Med Parasitol 58:116–118

Forbes LS (1964b) The relation between method of administration, route of absorption, inhibitory actions and acute toxicity of arecoline hydrobromide in dogs. Ann Trop Med Parasitol 58:119–131

Forbes LS (1966) The efficiency of bunamidine hydrochloride against young *Echinococcus granulosus* infection in dogs. Vet Rec 79:306–307

Forbes LS (1971) Anthelmintic toxicity, administration technique and routes of absorption. Aust Vet J 47:601–602

Forbes LS, Whitten LK (1961) Arecoline hydrobromide as a purgative in dogs: the effect of method of administration on its speed of action. NZ Vet J 9:101–104

Frost C (1951) A new taeniacide for dogs. Vet Rec 63:28

Fry JL, Wilson HR (1967) Studies on dietary piperazine, phenothiazine, and dibutyltin dilaurate 2. Yolk mottling and other egg quality characteristics. Poult Sci 46:319–322

Gallie GJ, Sewell MM (1978) Efficacy of praziquantel against the cysticerci of *T. saginata* in calves. Trop Anim Health Prod 10:36–38

Gemmell MA (1958a) Arecoline hydrobromide as a taeniafuge in dogs, with special reference to its use in controlling hydatid disease. Aust Vet J 34:207–212

Gemmell MA (1958b) The efficiency of dichlorophen (2,2′-dihydroxy-5,5′-dichloro-diphenyl methane) against *Echinococcus granulosus* infestation in dogs. Aust Vet J 34:249–252

Gemmell MA (1968) The Styx Field-Trial. A study on the application of control measures against hydatid disease caused by *Echinococcus granulosus*. Bull WHO 39:73–100

Gemmell MA, Johnstone PD (1981) Cestodes. Antibiotics Chemother 30:54–114

Gemmell MA, Oudemans G (1974) The treatment of *Echinococcus granulosus* and *Taenia hydatigena* in dogs with bunamidine hydroxynaphthoate in a prepared food. Res Vet Sci 16:85–88

Gemmell MA, Oudemans G (1975a) Treatment of *Taenia hydatigena* infections in dogs with bunamidine hydroxynaphthoate incorporated in food. NZ Vet J 23:142–144

Gemmell MA, Oudemans G (1975b) The effect of nitroscanate on *Echinococcus granulosus* and *Taenia hydatigena* infection in dogs. Res Vet Sci 19:217–219

Gemmell MA, Oudemans G (1975c) The effect of fospirate on *Echinococcus granulosus* and *Taenia hydatigena* infections in dogs. Res Vet Sci 19:216–217

Gemmell MA, Shearer GC (1968) Bunamidine hydrochloride: its efficiency against *Echinococcus granulosus*. Vet Rec 82:252–256

Gemmel MA, Johnstone PD, Oudemans G (1975) The effect of mebendazole on *Echinococcus granulosus* and *Taenia hydatigena* infection in dogs. Res Vet Sci 19:229–230

Gemmell MA, Johnstone PD, Oudemans G (1977a) The effect of niclosamide on *Echinococcus granulosus, Taenia hydatigena* and *Taenia ovis* infection in dogs. Res Vet Sci 22:389–391

Gemmell MA, Johnstone PD, Oudemans G (1977b) The effect of praziquantel on *Echinococcus granulosus, Taenia hydatigena* and *Taenia ovis* infection in dogs. Res Vet Sci 23:121–123

Gemmell MA, Johnstone PD, Oudemans G (1977c) The effect of micronised nitroscanate on *Echinococcus granulosus* and *Taenia hydatigena* infection in dogs. Res Vet Sci 22:391–392

Gemmell MA, Johnstone PD, Oudemans G (1977d) The lethal effect of some benzimidazole on *Taenia hydatigena* in dogs. Res Vet Sci 23:115–116

Gemmell MA, Johnstone PD, Oudemans G (1978a) The effect of diuredosan on *Echinococcus granulosus* and *Taenia hydatigena* infection in dogs. Res Vet Sci 25:111–112
Gemmell MA, Johnstone PD, Oudemans G (1978b) The effect of an antibiotic of the streptothricin family against *Echinococcus granulosus* and *Taenia hydatigena* infections in dogs. Res Vet Sci 25:109–110
Gemmell MA, Johnstone PD, Oudemans G (1978c) The effect of mebendazole in food on *Echinococcus granulosus* and *Taenia hydatigena* infections in dogs. Res Vet Sci 25:107–108
Gemmell MA, Johnstone PD, Oudemans G (1979a) The effect of nitroscanate tablets on *Echinococcus granulosus* and *Taenia hydatigena* infections in dogs. Res Vet Sci 27:255–257
Gemmell MA, Johnstone PD, Oudemans G (1979b) The effect of oxfendazole on *Echinococcus granulosus* and *Taenia hydatigena* infections in dogs. Res Vet Sci 26:389–390
Gemmell MA, Johnstone PD, Oudemans G (1980) The effect of route of administration on the efficacy of praziquantel against *Echinococcus granulosus* infections in dogs. Res Vet Sci 29:131–132
Gibbs HC, Gupta RP (1972) The anthelmintic activity of cambendazole in calves and lambs. Can J Comp Med 36:108–115
Gibson TE (1975) Veterinary anthelmintic medication, 3rd edn. Tech Comm No. 33, Comm Inst Helminthol, St. Albans
Gleason NN, Healy GR (1967) Report of a case of *Mesocestoides* (Cestoda) in a child in Missouri. J Parasitol 53:83–84
Gnezdilov VG (1957) The hamster (*Mesocricetus auratus*) as potential definitive host of the dog tapeworm (*Diphyllobothrium latum*). Dokl Akad Nauk SSSR (Otd Biol) 114:1328–1330
Graber M, Gras R (1962) Études de l'activité anthelminthique et de la toxicité du dilaurate d'etain dibutyle chez le poulet. Rev Elev Med Vet Pays Trop 15:411–426
Greenberg AE, Dean BH (1958) The beef tapeworm, measly beef and sewage – a review. Sewage Ind Wastes 30:262–269
Gregor WW (1963) A clinical assessment of 5-chloro-*N*-(2-chloro-4-nitrophenyl) salicylamide as a taeniacide for dogs and cats. Vet Rec 75:1421–1422
Gregory GG (1976) Fecundity and proglottid release of *Taenia ovis* and *T. hydatigena*. Aust Vet J 52:277–279
Guralp N, Tigin Y (1966) Anthelmintic efficiency of Yomesan against tapeworms in dogs and cats. Vet Fak Derg, Ankara Univ 13:253–267
Guralp N, Tigin Y (1971) Kopeklerdeki *Taenia hydatigena* enfeksionlarina bunamidine hydrochloride in etkisi. Vet Fak Derg, Ankara Univ 18:1–7. From Vet Bull 42:4696 (1972) (abstract)
Guralp N, Tigin Y, Oguz T, Tinar R, Burgu A (1976) Preliminary studies on the effect of Droncit against different tapeworms in dogs and cats. Vet Med Rev 2:129–133
Guthrie JE, Harwood PD (1941) Use of tin preparations for the treatment of chickens experimentally infected with tapeworms. Am J Vet Res 2:108–116
Hall CA (1966) Mansonil, a new cestocide for sheep. Vet Med Rev 1:59–66
Hall MC, Shillinger JE (1923) Some critical tests of arecoline hydrobromide as an anthelmintic. J Am Vet Med Assoc 63:454–463
Hart RJ, Turner R, Wilson RG (1977) A biochemical and ultrastructural study on the mode of action of bunamidine against *Hymenolepis nana*. Int J Parasitol 7:129–134
Hatch C, Smyth JD (1975) Attempted infection of sheep with *Echinococcus granulosus equinus*. Res Vet Sci 19:340
Hatton CJ (1965) A new taeniacide, bunamidine hydrochloride: its efficiency against *Taenia pisiformis* and *Dipylidium caninum* in the dog and *Hydatigera taeniaeformis* in the cat. Vet Rec 77:408–411
Hatton CJ (1967) Efficiency of bunamidine salts against tapeworms. Vet Rec 81:104–106
Heath DD (1970) The development of *Echinococcus granulosus* larvae in laboratory animals. Parasitology 60:449–456

Heath DD, Chevis RAF (1974) Mebendazole and hydatid cysts. Lancet 2:218–219
Heath DD, Lawrence SB (1976) *Echinococcus granulosus:* development in vitro from oncosphere to immature hydatid cyst. Parasitology 73:417–423
Heath DD, Lawrence SB (1978) The effect of mebendazole and praziquantel on the cysts of *Echinococcus granulosus, Taenia hydatigena* and *T. ovis* in sheep. NZ Vet J 26:11–15
Heath DD, Osborn PJ (1976) Formation of *Echinococcus granulosus* laminated membrane in a defined medium. Int J Parasitol 6:467–471
Heath DD, Christie MJ, Chevis RAF (1975) The lethal effect of mebendazole on secondary *Echinococcus granulosus,* cysticerci of *Taenia pisiformis* and tetrathyridia of *Mesocestoides corti.* Parasitology 70:273–285
Hecht G von, Gloxhuber C (1960) Experimental studies on *N*(2′-chloro-4′-nitrophenyl)-5-chloro-salicylamide, a new taeniacide. Arzneimittelforsch 10:884–885
Henderson GLB (1951) A new taeniacide for dogs. Vet Rec 63:12
Hopkins AC (1970) Diurnal movement of *Hymenolepis diminuta* in the rat. Parasitology 60:255–271
Horak IG (1964) Studies on paramphistomiasis VI. The anthelmintic efficiency of Lintex and Freon against *Paramphistomum* spp. in sheep and cattle. J S Afr Vet Assoc 35:161–166
Horak IG, Snijders AJ, Pienaar I (1972) The efficacy of cambendazole against cestode and nematode infestations in sheep and cattle. J S Afr Vet Assoc 43:101–106
Hromatka L von, Kutzer E, Stettner W (1966) Versuche mit dem Bandwurmmittel Scolaban beim Hund. Wien Tieraerztl Monatschr 9:616–617
Humes AG (1950) Experimental copepod hosts of the broad tapeworm of man, *Dibothriocephalus latus* (L.). J Parasitol 36:541–547
Humke R, Tiefenbach B, Düwel D (1970) Erfahrungen mit Terend bei der Bekämpfung des Bandwurmbefalls der Schafe. Tieraerztl Umschau 25:185–191
Jackson PJ, Arundel JH (1971) The incidence of tapeworms in rural dogs in Victoria. Aust Vet J 47:46–53
Johns DJ, Philip JR (1977) Albendazole: safety in sheep. Proc 8th Int Conf World Assoc Adv Vet Parasitol, Sydney
Kammerer WS, Judge DM (1976) Chemotherapy of hydatid disease (*Echinococcus granulosus*) in mice with mebendazole and bithionol. Am J Trop Med Hyg 25:714–717
Kartsonis PL, Austin JA (1950) Anthelin – a new compound for removing tapeworms and roundworms from dogs. J Am Vet Med Assoc 116:301–308
Kassai T, Redl P, Takats C, Hollo F, Magyar K, Gyenes J (1975) Investigations on the efficacy of some anticestode compounds against *Echinococcus granulosus* in the dog. Parasitol Hung 8:29–35
Katiyar JD, Garg RK (1966) Anthelmintic efficacy of Yomesan against tapeworms in sheep. Indian Vet J 43:310–314
Kelly JD, Bain SA (1975) Critical test evaluation of micronised mebendazole against *Anoplocephala perfoliata* in the horse. NZ Vet J 23:229–232
Kerr KB (1952) Butyronate, an effective and safe substance for the removal of *Raillietina cesticillus* from chickens. Poult Sci 41:1358–1360
Klein JB, Bradley RE Sr (1976) Critical testing of Sansalid against intestinal helminths in dogs and cats. Vet Med Small Anim Clin 71:598–599
Korkhaus R (1933) Zur parasitologisch-klinischen Bewertung einer Anthelmintika II. Arecolinum Hydrobromicum bei Hunden und Katzen. Tieraerztl Rundschau 39:794–799
Kuhlow F (1953) Untersuchungen über die Entwicklung des Breiten Bandwurmes (*Diphyllobothrium latum*). Z Tropenmed Parasitol 6:213–225
Kumratilake LM, Thompson RCA, Dunsmore JD (1979) Intraspecific variation in *Echinococcus:* a biochemical approach. Z Parasitenkd 60:291–294
Kurelec B, Rijavec M (1961) "Yomesan" an anthelmintic for dog and poultry tapeworm. Vet Glasn 15:602–606
Laws GF (1968 a) The hatching of taeniid eggs. Exp Parasitol 23:1–10
Laws GF (1968 b) Physical factors influencing survival of taeniid eggs. Exp Parasitol 22:227–239
Lentz WJ (1921) Treatment for tapeworms in dogs. Bull Univ Pa 21:2–3

LeRiche PD, Sewell MMH (1978) Identification of *Echinococcus granulosus* strains by enzyme electrophoresis. Res Vet Sci 25:247–248

Levine ND (1978) Textbook of veterinary parasitology. Burgess, Minneapolis

Link RP (1965) Anticestodal drugs. In: Jones LM (ed) Veterinary pharmacology and therapeutics, 3rd edn. Iowa State Univ Press, Ames, p 652

Liu IK, Schwabe CW, Schantz PM, Allison MN (1970) The occurrence of *Echinococcus granulosus* in coyotes (*Canis latrans*) in the central valley of California. J Parasitol 56:1135–1137

Lloyd S, Soulsby EJL, Theodorides VJ (1978) Effect of albendazole on the metacestodes of *Taenia saginata* in calves. Experientia 34:723–724

Lungu T, Milla C, Barbarosa E (1965) Observatii terapeutice in cestodozele gainilor. Revta Zooteh Med Vet Bucaresti 15:74–77

Lyons ET, Drudge JH, Tolliver SC (1977) Critical tests of oxfendazole against internal parasites of horses. Am J Vet Res 38:2049–2053

McAninch NH (1974) An outbreak of cysticercosis in feedlot cattle. Can Vet J 15:120–122

McManus DP, Smyth JD (1978) Differences in the chemical composition and carbohydrate metabolism of *Echinococcus granulosus* (horse and sheep strains) and *E. multilocularis*. Parasitology 77:103–109

MacNair AL (1980) Mebendazole and hydatid disease. Br Med J 280:1055

McBeath DG, Best JMJ, Preston NK (1977) Efficacy of fenbendazole against naturally acquired *M. expansa* infections in lambs. Vet Rec 101:408–409

McCulloch B, Kasimbala S (1967) The efficiency of bunamidine hydroxynaphthoate in poultry. Vet Rec 81:226–230

Malan FS (1980) Anthelmintic efficacy of fenbendazole against cestodes in sheep and cattle. J S Afr Vet Assoc 51:25–26

Matoff K, Kolev G (1963) Efficacy of the antimony compound Anthelin against *Echinococcus* in dogs. Agnew Parasitol 4:36–39

Matossian RM, Rickard MD, Smyth JD (1977) Hydatidosis: a global problem of increasing importance. Bull WHO 55:499–507

Menrath RLE, Sharard A, Gray KW, Cameron CW (1973) Toxicity of bunamidine 2. Metabolic effects. NZ Vet J 21:212–215

Michael SA, El-Refaii AH, Mansour WH, Selim MK, Higgins AJ (1979) Efficacy of oxfendazole against natural infestations of nematodes and cestodes in sheep in Egypt. Vet Rec 104:338–340

Morseth DJ (1966) Chemical composition of embryophoric blocks of *Taenia hydatigena, Taenia ovis* and *Taenia pisiformis* eggs. Exp Parasitol 18:347–354

Mueller JF (1938) The life history of *Diphyllobothrium mansonoides* Mueller, 1935, and some considerations with regard to sparganosis in the United States. Am J Trop Med 18:41–66

Mueller JF (1963) Parasite-induced weight gain in mice. Ann NY Acad Sci 113:217–233

Mueller JF (1965) Further studies on parasitic obesity in mice, deer mice, and hampsters. J Parasitol 51:523–531

Mueller JF (1970) Comparison of the growth-promoting effect of *Spirometra mansonoides* vs. three oriental forms in intact mice and hypophysectomized rats. J Parasitol 56:842–844

Mueller JF (1972) Survival and longevity of *Mesocestoides* tetrathyridia under adverse conditions. J Parasitol 58:228

Mueller JF (1974) The biology of Spirometra. J Parasitol 60:3–14

Mueller JF, Strano AJ (1974) *Sparganum proliferum,* a sparganum infected with a virus? J Parasitol 60:15–19

Muermann P, Eberstein M von, Frohberg H (1976) Notes on the tolerance of droncit. Vet Med Rev 2:142–153

Nadakal AM, Muraleedharan K, John KO, Mohandas A (1971) Resistance potential of certain breeds of domestic fowl exposed to *Raillietina tetragona* infections V. Pathogenic effects of the cestode on growing chickens. Jpn J Parasitol 20:433–438

Nelson GS, Pester FRN, Rickman R (1965) The significance of wild animals in the transmission of cestodes of medical importance in Kenya. Trans R Soc Trop Med Hyg 59:507–524

Novak M (1977) Efficacy of a new cestocide, praziquantel, against larval *Mesocestoides corti* and *Taenia crassiceps* in mice. J Parasitol 63:949–950

Nugara D (1963) The efficacy of Yomesan in removing *Moniezia* spp. and *Avitellina* spp. of tapeworms from goats. Ceylon Vet J 11:91–92

Nugara D, Reid WM (1962) Some drug treatments for the turkey tapeworm, *Raillietina georgiensis*. Poult Sci 41:674–675

Olsen OW (1953) An evaluation of medicaments, with special reference to Teniatol for removing fringed tapeworms (*Thysanosoma actinioides*) from the livers of sheep. Am J Vet Res 14:616–620

Opuni EK, Muller RL (1974) Studies on *Spirometra theileri* (Baer 1925) n. comb. I. Identification and biology in the laboratory. J Helminthol 48:15–23

Pagani GL, Agosti M (1969) The piperazine salt of *N*-(2′-chloro-4′-nitrophenyl)-5-chlorosalicylamide for the treatment of tapeworm infestation of the dog. Prog VIIIth Congress Ass Sci An Vet, San Remo. From Vet Med Rev 3:235–236 (1970) (abstract)

Pawlowski Z, Kozakiewicz B, Zatonski J (1976a) Effect of mebendazole on hydatid cysts in pigs. Vet Parasitol 2:299–302

Pawlowski Z, Kozakiewicz B, Wroblewski H (1976b) Effect of intraperitoneal inoculation of mebendazole on *Taenia saginata* cysticercosis in calves. Vet Parasitol 2:303–306

Pawlowski Z, Kozakiewicz B, Wroblewski H (1978) The efficiency of mebendazole and praziquantel against *Taenia saginata* cysticercosis in cattle. Vet Sci Comm 2:137–139

Perez-Esandi MV, Colli CW, Schantz PM (1974) The ovicidal effect of selected chemicals against eggs of *Echinococcus granulosus*. Bull WHO 51:550–551

Pfeiffer A (1970) Untersuchungen mit Terenol zur Bandwurmbehandlung bei Schafen. DTW 77:104–107

Piercy DWT, Reynolds J, Brown PRM (1979) Reproductive safety studies of oxfendazole in sheep and cattle. Br Vet J 135:405–410

Poole JB, Dooley KL, Rollins LD (1971) Efficacy of niclosamide for the removal of tapeworms (*Dipylidium caninum* and *Taenia pisiformis*) from dogs. J Am Vet Med Assoc 159:78–80

Popescu F, Mironescu DM (1934) Cercetari experimentale pentru stabilirea proprietatii teniifuge, la caini, a produsului nemural. Arh Vet 26:216–224

Prichard RK (1978) Anthelmintics. In: Proceedings No. 39. The therapeutic jungle. Post Grad Comm Vet Sci, Sydney, pp 421–463

Prichard RK, Hennessy DR, Steel JW (1977) Prolonged administration: a new concept for increasing the spectrum and effectiveness of anthelmintics. Proc 8th Int Conf World Assoc Adv Vet Parasitol, Sydney

Prieto R (1971) Efficacia de le niclosamida en el tratamiento de la monieziosis en bovinos y ovinos jovenes. Rev Cubana Cienc Vet 2:69–75

Radionov PV, Kemel'Bekov NK (1977) The role of the components of the intestinal parasitocoenosis in the pathogenesis of infective enterotoxaemia in sheep. Vestnik Sel'skokhozyaĭstvennoĭ Nauki Zazakhstana (Kazakstan Auyl Sharuashylyk Gylymynyn Habarshysy) 8:64–67. From Helminthol Abstr Series A 47:4573 (1978) (abstract)

Ranatunga P (1971) The efficacy of bunamidine hydroxynaphthoate for removing *Moniezia expansa* in goats. Preliminary examination. Ceylon Vet J 19:13–14

Rausch RL, Bernstein JJ (1972) *Echinococcus vogeli* sp. n. (Cestoda: Taeniidae) from the bush dog *Speothus venaticus* (Lund.). Z Tropenmed Parasitol 23:25–34

Read CP, Kilejian AZ (1969) Circadian migratory behaviour of a cestode symbiote in rat host. J Parasitol 55:574–578

Reid JF, Armour J (1978) An economic appraisal of helminth parasites in sheep. Vet Rec 102:4–7

Reinhardt R (1933) Arekolin als Antitaenikum. Berl Munch Tierarztl Wochenschr 49:129

Reisin IL, Rabito CA, Rotunno CA, Cereijido M (1977) The permeability of the membranes of experimental secondary cysts of *Echinococcus granulosus* to [^{14}C] mebendazole. Int J Parasitol 7:189–194

Richards RJ, Somerville JM (1980) Field trials with nitroscanate against cestodes and nematodes in dogs. Vet Rec 106:332–335

Rickard MD, Adolph AJ (1977) The prevalence of cysticerci of *Taenia saginata* in cattle reared on sewage-irrigated pasture. Med J Aust 1:525–527

Rickard MD, Arundel JH, Adolph AJ (1981) A preliminary field trial to evaluate the use of immunisation for the control of naturally acquired *Taenia saginata* infection in cattle. Res Vet Sci 30:104–108

Roberson EL (1976) Comparative effects of uredofos, niclosamide, and bunamidine hydrochloride against tapeworm infections in dogs. Am J Vet Res 37:1483–1484

Roberson EL (1977) Anticestodal and antitrematodal drugs. In: Jones LM, Booth NH, McDonald LE (eds) Veterinary pharmacology and therapeutics, 4th edn. The Iowa State University Press, Ames, Iowa, pp 1052–1078

Roberson EL, Ager AL (1976) Uredofos: anthelmintic activity against nematodes and cestodes in dogs with naturally occurring infections. Am J Vet Res 37:1479–1482

Roberson EL, Burke TM (1980) Evaluation of granulated fenbendazole (22.2%) against induced and naturally occurring helminth infection in cats. Am J Vet Res 41:1499–1502

Rommel M, Grelck H, Horchner F (1976) The efficacy of praziquantel against tapeworms in experimentally infected dogs and cats. Berl Munch Tierarztl Wochenschr 89:255–257

Ross IC (1924) The possible use of arecoline hydrobromide as an anthelmintic. J Comp Pathol 37:246–259

Ross IC (1936) A note on the development of *Echinococcus granulosus*. J Counc Sci Ind Res 9:67

Safaev YaS (1972) Efficacy of phenasal against anoplocephalids in horses. Veterinariya, Moscow 49:68–69

Sakamoto T (1977a) The anthelmintic effect of Droncit on adult tapeworms of *Hydatigera taeniaeformis, Mesocestoides corti, Echinococcus multilocularis, Diphyllobothrium erinacei* and *D. latum*. Vet Med Rev 1:64–74

Sakamoto T (1977b) The cestocidal effect of praziquantel on the larval stages of *Hydatigera taeniaeformis, Mesocestoides corti* and *Echinococcus multilocularis* in laboratory animals. Vet Med Rev 2:153–162

Sakamoto T, Orihara M, Sarashina T, Ishimoto Y, Kamiya H (1971) Studies on pharmocotherapy against larval and adult multilocular echinococcoses I. Anthelmintic and ovicidal effects of drugs against adult *Echinococcus multilocularis*. Jpn J Parasitol 20:120–131

Salem HH, El-Allaf G (1969) Treatment of *Taenia saginata* and *Hymenolepis nana* infections with paromomycin. Trans R Soc Trop Med Hyg 63:833–836

Salminen K (1970) The effect of high and low temperature treatments on the infestiveness of *Diphyllobothrium latum* with regard to public health. Acta Vet Scand [Suppl] 32:29

Sawada I (1963) The effect of butyronate preparation on egg production in laying hens. Jpn J Parasitol 12:379–381

Sawada I (1965a) Experimental removal of *Raillietina kashiwarensis* with Bayer 2353 (Yomesan). Jpn J Parasitol 14:189–191

Sawada I (1965b) Anthelmintic activity of Yomesan (75% powder) against *Raillietina cesticillus*. Jpn J Parasitol 14:220–221

Schalkwyk PC van, Geyser TL, Recio M, Erasmus FPG (1979) The anthelmintic efficiency of albendazole against gastro-intestinal roundworms, tapeworms, lungworms and liver fluke in sheep. J S Afr Vet Assoc 50:31–35

Schantz PM, Prezioso U (1976) Efficacy of divided doses of fospirate against immature *Echinococcus granulosus* infection in dogs. Am J Vet Res 37:619–620

Schantz PM, Prezioso U, Marchevsky N (1976) Efficacy of divided doses of GS 23654 against immature *Echinococcus granulosus* infection in dogs. Am J Vet Res 37:621–622

Schillings RT, Schaffner CP (1961) Differentiation of catenulin-neomycin antibiotics, identity of catenulin, paromomycin, hydroxymycin and amminosidin. Antimicrob Agents Chemother, 274–285

Schmidt JM, Todd KS (1978) Life cycle of *Mesocestoides corti* in the dog (*Canis familiaris*). Am J Vet Res 39:1490–1493

Sharp ML, Sepesi J, Collins JA (1973) A comparative critical assay on canine anthelmintics. Vet Med Small Anim Clin 68:131–132
Shearer GC, Gemmell MA (1969) The efficiency of bunamidine hydroxynaphthoate against *Echinococcus granulosus* in dogs. Res Vet Sci 10:296–299
Siedel MC, Kilbourne EE, Peardon DL, Tetzlaff RD, Weiler ED, Weir WD (1975) A new broad spectrum anthelmintic for dogs and cats. Proc 20th World Vet Congress, Thessalonika
Singh BB, Rao BV (1967) Chemotherapeutic trials with Nemural and Yomesan in experimental *Taenia taeniaeformis* infection in cats. Indian Vet J 44:208–212
Slais J (1970) The morphology and pathogenicity of the Bladder worms *Cysticercus cellulosae* and *Cysticercus bovis*. Junk, The Hague
Slais J, Mann I (1976) Morphological determination of the age of *Cysticercus bovis* in very young calves with cysticercosis. Folia Parasitol (Praha) 23:321–326
Slonka GF, Matulich W, Morphet E, Miller CW, Bayer EV (1978) An outbreak of bovine cysticercosis in California. Am J Trop Med Hyg 27:101–105
Smyth JD (1969) The physiology of cestodes. Oliver and Boyd, Edinburgh
Smyth JD, Davies Z (1974a) Occurrence of physiological strains of *Echinococcus granulosus* demonstrated by in vitro culture of protoscoleces from sheep and horse hydatid cysts. Int J Parasitol 4:443–445
Smyth JD, Davies Z (1974b) In vitro culture of the strobilar stage of *Echinococcus granulosus* (sheep strain): a review of basic problems and results. Int J Parasitol 4:631–644
Smyth JD, Heath DD (1970) Pathogenesis of larval cestodes in mammals. Helminthol Abstr Series A 39:1–23
Soldatova AP (1944) A contribution to the study of the development cycle in the cestode *Mesocestoides lineatus* (Goeze 1782), parasitic in carnivorous mammals. Dokl Akad Nauk SSSR 45:310–312
Soulsby EJL (1965) Textbook of veterinary clinical parasitology, Vol I, Helminths. Blackwell, London
Soulsby EJL (1968) Helminths, arthropods and protozoa of domesticated animals (Sixth edition of Monnigs veterinary helminthology and entomology), Bailliere Tindall and Cassell, London)
Specht D, Voge M (1965) Asexual multiplication of *Mesocestoides* tetrathyridia in laboratory animals. J Parasitol 51:268–272
Speckman G, Webster WA (1975) Natural infection and treatment of a dog with *Mesocestoides* tapeworms. Can Vet J 16:26–27
Stampa S (1967) A contribution towards the influence of tapeworms on life weights of lambs. Vet Med Rev 1:81–85
Stampa S, Terblanche HJJ (1961) Trials with Bayer 2353 and other drugs as cestocides for ruminants. J S Afr Vet Assoc 32:367–371
Standen OD (1963) Chemotherapy of helminthic infections. In: Schnitzer RJ, Hawking F (eds) Experimental chemotherapy, vol 1. Academic, New York, London, p 716
Stetter R (1933) „Nemural“, ein neues Bandwurmmittel für Hunde und Katzen. MTW 84:385–389
Strufe R, Gonnert R (1967) Über die Beeinflussung des Bandwurmstoffwechsels durch Arzneimittel. Z Tropenmed Parasitol 18:193–202
Stunkard HW (1937) The life-cycle of *Moniezia expansa*. Science 186:312
Sweatman GK, Williams RJ (1963) The significance of the distribution and fluorescence of *Taenia ovis* in sheep in meat inspection procedure. Res Vet Sci 4:359–366
Szanto J, Lillis WG, Brown WE, Sutphin CF, Maplesden DC (1979) Critical evaluation of taeniacidal antibiotic S 15-1 (SQ 21,704) for removal of natural tapeworm infections in dogs and cats. Am J Vet Res 40:673–675
Teichert HG (1963) Versuche mit dem Bandwurmmittel „Yomesan“ bei Schafen. Wien Tierarztl Monatsschr 50:1023–1027
Terblanche HJJ (1966) Control of pigeon tapeworm with Lintex. Vet Med Rev 1:55–59
Thakur AS, Prezioso U, Marchevsky N (1978) Efficacy of Droncit against *Echinococcus granulosus* in dogs. Am J Vet Res 39:859–860

Thakur AS, Prezioso U, Marchevsky N (1979) *Echinococcus granulosus:* ovicidal activity of praziquantel and bunamidine hydrochloride. Exp Parasitol 47:131–133
Theodorides VJ, Gyurik RJ, Kingsbury WD, Parish RC (1976a) Anthelmintic activity of albendazole against liver flukes, tapeworms, lung and gastro-intestinal roundworms. Experientia 32:702
Theodorides VJ, Nawalinski T, Chang J (1976b) Efficacy of albendazole against *Haemonchus, Nematodirus, Dictyocaulus* and *Moniezia* of sheep. Am J Vet Res 37:1515–1516
Thienpont D, Vanparijs O, Hermans L (1974) Anthelmintic activity of mebendazole against *Cysticercus fasciolaris.* J Parasitol 60:1052–1053
Thomas H, Gonnert R (1977) The efficacy of praziquantel against cestodes in animals. Z Parasitenkd 52:117–127
Thomas H, Gonnert R (1978a) The efficacy of praziquantel against cestodes in cats, dogs and sheep. Res Vet Sci 24:20–25
Thomas G, Gonnert R (1978b) The efficacy of praziquantel against experimental cysticercosis and hydatidosis. Z Parasitenkd 55:165–179
Thomas H, Gonnert R, Pohlke R, Seubert J (1975) Experimental and clinical studies with a new compound against adult tapeworms. Proc 7th Conf World Assoc Adv Vet Parasitol, Thessalonika
Thompson RCA (1976a) The occurrence of *Mesocestoides* sp. in British wild red foxes (*Vulpes vulpes crucigera*). J Helminthol 50:91–94
Thompson RCA (1976b) The development of brood capsules and protoscoleces in secondary hydatid cysts of *Echinococcus granulosus:* a histological study. Z Parasitenkd 51:31–36
Thompson RCA (1978) Aspects of speciation in *Echinococcus granulosus.* Vet Parasitol 4:121–125
Todd KS Jr (1978) Albendazole in treatment of *Mesocestoides corti* (Cestoda) infections in dogs. Vet Med Small Anim Clin 73:453–454
Todd KS Jr, Yates RL (1976) Anthelmintic activity of diuredosan in dogs experimentally infected with *Ancylostoma caninum* and *Trichuris vulpis.* Am J Vet Res 37:1329–1330
Todd KS Jr, Howland TP, Woerpel RW (1978) The activity of uredofos, niclosamide, bunamidine hydrochloride, and arecoline hydrobromide against *Mesocestoides corti* in experimentally infected dogs. Am J Vet Res 39:315–316
Townsend RB, Kelly JD, James R, Weston I (1977) The anthelmintic efficacy of fenbendazole in the control of *Moniezia expansa* and *Trichuris ovis* in sheep. Res Vet Sci 23:385–386
Trejos A, Szyfres B, Marchevsky N (1975) Comparative value of arecoline hydrobromide and bunamidine hydrochloride for the treatment of *Echinococcus granulosus* in dogs. Res Vet Sci 19:212–213
Ulivelli A (1963) Terapia antibiotica della teniasi (Primi favorevoli risultati del trattamento con paromomicini). Riv Clin Pediatr 72:371–383
Vanden Bossche H (1972) Biochemical effects of the anthelmintic drug mebendazole. In: Van den Bossche (ed) Comparative biochemistry of parasites. Academic, New York, pp 139–157
Vanparijs O, Thienpont D (1973) Anthelmintic activity of mebendazole against nematodes and cestodes in dogs. DTW 80:320–322
Vassilev I, Denev J, Kostov R (1977) Trials regarding the anticestodal activity of Droncit in poultry. Vet Met Rev 2:149–152
Verster A (1969) A taxonomic revision of the genus *Taenia* Linnaeus, 1758 S. Str. Onderstepoort J Vet Res 36:3–58
Verster A, Tustin RC, Reinecke RK (1978) An attempt to treat the larval stage of *Taenia multiceps* and a resumé of its neural and extraneural distribution in sheep. Onderstepoort J Vet Res 45:257–259
Vibe PP (1976) Parasitic coenoses in sheep. Veterinariya, Moscow 6:58–60
Vik R (1964) The genus *Diphyllobothrium.* An example of the interdependence of systematics and experimental biology. Exp Parasitol 15:261–380
Virji AS, Laverty R (1972) Bunamidine uptake and distribution in rats and dogs. Aust J Exp Biol Med Sci 50:209–215

von Bornsdorff B (1978) The broad tapeworm story. Acta Med Scand 204:241–247
Waitz JA, McClay P, Thompson PE (1966) Effects of Paromomycin on tapeworms of mice, rats and cats. J Parasitol 52:830–831
Walther M, Koske JK (1979) The efficacy of praziquantel against *Taenia saginata* cysticercosis in naturally affected calves. Tropenmed Parasitol 30:401–403
Wardle RA, McLeod JA (1952) The zoology of tapeworms. Hafner, New York
Wardle RA, McLeod JA, Radinovsky S (1974) Advances in the zoology of tapeworms. University of Minnesota Press, Minneapolis
Wescott RB (1967) Efficacy of niclosamide in the treatment of *Taenia taeniaeformis* infection in cats. Am J Vet Res 28:1475–1477
Whitten LK (1951) A new taeniacide for dogs. Vet Rec 63:381
Whitten LK (1956) The treatment of tapeworm infestations in man and animals. Vet Rev Annot 2:1–24
Williams JF, Keahey KK (1976) Sudden death associated with treatment of three dogs with bunamidine hydrochloride. J Am Vet Med Assoc 168:689–691
Williams JF, Trejos A (1970) The influence of gelatine capsules upon the activity of bunamidine hydrochloride against *Echinococcus granulosus* in dogs. Res Vet Sci 11:392–394
Williams JF, Colli CW, Leid RW, MacArthur R (1973) The effects of bunamidine hydrochloride on the infectivity of Taeniid ova. J Parasitol 59:1141–1144
Williams JF, Westheimer J, Banman WR (1975) *Mesocestoides* infection in the dog. J Am Vet Med Assoc 166:996–998
Williams JF, Sheehan D, Fuselier RH (1977) Effect of albendazole on gastro-intestinal parasites of cattle. Am J Vet Res 38:2037–2038
Wilson HR, Fry JL, Jones JE (1967) Studies on dietary piperazine, phenothiazine and dibutyl tin dilaurate I. Fertility, hatchability and egg production. Poult Sci 46:304–309
Wilson JF, Diddams AC, Rausch RL (1968) Cystic hydatid disease in Alaska. Am Rev Respir Dis 98:1–15
Witenburg G (1934) Studies on the cestode genus *Mesocestoides*. Arch Zool Ital 20:467–509
Yamaguti S (1959) Systema Helminthum, vol II. The cestodes of vertebrates. Interscience, New York
Zettl K (1965) Erfahrungsbericht über den Einsatz von Mansonil und Maretin bei Band-, Magen- und Darmwurmbefall von Schafen. Vet Med Nachrichten 3:193–200

CHAPTER 14

Chemotherapy of Tapeworm Infections in Man

W. S. KAMMERER

A. Introduction

In the past 20 years, three new compounds, niclosamide, mebendazole, and praziquantel, have emerged to replace the innumerable organic and inorganic products and potions previously available for the treatment of human cestode infections. In terms of efficacy, safety, and ease of administration, they are far superior to their predecessors. The clinical use and chemistry of these older compounds (i.e., aspidium oleoresin, quinicrine, dichlorophen, and various tin, arsenical, lead, copper, and other inorganic elements) have been extensively reviewed, and, as they have been almost entirely replaced in human therapeutics, they will not be further examined here. While demonstrably better than our previous remedies for adult cestode infections, these three new compounds are not without their own problems in clinical use. Major advances in drug therapy for larval cestode infections in man have also been made, but much remains to be done before it reaches the effectiveness we currently can achieve with adult infections.

B. General Features of Human Cestode Infections

While found worldwide (Table 1), the distribution of human cestode infections is by no means uniform. Agricultural factors, food preparation and preferences, general hygienic practices, and the distribution and types of intermediate hosts, along with multiple other considerations, influence the presence and intensity of the various infections found in man.

Table 1. Number of human tapeworm infections in millions [as compiled by GÖNNERT (1974) and DE CARNERI and VITA (1973)]

Tapeworm	Europe	Asia	Africa	North America	Central and South America	Australia, New Zealand	Total
Diphyllobothrium latum	5	4	< 0.1	<0.1	–	–	9
Taenia saginata	11	15	18.1	0.1	0.7	0.1	45
T. solium	0.4	1.6	0.9	0.5	0.1	<0.1	3
Echinococcus	< 0.1	< 0.1	< 0.1	<0.1	<0.1	<0.1	0
Hymenolepis nana	4	30	5.5	0.5	4	<0.1	44

Table 2. Human cestode infections

Only adult in man	Adult and larva in man	Only larva in man
Diphyllobothrium latum	*Taenia solium*	*Taenia multiceps* *T. crassiceps*
D. pacificum	*T. saginata*	*Echinococcus granulosus*
Dipylidium caninum	*Hymenolepis nana*	*E. multilocularis*
	H. diminuta	*E. vogeli* *Spirometra mansonoides* *S. proliferum*

In general, the tapeworm infections of man can be broadly grouped into three categories: (1) only adults found in man (man serves as the definitive host); (2) only larvae found in man (man an aberrant intermediate host – anthropozoonotic infections); and (3) both adults and larvae found in man (Table 2).

Adult tapeworms in man range in length from the diminutive dwarf tapeworm, *Hymenolepis nana,* approximately 2.5–4 cm, to the enormous fish tapeworm, *Diphyllobothrium latum,* reaching up to 10 or more meters in length. Larval stages in man progress in complexity from the rudimentarily simple sparganum (Pseudophyllidae) through progressively more organized structures, i.e., cysticercoids (e.g., *H. nana*), cysticercus (e.g., *Taenia solium*), coenurus (e.g., *T. multiceps*), and hydatids (*Echinococcus* species). Details of life cycles and epidemiological considerations pertinent to the treatment of these various infections will be discussed with clinical results of drug therapy.

C. Niclosamide

Niclosamide was introduced into medicine in 1960. A nucleoside analogue (JAFFE 1975), niclosamide is classified as a hydrogen ionophore (VANDEN BOSSCHE et al. 1979; VAN DEN BOSSCHE 1980) capable of translocating protons through the inner mitochondrial membrane and inhibiting oxidative phosphorylation in the mitochondria. In susceptible adult tapeworms uptake of oxygen and glucose is blocked, killing them on contact, both in vivo and in vitro. Its major action takes place in the scolex and proximal segments, with the more distal gravid segments unaffected (PAWLOWSKI and SCHULTZ 1972).

Studies with radio-labeled niclosamide demonstrate that 25%–30% of the orally administered compound is rapidly excreted in the urine, almost entirely as metabolites, and that the remainder is excreted in the feces. There is no evidence of accumulation in body fluids or tissue (PAWLOWSKI and SCHULTZ 1972).

Results in Clinical Trials – Adult Cestode Infections

Numerous worldwide studies have demonstrated the efficacy and safety of niclosamide for human intestinal infections with *T. saginata, T. solium, H. nana,* and *D.*

Table 3. Composite results for niclosamide treatment in man

Tapeworm	% cured
Taenia saginata	85–97
T. solium	81–86
Hymenolepis nana	84–98
H. diminata	89
Diphyllobothrium latum	83–87
Dipylidium caninum	100

latum. Fewer, but similar, results are also available for infections with *H. diminuta* and *Dipylidium caninum* (JONES 1979). The great majority of these studies have been compiled and commented upon in recent revies (STANDEN 1963; KEELING 1968; DAVIS 1973; PAWLOWSKI and SCHULTZ 1972; ANONYMOUS 1970; JONES 1978; PERERA et al. 1970; EL-MASRY et al. 1974; KAHRA and VEHARANTA 1963). Overall, a greater than 80% cure rate can be expected with a single course of treatment with niclosamide (Table 3).

Niclosamide is supplied in 0.5-g chewable tablets. The adult dose for all but *Hymenolepis* infections is 2 g, thoroughly chewed, as a single oral dose. No special precautions or purges are required, although the drug is generally administered after an overnight fast and with only a small amount of water. Normal activity and light meals may commence 2–4 h afterward. Children between the ages of 2 and 6 years are given 500 mg; from age of 6 years up to 34 kg body weight, 1 g; and 34–45 kg body weight, 1.5 g (ANONYMOUS-CDC 1970; KEAN 1976).

Due to the fact that *H. nana* and *H. diminuta* can complete their life cycles entirely within the human gastrointestinal tract over a 1- to 2-week period, therapy for this infection differs from the others. A loading dose of 40–80 mg/kg (or 1–2 g) is given on the 1st day, followed by 20 mg/kg per day (or 0.5–1 g) for 5–7 days. If still infected 2 weeks later, the course is repeated. Niclosamide is without effect on any of the cestode larval stages.

Many of the earlier less impressive results with niclosamide were probably due to the use of drug preparation with a particle size greater than the optimal 2–6 μm (PAWLOWSKI and SCHULTZ 1972).

A practical problem with niclosamide therapy is the inability to establish a parasitological cure for up to 3 months after treatment. The adult worms are killed by the drug and are digested during their expulsion from the gastrointestinal tract, usually making identification of the scolex impossible. In addition, niclosamide is not ovicidal. Theoretically, therefore, especially with *T. solium* infections, if vomiting were to follow treatment, eggs liberated from the gravid segments could be swallowed and could hatch, penetrate the intestinal mucosa, and develop into larval cysts (cysticercosis). While no such cases have yet been documented, every effort should be taken to prevent vomiting following therapy.

Patients infected with *Diphyllobothrium latum,* especially in Scandinavia, are often found to have a megaloblastic anemia. This has been related to a "steal" phenomenon of vitamin B_{12} and intrinsic factor by the worm (ANONYMOUS 1977).

Curiously, this is rarely seen outside of Scandinavia and may be related to strain differences in the worm (ANONYMOUS 1976). I am also aware of a case where orally administered radio-labelled digoxin was similarly "stolen" by *D. latum* (J. W. Burnside, M. D. Hershey, Pennsylvania 1978, personal communication). Whether other drugs can be absorbed by *D. latum,* or other adult cestodes in the human intestine, has not yet been studied but seems possible.

D. Mebendazole

Mebendazole, a broad-spectrum intestinal anthelminthic, is one of a series of benzimidazole derivatives developed over the past 10 years. Information on its chemistry, mode of action, pharmacokinetics, and toxicity can be found in Chap. 4.

Two liquid chromatographic techniques have been described to measure plasma concentrations of mebendazole. ALTON et al. (1979), using repeated extractions with ethyl acetate and petroleum ether, measured plasma mebendazole with a reversed phase column and UV detection at 313 nm. This method is sensitive to a level of 10 ng/ml with an average recovery of 75($\pm$3.8 SD)%. KARLAGANIS et al. (1979), using high-pressure liquid chromatography and a single extraction of plasma with chloroform at pH 11, measured plasma mebendazole spectrophotometrically at 307 nm. They report this method accurate between 20 and 200 ng/ml. Average recovery from plasma varied from 70% to 80%. A radioimmune assay sensitive to 0.2 ng mebendazole/ml plasma has been reported by MICHIELS et al. (1978).

In approximately 500 human cases of echinococcosis either reported in the literature or for whom adequate records exist, treatment with mebendazole or flubendazole for weeks to years with 25–200 mg/kg per day resulted in relatively little toxicity. Three cases of agranulocytosis have occurred with mebendazole, two of them reversible (WILSON and RAUSCH 1980; MISKOVITZ and JAVITT 1980; KERN 1980). Several cases of a reversible, partial to total alopecia have been reported (BEARD et al. 1978; KERN 1980). In five fatal African cases of *Echinococcus granulosus,* a mild membraneous glomerulonephritis was found, but was not thought to be related to the patients' demise (FRENCH 1980). No urinary or renal abnormalities have been reported from elsewhere.

Transient mild elevations of hepatic enzymes have occasionally been noted during long-term mebendazole therapy (BRAITHWAITE, 1980; SABRIE et al. 1980), returning to normal when it was stopped. In rats and rabbits given one oral dose of 2,650 mg/kg (the LD_{50}) flubendazole, hepatocyte mitochondrial cristae and microvilli in bile canaliculi were disrupted but usually resolved within 1–6 days (KANG et al. 1978). However, no changes in hepatic enzymes were observed in the rabbits, and only minimal elevations of serum glutamic oxaloacetic transaminase (SGOT) and alkaline phosphatase in the rats.

Much concern has been expressed over the possibility of anaphylactic reactions occurring if hydatid cysts were to rupture or leak with mebendazole therapy (KAMMERER and JUDGE 1976). A number of case reports of prolonged fevers, hypotension, wheezing, urticaria, pain over the cyst site, etc. have suggested that this does occur (WERCZBERGER et al. 1979; KERN et al. 1979; KAYSER

1980; BRYCESON 1980a). As yet however, no human fatalities have been related to anaphylactic reactions during mebendazole therapy. Women who have taken mebendazole in early pregnancy have not had any increase in fetal abnormalities or loss, suggesting that humans are less susceptible than rats to the embryotoxicity of mebendazole (Brugmans 1978, personal communication).

In summary, mebendazole, in doses of 40–200 mg/kg per day for weeks to years appears to be well tolerated by humans. However, three cases of agranulocytosis have been associated with the use of high doses of mebendazole and blood counts should be carefully monitored. In addition, the possibility of anaphylactic reactions due to degenerating cysts should be kept in mind and patients appropriately forewarned and closely followed. Because of limited human data and of embryotoxicity in rats, mebendazole should not be given during pregnancy.

Flubendazole is the only other benzimidazole derivative to have been used to any degree in humans (SCHENONE et al. 1977b; QUILICI et al. 1979; DANIS et al. 1977). In France, flubendazole was used for a time to treat human hyatid disease. It is less well absorbed than mebendazole and has a shorter plasma half-life (MICHIELS 1980). Acute and chronic toxicity studies reveal it to be better tolerated than mebendazole in the most sensitive test animal the rat, with no evidence of embryotoxicity or effect on fertility (THIENPONT et al. 1978).

Results in Clinical Trials

1. Adult Cestode Infections

Mebendazole has been shown to be effective against *T. solium*, *T. saginata*, and *H. nana* infections in man. While excellent results have been reported with *T. solium*, *T. saginata* seems more resistant. PEÑA-CHAVARRIA et al. (1977) in Costa Rica, reported a 100% cure rate for *T. solium* and *T. saginata* after a 4- to 5-month follow-up period when mebendazole was administered at 300 mg b.i.d. for 3 days. However, at doses of 100–200 mg b.i.d. for 4–6 days, cure rates of only 50%–80% were found. They also state that *T. saginata* was relatively more resistant than *T. solium*. Furthermore, VAKIL et al. (1975) in India reported no cures in ten patients with *T. saginata* infections after a 3-month follow-up period following treatment with 100–300 mg mebendazole b.i.d. for 4 days (Table 4).

PEÑA-CHAVARRIA et al. also report that many of their patients passed intact but immobile proglottids of *T. solium* after mebendazole treatment. This would have important therapeutic implications regarding the possibility of autoinfection (cysticercosis) developing from regurgitated eggs (as discussed earlier with ni-

Table 4. Composite results of mebendazole treatment of adult cestode infections in man

Tapeworm	% cured
Taenia solium	50–100
T. saginata	0–100
Hymenolepis nana	18– 50

closamide therapy; see also KEAN and HOPKINS 1980), suggesting that mebendazole be used in preference to niclosamide for *T. solium* infections. However, OLIVEIRA-GOMES (1973) reports in his series that proglottids were completely disintegrated after mebendazole therapy. Also, it may be possible that mebendazole has ovicidal properties for *T. solium* eggs, as has been reported for the eggs of *Trichuris trichiura* and *Necator americanus* (WAGNER and PEÑA-CHAVARRIA 1974 a, b). Further clarification of these issues is needed.

Two studies with a total of 38 cases of *H. nana* treated with 100 mg mebendazole twice a day for 3 days found a 40% cure rate (GOLDSMID 1974; HUTCHISON et al. 1975). However, *H. nana* has at least a 4- to 5-day larval development phase (cysticeroid) in the intestinal submucosa, which apparently is not effected by mebendazole. Therefore, a more prolonged course of 7 days (as for niclosamide) would be expected to produce better results (KEYSTONE and MURDOCH 1979).

2. Larval Infections

With the development in the 1960s (LUBINSKY 1964; SCHWABE et al. 1970; WILLIAMS and COLLI 1970; HEATH 1970) of laboratory animal models of infection for *E. granulosus* and *E. multilocularis* and the characterization of the usual course of these infections, it was possible to discount scientifically many of the claims of effectiveness made for older drugs (e.g., iodinized oil of thymol and chloroguanide) and to carry out efficient and relatively rapid screening programs with promising new drugs (KAMMERER et al. 1973). In 1974, the effectiveness of mebendazole against larval infections of *E. granulosus* and *E. multilocularis* in mice and jirds was reported almost simultaneously from Russia (KROTOV et al. 1974), the United States (CAMPBELL et al. 1975), and Australia (HEATH et al. 1975). In the subsequent 7 years, several series and numerous case reports and letters have appeared recounting the results of mebendazole therapy of *E. granulosus* and *E. multilocularis* infections in uncontrolled clinical trials in man. In November, 1980, most of the investigators involved in clinical therapy trials in humans in Europe, Australia, United States, Kenya, and South America met at a workshop on "Chemotherapy of Larval Echinococcosis" in Beerse, Belgium. The results of the unpublished reports have permitted us to draw some preliminary conclusions regarding the use of mebendazole for human hyatid disease. (A summary of this workshop has been published by SCHANTZ et al. (1982.)

3. Hydatid Disease Caused by *Echinococcus granulosus*

In 1977, BEKHTI et al. reported their results in four patients with hepatic cysts (2–5 cm in diameter) treated with 16–35 mg/kg per day mebendazole for 21–30 days. Three of the four patients received more than one course of treatment. The cysts regressed and all eventually disappeared over 4–13 months. In subsequent follow-up reports (BEKHTI 1980; BEKHTI et al. 1980), it was noted that six of eight patients treated at these doses cleared their infections initially but that two relapsed within 3 years. In eight further cases treated with 50 mg/kg per day for 3 months, six improved, with hepatic cysts of less than 5 cm in diameter disappearing in two of these patients. Of note was that lung cysts in three patients ruptured within 1 month of beginning treatment. There was no evidence of recurrence, however, after a follow-up of 12–23 months.

BEARD et al. (1978) in Australia confirmed the favorable results of BEKHTI et al. in 35 of 37 cases of hepatic, pulmonary, and bone cysts. Details of therapy are not given but most patients received 40 mg/kg per day for 3 months (P. Schantz 1979, personal communication). A number of these patients received multiple courses of therapy before optimal results were obtained. No mention is made of rupture of pulmonary cysts after initiation of therapy.

KERN et al. (1979) report that of 15 patients treated with 50 mg/kg per day for 1 month, seven improved, although the course of therapy had to be repeated up to five times in some patients before maximal benefit was obtained. There were three cases of rupture of lung cysts and one of rupture of a hepatic cyst after beginning mebendazole therapy (KERN 1980).

In further reports from Sardinia (SABRIE et al. 1980), Lebanon (NASSAR 1980), Spain (BARTLETT 1980), Netherlands (DEBOER 1980), Kenya (FRENCH 1980), Argentina (REISIN 1980), Tasmania (BRAITHWAITE 1980), Switzerland (AMMANN 1980), the United States (KAMMERER 1980), Great Britain (BRYCESON 1980 b), and South Africa (KAYSER 1980), a total of 365 patients were treated with from 25 to 200 mg/kg per day for periods of 1–3 months, with many receiving more than one course of therapy. While almost all patients reported an initial subjective improvement, objective improvement varied from 10% to 100%. Pulmonary cysts and hepatic cysts of less than 5 cm in diameter were the most likely to respond, whereas bone cysts seemed particularly resistant. A higher than expected number (more than 75% in some series) of pulmonary cysts ruptured soon after beginning mebendazole therapy, but in none were secondary infections reported, with follow-ups of up to 3 years reported. A number of patients subsequently underwent surgery due to a failure to respond and in many of these viable protoscoleces have been found.

Due to the uncontrolled nature of these trials, and because of an incomplete understanding of the natural history of the disease, it is difficult to draw firm conclusions from these studies (SCHANTZ et al. 1982). Dosage, administration, and duration of mebendazole therapy varied from study to study and from patient to patient. Results varied from country to country, suggesting differing degrees of susceptibility.

From the few published studies available, we do know that untreated, symptomatic patients do less well than asymptomatic patients. In Iran, 60% of symptomatic patients not operated upon died (AMIR-JAHED et al. 1975). In China, in a group of patients with pulmonary cysts who refused surgery, 6% died after an average of 3 years, 19% returned subsequently for surgery, in 33% the cysts spontaneously disappeared after an average of 4 years, and in the remainder (42%) the infection persisted after an average follow-up of 8 years (ZHONGXI et al. 1980). In Alaska and Canada in patients with the classical pastural type of cystic hydatid disease due to *E. granulosus*, 20%–33% of symptomatic patients experienced a spontaneous rupture of their cysts, with 2%–20% of these developing secondary infections (WILSON et al. 1968). Six percent were spontaneously cured. Total mortality in untreated cases over a 15-year follow-up was 2%–10%. Bearing these facts in mind, most experienced clinicians feel that mebendazole does have a therapeutic effect in human hydatid disease, although variable and somewhat unpredictable. The current consensus is to treat inoperable cases with 50–200 mg/kg per day, given in divided doses with a fatty meal, for 2–3 months, and to repeat as necessary until optimal results are obtained. Whenever possible, the dosage should be adjusted in order to obtain a peak serum level of 100–200 ng/ml.

4. Hydatid Disease Caused by *Echinococcus multilocularis*

Hydatid disease caused by *E. multilocularis* follows a more predictable and relentless course than that due to *E. granulosus*. In untreated cases, 5-year survival from the time of diagnosis has been reported to be 50% and 10-year survival, 10% (WILSON-AMMANN 1980). In several reported studies (WILSON et al. 1978; KERN 1980; AMMANN 1980; PANADES et al. 1980; LUDIN and GYR 1977), continuous long-term therapy with 40 mg/kg per day for up to 5 years appears capable of arresting the disease and providing symptomatic relief, but no cures have been established. Whenever subsequent surgery has been undertaken, the cyst has been shown to be still viable by animal inoculation studies. Similar results have been obtained in Russia with lower doses combined with levamisole (TUMOLSKAIA and OZERETSKOVSKAIA 1979). LUBENSKI and LIUDKOVA (1980) also report some objective improvement with the long-term use of sarcolysine given by transumbilical vein infusion.

5. Cysticercosis

No published studies exist regarding the effectiveness of mebendazole for cysticercosis in man. However, informal anecdotal information would suggest that it is without effect. In calves with experimental cysticercosis (*Taenia saginata*) given one to two treatments of 100 mg/kg mebendazole intraperitoneally 4 and 12 weeks after infection, no effect was found on either the number or the percentage of viable cysts compared with untreated controls (GALLIE and SEWELL 1977).

E. Praziquantel

Since the first report of the effectiveness of praziquantel against adult and larval cestode infections in laboratory animals in 1975 (THOMAS et al. 1975 a, b), it has been found to have an astonishingly broad therapeutic spectrum against numerous adult cestodes, as well as against cysticercosis cellulosae, in man.

The mechamisms of action and gross effects of praziquantel on both adult and larval cestodes in vitro and in vivo have been well summarized by THOMAS (1977), VANDEN BOSSCHE (1980), and ANDREWS et al. (1983). Details are given in Chap. 4 of this volume.

Praziquantel rapidly enters isolated adult *H. nana* but is not metabolized (ANDREWS et al. 1980). It penetrates into cysts of *T. taeniaformis* to a much lesser degree, where its greatest concentration was found in the cyst wall itself.

Praziquantel is rapidly absorbed from the stomach and small intestine. In rats, dogs, rhesus monkeys, sheep, and man, peak serum levels after an oral dose of 10 mg/kg are achieved in ½–3 h (STEINER et al. 1976; LEOPOLD et al. 1978). Absorption of the orally administered drug varies between 80% and 100%. Eighty percent of the drug found in the plasma is protein bound. It is rapidly metabolized in the liver (a very high "first-pass effect") to inactive metabolites, primarily mono- and poly-hydroxylated products (BUHRING et al. 1978). The half-life of praziquantel itself is 2–4 h, and for the drug plus metabolites, 6–8 h. Eighty-five percent is excreted by the kidneys, 15% in the bile, all of it as metabolites, with over 80% of the administered dose being eliminated in the first 24 h. There is no evidence of accumulation in body tissues.

A thin-layer gas-chromatographic assay has been reported (DIEKMANN and BUHRING 1976; LEOPOLD et al. 1978; FROHBERG and SCHULZE SCHENCKING 1981). Using the cycloheptylcarbonyl homologue of praziquantel, the detection limit in serum is approximately 5 ng/ml.

Toxicity studies in animals (MUERMANN et al. 1978) and man (LEOPOLD et al. 1978) have demonstrated a wide margin of safety. The LD_{50} for orally administered praziquantel in rats and mice is between 2,000 and 3,000 mg/kg and in rabbits, approximately 1,000 mg/kg. The subcutaneous LD_{50} is much higher (> 16,000 mg/kg) due to its slow absorption via this route. In dogs fed 180 mg/kg per day for 4 weeks the drug was well tolerated and produced no abnormalities. In doses of 30–300 mg/kg per day from days 6–15 of gestation in rats and from days 6–18 in rabbits there was no evidence of embryotoxicity or teratogenicity. However, there are no specific data available for pregnant women and all human clinical trials to date have excluded them from the studies. In healthy men given up to 25 mg/kg three times a day with meals there were no clinical or laboratory abnormalities, with the exception of several cases of vague unease and transient drowsiness. This same general safety has been duplicated in a number of clinical trials in man (THOMAS 1977), where the only adverse effects reported were occasional abdominal cramps and transient drowsiness. Because of its marked "first-pass" hepatic metabolism, concern has been expressed regarding possible increased toxicity in patients with hepatic fibrosis and portocaval shunting (LEOPOLD et al. 1978). However, in the multinational schistosomiasis treatment project (DAVIS and WEGNER 1979) only similar very mild toxicity has been observed. In addition, praziquantel is not sensitizing to animal or human skin after repeated applications.

Results in Clinical Trials

For a review of clinical trials with praziquantel, see ANDREWS et al. (1983)

1. Adult Cestode Infections

Because of its pronounced lethal effect on a wide variety of adult cestodes in laboratory and domestic animals, a clinically controlled multicenter trial in South America and Finland was undertaken. The results were truly spectacular. In all patients with *H. nana, T. saginata, T. solium, D. latum,* and *D. pacificum* infections, praziquantel in a single oral dose of 5–25 mg/kg was completely successful in eradicating every infection (GROLL 1977; APAJALAHTI 1977; CANZONIERI et al. 1977; ESPEJO 1977; BARANSKI 1977; PAZ 1977; SCHENONE et al. 1977 a) (Table 5).

Table 5. Results of praziquantel treatment of adult cestode infections in man

Tapeworm	Dose (mg/kg)	% cured
Taenia saginata	5–10	100
T. solium	10	100
Hymenolepis nana	20–25	91–99
Diphyllobothrium latum	25	100
D. pacificum	10	100

However, praziquantel in usual doses is not generally effective against cysticeroids of *H. nana* of less than 48 h of developmental age (THOMAS 1977). Therefore, occasional treatment failures are to be expected and a second course of therapy would be necessary in these patients (SCHENONE 1980).

In most patients intact proglottids are not found after treatment. Whether praziquantel is ovicidal for *T. solium* or other cestode eggs has not been clearly established in man. However, PAZ (1978) has noted a fragmentation and disruption of the egg membrane following treatment of *T. saginata* infections, indicating a possible lethal effect.

There are no reports in man regarding the effectiveness of praziquantel for *Dipylidium caninum* infections. However, in dogs (THOMAS and GONNERT 1977) praziquantel administered orally was 100% effective.

2. Larval Cestode Infection

Following the demonstration of its effectiveness against *Cysticercus bovis* in cattle (THOMAS 1977; THOMAS and GONNERT 1978; THOMAS et al. 1975a; ANDREWS et al. 1983) at from 10 mg/kg per day for 4 days to 50 mg/kg in one dose, and against *C. cellulosae* in pigs (CHAVARRIA and GONZALEZ 1979) at 50 mg/kg per day for 15 days, and because of its minimal toxicity for man, clinical trials in man with praziquantel for the treatment of *C. cellulosae* were undertaken. RIM et al. (1980) in South Korea report that in 20 patients with subcutaneous cysts treated with 25 mg/kg, p.o. t.i.d. for 3–5 days, that most cysts had disappeared by 2–6 months. However 7 of these 20 still had a few cysts remaining 1 year after therapy. Biopsies 2 weeks after completing treatment revealed a disappearance of mitrotriches and vacuolization and degeneration of the cyst tegument. At 1 month, frank necrosis was found. Eight of these 20 patients also had symptomatic cerebral cysticercosis and four became symptom free by 6 months. Four had to be retreated at 6 months because of persistence of seizures. They all responded and remained symptom free 1 year later.

ROBLES and CHAVARRIA (1979) in Mexico reported the successful treatment of a 6-year-old boy with severe cerebral cysticercosis with praziquantel, 50 mg/kg per day, in three divided doses for 15 days. Clinical improvement was complete after 3 months of follow-up and all traces of the cysts disappeared on cranial computed tomography. They also stressed the need for concomitant corticosteroid therapy to prevent immunological reactions to degenerating cysts in the central nervous system. ANDREWS et al. (1983), at the end of their review on the activity of praziquantel in neurocysticercosis, write that at present "praziquantel should be used in patients, only by an expert neurologist, and it is strongly recommended that additional corticosteroid treatment be given in order to prevent development of endocranial hypertension, which may result as a reaction to disintegrating cerebral cysts."

BOTERO and CASTAÑO (1980) report the successful outcome of nine further cases, two with subcutaneous cysts and seven with cerebral cysticercosis, using a dose of 10 mg/kg, three times a day for 6 days, repeated after 1–2 months for the patients with cerebral disease. In all cerebral cases cranial computed tomography had become negative by 3 months after therapy. Subcutaneous cysts had disappeared by 2 months after therapy.

In none of the above cases were any significant clinical or laboratory adverse effects or abnormalities due to praziquantel noted.

BYLUND et al. (1977) report that plerocercoids of *Diphyllobothrium latum* in vitro tolerated incubation with up to 300 μg praziquantel/ml fairly well. At 600–700 μg/ml, however, 45%–85% of the larvae were killed after 24 h. As yet, no information is available on the use of praziquantel for sparganosis in man.

Unfortunately, praziquantel has been ineffective against hydatid cysts of *E. multilocularis* in mice (THOMAS and GONNERT 1975b) at 50–250 mg/kg, p.o. or subcutaneously × 1 or intraperitoneally × 2, or of *E. granulosus* in sheep (HEATH and LAWRENCE 1978) at 50 mg/kg, given once subcutaneously.

F. Summary

While great progress has been made in the treatment of adult and larval cestode infections in man with the introduction of niclosamide, mebendazole, and praziquantel, several problems remain.

It is not clear whether any of these drugs are ovicidal. Thus, extreme caution must continue to be exercised, especially with *T. solium* infections, to prevent vomiting and the possible development of cysticercosis. Studies in swine to resolve this issue could be of critical importance in choosing the drug of choice for the treatment of *T. solium* infections in man.

Mebendazole has proved to be our first breakthrough in the medical treatment of hydatid disease. Yet its poor solubility and inconsistent absorption greatly hinder its practical usefulness. Also, increasingly frequent reports of drug toxicity with the use of high concentrations for prolonged periods and also of troublesome and potentially lethal anaphylactic reactions to degenerating cysts further complicate its clinical use. A better absorbed or parenteral formulation allowing for shorter treatment courses during which the patient could be more closely monitored under controlled conditions would be a major advance in safety for the patient and, perhaps also, in overall efficacy, especially as related to multiple organ infections and for cysts located in the brain or bone.

Praziquantel has proven to be a resounding success for the treatment of all adult tapeworm infections for which it has been tried in man, as well as for subcutaneous and cerebral *C. cellulosae* infections, at least in the preliminary reports now available. However, experience with cysticercosis patients remains limited

Table 6. Current recommendations for the treatment of cestode infections in Man

Adult	Drug	Dose	Approximate % cured
Taenia saginata	Praziquantel	10 mg/kg, p.o., ×1 [a]	100
T. solium	Niclosamide	2 g, p.o., ×1 [b]	80–95
Hymenolepis nana	Praziquantel	25 mg/kg, p.o., ×1 [c]	95
	Niclosamide	1–2 g, p.o., ×1, then 0.5–1 g, q.d., ×6	85–98
H. diminuta	Niclosamide	2 g. p.o., ×1, then 1 g, p.d., ×6	90
Diphyllobothrium latum	Praziquantel	25 mg/kg, p.o., ×1 [c]	95
	Niclosamide	2 g, p.o., ×1	85
D. pacificum	Praziquantel	10 mg/kg, p.o., ×1 [a]	100
Dipylidium caninum	Niclosamide	2 g, p.o., ×1	100
Larvae			
Echinococcus granulosus	Mebendazole	50–200 mg/kg/day, p.o., ×3 months, (repeat in 3–6 months)	10–100 (average, 50–60, see text)
E. multilocularis	Mebendazole	40–50 mg/kg/day, p.o., ×years	0 (90% stabilized and clinically improved)
Cysticercus cellulosae	Praziquantel	10–50 mg/kg/day, p.o., ×6–15 days (repeat in 2–6 months)	90–100 (cerebral and subcutaneous)
Coenurus (*T. multiceps*)	Praziquantel [d]		

[a] Doses recommended for the treatment of human tapeworm infections [% efficacy according to ANDREWS et al. (1983) is 100% for *T. solium* and 96% for *T. saginata*]
[b] Less for children (see text)
[c] Highest dose tested (ANDREWS et al. 1983)
[d] An oral dose of 2×50 mg/kg is recommended for use in sheep (ANDREWS et al. 1983)

and clinical follow-up has been relatively brief. With further experience we should gain a better appreciation of its ultimate effectiveness and of any delayed toxicity. As yet, its effectiveness in the treatment of ocular cysticercosis is not known.

While initial short-term treatment of hydatid disease in animals with praziquantel has not been successful, it is possible that, as with mebendazole, longer courses with high doses might be of benefit.

No information is available yet for the treatment of coenurus (*Taenia multiceps*) infections in man, but, because of its effectiveness in similar larval cestode infections in animals, praziquantel may be effective.

Current recommendations for the treatment of adult and larval cestode infections in man are summarized in Table 6.

References

Amir-Jahed AK, Fardin R, Farzad A, Bakshandeh K (19/5) Clinical echinococcosis. Ann Surg 182:541–546
Ammann RW (1980) Experiences with mebendazole treatment in Switzerland. Chemotherapy of larval echinococcosis: report of a workshop. Z Parasitenkd 67[1]
Andrews P, Thomas H, Weber H (1980) The in vitro uptake of ^{14}C-praziquantel by cestodes, trematodes, and a nematode. J Parasitol 66:920–925
Andrews P, Thomas H, Pohlke R, Seubert J (1983) Praziquantel. Med Res Rev 3:147–200
Anonymous (1970) Information material – Yomesan® (niclosamide). Center for Disease Control, Department of Health, Education and Welfare, Atlanta, Georgia
Anonymous (1976) Pathogenesis of the tapeworm anaemia. Br Med J 2:1028
Anonymous (1977) Anaemia and the fish tapeworm. Lancet 1:292
Anonymous (1979) Medical treatment fo hydatid disease? Br Med J 2:563
Apajalahti J (1977) Tratamiento de infecciones por *Diphyllobothrium latum* con una dosis oral unica de praziquantel. Bol Chil Parasitol 32:43
Baranski MC (1977) Tratamiento de teniasis e himenolepiasis humanas con praziquantel (Embay 8440). Bol Chil Parasitol 32:37–39
Bartlett A (1980) Experiences with mebendazole therapy in hydatid disease in Spain. Chemotherapy of larval echinococcosis: report of a workshop. Z Parasitenkd 67[1]
Beard TC, Rickard MD, Goodman HT (1978) Medical treatment for hydatids. Med J Aust 1:633–635
Bekhti A (1980) Experience with mebendazole therapy in hydatid disease in Belgium. Chemotherapy of larval echinococcosis: report of a workshop. Z Parasitenkd 67[1]
Bekhti A, Schaaps J-P, Capron M, Dessaint J-P, Santoro F, Capron A (1977) Treatment of hepatic hydatid disease with mebendazole: preliminary results in four cases. Br Med J 2:1047–1051
Bekhti A, Nizet M, Capron M, Dessaint J-P, Santoro F, Capron A (1980) Chemotherapy of human hydatid disease with mebendazole. Acta Gastroentol Belg 43:48–65
Botero D, Castaño S (1980) Treatment of human cysticercosis with praziquantel (preliminary report) (Abstract 270). International congress on tropical medicine, Manila. Available from Dr David Botero, Antioqua University, Medelline, Columbia, South Africa
Braithwaite PA (1980) Clinical results obtained in the treatment of hydatid disease with mebendazole in Tasmania (Australia). Chemotherapy of larval echinococcosis: report of a workshop. Z Parasitenkd 67[1]
Bryceson A (1980 a) Mebendazole and hydatid disease. Br Med J 1:796
Bryceson A (1980 b) The clinical results obtained in hydatid disease after mebendazole treatment in the UK. Chemotherapy of larval echinococcosis: report of a workshop. Z Parasitenkd 67[1]
Buhring KU, Diekmann HW, Garbe A, Nowak H (1978) Metabolism of praziquantel in man. Eur J Drug Metabol Pharmacokinet 3:179–190
Bylund G, Bang B, Wikgren K (1977) Evaluacion experimental del efecto de praziquantel contra *Diphyllobothrium latum* in vivo e in vitro. Bol Chil Parasitol 32:7–16
Campbell WC, McCracken RO, Blair LS (1975) Effect of parenterally injected benzimidazole compounds on *Echinococcus multilocularis* and *Taenia crassiceps* metacestodes in laboratory animals. J Parasitol 61:844–852
Canzonieri CJ, Rodriquez RB, Castillo HE, Balella CI de, Lucena M (1977) Ensayos terapeuticos con praziquantel en infecciones por *Taenia saginata* e *Hymenolepis nana*. Bol Chil Parasitol 32:41–42
Chavarria M, Gonzalez D (1979) Droncit en el tratamiento de la cisticercosis porcina. Esp Vet 1:160–165
Danis M, Brucker G, Gentilini M, Richard-Lenoble D, Smith M (1977) Treatment of hepatic hydatid disease. Br Med J 2:1356
Davis A (1973) Drugs for cestodiasis. In: Davis A Drug treatment in intestinal helminthiasis. WHO, Geneva

1 See Schantz et al. (1982)

Davis A, Wegner DHG (1979) Multicentre trials of praziquantel in human schistosomiasis. Bull WHO 57:767–800
DeBoer H (1980) Experiences with the high-dose mebendazole treatment in echinococcosis in the Netherlands. Chemotherapy in larval echinococcosis: report of a workshop. Z Parasitenkd 67[1]
DeCarneri I, Vita G (1973) Drugs used in cestode diseases. In: Cavier R (ed) International encyclopedia of pharmacology and therapeutics, sect 64. Pergamon, New York, pp 145–213
Diekmann HW, Buhring KU (1976) The fate of praziquantel in the organism III. Metabolism in rat, beagle dog, and rhesus monkey. Eur J Drug Metabol Pharmacokinet 2:107–112
El-Masry NA, Farid Z, Bassily S (1974) Treatment of *Hymenolepis nana* with niclosamide, mepacrine and thiabendazole. East Afr Med J 51:532–535
Espejo H (1977) Tratamiento de infecciones por *Hymenolepis nana, Taenia saginata, Taenia solium* y *Diphyllobothrium pacificum* con praziquantel. Bol Chil Parasitol 32:39–40
French M (1980) Experience with mebendazole therapy of hydatid disease in Kenya. Workshop: chemotherapy of larval echinococcosis. Beerse, Belgium[1]
Frohberg H, Schulze Schencking M (1981) Toxicological profile of praziquantel, a new drug against cestode and schistosome infections, as compared to some other schistosomicides. Arzneimittelforsch 31:555–565
Gallie GJ, Sewell MM (1977) The effect of mebendazole on the cysticerci of *Taenia saginata* in calves. Trop Amin Health Prod 9:24
Gönnert R (1974) Die Bandwurm-Infektionen des Menschen und ihre Behandlung. MMW 116:1531–1538
Goldsmid JM (1974) The use of mebendazole as a broad-spectrum anthelmintic in Rhodesia. S Afr Med J 48:2265–2266
Groll E (1977) Panorama general del tratamiento de las infecciones humanas por cestodes con praziquantel. Bol Chil Parasitol 32:27–31
Heath DD (1970) The development of *Echinococcus granulosus* larvae in laboratory animals. Parasitology 60:449–456
Heath DD, Lawrence SB (1978) The effect of mebendazole and praziquantel on the cysts of *Echinococcus granulosus, Taenia hydatigena* and *T. ovis* in sheep. NZ Vet J 25:11–15
Heath DD, Christie MJ, Chevis RAF (1975) The lethal effect of mebendazole on secondary *Echinococcus granulosus,* cysticerci of *Taenia pisiformis* and tetrathyridia of *Mescocestoides corti.* Parasitology 70:273–285
Hutchinson JCP, Johnston NM, Plevey MVP, Thankgkhiew I, Aidney C (1975) Clinical trial of mebendazole, a broad-spectrum anthelmintic. Br Med J 2:309–310
Jaffe JJ (1975) Nucleoside analogs as antiparasitic agents. Ann NY Acad Sci 255:306–316
Jones TC (1978) Cestodes. Cli Gastroenterol 7:105–128
Jones WE (1979) Niclosamide as a treatment of *Hymenolepis diminuta* and *Dipylidium caninum* infection in man. Am J Trop Med Hyg 28:300–302
Kahra A, Veharanta T (1963) Expulsion of tapeworms with yomesan. Suom Loak 18:325–327
Kammerer WS (1980) Treatment of human hydatid disease (*Echinococcus granulosus*) with a high-dose mebendazole regimen. Chemotherapy of larval echinococcosis: report of a workshop. Z Parasitenkd 67[1]
Kammerer WS, Judge DM (1976) Chemotherapy of hydatid disease (*Echinococcus granulosus*) in mice with mebendazole and bithionol. Am J Trop Med Hyg 52:714–717
Kammerer WS, Perez-Esandi MV (1973) The current status of the chemotherapy of hydatid disease. Bull Pan Am Health Organ 7:47–52
Kammerer WS, Miller KL (1981) *Echinococcus granulosus:* permeability of hydatid cysts to mebendazole in mice. Int J Parasitol 11(3):183–185
Kang HC, Min DY, Soh C-T (1978) Changes of liver cells of animals with administration of flubendazole. Yonsei Rep Trop Med 9:11–22
Kayser HJS (1980) Treatment of hydatid disease with mebendazole at Frere Hospital, East London. S Afr Med J 58:560–563
Kean BH (1976) How to treat tapeworm infections in humans. Consultant 9:82–87

Kean BH, Hopkins D (1981) Intestinal parasitism, tapeworm infection. In: Conn HF (ed) Drugs of choice. Saunders, Philadelphia, pp 365–367

Keeling JED (1968) The chemotherapy of cestode infections. Adv Chemotherapy 3:109–152

Kern P (1980) Follow-up observations of patients with advanced cystic or alveolar echinococcosis with mebendazole. Chemotherapy of larval echinococcosis: report of a workshop. Z Parasitenkd[1]

Kern P, Dietrich M, Volkmer K-J (1979) Chemotherapy of echinococcosis with mebendazole – clinical observation of 7 patients. Tropenmed Parasitol 30:65–72

Keystone JS, Murdoch JK (1979) Diagnosis and treatment – drugs five years later – mebendazole. Ann Intern Med 91:582–586

Krotov AI, Tchernaev AI, Kovalenko FP, Bajandino DG (1974) Experimental therapy of alveococcosis. II. Effectivity of some defensive remedies against alveococcosis of laboratory animals (in Russian). Med Parasitol 43:314–321

Leopold G, Ungethum W, Groll E, Diekmann HW, Nowak H, Wegner DHG (1978) Clinical pharmacology in normal volunteers of praziquantel, a new drug against schistosomes and cestodes. Eur J Clin Pharmacol 14:281–291

Lubenski AU, Liudkova VM (1980) Chemotherapy of inoperable forms of hepatic alveolar hydatid disease. Khirugiia (Mosk) 6:68–71

Lubinsky G (1964) Growth of the vegetatively propagated strain of larval *Echinococcus multilocularis* in some strains of Jackson mice and in their hybrids. Can J Zool 42:1099–1013

Ludin CE, Gyr K (1977) Therapy of alveococcosis in man. J Int Med Res 5:367–368

Michiels M (1980) Pharmacokinetics of mebendazole and flubendazole in animals and man. Chemotherapy of larval echinococcosis: report of a workshop. Z Parasitenkd 67[1]

Miskovitz PF, Javitt NB (1980) Leukopenia associated with mebendazole therapy of hydatid disease. Am J Trop Med Hyg 29:1356–1358

Muermann P, Eberstein MV, Frohberg H (1976) Notes on the tolerance of droncit – summary of trial results. Vet Med Rev 2:142–153

Murray-Lyon IM, Reynolds KW (1979) Complication of mebendazole treatment for hydatid disease. Br Med J 2:1111–1112

Nassar N (1980) Clinical results with high-dose mebendazole treatment of hydatid disease in Lebanon. Chemotherapy of larval echinococcosis: report of a workshop. Z Parasitenkd 67

Oliviera Gomes MC (1973) The treatment of taeniasis with mebendazole. Folha Med 66:87–95

Panadas RN, Salas MN, Lerma FA, Rodrizuez T (1980) Tratamiento de la hidatidosis microvesicular con mebendazol. Rev Clin Esp 156:295–303

Pawlowski Z, Schultz MG (1972) Taeniasis and cysticercosis (*Taenia saginata*). Adv Parasit 10:269–343

Paz G (1977) Tratamiento de teniasis saginata con praziquantel. Bol Chil Parasitol 32:14–16

Peña Chavarria A, Villarejos VM, Zeledon R (1977) Mebendazole in the treatment of taeniasis solium and taeniasis saginata. Am J Trop Med Hyg 26:118–120

Perera DR, Western KA, Schultz MG (1970) Niclosamide treatment of cestodiasis – clinical trials in the United States. Am J Trop Med Hyg 19:610–612

Quilici M, Dumon H, Rampal M, Alimi JC (1979) Hydatidosis: traitement preoperatoire par fluoromebendazole. Nouv Presse Med 8(7):524

Reisin IL (1980) Experience with mebendazole therapy of hydatid disease in Argentina. Chemotherapy of larval echinococcosis: report of a workshop. Z Parasitenkd 67[1]

Reisin IL, Rabito CA, Rotunno CA, Cereijido M (1977) The permeability of the membranes of experimental secondary cysts of *Echinococcus granulosus* to ^{14}C mebendazole. Int J Parasitol 7:189–194

Rim H-J, Won C-R, Hyun I (1980) Therapeutic trial on the human cysticercosis with praziquantel. International congress on tropical medicine, Manila. Abstract 271

Robles C, Chavarria MC (1979) Presentacion de un caso clinico de cisticercosis cerebral tratado medicamente con un nuevo farmaco: praziquantel. Salud Publica Mex 21:603–618

Sabrie A, Brandimarte C, Ferretti G (1980) Experience with mebendazole therapy in hydatid disease in Italy. Workshop: chemotherapy of larval echinococcosis. Beerse, Belgium. Z Parasitenkd 67[1]

Schantz PM, Vanden Bossche H, Eckert J (1982) Chemotherapy for larval *Echinococcosis* in animals and humans: report of a workshop: Z Parasitenkd 67:5–26

Schenone H (1980) Praziquantel in the treatment of *Hymenolepis nana* infections in children. Am J Trop Med Hyg 29:320–321

Schenone H, Galdames M, Rivadeneira A, Morales E, Hoffmann M, Asalgado N, Meneses G, Mora M, Cabrera G (1977a) Tratamiento de las infecciones por *Hymenolepis nana* en ninos con una dosis oral unica de praziquantel. Bol Chil Parasitol 32:11–12

Schenone H, Galdames M, Inzunza E, Jimenez M, Romero E, Bloomfield E (1977b) Flubendazol en el tratamiento de infecciones por nematodes intestinales en ninos. Bol Chil Parasitol 32:85–86

Schwabe CW, Kilejian A, Lainas G (1970) The propagation of secondary cysts of *Echinococcus granulosus* in the mongolian jird, *Meriones unguiculatus*. J Parasitol 56:80–83

Seiler JP (1975) Toxicology and genetic effects of benzimidazole compounds. Mutat Res 32:151–168

Standen OD (1963) Chemotherapy of cestode infections. In: Schnitzer RJ, Hawking F (eds) Experimental chemotherapy. Academic, New York, pp 716–740

Steiner K, Garbe A, Diekmann HW, Nowak H (1976) The fate of praziquantel in the organism I. pharmacokinetics in animals. Eur J Drug Metabol Pharmacokinet 2:85–95

Thienpont D, Vanparijs O, Niemegeers C, Marsboom R (1978) Biological and pharmacological properties of flubendazole. Arzneimittelforsch 28:605–612

Thomas H (1977) Experimental results with praziquantel in cestodiasis and cysticercosis. Bol Chil Parasitol 32:2–5

Thomas H, Gonnert R (1977) The efficacy of praziquantel against cestodes in animals. Z Parasitenkd 52:117–127

Thomas H, Gonnert R (1978) The efficacy of praziquantel against experimental cysticercosis and hydatidosis. Z Parasitenkd 55:165–179

Thomas H, Gonnert R, Pohlke R, Seubert J (1975a) Experiences with a new compound against larval cestodes. Second European multi-colloquy of parasitology, Trogir, Yugoslavia. Available from: Institute of chemotherapy, Bayer AG, Wuppertal-1, West Germany

Thomas H, Gonnert R, Pohlke R, Seubert J (1975b) Experimental and clinical studies with a new compound against tapeworms. Second European multi-colloquy of parasitology, Trogir, Yugoslavia. Available from: Institute of chemotherapy, Bayer AG, Wuppertal-1, West Germany

Tumol'skaia NI, Ozeretskovskaia NN (1979) Mebendazole in the treatment of acute and chronic stages of helminthiases. II. Mebendazole (Vermox) in the treatment of alveolar hydatid disease and echinococcosis (in Russian). Med Parazitol (Mosk) 48:17–24

Vakil BJ, Dalal NJ, Enjetti E (1975) Clinical trials with mebendazole – a new broad spectrum anthelmintic. J Trop Med Hyg 78:154–158

Vanden Bossche H (1980) Commentary – peculiar targets in anthelmintic chemotherapy. Biochem Pharmacol 29:1981–1990

Vanden Bossche H, Verhoeven H, Vanparijs O, Lauwers H, Thienpont D (1979) Closantel, a new antiparasitic hydrogen ionophore. Arch Int Physiol Biochim 87:851–852

Wagner ED, Peña Chavarria A (1974a) In vivo effects of a new anthelmintic mebendazole (R 17635) on the eggs of *Trichuris trichiura* and hookworm. Am J Trop Med Hyg 23:151–153

Wagner ED, Peña Chavarria A (1974b) Morphologically altered eggs of *Trichuris trichiura* following treatment with mebendazole. Am J Trop Med Hyg 23:154–157

Werczberger A, Golhman J, Wertheim G, Gunders A, Chowers I (1979) Disseminated echinococcosis with repeated anaphylactic shock treated with mebendazole. Chest 76:482–484
Williams JF, Colli Christina W (1970) Primary cystic infection with *Echinococcus granulosus* and *Taenia hydatigena* in *Meriones unguiculatus*. J Parasitol 56:509–513
Wilson JF (1980) Alveolar hydatid disease: a review of clinical features of 33 indigenous cases of *Echinococcus multilocularis* infection in Alaskan eskimos. Chemotherapy of larval echinococcosis: report of a workshop. Z Parasitenkd 67
Wilson JF, Rausch RL (1980) Alveolar hydatid disease – a review of clinical features of 33 indigenous cases of *Echinococcus multilocularis* infection in Alaskan eskimos. Am J Trop Med Hyg 29:1340–1355
Wilson JF, Diddams AC, Rausch RL (1968) Cystic hydatid disease in Alaska. Am Rev Respir Dis 98:1–15
Wilson JF, Davidson M, Rausch RL (1978) A clinical trial of mebendazole in the treatment of alveolar hydatid disease. Am Rev Respir Dis 118:747–757
Zhongxi Q, Shuiyuan G, Guoxue T, Ruilin L, Mingbai W, Jun Q, Kurban (1980) Immediate and long-term results of surgical treatment of intrathoracic hydatid cysts. Chin Med J 93:569–572

CHAPTER 15

Mass Treatment

P. G. JANSSENS and A. DE MUYNCK

"The supply of appropriate pharmaceutical products should be seen as fundamental requirement of public health care, like the supply of clear water, sanitation, adequate food and basic education."

D. Taylor – *Medicines, health and the poor world* – London (1982).

A. Introduction

In countries with poor "health" facilities the control or eradication of communicable diseases is often limited to community-wide "medical" measures aiming at arresting the infection(s) collectively. Such mass campaign schemes have to be carried out by operational systems with such an objective. The great diversity of health-care circumstances implies an even greater variety of activities.

A vaccination program at the population level is one good example. It can achieve a solid collective immunity even with a 70%–80% coverage. Smallpox, poliomyelitis, and measles are examples of diseases which have been successfully vaccinated against. Antimalarial suppressive treatment or chemoprophylaxis reduces the infection to a subclinical level and induces resistance to reinfection in a number of individuals. On a community level this technique limits the pool of infective organisms and reduces the risks in the more susceptible groups. Chemoprophylaxis can in the same way be helpful in limiting the extension of epidemics of cerebrospinal meningitis, pulmonary plague, and cholera, when administered to persons in contact with the sick. Reliable methods for rapid and specific detection of masked or overt leprosy and tuberculosis in a community may be followed by individual treatment, which in turn will protect the community concerned by limiting the number of bacteria carriers. Generalized mass treatment for yaws with repository penicillin (if the prevalence is higher than 10%) or selective treatment of all household or obvious contacts (when the prevalence is below 5%) has proven its value. Periodic deworming is a further example of mass treatment. It has been tried out with different drugs: carbon tetrachloride against hookworms – too toxic and of historical interest only; piperazine salts (1950) against Ascaris – cheap but cure rate too low; bephenium hydroxynaphthoate (1958) – mainly active against *Ancylostoma duodenale*, too expansive; tiabendazole (1959) – broad spectrum, too many side effects; levamisole (1965), mebendazole (1971), and pyrantel (1971) are taking over – broad spectrum, not expensive.

All of these procedures need professional knowledge, development of effective distribution and administration techniques, and a careful study of the problems arising in connection with the program. Peroral or parenteral administration on a community- or population-wide base of biological or chemical substances will bring down the degree of infection, but more often than not only temporarily. The administration will have to be repeated periodically, at intervals, keeping the transmission level sufficiently low to guarantee a steady decrease of the infective mass and thus achieve good control or, if one is lucky, a breakdown of the transmission chain and thus leading toward eradication.

The main obstacle for permanent success is the continuous presence of infective eggs or larvae in the tropical environment, the main reservoir of worms. This situation is unlikely to improve for many years to come. The kinetics behind this permanent challenge must be taken carefully into consideration. The infective larvae are either in embryonated eggs (e.g., *Ascaris, Trichuris*) or free living in the environment (e.g., hookworm, *Strongyloides*) and penetrate the host orally or parenterally. They may remain dormant in some hosts before coming free in the intestine. These larvae will be involved in a systemic cycle and may produce sensitization, and allergic and other pathogenic reactions. The larval stage is the most pathogenic. The adult worms cause limited lesions, but if only present in a limited number the host may remain symptom free.

I. Standpoints and Prejudices

Man, even the most primitive, is familiar with worms such as *Ascaris* and *Taenia*. He wishes to get rid of these undesired commensals. He engages in self-treatment, using traditional and/or modern drugs. His trust in the efficacy of modern drugs results from the reliability of health services. Such a positive attitude is an efficient entry point for other health measures and programs. Moreover, the intestinal helminthiases markedly increase expenditure on health: an striking number of outpatients and a fair amount of inpatients seek help in relation to worms.

Doctors and health personnel generally have a simplistic view on helminthiases. The detection of a worm egg and the spontaneous expulsion of a worm rouses a therapeutic reflex and generates the satisfaction of the use of an efficient drug when available. A broader vision is often missing.

The tropical doctor looks at the wormy stock of his consultants as part of a normal burden arising from the deplorable sanitation and the tropical environment. Anthelminthics are distributed, if available, to those asking for treatment. Few will engage in selective mass treatment of the most exposed groups: infants, schoolchildren, and pregnant or lactating women. Depending on the selected drug and on the frequency of its administration, the attendance rate will decrease progressively and concomitantly the active concern of the medical profession.

The public health authorities have the duty to assess the importance of all health problems. Among them the parasitoses occupy a not insignificant place. Ascariasis and ancylostomiasis rank high among the infections of man and, together with trichuriasis, amoebiasis, giardiasis, they are in the top twenty. But high prevalence, without dramatic epidemics, is not a sufficient incentive for the public health decision makers. This lack of insight will preclude the will to solve the problem.

As a matter of fact, control of the major intestinal helminthiases has been, since the Rockefeller control campaign against ancylostomiasis, off and on in the forefront of the minds of the public health authorities. But only very few campaigns have been successful. The failures were due to the absence of the much-needed basic conditions. Nowadays serious diagnostic problems no longer hamper such programs and efficient anthelminthics are available, sometimes in a confusing variety. The time is ripe to consider seriously the reduction of the worm burden in hundreds of millions of people to a tolerable level. However, the authorities will have to be confronted first by hard pathological and epidemiological facts.

II. Pathogenicity

The consequences of the intestinal parasitoses for their hosts need a critical assessment. Much of the accepted opinions are mere presumptions backed up by analogies to the facts known from animal-breeding problems. In depth studies are needed about the occurrence and importance of biological loss, diarrhea, anemia, malabsorption, malnutrition, retardation in growth, lowered resistance to infections, disturbed immunogenicity, hypersensitivity to potent specific allergens, disability, reduced lactation, vitamin and enzyme deficiencies, etc.

The pathological symptoms and consequences, as described, result too often from anecdotal publications. The existence of serious disturbances of the intestine, lungs, and other organs, and obstructions and other complications resulting from the presence of worms and/or larvae are well known, but not their frequency. A single *Ascaris* can obstruct a vital duct and become life threatening.

In a given "wormy" community symptomatic carriers and diseased persons are present simultaneously. This coexistence depends on the degree and duration of exposure and on the resistance of the host. With these data in mind it becomes impossible to distinguish between cure with reinfection and suppression with relapse.

With the exception of *Strongyloides stercoralis, Capillaria philippinensis,* and *Enterobius vermicularis,* which are capable of autoinfection mechanisms or retroinfection possibilities, intestinal helminths do not multiply within their hosts.

B. Epidemiology

A reliable and broad epidemiological knowledge about intestinal helminthiasis is lacking. Epizootiological data have been carefully gathered by veterinarians. They indeed have a strong incentive for engaging in this research in order to avoid unnecessary economic losses in cattle, sheep, and pig breeding. Being in touch with the ups and downs of daily animal management they have started by taking a good look at the real situation. Sophisticated experiments on survival, development, dissemination, availability of worms, free-living infective stages, intermediate hosts – pet subjects for research in human parasitology – are less rewarding than the direct observation of real situations, supplemented and illustrated by complementary experiments. Experimental and natural infections are in essence different.

Some parasitoses of man being zoonotic, information is readily available for those. Many of the strong points in the veterinarian approach to the population dynamics of the host-worm systems are at a low pitch or lacking in the study of human helminthiases: spontaneous regulation of worm populations; the existence of strains of helminths; seasonal fluctuations; loss of worms; self-cure; tolerated level; arrested and retarded development (hypobiosis); the effect of parturition, lactation, and intercurrent infections; the role of diet, especially mineral and trace element deficiencies; the role of steroids; and the influence of human behavior and sociocultural and educational level.

The buildup of a worm population in a living host is not a linear accumulation, but a dynamic process. The intruder encounters a variable susceptibility or resistance in the host. Innate resistance is based on a reaction of the host whereby the infective larvae are prevented from reaching a stage at which development could be achieved. This innate resistance shows variations of a genetic nature within the host: sex, hemoglobin type, amount of plasma IgA, etc. and also with the strain of the worm.

Acquired resistance is a progressive protection following simple or repeated infections, preventing the bulk of the new infective larvae from reaching maturity. Thus old worms are lost and new ones acquired within a level below the threshold of disease. This protracted loss opposes severe infections.

Sometimes the primary infection is terminated spontaneously by the sudden expulsion of the worms. It is attributed to the presence of a critical biomass, but in fact this "self-cure" mechanism is not well understood.

Acquired resistance is not necessarily permanent. Susceptibility may be altered by a decrease of immune vigilance accompanying late pregnancy and lactation, by intercurrent infections which may impair immune regulations, e.g., trypanosomes and helminths, by normal or therapeutic increase of the steroid concentration which depresses immunity and increases the worm metabolism (or both combined), by a change in diet increasing the carbohydrate intake, or by depletion of mineral and trace elements, e.g., P, Ca, and Co.

Another interesting phenomenon, which has not recieved proper attention in human helminthiasis, is the arrested development or "hypobiosis" in one or more organs, especially lung tissue. Infective larvae are interrupted in their development in the host following some signals, host resistance (but it happens also in susceptible hosts) or climatic or seasonal conditions as such, or through the endocrine system regulation of the host. There may be more than one mechanism for this biological clock.

This interruption in the biological cycle, which coincides with the onset of environmental conditions adverse for free-living nematodes (winter, arid conditions), serves the purpose of synchronizing development with environmental events. The postponement of development during an unfavorable period, followed in due time by resumption of development, guarantees survival through unfavorable periods. The possible role of endocrinal signals is clearly demonstrated by *Toxocara canis* infection in adult bitches. This animal becomes a kind of temporary paratenic host and the somatic larvae are mobilized in the case of pregnancy and infect the pups via the placenta and the colostrum, while the pregnant bitch will pass eggs in the feces. In humans a seasonal induced arrest has been observed for *Ancylostoma duodenale,* with possible transmission by infective larvae in the colostrum. The maturation of hypobiotic larvae plays an important epidemiological role. It increases transmission at a period when the environment is ripe for free-living development. It is well-known that in a resistant host, e.g., having acquired age immunity in an endemic environment, the worms grow more slowly, reach a smaller size, and the female contains less eggs: egg output is depressed and prepatent period is prolonged. But age resistance is not absolute; helminth-naive adults, i.e., with no previous contact, can develop an acute infection.

Worms presenting retarded development are difficult to distinguish from aging, less fertile worms. The survival and development of eggs and larvae occur in a complex ecosystem, first in feces and afterwards in soil. The latter microhabitat must supply adequate temperature, moisture, and aeration. The eggs and larvae must compete with bacteria, viruses, fungi, free-living nematodes, and predatory fauna, e.g., dung beetles.

The critical temperatures may vary, with an optimum as the most important parameter. All larval stages, except embryonated eggs (*Ascaris, Trichuris*), are susceptible to desiccation: some feces dry out quickly. The development time fluctuates between weeks and months. Longevity is variable since at a high temperature the larvae are more active, exhaust their food reserves more quickly, and shorten their survival period.

Seasonal fluctuations are a fact, but the signals are not always the same. They play an important role in the reinfection peak pattern, both in humans and animals. For the latter, prediction models of seasonal increase are extremely useful. In humans it is more a matter of understanding decrease or increase of the worm burden.

In moderate and tropical climates, the adverse role of environmental conditions on the free-living stages is obvious. In equatorial regions, without real seasons, such situations do not occur. However, the role of temperature should not be overestimated as the arrest of development in late summer is conditioned during the hottest part of the year.

Even our limited knowledge of the epidemiology and the prevalence of parasitoses underlines the magnitude of the problems on a worldwide basis and the necessity of undertaking serious studies of the prevailing situation.

C. A Mass Treatment Campaign

I. Definition

"Mass campaign" is a term covering every "scheme for control or eradication of a particular comunicable disease on a community-wide basis, carried out by machinery operating with that precise objective" (WHO Study Group 1965). "Collective or mass treatment" refers specifically to the oral or parenteral administration of biological or chemical substances to more or less large communities or the whole population with regard to the control or the eradication of a communicable disease.

Mass treatment is hence currently applied to the anthelminthic control programs of periodic deworming. This is usually a blanket treatment and as such implicates ethical problems. Can noninfected persons be treated for the benefit of the community? It is admissible to administer drugs to pregnant women? Given the use of safe drugs and the voluntary participation of a duly informed and consenting community, there is no real problem. In any case "an incidental infringement of individual liberties will be outweighted by the benefit to the community as a whole." Furthermore the presumed negative persons are more often than not undiagnosed worm-bearers and it has been proved that deworming of pregnant women is beneficial for them and for their progency. It should be reminded that *Strongyloides* and hookworm infections can be transmitted by the colostrum.

II. Organization

1. Basic Principles

Whenever the public health authorities decide to consider the organization of a mass campaign either spontaneously, or under pressure from local health services, public opinion, and/or international organizations, the following steps will be taken:

1. A preliminary reconnaissance of the extent of the problem. This involves a correct assessment of the prevalence and incidence, risk factors, and high-risk groups.
2. A preplanning stage is undertaken to make explicit the available solutions for the problem, if the program appears worthwhile from the reconnaissance. The available solutions are investigated more in depth in relation to a large-scale operation. This stage will include the *recruitment* and *training* of an executive nucleus. A *pilot run* will enable the practical implications of the project to be tested.
3. The planning stage includes a careful assessment of all available data and factors, including the results of the preliminary surveys, the feedback of the pilot trial, and all other relevant information.
4. The execution of the mass campaign consists in an *attack* phase (=implementation of the program) and a final *consolidation* phase.

2. Organization at the Central Level and Training

At the central level the department of epidemiology or its substitute are the *de facto* headquarters of the program.

The person in charge should be a public health specialist with field experience and a fair knowledge of epidemiology, biostatistics, operational research and with managerial capacities, including a talent for team leadership. At the heart of the organization the person in charge should be seconded by local or external advisors and/or consultants in the fields concerned and in health education, sociology, geography, and economy. Such a multidisciplinary approach, at least during the planning, preparatory, and early execution stages, is not only desirable, but indispensable.

The team for a pilot run will be the nucleus for a master strategy, ready for progressive extension if a long-range program comes into being. Next to adequate training, management and supervison are primordial. A clear understanding of all elements involved in a regular servicing of the periphery, carefully related to the real needs, will result in good logistics. Drug purchase, conditioning, central storage, distribution channels, local availability of a properly stored minimum stock, timing of delivery, feedback mechanisms, and regular supervision must all receive serious attention.

The duties of the administration officer may, at the incipient stage, be combined with those of team leader. They will also include the financing of the whole operation staff and manpower, equipment, supplies, transportation, accommodation, and extra allowances, etc.

The manpower recruitment will be much facilitated whenever there are mobile teams in charge of the control of endemoepidemic diseases, extended vaccination programs, and mother and child health promotion of other similar activities. Such teams consist of nurses, microscopists, sanitarians, clerks, and drivers. They will of course have to be retrained in view of the new approach and novel activities: collection of stools (specimens and worms), of blood (parasitological and serological examinations), and of urine; the microscopic identification of parasites and adult worms; the use of WHO and/or other diagnostic kits; the performance of simple, serological tests; the crude hemoglobin concentration; the assessment of nutritional status; and, not least, the regular, correct entering of the records.

At first sight this enumeration of duties might give the impression of an overloading, impracticable program. It becomes easily manageable, however, by distributing the duties over well-defined tasks assigned to specific team members.

The training should be carried out with the utmost care. In addition to the technical building up of the indispensable know-how, an understanding of the importance of the team members' specific input toward the achievement of the program as a whole should be roused. Every team member should be aware of the value of his or her own commitment and become proud of participating in a common endeavour toward a better health of the population concerned.

The propensity of the team members to become in turn enthusiastic teachers should be taken seriously into consideration for the final selection. They will indeed be in charge of the teaching and motivation at the peripheral level. Education and training are without an end point. The needs for and timing of a partial or more extensive retraining will be determined by regular supervision and feedback mechanisms. Vigilance should never slacken.

3. Community Participation

The bulk of the mass treatment activities take place at the community level. The planning, programming, budgeting, performing, supervision, and evaluation are duties to be dealt with at a central level. A prerequisite for success is a permanent and efficient interaction between both levels.

On the periphery a number of health facilities are, or should be, present: health posts, dispensaries, health centers. They are served by health personnel of variable local denominations. Any attempt at uniformization would be a futile exercise; phraseology does not pay off. This manpower is made up by professionals and/or auxiliares belonging to the governmental health services or voluntary agencies. Their equipment and capacities are variable. Some may have a microscope and be able to use it.

Such regular health personnel and voluntary aids must be directly involved in the program. The first step will be to inform them about the possible impact of some parasitoses prevailing in their community and about the important role that they might play in the proposed attempt to control such a bane. Emphasis should be put on the expected benefit for the health of the community under their care.

Proper attention should be paid not to overrule the authority of the local health personnel in the proposed carrying out of the program. They should instead become convinced that their active participation in such a health program will increase both the efficacy of their work and their prestige. It should become the duty of the local health personnel to motivate the political, administrative, ethnical, religious authorities, and the population, and to obtain their wholehearted participation. They are on the spot, live in the community, and are generally trusted. They will therefore be invaluable help in easing the contacts between the promoters and the local authorities and persons concerned, relations which are not always frictionless. Likewise they might provide indispensable information for avoiding psychological and other mistakes, which for otherwise unforeseeable reasons often suddenly block the best programs. They will be just as useful for tearing down some walls and for advising in the handling of unforeseen situations or too strict rules with some flexibility.

4. Health Education

Health education must be an integral part of any mass campaign, not only to improve coverage and to increase the participation of the people, but also to induce long-term changes in attitude toward the problem and in practices favorable for better sanitation and to make provision for consent. The acceptance of compulsory drug administration or other prophylactic measures may arouse some apprehension concerning risks, hypothetical or apparent, which can easily be prevented. Adequate information corroborated by some health improvement as such may be "health education." In a study by LECHAT et al. (1974) it was shown that 1 year after a single mass treatment with follow-up, the prevalence rate was lowered, even in the control placebo group; the logical hypothesis of this observation being that a mass campaign in itself has an educational value, contributing to a better hygiene and improved sanitation.

5. Informed Consent

For ethical but also for operational reasons, informed consent of the community and its individual members is a must. It presumes correct information of the community through its natural and official leaders about the objectives of the mass treatment: the alleviation of the parasitological burden and the prospects of health and work capacity improvement. Furthermore, it supposes an awareness of the problem and of its solutions and a motivation to join hands (community and health team) to solve the problem.

III. Preliminary Survey

The decision to undertake a preliminary investigation shows at an early stage the expression of a political will to organize, if it seems necessary, a mass treatment program. But the identification of such a parasitological objective is only a preliminary item for consideration. In order to substantiate such a project a good balanced view of this multifactorial problem has to be taken.

To assess the importance of the prevailing parasitosis, the logical procedure is to start with a very carefully and technically soundly prepared survey. The latter should not be limited to case detection, but should also include quantified measurements.

The identification of the problem must be faultless and its involvement in a complex situation must be assessed correctly. A systematic overview of the situation implies the search of all of the worm species involved; the worm load by species; and the distribution according to determining factors such as age, sex, race, occupation, degree of exposure, etc. It might produce evidence about the groups at high risk and the existence of heavy worm bearers.

The coexistence of other infections and diarrheal diseases, caused by protozoa (e.g., *Plasmodium, Entamoeba*), bacteria (e.g., *Salmonella, Shigella, Vibrio*), viruses (e.g., rotaviruses), or yeast (*Candida*), which may play a role in the morbidity and in the response to anthelmintics must be explored. The existence of hemoglobinopathia and enzymopathia, which may produce anemia and other deficiencies, and the nutritional status must be investigated.

The morbidity pattern must be checked. So many clinical and subclinical situations may complicate the picture. It is always preferable to have a reasonable view of the real benefits that can be expected from a proposed program, than to start by claiming unattainable benefits.

The felt needs and the expected participation of those concerned has to be investigated, as well as the health infrastructure and manpower. The preliminary survey should assess the general sanitation (water, waste disposal, housing), the educational status of children and adults, the migration of the population, the sociocultural environment, and the attitude with regard to change.

The sample of the population to be examined must be representative of all major demographic strata (all age groups, both sexes, major ethnic groups, socioeconomic-cultural classes). The sample size in each stratum has to be large enough to allow for precise inference, e.g., for an estimated prevalence rate of 50%, an error of 5%, and confidence intervals of at most 10%, the maximum sample size per stratum should be about 100 persons. In each stratum the selected people must be representative of the total eligible population; therefore probability samples have to be taken. The dynamics of the endemicity must be studied, by means of at least one follow-up survey: all the persons examined initially (= at the moment of the prevalence survey), be they parasitologically positive or negative, must be examined some months later. The conversion of the negative individuals gives an estimate of the general and species specific incidence; the evolution of the worm burden in the positive examinees enables the dynamics of the endemicity to be quantified.

Country-wide similar but well-coordinated inquiries into the different prevailing ecological situations might be indicated before the next stage can be entered.

IV. Preplanning Stage

1. Rationale for Periodic Mass Treatment

When community-wide treatment for helminthiasis has been decided upon after a careful assessment of all the factors involved, its design will be based on a periodic mass treatment or deworming.

The same drugs are available for individual and mass treatment. But while the person seeking medical advice is prepared to accept diagnosis and treatment, a community is only exceptionally concerned about the presence of intestinal helminths and will not ask spontaneously for help.

Experiments have been tried out in several closed and open communities with thymol, tetrachloroethylene, bephenium, piperazine, levamisole, mebendazole, flubendazole, pyrantel, tiabendazole, and recently albendazole. All have confirmed the experience acquired in livestock: complete elimination of all parasitic worms is an unattainable goal. Even in countries with high levels of sanitation such as Japan, the United States, and the USSR, the worm burden has been successfully lowered to below a public health problem level, but never eliminated. A successful selective approach, consisting in the biannual treatment, for 4–5 years, of all the parasite bearers, irrespective of age and worm burden (KATO and MIURA 1954), has been possible in Japan, due to its well-organized health system, but it is by far too expensive and operationally too difficult to be carried out in less-developed countries.

In developing countries, the reasons for partial or transient results are manifold: environmental hazards remain unchanged; poor sanitation such as ill-maintained toilets favors the maintenance of parasites in the soil and ensures the contact with the thus infected ground; the behavior of man remains unhygienic (dirty fingers and hands, improper food preparation, disorderly excreta disposal, etc.); the people showing a low level of resistance continue to act as a reservoir and the reproductive potential of the worms takes care of a permanent reproductive potential.

The persistence of the infection in the community is related to the risk of permanent reinfection. Sanitation has only limited impact on the soil-transmitted helminths until a high degree of hygiene has been achieved. Other infections are maintained by intermediate hosts, such as mollusks, which are quite resistant to the available control methods. Some are simply carried by transport hosts, pulvillae and other parts of *Musca, Lucilia,* or *Calliphorina,* or by paratenic hosts in which the parasite survives without undergoing further development. Man is such a host for *Toxocara cati* and *T. canis,* as rodents are for *Toxascaris leonina.* One should keep in mind that natural hosts can also become infected before birth by the mother, who harbours larvae.

2. Choice of Drugs and Treatment Schedules

The choice of drug must obviously take into account the most threatening helminth, but a broader spectrum, a lesser risk for side effects, and a lower cost price are among the many elements pertaining to a judicious choice.

The selection of a drug – old or new – for mass treatment needs for obvious reasons to fulfil more prerequisites than for individual therapy. Preference should be given to drugs which produce the expulsion of adult worms and are also ovicidal and larvicidal. The degree of safety must be high enough to avoid a high percentage of side effects: gastric discomfort, gastrointestinal intolerance, dermatological reactions, hematological, neurological, or other disorders.

In developing countries only the cheapest drugs are economically and budgetarily accessible. Besides, the drug must be easy to keep and stable in a tropical or equatorial environment and easy to administer under mass treatment conditions. The peremption period should not be too short. The supply, distribution chain, and storage facilities must be ensured. The drug should not produce resistance of the parasite. The administration should be easy, preferably oral, not requiring preparation or purgation.

The dosage requirement should allow an indiscriminate distribution of a common dose independent of age or weight, preferably single in accordance with the dictum "one dose – one day." If a multidose administration is unavoidable, the rhythm, frequency, and timing should cause as little disturbance as possible for the community. The control of the intake should be easy.

In order to acquire some rational basis for the choice of drug suitable for mass application, STÜRCHLER (1982) proposed a score system, which can be easily adopted as a model for the more limited problem of mass chemotherapy for intestinal nematodes (Table 1).

In spite of the limited number of parameters and of the strong subjective input in the selection of criteria for scoring, this system of assessment is often very helpful. Other criteria such as acceptability by the people from the endemic areas and teratogenic effects could be incorporated in this assessment score.

The trend in the past to use drug combinations aimed at widening the spectrum of activity, e.g., tetrachloroethylene and bephenium salt, is seemingly anew in fashion. Combinations of poorly and readily absorbed compounds, which may act on both adults and circulating larvae, e.g., levamisole and mebendazole, or may unite a paralyzing and a killing compound, e.g., pyrantel and mebendazole,

Table 1. Evaluation of anthelminthics for mass application (heuristic method)

Drug	Efficacy[a]	Length of treatment[b]	Side effects[c]	Cost[d]	Total
Albendazole	7	11	−8	?	(10?)
Bephenium	4	8	−6	0	6
Levamisole	5	11	0	0	16
Mebendazole	7	11	0	0	18
Piperazine	2	1	−5	0	−2
Pyrantel	6	14	0	−2	18
Tetrachloroethylene	2	6	−5	0	4
Tiabendazole	7	12	−12	−2	5

[a] One point for each worm and an additional point for efficacy >90%
[b] In a single dose, 3 points; 3 days protocol, 1 point; >3 days, 0
[c] Only frequent and severe side effects, −1 point for each
[d] Prices according to Medeor, Mission Pharma

are a few of the more recent examples. In so far as the combinations are logical, they may improve the possibilities and sometimes lower the risk.

As the one-dose, cheap, all-embracing wonderdrug does not yet exist, an important item is the spacing of the administration. An optimal spacing does not exist. The timing will vary with geographical, climatological, environmental, and epidemiological factors such as the persistent contamination risk and the prepatent period. Overseas a 3-monthly interval has been selected most frequently. However, no agreement has been achieved on the appropriate number of campaigns: two or three or more.

GATTI et al. (1972) and ARFAA and GHADIRIAN (1978) stopped after three administrations and observed a slow reincrease of prevalence rates. In the Zaire testing, prevalence was still low after 6 months and in Iran after 1 year. These data confirm the observations made after 5–6 months by CHAIA and DA CUNHA (1971).

In accordance with many experiences, it seems an acceptable proposition to select, in heavily infected communities, as a basic rhythm 3 months or in any case not longer than 4 months. A more logical complementary approach is to make provision for a second administration after the prepatent period of the worm concerned, which will be followed by a 3- or 4-monthly or longer interval, in accordance with the local seasonal variations in the transmission period, covering a full year. To guarantee a more lasting result, the administration should be resumed after 6 months or 1 year. To establish on objective grounds the interactive rhythm, it is imperative to try it out with the chosen drug in a pilot run.

A great number of interesting and orientating studies have been published by ARFAA et al. (1977), ARFAA and GHADIRIAN (1978), BOTERO (1979), CABRERA et al. (1975, 1980), CAMPBELL (1977), GATTI et al. (1972), GAXOTTE and ROSIN (1975), GERWEL et al. (1970), GUPTA et al. (1976), KABA et al. (1978), JANCLOES et al. (1979), KRUBWA et al. (1974), DE OLIVEIRA (1970), POND et al. (1970), PURNOMO et al. (1980), RIPERT et al. (1978), and STÜRCHLER et al. (1980).

3. **Pilot Run** (Field testing)

Control of parasitosis is always in need of clearly defined objectives and this for every step of the program. Before engaging in a vast field program of massive treatment, every aspect of the program should be tried out to assess the attainability of the objectives: are they realistic and acceptable to the community concerned and local health teams; what are the operational and logistical constraints? In order to assess every phase and activity of the program a pilot run is indicated.

A pilot run is very convenient to cover the needs for operational research, to ascertain the logistics, and to watch the planned schedule of the drug administration, the checking of the optimal dosage, the effective delivery, the availability of supplies, the acceptability of the taste, and the presentation of the drug.

The planned schedules are often met only partially and coverage is frequently inadequate. This is caused by poor cooperation of the population and a reluctant attitude of the authorities. To anticipate this underhand opposition, great care must be taken not to interfere uselessly with the way of life, occupations, and sociocultural and political structures. Given an adequate approach this knowledge may by very helpful.

The pilot run will offer a real possibility to try out diversified coverage protocols of drug administration such as: blanket treatment of the whole population, treatment of the screened positive individuals, treatment limited to the persons with high worm load, and treatment limited with or without screening to "high-risk" groups: infants, schoolchildren, pregnant women, and lactating mothers. A pilot run will also be useful in establishing a reliable follow-up schedule according to the reappearance of eggs after temporary suppression in different target groups, by means of the indicative cure rate (CR) and egg reduction rate (ERR) values.

Such a small-scale trial will be necessary for the tuning up of the logistics involved in a full-scale realization, and for assessing the efficacy and acceptability of the selected drug. The pilot test will also provide reliable data on eggs per gram (EPG), CR, ERR, rupture of the transmission chain, duration of the improvement, rate of reappearance of eggs after treatment, slowing down of reinfection, impact on most heavily infected individuals, coverage, and surveillance for reinfection.

A pilot run is a well-chosen opportunity to decide on the use of professional, auxiliary, or primary health care (PHC) personnel and the use of local static or mobile teams intended for uni- or polyvalent activities, to recycle the health personnel, to train auxiliaries and to motivate all of them. In default of a pilot run, the majority of the mass treatment trials will end up in being only attempts of mono- or polyvalent chemotherapy with a more or less extended follow-up aiming at assessing the appearance of a reinfection, but without any continuity.

Practical Organization

The organization of a pilot run depends largely on the population target group (urban-versus rural population, special risk groups, total population). The general principles set forward here concern a total population treatment, but they can easily be adapted to special target groups.

The people sampled for the pilot run must be representative of the total population eligible for mass treatment. Lack of representativeness induces selection biases, these have to be avoided at any cost, because the results obtained from the pilot sample have to be inferred to the parent population and also the lessons learnt from that pilot experience have to be taken into account in the planning of the mass treatment campaign.

A probability sample is obtained from a reliable population list. Generally these lists are rare. A more realistic approach is to start with a list of dwellings. If such a list does not exist, it is not impossible, even for a medical team, to prepare one correctly in a limited time span. Consequently the survey unit should be a house, serving as a proxy for a family. All the permanent members of the family are eligible for selection in a total population mass treatment scheme. There are different types of probability samples, but the best simulation of the mass treatment situation is given by a total cluster sampling. The procedure consists of dividing the area into geographically distinct clusters. If by demographic standards, the clusters are not homogeneous, strata are formed and within the strata the clusters are delineated. Inside the strata the clusters are randomly sampled, and all the families of the sampled clusters are examined and treated. A map of the dwellings in the sample area is drawn and each house and family is localized on the map (BROWN and BROWN 1975). The total sample size depends on the desired precision of the estimates and the prevalence rates. For example for an error of 5%, confidence intervals of 5%, and a prevalence rate of 50%, the total sample size should at least be 384.

The people must be informed not only of the objectives of the trial, but also of the operational details. During the trial the necessary contacts must be maintained with the population. The necessity of good contact with the population cannot be stressed enough, because *lack of cooperation* in a prospective study is *the* major source of biases results.

A mass campaign probably has to be held on a house-to-house basis; however, in the context of an extremely well developed community organization, the pilot study (and the mass campaign also) could be based on the health center. Depending on the target groups and the local community organizations, other bases could be chosen too; e.g., STEPHENSON et al. (1983) reported a mass campaign trial, directed at preschool and school-age children, which was school based.

Supervision of the intake of the drugs is indispensable, at least during the pilot study. Volunteer health promoters can be incorporated in the team to advantage but they need to be very well supervised. The pilot study starts with a census of the selected clusters of families. For that a locally workable definition of "permanent inhabitant" has to be made.

A questionnaire must be developed, a sample of which is given in Appendix A. When the language of the local people is different from that of the interviewers, the questionnaire should be translated into local language and terminology. The questions should always be put to the same family member. The choice is defined on anthropological criteria. Before the start of the pilot study, a small-scale trial should be carried out to train the staff and to assess the operational feasibility and acceptability of the pilot study. The whole chain of activities must be checked, and special attention must be given to possible fecal taboos, because they might account for a large nonresponse. [In a prevalence survey of intestinal parasitosis carried out in Yapacany, Bolivia, 20% of the schoolchildren refused to participate; an anthropologist found out that this was due to unrecognized fecal taboos (DE MUYNCK et al. 1976).] Such a test must be done in a region similar to the pilot area, but should not be held in the latter area. The whole staff should participate, and the size of the sample may be small: some five to ten families.

It is highly desirable to register the side effects of the administered drugs. Therefore the team should systematically visit the participating families; by doing so the team keeps in touch with the population. This is important for further compliance of the community. The drugs should be taken under supervision, and one should record whether the drug was vomited or not swallowed. It has to be remembered that drinkable water is a problem in many areas; therefore an on hand supply of lemonade can be an important help.

A pilot study addresses the question of the interval between the consecutive treatments. Different schemes should be tried out: on a periodic basis or adjusted to the epidemiology of the worm(s) concerned.

A biostatistician with a good knowledge of survey methodology should be an integral member of the staff, from the design stage on. During the campaign he must watch for missing items on the questionnaire and for missing records. Missing items can be avoided by careful supervision of each record and consequent return to the interviewee to complete the record, and also by detailed checking of the phrasing and understanding of the questions by interviewer and interviewees during the test session. Missing items are a parameter of the quality of the team. Missing records are a much more difficult question to deal with. They are essentially of two kinds: physical absence of the interviewee when the team passes (this is nearly always a problem for the male adults during weekdays; the working hours of the team have to be adapted to the presence of the people at home) and secondly lack of desire to cooperate or even frank refusal. This very negative element can be diminished in importance by a good preparation and by having the support of the leaders of the community. At least two calls should be made to the missing family members to participate. The data should be accessible to the curative staff of the local health team.

V. Planning Stage

After the results of the pilot run are known and assessed, and based on epidemiological evidence of prevalences and incidences of intestinal parasites in the different ecological settings, the decision on the justification of the mass campaign and its operational modalities must be made.

Collected data and accompanying comments must be reported to the authorities with regard to an accurately informed final decision. The report of the planning stage must involve a critical survey of the problems in the census-taking, mobility of the population, and percentage of dropouts and absentees; the number of parasite species, their mode of transmission, and seasonal variations if any; the collection of feces and other specimens; the reliability of the microscopic and other examinations; the drug, broad spectrum and single dose if possible; the administration of the drug and complaints about side effects; the different schedules; and the relative benefits of a simultaneous or progressive blanket treatment or of a distribution limited to certain groups at risk or only to the infected persons.

It will also cover the quality of the professional, auxiliary, and voluntary personnel, their specific training and retraining needs, and the composition and qualification of the basic team, both central and peripheral.

VI. Execution Stage

After the final decision has been made by the national authorities to start a mass campaign, and after provision has been made for the indispensable funds, basic logistics, and continuous availability of the drugs, the field operations are started by training the local field personnel and by informing the local communities concerned. Only thereafter may the field operations, consisting of the distribution of the drugs, be started. During the execution of the mass campaign no systematic assessment of the endemicity is necessary. However, the evolution of the endemicity should be followed and assessed periodically, on a representative sample.

In the execution two distinct phases can be distinguished:

1. Attack Stage

The attack stage will follow the decision to implement the program. The duration and timing of the drug administration should take into account that, due to the possibilities of reinfection, as a rule a return to the previous situation is reached 1 year after a single drug administration.

2. Consolidation Stage

The consolidation stage follows in order to lessen the worm burden to a tolerable level if the exhaustion of the environmental infective reservoir cannot be achieved and reinfection stopped. The time to reach transmission breaking point depends on the survival time of infective larvae in the environment (2–5 or even 10 years). No model program can be advised due to the many variations in prevalence, intensity, local conditions, seasonal changes, and participation of population.

The population should be kept informed about the decisions taken and also about the real impact of the prevailing parasitosis on their health. The coverage may be hampered by absenteeism and dropping out and will therefore in general be inadequate in the absence of a regularly stimulated motivation.

This applies just as well to the political, administrative, ethnic, and religious authorities: if their sense of responsibility is not reawakened in due course, they are mostly uninterested.

D. Alternative Control Measures

The survey and the decision-making process of mass treatment should always turn a keen eye to the sanitation level and should involve an accurate insight into the educational degree and the sociocultural background. The results will usually be rather disappointing or even depressing.

Sanitation can indeed play a role in the control of soil-transmitted helminths such as the **"worm trinity"** – *Ascaris,* hookworm, *Trichuris* – and a few others, such as *Trichostrongylus* and *Ternidens,* by breaking up or limiting the feces-soil contact. This is readily achieved by rehousing, proper sewage disposal, water supply as demonstrated brilliantly by the multistore flats in Singapore. But in tropical rural and periurban areas the proper use of latrines is exceptional and sanitation is difficult, too expensive, and of doubtful value. The situation is unmanageable when nightsoil is used as fertilizer in vegetable gardens.

Allowance should be made for the fact that the degree of sanitation achieved after building latrines may be a worsened one. Indiscriminate defecation in the fields is neutralized by the sterilizing rays of the sun. Ill-maintained and faultily used toilets, moreover, covered by a roof hampering the sterilizing capacity of the sun, favor in fact the multiplication of parasites in the soil and ensure regular contact with permanently infected ground. All the serious investigations about the results of the construction of latrines have made it clear that a "status quo" is the best than can be achieved.

Education is another widely advocated tool. Nobody will challenge the assertion that properly educated people are able to solve their own sanitation problems. However, education and especially health education cannot be built on a vacuum. Health education is an arduous undertaking even in a developmed community. In an underdeveloped world it becomes an impossible, extremely frustrating, and by nature fugitive engagement if it cannot be supported by perceptible and concrete results in solving felt needs.

The interference of the sociocultural background may also be anticipated: customs, taboos, and prohibitions, which are not easily overcome. The way of life, harvests, markets, fairs, etc. has an influence on day-to-day attendance.

In all of these matters a compromise has to be sought in consultation and in agreement with those involved. In other words, socioeconomic improvement is an important, but not a decisive, method. Sanitation and health education are not to be seen as easy or temporary substitutes for health improvement, but as integrated parts of an overall health promotion program. To expect a speedy return from improved sanitation, water supply, and health education is as irrealistic as to plan the destruction of the parasites in the soil, which is also theoretically feasible. Thus the only way to control the soil-transmitted helminths is their destruction in the only readily accessible location: the human host. Drugs remove worms, prevent the dispersal of eggs, and thus provide immediate results.

E. Conclusion

Intestinal worms constitute an important problem for public health in developing countries. They can be controlled if correct use is made of the modern antihelmintic drugs in a prolonged community effort. Such mass campaigns must well-designed, planned, and executed together with the local authorities and health staff.

Appendix A: Questionnaire[1]

ID No. | 1 | 2 | 3 |

Identification

Name of head of family: .... First wife | 4 |

Second wife

Third wife

House No.: ....

Block or street: ....

Village or

suburb: .... | 5 |

Specific details: ....

1 The questionnaire has been prepared for processing by computer

Interviewer: ....

Time of start of interview: day + hour + minutes: ....

Family composition

No.	Name	Sex	Age	Race	Shoes	Schooling							
1	Father						6	7	8	9	10	11	12
2	Mother						13	14	15	16	17	18	19
3							20	21	22	23	24	25	26
4							27	28	29	30	31	32	33
5							34	35	36	37	38	39	40
6							41	42	43	44	45	46	47
7							48	49	50	51	52	53	54
8							55	56	57	58	59	60	61
9							62	63	64	65	66	67	68
10							69	70	71	72	73	74	75

Father: Profession 76

Religion 77

Has lived in the area since 78

Mother: No. of pregnancies 79

No. of children born alive 80

No. of children alive today 81

Family data

House

Walls: materials 82

Floor in living room ☐ earthen ☐ other 83

Materials of roof: 84

Ceiling ☐ present ☐ absent 85

Rooms: No. 86

Beds ☐ yes ☐ no 87

if yes, No. ☐

Ownership of house		☐ yes	no	88
Refrigerator		☐ yes	☐ no	89
Electricity		☐ yes	☐ no	90
Radio		☐ yes	☐ no	91
Books and/or newspapers		☐ present	☐ absent	92
Bicycle		☐ present	☐ absent	93
Sewing machine		☐ present	☐ absent	94
Cleanliness		☐ good ☐ moderate ☐ poor		95
Water supply		☐ running water ☐ other drinkable water ☐ no clear water		96
Latrine		☐ own latrine ☐ communitarian latrine ☐ absent		97
Domestic animals	Cats	☐ present	☐ absent	98
	Dogs	☐ present	☐ absent	91
	Cows	☐ present	☐ absent	100
	Sheep	☐ present	☐ absent	101
	Goats	☐ present	☐ absent	102
	Fowl	☐ present	☐ absent	103
Meals:				
Does the family consume meat		☐ yes	☐ no	104
Does the family produce crops		☐ yes	☐ no	105

If yes which: ....

End of interview: hour: ....

Appendix B: Stool Examination

Name: .... ID No.

1	2	3	4	5

Date of stool collection

year	month	day

Date of stool examination

year	month	day

Parasites Methods EPG

	Direct smear	Kato method	Concen-tration	
Ascaris				
Ancylostoma				
Necator (Hookworm)				
Trichuris				
Strongyloides				

Lab technician Lab supervisor

....

Appendix C: Clinical Examination

ID No. | | | | |

No	Weight	Height	Skin-fold	Fever	Cough >15 days	Presence of diarrhea	Skin lesions +hair	Anemia: "paleness of mucosae"	Health status

Appendix D: Instructions for the File

House No.: enter the number of the house.

Name of head of family: enter the name of the person in charge of the family. If the man is polygamous, prepare a file for each wife and her children if they live in a separate house (or apartment). Keep the same ID No. for the polygamous family, but indicate to which wife the children belong.

Specific details: indicate any details which would enable the family to be easily located for a further visit.

Interviewer: name and signature of the interviewer. Time of start of interview: the exact time of the start of the interview should be entered, e.g., 8:30 a.m.

Age: > 15 years: if the age is not known exactly, enter AD (adult). 5–14 years: enter the age in years. < 5 years: enter the date of birth.

Shoes: did the interviewee wear shoes at the time of the interview? Enter the observation.

Schooling: enter the years of formal education.

Family composition: rank the children according to age in ascending order, starting with the youngest child, e.g., No. 3 = youngest child.

Definition of family (extended family): "all the family members (+relatives) living in the same house and participating in the meals."

Father: enter his main profession.

House
Refrigerator: enter "yes" if the refrigerator is seen.
Electricity: enter "yes" if a light bulb is seen.
Radio: enter "yes" if a radio is shown or any other evidence can be observed.
Books or newspapers: enter "yes" if there is evidence of written texts in the house at the time of the interview.
Bicycle: ask if the father owns a bicycle.
Sewing machine: enter "yes" if evidence is observed.
Cleanliness: compare the house with the local standard of a moderately clean house: if this house is similar, enter ☐ moderate; if this house is assessed better, enter ☐ good; if this house is assessed worse, enter ☐ poor.

Water supply: by "other drinkable water", all the water that is treated by boiling, by filtration, or chemically is meant.

Latrine: if the family owns of a latrine cross the box "own latrine"; if the family uses a communitarian latrine enter a cross in the corresponding box; otherwise cross "absent".

Domestic animals: enter a cross in the "present" box only if some evidence is observed.

End of interview: enter exact time of the end of interview.

Stool Examination

ID No. Enter the ID No. of the questionnaire. Enter in box No. 5 the corresponding number from the family composition, e.g., the mother of family 12 if the family is monogamous = | 0 | 1 | 2 | 1 | 2 |. 012 = 12th family; 1 = first wife; 2–second on the list of family composition.

The EPG (egg count per gram) is entered in absolute numbers. The score for the results of the three methods is entered in the following manner: 0 = absence of eggs or larvae; 1 = + (low); 2 = ++ (moderate); 3 = +++ (high).

The lab technician must fill in his name and the lab supervisor must indicate he has checked the results.

Note: 1. The same basic methods, carried out with the same methodology, must always be applied through the pilot run. 2. The stool examination is indicated at: t_0 = the moment of the intake of the drug; t_{2-3} = 2–3 weeks after the first intake; and t_X = afterwards at the moment of the intake of the drug.

Clinical Examination

The clinical examination must be carried out by a person with a certain level of diagnostic skills. Therefore the people are required to come to a central place (health post or center or any accessible place).

Weight: measure to the nearest ½ kg in adults. The estimated weight of the clothes must be taken into account. For underfive's the weight should be measured to the nearest 0.1 kg.

Height: for very small children the height must be taken when the child is lying down on a special measurement scale. For bigger children and adults the measurements are taken standing; and be given to the nearest 0.5 cm. Skin fold: this is determined with a pair of callipers. Arm circumference: this is taken by means of flexible meter placed carefully in the middle of the left upper arm.

Cough: by anamnesis.
Diarrhea: by anamnesis.
Anemia: observation of color of conjunctival mucosae and tongue: if pale = anemia.
Health status: subjective impression by the examiner.

Note: the same ID No. should be entered on this clinical examination list.

References

Arfaa F, Ghadirian E (1977) Epidemiology and mass treatment of ascariasis in six rural communities in central Iran. Am J Trop Med Hyg 26:866–871

Arfaa F, Ghadirian E (1978) The effect of mass treatment in the control of helminthiasis in Ispahan, central Iran. Iran J Publ Health 7:100–114

Arfaa F, Sahba GH, Farahmandian I, Jalali I (1977) Evaluation of the effect of different methods of control of soil-transmitted helminths in Khuzestan, Southwest Iran. Am J Trop Med Hyg 26:230–232

Botera D (1979) Possibilities of controlling soil transmitted helminths by mass treatment. Bol Chil Parasitol 34:39–43

Brown J, Brown R (1975) The community census as a basis for health programmers. J Trop Paediatr Environ Child Health 315–320

Cabrera BD, Arambulo III PV, Portillo GG (1975) Ascariasis control and/or eradication in a rural community in the Philippines. SE Asian J Trop Med Public Health 6:510–518

Cabrera B, Valdez EV, Go T (1980) Clinical field trials of broad spectrum anthelmintics against soil-transmitted helminthiasis. SE Asian J Trop Med Public Health 11:502–506

Campbell WC (1977) The control of parasites: the role of drugs. The Helminthol Soc Wash 44:17–28

Chaia G, Da Cunha AH (1971) Therapeutic action of mebendazole (R17635) against human helminthiasis. Folha Med 63:67–76

De Muynck A, Silva de Lagrave M (1976) Encuesta sobre parasitosis intestinal en y apacini. Bol Inf Cenetrop 2:29–38

De Oliveira AB (1970) Eradication in mass of *Ascaris lumbricoides* in a small and isolated community. Consecutive monthly treatment. Rev Bras Med 27:173–189

Faust EC, Beaver PG, Juno RC (1975) Parasitologic diagnosis in animal agents. In: Animal agents and vectors of human disease. Lea and Febinger, Philadelphia, pp 421–441

Gatti F, Krubwa F, Vandepitte J, Thienpont D (1972) Control of intestinal nematodes in African schoolchildren by the trimestrial administration of levamisole. Ann Soc Belge Med Trop 52:19–32

Gaxotte P, Rosin G (1975) Activité anthelminthique du pyrantel pamoate administré en traitement de masse dans une population isolée du Pacifique Sud. Bull Soc Pathol Exot 68:491–496

Gerwel C, Pawlowski Z, Chuirot E (1970) The usefulness of thiabendazole, bephenium and piperazine of mass control of ascariasis and anafortomiasis. Wiad Parazytol 16:393–399

Gupta MC, Mithal S, Tandon BN (1976) Use of tetramisole for mass deworming in a community with heavy ascaris infection. J Indian Med Assoc 67:180–182

Gupta MC, Mithal S, Arora KL, Tandon BN (1977) Effect of periodic deworming on nutritional status of *Ascaris*-infected preschool children receiving supplementary food. Lancet II:108–110

Jancloes MF, Jancloes-Diepart M (1981) Campagnes periodiques d'assainissement et de chimiotherapie de masse contre les nematodes intestinaux, appliquées isolement et en combinason, au Bas-Zaire. Ann Soc Belge Med Trop 61:111–118

Jancloes MF, Cornet P, Thienpont D (1979) Mass control of ascariasis with single oral doses of levamisole. A controlled comparison of 3,056 subjects between three incomplete population coverages. Trop Geogr Med 31:111–122

Kaba AS, Luvwezo M, Nzuzi K, Thienpont D (1978) Le traitement anthelminthique périodique d'enfants d'àge scolaire au Zaïre. Ann Soc Belge Med Trop 58:241–249

Krubwa F, Gatti F, Lontie M, Nguete K, Vandepitte J, Thienpont D (1974) Administration trimestrielle de mebendazole en mileu scolaire suburbain. Med Trop 34:679–687

Lechat MF, Jancloes MF, Galambos FG, Cornet P, Thienpont D (1974) Control by levamisole of ascariasis and ancylostomiasis in rural areas. Trop Geogr Med 26:441–445

Pond HS, Bokat RD, Johnson JP, Knight JL, Healey GR, Gleason NN, Hall EC (1970) Mass treatment for ascariasis: value of prophylactic use of piperazine in groups heavily infected with *Ascaris lumbricoides*. South Med J 62:599–602

Purnomo, Partono F, Soewarta A (1980) Human intestinal parasites in Karakuak. West Flores, Indonesia and the effect of treatment with mebendazole and pyrantel pamoate. Southeast Asian J Trop Med Public Health 11:324–331

Ripert C, Durand B, Carrie J, Riedel D, Bray-Zorra D (1978) Etude épidémiologique des nématodoses intestinales dans cinq villages de la vallée de la Sanaga (Cameroun). Bull Soc Pathol Biol 71:361–369

Stephenson L, Crompton D, Latham M, Arnold S, Jansen A (1983) Evaluation of a four year project to control *Ascaris* infection in children in two Kenyan villages. J. Trop Pediatr 29:175–184

Stürchler D (1982) Chemotherapy of human intestinal helminthiasis: A review, with particular reference to community treatment. Adv Pharmacol Chemother 19:67–128

Stürchler D, Stahel E, Saladin K, Saladin B (1980) Inestinal parasitoses in eight Liberian settlements: prevalences and community anthelminthic chemotherapy. Tropenmed Parasitol 31:87–93

Taylor D (1982) Medicines, health and the poor world. Office of Health Economics, London

WHO Study Group (1965) Report on integration of mass campaigns against specific diseases into general health services. WHO Tech Rep Ser 294:5

Further Reading

Jelliffe D (1966) The assessment of the nutritional status of the community, WHO monograph series No 53. WHO, Geneva

Lutz W (1981) Planning and organizing a health survey. International Epidemiological Association Monograph, pp 1–112

Lutz W (1982) Sampling: how to select people, households, and places to study community health. International Epidemiological Association Monograph, pp 1–123

List of International Nonproprietary, United States Adopted, and Trade Names of Some Anthelmintics

International nonproprietary name	United States adopted name	Trade names
Acetarsol	–	Cestarsol, Nemoral, Nemural, Tenoban
Albendazole	Albendazole	Valbacen, Valbazen, Zentel
Amidantel	–	
Bephenium hydroxynaphthoate	–	Alcopar, Alcopara, Frantin
Bithionol	Bithionolate sodium	Actamer, Bitin, Lorothidol
Bitoscanate	–	Jonit
Bromoxanide	Bromoxanide	
Brotianide	–	
Bunamidine	Bunamidine hydrochloride	Ruban, Scolaban
Cambendazole	Cambendazole	Bonlam, Camben, Camdan, Equiben, Neminil, Porcam 5%
Ciclobendazole	Ciclobendazole	
Clioxanide	Clioxanide	Tremerad
Closantel	Closantel	Flukiver, Seponver
Coumafos	–	Asuntol, Baymix, Co-Ral, Meldane, Muscavox
Dichlorophen	–	Antiphen, Dicestal, Didroxone, Diphenthane-70, Parabis, Teniathane, Teniatol, Vermiplex
Dichlororphenol + bithionol	–	Trematol
Dichlorvos	–	Atgard, Dichlorman, Equigard, Equigel, Task, Tenac
Diethylcarbamazine	–	Caricide, Dirocide, Hetrazan
Difetarsone	–	Bemarsal
Dithiazanine iodide	–	Abminthic, Delvex, Deselmine, Dizan, Pankiller, Telmid
Erythromycine (= carbomycin)	Erythromycin estolate	Magnamycin
Febantel	Febantel	Rintal
Febantel + trichlorfon	–	Rintal-plus
Fenbendazole	Fenbendazole	Axilur, Panacur

(continued)

International nonproprietary name	United States adopted name	Trade names
Fenclofos	Ronnel	Dermaphos, Ectoral, Etrolene, Ronnel, Tro lene
Flubendazole	Flubendazole	Flubenol, Flumoxal, Flutelmium, Fluverma
Fospirate	Fospirate	Torelle
Haloxon	–	Cavoxon, Equivurm, Eustidil, Galloxon 77' Halox, Helmiren, Loxon, Verloxon
Hexachlorophene	–	Bilevon, Distocid, Distodin, Distophen, Fasciobitin, Fasciophene
Ivermectin	Ivermectin	Ivomec, Eqvalan
Levamisole	Levamisole hydrochloride	Anthelpor, Anthesol, Ascaridil, Ascaryl, Aviverm, Aviversol, Citarin-L, Concurat-Decaris, Decaris vet, Ergamisol, Getevern L, Istamicide, Ketrax, Levipor, Levoriper col, L-Narpenol, L-Ripercol, L-Spartakoı L-Tramisol, Nemaphenine, Nemicanisol, Nemicide, Nemisol, Nilverm, Nilzan, Pa-gliderm, Paglisol, Pig wormer, Riporon, Solaskil, Stimamizol, Tramisol, Tramizan Vermisol, Wormex
Mebendazole	Mebendazole	Antiox, Equiverm-plus, Fugacar, Gammax, Lomper, Mebatreat, Mebenav, Mebenvet, Multispec, Nemasole, Noverme, Ovitelmiı Pantelmin, Parmeben, Telmin, Telmin-KH Telmin RTL, Telmintic, Vermox, Vermox vet, Verpanil
Mebendazole + metrifonate	–	Trichlorfon-Telmin
Metyridine		Dekelmin, Mintic, Promintic
Metrifonate (trichlorfon)	–	Bilarcil, Combot, Dipterex, Ditrifon, Dylox, Dyrex, Foschlor, Neguvon, Tugon
Morantel	Morantel tartrate	Banminth II, Bovhelm, Expar, Glylox, Ibantic, Nemantel, Ovithelm, Paratect
Naftalofos	–	Amdax, Maretin, Rametin
Niclofolan	–	Bilevon, Dertil, Distolon
Niclosamide	Niclosamide	Cestocid, Devermin, Lintex, Mansonil, Phe-nasal, Radeverm, Sagimid, Tredemine, Vermitin, Yomesan
Nitrodan	Nitrodan	Everfree
Nitroscanate	Nitroscanate	Lopatol
Nitroxynil	–	Dovenix, Trodax
Oxantel	Oxantel pamoate	
Oxantel + pyrantel	–	Polbantrin, Quantrel
Oxfendazole	Oxfendazole	Synanthic, Systamex

(continued)

International nonproprietary name	United States adopted name	Trade names
Oxibendazole	Oxibendazole	AM 313, Bovinol, Equiminthe, Loditac, Neplon 100
Oxibendazole + dichlorvos	–	Equiminthe-plus
Oxibendazole + niclosamide	–	Polyverkan
Oxyclozanide	–	Diplin, Metiljin, Zanil
Oxytetracyline	–	Terramycin
Parbendazole	Parbendazole	Helmatax, Verminum, Wormguard
Paromomycin	–	Gabbromycin, Gabbroral, Humagel, Humatin
Phenothiazine	–	Contaverm, Coopazine, Helmitina, Phenobent, Phenovis
Piperazine		*Adipate:* Antivermin, Ascatrix, Coopane, Entacyl, Mapiprin, Pipadox, Piperfesa, Pipradin
		Citrate: Antelmin, Bryrel, Moncasan, Piperasol, Piprelix, Safersol
		Phosphate: Candizine, Piperazate
		Sebacate: Nematorazine
Praziquantel	Praziquantel	Biltricide, Cesol, Droncit
Promethazine	–	Phenergan
Pyrantel	Pyrantel pamoate	Antiminth, Combantrin, Strongig P
	Pyrantel tartrate	Banminth, Exhelm, Pyrequan, Strongid
Pyrantel + oxantel	–	Canex plus
Pyrvinium	–	*Pamoate:* Vanquin, Povan
Rafoxanide	Rafoxanide	Flukanide, Ranide
Resorantel	–	Terenol
Spiramycin	Spiramycin	Rovamycin
Stilbazium iodide	Stilbazium iodide	Monopar
Tetramisole	Tetramisole-hydrochloride	Anthelvet, Aviverm, Aviversol, Deltram, Imena, Nemicide, Nilverm, Nilzan, Pig wormer, Ripercol, Strongophenine, Vadephen, Vermium
Tetramisole + niclosamide	–	Aritene, Stromiten
Thenium closylate + piperazine	–	Ancaris, Canopar
Tiabendazole	Thiabendazole	Bovizole, Coglazol, Equizole, Mintizol, Omnizole, Thibenzole

(continued)

International nonproprietary name	United States adopted name	Trade names
Tiabendazole + piperazine	–	Equizole A
Ticarbodine	Ticarbodine	
Tioxidazole	Tioxidazole	
Uredofos	Uredofos	Sansalid
Vincofos	Vincofos	

Subject Index

Handbook of Experimental Pharmacology

Continuation of "Handbuch der experimentellen Pharmakologie"

Springer-Verlag
Berlin
Heidelberg
New York
Tokyo

Volume 37
Angiotensin

Volume 38: Part 1
Antineoplastic and Immunosuppressive Agents I

Part 2
Antineoplastic and Immunosuppressive Agents II

Volume 39
Antihypertensive Agents

Volume 40
Organic Nitrates

Volume 41
Hypolipidemic Agents

Volume 42
Neuromuscular Junction

Volume 43
Anabolic-Androgenic Steroids

Volume 44
Heme and Hemoproteins

Volume 45: Part 1
Drug Addiction I

Part 2
Drug Addiction II

Volume 46
Fibrinolytics and Antifibronolytics

Volume 47
Kinetics of Drug Action

Volume 48
Arthropod Venoms

Volume 49
Ergot Alkaloids and Related Compounds

Volume 50: Part 1
Inflammation

Part 2
Anti-Inflammatory Drugs

Volume 51
Uric Acid

Volume 52
Snake Venoms

Volume 53
Pharmacology of Ganglionic Transmission

Volume 54: Part 1
Adrenergic Activators and Inhibitors I

Part 2
Adrenergic Activators and Inhibitors II

Volume 55
Psychotropic Agents

Part 1
Antipsychotics and Antidepressants

Part 2
Anxiolytics, Gerontopsychopharmacological Agents and Psychomotor Stimulants

Part 3
Alcohol and Psychotomimetics, Psychotropic Effects of Central Acting Drugs

Handbook of Experimental Pharmacology

Continuation of
"Handbuch der experimentellen Pharmakologie"

Volume 56, Part 1+2
Cardiac Glycosides

Volume 57
Tissue Growth Factors

Volume 58
Cyclic Nucleotides

Part 1: **Biochemistry**

Part 2: **Physiology and Pharmacology**

Volume 59
Mediators and Drugs in Gastrointestinal Motility

Part 1: **Morphological Basis and Neuro-physiological Control**

Part 2: **Endogenous and Exogenous Agents**

Volume 60
Pyretics and Antipyretics

Volume 61
Chemotherapy of Viral Infections

Volume 62
Aminoglycoside Antibiotics

Volume 63
Allergic Reactions to Drugs

Volume 64
Inhibition of Folate Metabolism in Chemotherapy

Volume 65
Teratogenesis and Reproductive Toxicology

Volume 66
Part 1: **Glucagon I**

Part 2: **Glucagon II**

Volume 67
Part 1
Antibiotics Containing the Beta-Lactam Structure I

Part 2
Antibiotics Containing the Beta-Lactam Structure II

Volume 68, Part 1+2
Antimalarial Drugs

Volume 69
Pharmacology of the Eye

Volume 70
Part 1
Pharmacology of Intestinal Permeation I

Part 2
Pharmacology of Intestinal Permeation II

Volume 71
Interferons and Their Applications

Volume 72
Antitumor Drug Resistance

Volume 73
Radiocontrast Agents

Volume 74
Antieliptic Drugs

Volume 75
Toxicology of Inhaled Materials

Volume 76
Antiangial Drugs

Springer-Verlag
Berlin
Heidelberg
New York
Tokyo

MIX
Papier aus verantwortungsvollen Quellen
Paper from responsible sources
FSC® C105338

If you have any concerns about our products,
you can contact us on
ProductSafety@springernature.com

In case Publisher is established outside the EU,
the EU authorized representative is:
Springer Nature Customer Service Center GmbH
Europaplatz 3, 69115 Heidelberg, Germany

Printed by Libri Plureos GmbH
in Hamburg, Germany